D0841737

Download Your Included Ebook Today!

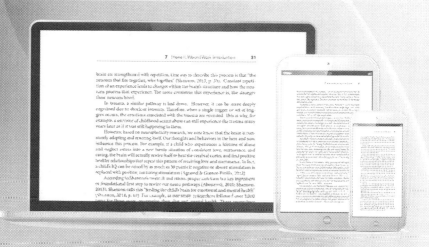

Your print purchase of *Complementary and Alternative Therapies in Nursing,* eighth edition, **includes an ebook download** to the device of your choice—increasing accessibility, portability, and searchability!

Download your ebook today at http://spubonline.com/cat and enter the access code below:

1NL9NP96C

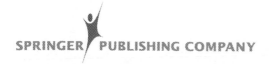

SPRINGER PUBLISHING COMPANY

SPC

Ruth Lindquist, PhD, RN, FAHA, FAAN, is professor of nursing and a graduate faculty member of the Earl E. Bakken Center for Spirituality and Healing in the Academic Health Center at the University of Minnesota. She is a member of the University of Minnesota Academy of Distinguished Teachers, a fellow of the American Academy of Nursing, and a fellow of the Stroke Council and Council on Cardiovascular and Stroke Nursing of the American Heart Association. Dr. Lindquist uses evidence-based complementary therapies and behavioral strategies in her research to reduce cardiovascular disease risk and improve an individual's health-related quality of life. She is cofounder of an innovative women's-only cardiac support group designed to enhance self-care and transform lifestyles to reduce heart disease risks. As a Densford Scholar in the Katharine J. Densford International Center for Nursing Leadership, she conducted a national survey of critical care nurses' attitudes toward and use of complementary and alternative therapies.

Mary Fran Tracy, PhD, RN, APRN, CNS, FAAN, is in a joint position as associate professor, University of Minnesota School of Nursing, and nurse scientist, University of Minnesota Medical Center, MHealth. She is also adjunct assistant professor, University of Minnesota School of Medicine. Dr. Tracy has been the principal investigator (PI) or co-PI on eight funded research projects, some of which focused on nurse use of complementary therapy interventions in critical care. She conducted a national survey of critical care nurses' attitudes toward and use of complementary therapies, and this survey has been further used by researchers in more than 15 additional countries. Dr. Tracy has published numerous papers and book chapters, including several in the current and past editions of Lindquist/Snyder, *Complementary & Alternative Therapies in Nursing*.

Mariah Snyder, PhD, RN, is professor emerita, University of Minnesota School of Nursing. Independent nursing interventions and complementary therapies have been the focus of her career. Dr. Snyder studied the effects of complementary therapies in promoting the health and well-being of elders, particularly those with dementia. She was a founding member of the Earl E. Bakken Center for Spirituality and Healing at the University of Minnesota and instrumental in the establishment of the center's graduate interdisciplinary minor. In retirement, she continues to incorporate complementary therapies in her volunteer activities with women in recovery programs, elders, and in her personal wellness.

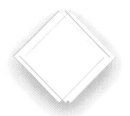

Complementary and Alternative Therapies in Nursing

Eighth Edition

Ruth Lindquist, PhD, RN, FAHA, FAAN

Mary Fran Tracy, PhD, RN, APRN, CNS, FAAN

Mariah Snyder, PhD, RN

Editors

SPRINGER PUBLISHING COMPANY

Springer Publishing Company, LLC
11 West 42nd Street
New York, NY 10036
www.springerpub.com

Acquisitions Editor: Margaret Zuccarini
Compositor: diacriTech

ISBN: 978-0-8261-4433-1
ebook ISBN: 978-0-8261-4434-8

18 19 20 21 / 5 4 3 2 1

The author and the publisher of this Work have made every effort to use sources believed to be reliable to provide information that is accurate and compatible with the standards generally accepted at the time of publication. Because medical science is continually advancing, our knowledge base continues to expand. Therefore, as new information becomes available, changes in procedures become necessary. We recommend that the reader always consult current research and specific institutional policies before performing any clinical procedure. The author and publisher shall not be liable for any special, consequential, or exemplary damages resulting, in whole or in part, from the readers' use of, or reliance on, the information contained in this book. The publisher has no responsibility for the persistence or accuracy of URLs for external or third-party Internet websites referred to in this publication and does not guarantee that any content on such websites is, or will remain, accurate or appropriate.

Library of Congress Cataloging-in-Publication Data
Names: Lindquist, Ruth (Professor of nursing), editor. | Tracy, Mary Fran, editor. | Snyder, Mariah, editor.
Title: Complementary and alternative therapies in nursing / Ruth Lindquist, Mary Frances Tracy, Mariah Snyder, editors.
Other titles: Complementary & alternative therapies in nursing.
Description: Eighth edition. | New York, NY : Springer Publishing Company, LLC, [2018] | Preceded by: Complementary & alternative therapies in nursing / [edited by] Ruth Lindquist, Mariah Snyder, Mary Fran Tracy. Seventh edition. 2014. | Includes bibliographical references and index.
Identifiers: LCCN 2017052269| ISBN 9780826144331 | ISBN 9780826144348 (ebook)
Subjects: | MESH: Holistic Nursing | Complementary Therapies—nursing
Classification: LCC RT41 | NLM WY 86.5 | DDC 610.73—dc23 LC record available at https://lccn .loc.gov/2017052269

Contact us to receive discount rates on bulk purchases.
We can also customize our books to meet your needs.
For more information please contact: sales@springerpub.com

Printed in the United States of America.

*To practicing nurses around the world who strive every day to
use the best evidence in delivering the highest quality care and comfort
to patients. To nurses who are pathfinders, breaking new ground
in ways to make us whole. To teachers and students in whose hands
is held the promise of a bright future for human health.*

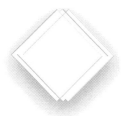

Contents

PART III MANIPULATIVE AND BODY-BASED THERAPIES

PART IV BIOLOGICALLY BASED THERAPIES

PART V   ENERGY THERAPIES

PART VI   EDUCATION, PRACTICE, RESEARCH, AND PERSONAL USE

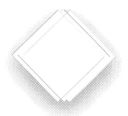

Contributors

Susan M. Bee, MS, RN, PMHCNS-BC
Clinical Nurse Specialist
Pain Rehabilitation Center
Mayo Clinic
Rochester, Minnesota

Carie A. Braun, PhD, RN
Professor, Department of Nursing
College of Saint Benedict/Saint John's University
Saint Joseph, Minnesota

Ulf G. Bronäs, PhD, ATC, FSVM, FAHA
Associate Professor
The University of Illinois at Chicago
College of Nursing
Chicago, Illinois

Miriam E. Cameron, PhD, MS, MA, RN
Graduate Faculty and Lead Faculty, Tibetan Healing Initiative
Earl E. Bakken Center for Spirituality and Healing
Academic Health Center
University of Minnesota
Minneapolis, Minnesota

Kuei-Min Chen, PhD, RN, FAAN
Professor, College of Nursing
Director, Master Program of Long-Term Care in Aging
Director, Center for Long-Term Care Research
Kaohsiung Medical University
Kaohsiung, Taiwan

Corjena K. Cheung, PhD, MS, RN, FGSA
Assistant Professor
School of Nursing
University of Minnesota
Minneapolis, Minnesota
Program Director
Department of Nursing
Hong Kong Adventist College
Hong Kong

Linda L. Chlan, PhD, RN, FAAN
Associate Dean for Nursing Research
Nursing Research Division
Professor of Nursing
Mayo Clinic College of Medicine and Health Sciences
Mayo Clinic
Rochester, Minnesota

Michael S. Christopher, PhD
Associate Professor
School of Graduate Psychology
Pacific University
Forest Grove, Oregon

Susanne M. Cutshall, DNP, APRN, CNS, APHN-BC, HWNC-BC
Integrative Health Specialist
General Internal Medicine
Assistant Professor of Medicine and Nursing
Mayo Clinic
Rochester, Minnesota

Connie White Delaney, PhD, RN, FAAN, FACMI, FNAP
Professor and Dean
School of Nursing
University of Minnesota
Minneapolis, Minnesota
Adjunct Professor
Faculty of Nursing and Faculty of Medicine
University of Iceland
Reykjavik, Iceland

Michele M. Evans, MS, RN, PMHCNS-BC APNG
Clinical Nurse Specialist
Pain Rehabilitation Center
Mayo Clinic
Rochester, Minnesota

Maura Fitzgerald, MS, MA, APRN, CNS
Clinical Nurse Specialist
Pain Medicine, Palliative Care, and Integrative Medicine Program
Children's Hospitals and Clinics of Minnesota
Minneapolis/St. Paul, Minnesota

Melissa H. Frisvold, PhD, RN, CNM
Assistant Professor
School of Nursing & Health Sciences
Georgetown University
Washington, DC

Marion Good, PhD, RN, FAAN
Professor Emerita
Frances Payne Bolton School of Nursing
Case Western Reserve University
Cleveland, Ohio

Cynthia R. Gross, PhD
Professor Emerita
School of Nursing and College of Pharmacy
University of Minnesota
Minneapolis, Minnesota

Thóra Jenný Gunnarsdóttir, PhD, RN
Associate Professor
Faculty of Nursing
University of Iceland
Reykjavik, Iceland

Niloufar Niakosari Hadidi, PhD, RN, ACNS-BC, FAHA
Associate Professor
School of Nursing
University of Minnesota
Minneapolis, Minnesota

Linda L. Halcón, PhD, MPH, RN
Associate Professor Emerita
School of Nursing
Faculty
Earl E. Bakken Center for Spirituality and Healing
University of Minnesota
Minneapolis, Minnesota

Melodee Harris, PhD, APN, GNP-BC, NGNAF
Associate Professor
Carr College of Nursing
Harding University
Searcy, Arkansas

Annie Heiderscheit, PhD, MT-BC, LMFT
Director of Music Therapy
Assistant Professor of Music
Augsburg College
Minneapolis, Minnesota

Lauren Johnson, MS, RN, CHTP
Independent Practitioner
Richfield, Minnesota

Mary Jo Kreitzer, PhD, RN, FAAN
Director
Earl E. Bakken Center for Spirituality and Healing
Professor
School of Nursing
University of Minnesota
Minneapolis, Minnesota

Mary Langevin, MSN, RN, FNP-C, CPON
Cancer and Blood Disorders Clinic
Children's Hospitals and Clinics of Minnesota
Minneapolis, Minnesota

Sohye Lee, PhD, RN
Assistant Professor
The University of Memphis
Memphis, Tennessee

Barbara Leonard, PhD, RN, FAAN
Professor Emerita
School of Nursing
University of Minnesota
Minneapolis, Minnesota

Angela S. Lillehei, PhD, MPN, RN
Minnesota Personalized Medicine
Minneapolis, Minnesota

Ruth Lindquist, PhD, RN, FAHA, FAAN
Professor
School of Nursing
University of Minnesota
Minneapolis, Minnesota

Ryan J. Mays, PhD, MPH, MS
Assistant Professor
School of Nursing
University of Minnesota
Minneapolis, Minnesota

Margaret P. Moss, PhD, JD, RN, FAAN
Assistant Dean of Diversity and Inclusion
Three Affiliated Tribes of North Dakota
Associate Professor
School of Nursing
The State University of New York
Buffalo, New York

Susan O'Conner-Von, PhD, RN-BC, CHPPN, CNE
Associate Professor
School of Nursing
Director of Graduate Studies
Earl E. Bakken Center for Spirituality and Healing
University of Minnesota
Minneapolis, Minnesota

Elizabeth L. Pestka, MS, RN, PMHCNS-BC, AGN-BC
Clinical Nurse Specialist
Department of Psychiatry and Psychology
Mayo Clinic
Assistant Professor of Nursing
Mayo Clinic College of Medicine
Rochester, Minnesota

Gregory A. Plotnikoff, MD, MTS, FACP
Minnesota Personalized Medicine
Minneapolis, Minnesota

Maryanne Reilly-Spong, PhD
Integrative Behavioral Health Consultants, LLC
Minneapolis, Minnesota

Debbie Ringdahl, DNP, RN, CNM, Reiki Master
Clinical Associate Professor
School of Nursing
Earl E. Bakken Center for Spirituality and Healing
University of Minnesota
Minneapolis, Minnesota

Dereck L. Salisbury, PhD
Clinical Assistant Professor
School of Nursing
University of Minnesota
Minneapolis, Minnesota

Mariah Snyder, PhD, RN, FAAN
Professor Emerita
School of Nursing
University of Minnesota
Minneapolis, Minnesota

Yeoungsuk Song, PhD, RN, ACNP-BC
Associate Professor
College of Nursing
Kyungpook National University
Daegu, South Korea

Mary Fran Tracy, PhD, RN, APRN, CNS, FAAN
Associate Professor
University of Minnesota School of Nursing
Nurse Scientist
University of Minnesota Medical Center
Minneapolis, Minnesota

Diane Treat-Jacobson, PhD, RN, FAAN, FAHA
Professor and Cooperative Chair
Adult and Gerontological Nursing
School of Nursing
University of Minnesota
Minneapolis, Minnesota

Shirley K. Trout, PhD, Med
Faculty Development Consultant
Pedagogy of Engagement (pedENG)
Owner, Teachable Moments
Lincoln, Nebraska

Alexa W. Umbreit, MS, RN, CHTP, CCP
Independent Practitioner
St. Paul, Minnesota

Shigeaki Watanuki, PhD, RN
Professor of Gerontological Nursing
Faculty of Nursing/Graduate School of Nursing
National College of Nursing
Tokyo, Japan

Pamela Weiss-Farnan, PhD, MPH, RN, Dip.Ac., L.Ac
Acupuncturist
Penny George Institute for Health and Healing
Abbott Northwestern Hospital
Minneapolis, Minnesota

Jaclene A. Zauszniewski, PhD, RN-BC, FAAN
Kate Hanna Harvey Professor in Community Health Nursing
Frances Payne Bolton School of Nursing
Case Western Reserve University
Cleveland, Ohio

Terri Zborowsky, PhD, EDAC
Earl E. Bakken Center for Spirituality and Healing
University of Minnesota
Minneapolis, Minnesota

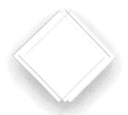

International Sidebar Contributors

Salahadin Abda
Senior student in Nursing
University of Minnesota
Bale-Robe Oromia, Ethiopia, Africa

Jehad Adwan, PhD, RN
Assistant Professor and Division Chair, Health Sciences
The Higher College of Technology
Sharjah Women's United Arab Emirates Campus
(Palestine and United Arab Emirates)

Eunice M. Areba, PhD, RN, PHN
Clinical Assistant Professor
School of Nursing
University of Minnesota
Minneapolis, Minnesota
Mombasa, Kenya

Karim Bauza, BSN, RN
Nursing Graduate
University of Minnesota
Minneapolis, Minnesota
Ciudad Mante, Tamaulipas, Mexico

Kesanee Boonyawatanangkool
Khon Kaen University
Thailand

Ulf G. Bronäs, PhD, ATC, FSVM, FAHA
Associate Professor
College of Nursing
The University of Illinois at Chicago
Chicago, Illinois
(Sweden)

Nutchanart Bunthumporn
Faculty of Nursing
Thammasat University
Thailand

Miryam Benites Cerna
Graduate Student in Nursing
Cesar Vallejo University
Trujillo, Peru

Sukjai Charoensuk, PhD, RN
Boromarajonani College of Nursing
Chon Buri, Thailand

Corjena K. Cheung, PhD, MS, RN, FGSA
Assistant Professor
School of Nursing
University of Minnesota
Minneapolis, Minnesota
Program Director
Hong Kong Adventist College
Department of Nursing
Hong Kong

Juliana Christina
PhD Candidate
Flinders University
Adelaide, Australia

Patrick J. Dean, EdD, RN, OSTJ
President, International Association for Human Caring
Clinical Associate Professor Ad Honorem
University of Minnesota School of Nursing
Minneapolis, Minnesota
Bath, United Kingdom

Marlene Dohm
Retired Clinical Nurse
Philippines

Trisha Dunning, PhD, RN, CDE, Med
Chair in Nursing, Faculty of Health
School of Nursing and Midwifery
Melbourne Burwood Campus
Barwon Health Deakin University
Victoria, Australia

Ikuko Ebihara, MBA
Third Degree Reiki Practitioner
NPO Reiki Association, Japanese Reiki Association
St. Paul, Minnesota
(Japan)

Leila Eriksen
Reflexologist, Complementary and Alternative Medicine Consultant
Denmark

Paula Eustáquio, Pedagogue
Hospital de Clinicas de Porto Alegre
Porto Alegre, Brazil

Theresa Fleming, PhD
Senior Lecturer
Department of Psychological Medicine
University of Auckland
Auckland, New Zealand
Senior Lecturer
Victoria University of Wellington
Wellington, New Zealand

Milena Flória-Santos, PhD, MS, RN
Assistant Professor
Ribeirão Preto College of Nursing
University of São Paulo
Nursing Research Development
São Paulo, Brazil

Karin Gerber, M. Cur, B.Cur, Dipl N Edu
Lecturer, Department of Nursing Science
Nelson Mandela Metropolitan University (NMMU)
Summerstrand, Port Elizabeth, South Africa

Nasra Giama, DNP, RN, PHN
Clinical Assistant Professor
University of Minnesota
Minneapolis, Minnesota
Balanbale, Somalia

Ioanna Gryllaki, BSN
Nursing Graduate
School of Nursing
University of Minnesota
Minneapolis, Minnesota
(Greece)

Mansour Hadidi MArch, MS in MIS
Information Technology Specialist
Minnesota Department of Health
Architect
Shiraz, Iran

Natalia Haire
Graduate Student
Georgetown University
Washington, DC
(Russia)

Larissa Hubbard, BSN, RN
Nursing Graduate
Carr College of Nursing
Harding University
Searcy, Arkansas
(Canada)

Sivchhun Hun, BSN, RN
Nursing Graduate
Carr College of Nursing
Harding University
Searcy, Arkansas
(Cambodia)

Gladys O. Igbo, MS, RN
Allina Health Systems
Founder-Synergy Wellness Boutique
Minneapolis/St. Paul, Minnesota
(Nigeria)

Sue Kagel, RN, BSN, HNB-BC, CHTP/I
Healing Touch Practice at Canyon Ranch Health Resort
Tucson Arizona
Adjunct Faculty
Arizona Center of Integrative Medicine
University of Arizona
(Ecuador)

Maria Tarlue Keita, MS, RN, CNS
Liberia, West Africa
Minneapolis, Minnesota

Sohye Lee, PhD, RN
Assistant Professor
The University of Memphis
Memphis, Tennessee
South Korea

Chris Lepoutre
Certified in Traditional Chinese Medicine Acupuncture
Energy Healing Therapist
North Oaks, Minnesota
(France)

Tashi Lhamo, BSN, RN, DTM
Tibetan Medicine Practitioner
Mercy Hospital
Unity Campus
Minneapolis, Minnesota
(Tibet)

Amália de Fátima Lucena, ScD, RN
Professor, Graduate Program in Nursing
Federal University of Rio Grande do Sul
Hospital de Clínicas de Porto Alegre
Grupo de Estudo e Pesquisa em Enfermagem no Cuidado ao Adulto e Idoso
(GEPECADI), Porto Alegre, RS, Brazil

Elizabeth McDonough, BS, RN, CPHON
Hematology/Infusion Center Nurse
Hematology/Oncology Clinic
Children's Hospitals and Clinics of Minnesota
Minneapolis, Minnesota

Naheed Meghani, MS, BSN, RN
PhD Candidate, University of Minnesota
The Aga Khan University Hospital
Karachi, Pakistan

Ingeborg Pedersen, PhD
Researcher
Department of Public Health Science
Norwegian University of Life Sciences
Ås, Norway

Azel Peralta, BSN, RN
Nursing Graduate
Carr College of Nursing
Harding University
Searcy, Arkansas
(Philippines)

Daniel J. Pesut, PhD, RN, FAAN
Professor of Nursing and Director
Katherine J. Densford International Center for Nursing Leadership
University of Minnesota School of Nursing
Minneapolis, Minnesota

Janice Post-White, PhD, RN, FAAN
International Research Consultant for Complementary Therapies in Oncology
Minneapolis, Minnesota, and Lanai, Hawaii

Lisiane Pruinelli, PhD, MS, RN
Assistant Professor, School of Nursing
University of Minnesota
Minneapolis, Minnesota
(Brazil)

Isabel Rossato
Physical Education
Hospital de Clinicas de Porto Alegre
Porto Alegre, Brazil

Matthew Shepherd, DClinPsy, PGH Cert HSc, BSW
Senior Lecturer in Social Work
University of Auckland
Auckland, New Zealand

Graeme D. Smith, PhD, BA, RN, FEANS
Professor, School of Nursing, Midwifery & Social Care
Edinburgh Napier University
Edinburgh, Scotland

Sumathy Sundar, PhD
Director, Chennai School of Music Therapy
Director, Center for Music Therapy Education and Research
Mahatma Gandhi Medical College and Research Institute
Sri Balaji Vidyapeeth University
Chair, Education and Training Commission
World Federation of Music Therapy
Founding Member
International Association for Music and Medicine
Pondicherry, India

Siok-Bee Tan, PhD, APN, RN
Deputy Director, Nursing
Advanced Practice Nurse
Singapore General Hospital
Republic of Singapore

Keiko Tanida, PhD, RN
Associate Professor
College of Nursing Art and Science
University of Hyogo, Japan

Jing-Jy Sellin Wang, PhD, RN
Professor and Chair
Department of Nursing, College of Medicine
National Cheng Kung University
Tainan City, Taiwan

Kenji Watanabe, MD, PhD
Keio University Center for Kampo Medicine
Shinjuku-ku, Japan

Shigeaki Watanuki, PhD, RN
Professor of Gerontological Nursing
Faculty of Nursing/Graduate School of Nursing
National College of Nursing
Tokyo, Japan

Esi Fosua Yeboah, BSN, RN, CCRN
Nursing Graduate
Carr College of Nursing
Harding University
Searcy, Arkansas
(Ghana)

Miaofen Yen, PhD, RN, FAAN
Professor and Director of International Studies
Department of Nursing, College of Medicine
National Cheng Kung University
Tainan City, Taiwan

Fang Yu, PhD, RN, GNP-BC, FGSA, FAAN
Associate Professor
School of Nursing
University of Minnesota
Minneapolis, Minnesota
Jilin Province, PR China

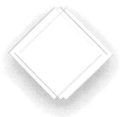

Foreword

Complementary and Alternative Therapies in Nursing, eighth edition, is launched into a world of prodigious and synergistic transformation and seismic opportunities for innovation using complementary therapies to provide comprehensive, patient-centered, high-quality nursing care. The powerful Meaningful Connections Lifting Up Leadership Elements of Mindfulness, Awareness, Intent, Vulnerability, Lovitude,[1] Transformation, and Transcendence (Pryor, Kasmirski, & Crandall 2017) can guide us in our opportunity to advance the use of complementary therapies, boldly lead education and discovery, and foster transcendence of health and healthcare challenges. Nursing education, informatics, technology, global nursing, and complementary therapies resonate with transformative energy, creating an enhanced context for integrative health approaches. The innovations range from use of complementary therapies to educational opportunities for complementary therapy professionals, health system reform, technological sea change, and planetary health.

The new edition of this text is unleashed within the context of increased use of complementary and alternative therapies while embracing integrative health and healing representing complementary therapies combined with other medical/health therapies. This awareness, intent, and actual adoption are distinct and vibrant (Freeman, 2003). In the United States alone, it was reported in data from the 2007 National Health Interview Survey (NHIS) that approximately 38% of adults (about four in 10) and approximately 12% of children (about one in nine) were using some form of complementary and alternative therapies (Barnes, Bloom, & Nahin, 2008). Over half (53%) of people aged 50 and older reported using complementary and alternative therapies at some point in their lives, and nearly as many (47%) reported using them in the past 12 months (Barnes et al., 2008). This use translates into approximately 354 million visits to complementary and alternative therapy practitioners, approximately 835 million purchases of complementary and alternative therapy products, and 83 million U.S. adults spending $33.9 billion out-of-pocket (11.2% of total out-of-pocket healthcare expenditures) on complementary and alternative therapy visits and related products (Nahin, Barnes, Stussman, & Bloom, 2009). The population clearly increasingly welcomes complementary and alternative therapies.

Today, nurses, physicians, and the full span of healthcare professionals embrace health and health reform anchored in personal and professional health and healing consciousness. This consciousness includes the physical, mental, emotional, social, and spiritual dimensions of human flourishing, holistic and integrated relationship-centered care, and optimal healing environments. In this pursuit, healthcare professionals embrace complementary and alternative therapies within each classification designated by the National Center for Complementary and Alternative Medicine (now known as the National Center for Complementary and Integrative Health [NCCIH]); these classifications continue to be used in the new edition of this text, including:

- Alternative or complete/whole medical systems
- Mind–body–spirit interventions
- Biologically based systems
- Manipulative and body-based methods
- Energy therapies

Healthcare professionals are greeted with increasing opportunities for the inclusion of complementary and alternative therapies in professional education. Indeed, even before the turn of the century, remarkably nearly 64% of U.S. medical schools offered courses inclusive of complementary and alternative therapies and integrative approaches (Wetzel, Eisenberg, & Kaptchuk, 1998). The University of Minnesota (UM) is one academy that concurs with the editors of this edition, who believe that the national climate in professional nursing demands that all nurses have a basic knowledge of complementary therapies since they undoubtedly will encounter their use by patients in the provision of care and there is greater demand by patients for the inclusion of these therapies in their care. As a member of the American Association of Colleges of Nursing (AACN) offering programs accredited by the Commission on Collegiate Nursing Education (CCNE), UM welcomes the chance to meet AACN criteria for knowledge of complementary therapies as essential content for BSN and post-BSN programs. The university offers exemplars that address increasing student and practitioner interest in exploring culture, spirituality, and healing options in complementary and alternative therapies/integrated health and healing practices. The Earl E. Bakken Center for Spirituality and Healing (n.d.) at UM offers an innovative, interdisciplinary postbaccalaureate graduate certificate in integrative therapies and healing practices. The UM School of Nursing, in partnership with the Earl E. Bakken Center for Spirituality and Healing, offers the only doctor of nursing practice degree in integrative health and healing in the United States (Regents of the University of Minnesota, n.d.).

The significance of the sweeping movement for integration of complementary and alternative therapies into all aspects of healthcare was a key driver behind the decision to require that all nurse practitioners pursuing the DNP degree meet integrative health and healing course requirements, and the school's commitment to weave integrative health throughout all curricula. Complementary and alternative therapies and integrative health approaches are likewise empowered through the National Center for Interprofessional Practice and Education, a unique public–private partnership that provides the leadership, evidence, and resources needed to guide the nation on the use of interprofessional education and collaborative practice as a way of enhancing the experience of healthcare, improving population health, and reducing the overall cost of care (National Center for Interprofessional Practice and Education, 2017).

This new edition is virtually embedded and immersed in the context of an emerging Learning Health System (LHS) that supports complementary and alternative therapies and healing practices, discovery, and education. The LHS is a system designed to generate and apply the best knowledge for the collaborative healthcare choices of each patient/person/family/community and provider; to drive the process of discovery as a natural outgrowth of healthcare; and to ensure innovation, quality, safety, and value in healthcare. The LHS includes enormous interdisciplinary and interprofessional opportunities for incorporating behavioral psychology, communication science, implementation science, behavioral economics, policy science and organizational theory, and all health sciences, including complementary and alternative therapies (Friedman, 2014). The LHS incorporates precision medicine that will enable treatments and prevention strategies to be tailored to people's unique characteristics, including their genome sequence, microbiome composition, and so on (The White House, President Barack Obama, n.d.). Precision health, additive to precision medicine, addresses tailored health-related treatments and prevention interventions that consider all dimensions of an individual's health and well-being: health history; lifestyle; diet; underlying psychological processes such as cognition, emotion, temperament, and motivation; biobehavioral interactions; sociocultural, socioeconomic, and sociodemographic status; biosocial interactions; and various levels of social context from small groups to complex cultural societal systems (Galli, 2016). Complementary and alternative therapies and integrative approaches are essential within all of these dimensions.

As healthcare providers, we are plunged into a time when there is design and redesign of supportive technical infrastructures ranging from electronic health and personal health records to the opportunities and vulnerabilities of interconnections among robust human to human (H2H), human to machine (H2M), machine to machine (M2M), Internet of Things (IoT), and the Internet of Robotics Things (IoRT). We embrace intercommunications and discovery through emerging technologies—including meditation apps, mindfulness groups online or on the phone, the energy of emotion, and the expanse of touch—to expand the reach of complementary and alternative therapies to meet health and human needs in crowded cities or desolate areas here and around the world. New data streams are emerging to represent complementary and alternative therapies and integrative healing approaches; new modalities for whole person/whole systems healing are continuing to unfold. Incorporation of these therapies into terminology (e.g., Systematized Nomenclature of Medicine [SNOMED]) and into the electronic health record (EHR) ensures the inclusion of complementary and alternative therapies in the provision of care and measures of quality, as well as expansion of their recognition and use across the globe. The "technorganic" evolution of endosymbiosis between electrochemical reactions in humans and the electromechanical nature of machines/robots continues at an unrelenting pace that virtually invites complementary and alternative therapies and integrative health and healing practices. Integrative informatics supports integrative health, including complementary and alternative therapies. We are cocreating, through practice and our research, the healthy synergy between integrative informatics and integrative health (Delaney, Westra, Dean, Leuning, & Monsen, 2014).

The publication of this eighth edition is well-timed: Its content envelopes and resonates with the World Health Organization's inclusivity of spiritual and emotional well-being. It is wrapped in the evolution of planetary health, which expands beyond the global health perspective and is rooted in understanding the interdependencies of human and natural systems and finding solutions to health risks posed by our poor stewardship of our planet. Planetary health is focused on national and international health approaches that better balance human advancement with environmental and biodiversity sustainability (The Rockefeller Foundation, n.d.).

This text invites *you,* as a unique care provider, learner, teacher, researcher, and human being. It beckons and welcomes the transformation of your practice and your self-care. An essential Lifting Up Leadership element for Transformation is Lovitude—the capacity for expressing gratitude and love. I invite you to the journey of choosing Lovitude. Can you share gratitude for the gift of this book? Gratitude for

- Serving as an exemplar of information from credible national and international web- and text-based sources
- Bringing the most prominent experts and current research and practice together
- Highlighting digital and technical advances that can help nurses stay informed and effectively apply the therapies to patient populations
- Focusing on nursing while maintaining robust interprofessional connections
- Concentrating on the capacity of complementary and alternative therapies to increase patients' well-being and satisfaction with care
- Understanding the power of complementary and alternative therapies to increase the health and well-being of the care provider
- Living risks and demonstrating vulnerability in independent personal use of complementary therapies
- Bringing to you less mainstream or less well-known therapies and strategies
- Inviting you to dream and envision plausible, colorful, imagined directions of the field along exciting possible future trajectories

It invites transformation:

- Launched into a world of prodigious and synergistic transformation and seismic opportunities for innovation
- Unleashed within the context of the increased use of complementary and alternative therapies
- Propelled into a world where nurses, physicians, and the full span of health professionals embrace health and health reform
- Greeted with increasing opportunities for complementary and alternative therapies and integrative healing practices within professional education
- Immersed in an emerging LHS that supports complementary and alternative therapies, discovery, and education
- Plunged into the design and reform of supportive technical infrastructures
- Wrapped into the evolution of planetary health

And finally, *Complementary and Alternative Therapies in Nursing* invites *you* to welcome transcendence. You are invited to engage the fullness of your individual leadership to transcend current practices; to introduce complementary therapies; and to expand what nurses offer to meet needs of the human condition, including loss, love, anxiety, pain, stress, and depression, through meditation, Reiki, deep listening, presence, humor, music intervention, relaxation therapies, healing touch, acupressure, light, animal therapy, storytelling, herbals, aromatherapy, and nutritional/nutraceutical therapies.

You are invited to Communitude.[2] Building on the Lifting Up Leadership model, Communitude invites *you* to expand beyond self, complementary and alternative interventions, and transformative implementations within organizations to establish communities, partnerships, and collectives to recreate/cocreate organizations, institutions, programs, whole systems, and global entities that exemplify the Lifting Up Leadership model and principles through their vision/mission; organizational configurations; governance; human capacity; space technologies; financial resources; engagement, inclusivity, and diversity; health and well-being; and organizational and planetary outcomes.

You are invited to dream, imagine, and envision plausible, colorful, future communities, partnerships, and collectives that undeniably deliver holistic health and healing consciousness, human health and well-being, and planetary health.

Connie White Delaney, PhD, RN, FAAN, FACMI, FNAP
Professor and Dean, School of Nursing
University of Minnesota
Minneapolis, Minnesota
Adjunct Professor, Faculty of Nursing and Faculty of Medicine
University of Iceland
Reykjavik, Iceland

NOTES

1. Lovitude® is a registered trademark by Anne Pryor.
2. Communitude™ is a trademark by Connie White Delaney, Anne Pryor, and Risë Kasmirski.

REFERENCES

Barnes, P. M., Bloom, B., & Nahin R. (2008). Complementary and alternative medicine use among adults and children: United States, 2007. *National Health Statistics Reports No. 12.* Hyattsville, MD: National Center for Health Statistics. Retrieved from https://www.cdc.gov/nchs/data/nhsr/nhsr012.pdf

Delaney, C., Westra, B., Dean, P., Leuning, C., & Monsen, K. (2014). Informatics & integrative healthcare. In M. J. Kreitzer & M. Koithan (Eds.), *Integrative nursing* (pp. 109–121). Cary, NC: Oxford University Press. ISBN: 9780199860739

Earl E. Bakken Center for Spirituality & Healing. (n.d.). Certificate in integrative therapies & healing practices. Retrieved from https://www.csh.umn.edu/education/certificate-integrative-therapies-healing-practices

Freeman, B. (2003). Philosophy of CAM. Retrieved from https://www.worldhealth.net/news/philosophy_of_cam

Friedman, C. (2014). *Toward complete & sustainable learning systems*. Retrieved from https://medicine.umich.edu/sites/default/files/2014_12_08-Friedman-IOM%20LHS.pdf

Galli, S. J. (2016). Toward precision medicine and health: Opportunities and challenges in allergic diseases. *Journal of Allergy & Clinical Immunology, 137*, 1289–1300. doi:10.1016/j.jaci.2016.03.006

Nahin, R. L., Barnes, P. M., Stussman, B. J., & Bloom, B. (2009). Costs of complementary and alternative medicine (CAM) and frequency of visits to CAM practitioners: United States, 2007. *National Health Statistics Reports No. 18*. Hyattsville, MD: National Center for Health Statistics. Retrieved from https://www.cdc.gov/nchs/data/nhsr/nhsr018.pdf

National Center for Interprofessional Practice and Education. (2017). *Home page*. Retrieved from https://nexusipe.org

Pryor, A., Kasmirski, R., & Crandall, K. (2017). Meaningful Connection's Lifting Up Leadership Model. Retrieved from https://www.slideshare.net/annepryor/meaningful-connections-lifting-up-leadership-methodology-by-anne-pryor-kathleen-crandall-rise-kasmirski

Regents of the University of Minnesota. (n.d.). Integrative health and healing DNP. Retrieved from https://www.nursing.umn.edu/degrees-programs/doctor-nursing-practice/post-baccalaureate/integrative-health-and-healing

The Rockefeller Foundation. (n.d.). Planetary health. Retrieved from https://www.rockefellerfoundation.org/our-work/initiatives/planetary-health

The White House, President Barack Obama. (n.d.). The precision medicine initiative [archive]. Retrieved from https://obamawhitehouse.archives.gov/node/333101

Wetzel, M. S., Eisenberg, D. M., & Kaptchuk, T. J. (1998). Courses involving complementary and alternative medicine at US medical schools. *Journal of the American Medical Association, 280*(9), 784–787. doi:10.1001/jama.280.9.784

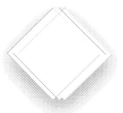

Preface

The eighth edition of this highly acclaimed book continues the legacy of the previous editions in offering the latest information on commonly used complementary therapies in a readily accessible manner for nurses; although the focus of the book is nursing, practitioners in other disciplines will also find the text helpful. The therapy chapters follow a consistent format that facilitates rapid access to the information under headings that include definition, scientific basis, intervention, measurement of outcomes, precautions, uses, cultural applications, and future research. The chapters contain practice protocols that describe an intervention along with a section on measurement of outcomes to help the reader more readily apply therapies in practice.

What contributes to the uniqueness of this book is that it is written with a specific focus on nurses. Along with definitions and descriptions of the selected therapies, the book provides a background for each therapy, as well as evidence for the use of therapies with a variety of specific patient populations in the delivery of patient-centered care. Credible information is needed to provide the safe and effective use of complementary therapies by consumers as well as practitioners. The book is a valuable resource that provides nurses with practical guidelines for using a wide range of complementary therapies to promote health and comfort while increasing patients' well-being and satisfaction with care.

We are pleased that the eighth edition features an expansion of the content of previous editions, including new approaches and applications of therapies in the care of patients. The text highlights the most recent and useful information from credible national and international web- and text-based sources and brings the most current research and practice together inside the covers of one book. Digital and technical advances that are included assist the reader in being informed and able to effectively apply the therapies in care situations. An important chapter focuses on integrating therapies, including institution- or organization-wide programs. This chapter provides useful strategies for nurses who wish to apply therapies in practice, as well as models that can serve as readily modifiable blueprints for their integration into healthcare settings.

The cultural and global perspectives provided in each chapter are essential in today's world in which immigration, refugees, and travel make it necessary to be aware of, open to, and knowledgeable about the health practices of other cultures. Nurses around the globe use complementary therapies. The international sidebars included in each chapter offer rich perspectives from some of these nurses regarding complementary therapy use in other countries and cultures. This sharing of stories and perspectives deepens our understanding of our diverse patients and fosters the delivery of more culturally sensitive care. The chapter contributors and sidebar authors together compose an amazing group of 96 contributing professionals representing perspectives from 39 countries and six continents.

This eighth edition of the text provides a description of key steps forward in the evolution and establishment of the National Center for Complementary and Integrative Health (NCCIH), including the current national agenda. A new chapter examines whole systems of care, especially focusing on Tibetan knowledge of health. In this edition, there is an updated discussion of legal concerns and information regarding regulation and credentialing. Once again, in this edition, there is carefully considered safety and precaution content, with helpful tips for selecting practitioners. There is also new and enhanced content on use of complementary therapies for nurse and patient self-care.

A decision always needs to be made regarding what therapies to include and exclude in the text. Countless complementary therapies exist and are used by people around the globe. The therapies selected for inclusion in this text were those that are commonly associated with the term *complementary therapies* and included on the NCCIH website (nccih.nih.gov). The decision was also based on the availability of scientific evidence for the use of any individual therapy and its promise for application to practice in a variety of settings and for a variety of health conditions. The selected therapies are viewed as adding value or quality to healthcare.

The urgency for research related to the use of complementary therapies is highlighted in the chapter on research, as well as in the assessment at the end of every chapter; more research is needed with larger samples and stronger designs. New designs are also needed to undergird and overcome the experimental challenges inherent in the research needed in this area, and to provide suitable controls.

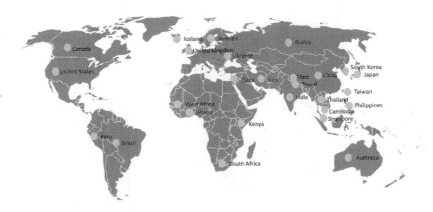

The afterword, "Creating a Preferred Future: Editors' Reflections" postulates plausible, colorful, imagined directions of the field along exciting possible future trajectories; it projects the modern-day trends forward into the future, extrapolating the realities of the day into an unknown future. The editors reflect on their own visions related to complementary therapies and urge the creation of a preferred future, one in which complementary therapies are available, selected, and used in an efficient and effective way that is well-informed by the evidence and available across the globe.

The text assists nursing educators in their important role of preparing 21st-century practitioners to provide holistic, culturally sensitive care to all patients. The content meets the American Association of Colleges of Nursing (AACN) requirements for BSN and post-BSN programs and will assist students in their preparation for the NCLEX-RN® examination (AACN, 2008; National Council of State Boards of Nursing, 2016). The text is a valuable resource for graduate and advanced practice registered nurses who desire to increase the use of complementary therapies to enhance the health of patients, to enhance quality of care, and to improve satisfaction outcomes. Directions for future research may prompt these practitioners to pursue studies that will add to the knowledge base about these therapies. Nursing students at all levels should be introduced to complementary therapies and integrative health approaches—care that can be used by nurses to meet "the needs of the whole person: Body, mind, emotion and spirit" (American Holistic Nurses Association, 2016).

The goal of the eighth edition is similar to the original goal set forth in the first edition in 1985 (Snyder, 1985). to enhance quality healthcare of people not only in the United States, but also across the globe through the inclusion of complementary therapies in plans of care. We, the editors, relying on the expertise of the many contributing authors and sidebar contributors, have faith that the eighth edition will not only help nurses and other practitioners to provide integrative care, but also allow you, the reader, to find content that piques your interest in delving deeper into these and other therapies. We encourage you to explore the use of these therapies as part of a self-care regimen or potential use in your professional practice.

Ruth Lindquist
Mary Fran Tracy
Mariah Snyder

REFERENCES

American Association of Colleges of Nursing. (2008). *The essentials of baccalaureate education for professional nursing practice.* Retrieved from http://www.aacnnursing.org/Portals/42/Publications/BaccEssentials08.pdf

American Holistic Nurses Association. (2016). *Position on the role of nurses in the practice of complementary and integrative health approaches (CIHA).* Retrieved from http://www.ahna.org/LinkClick.aspx?fileticket=Gdt_dxWvaqk%3D&portalid=66

National Council of State Boards of Nursing. (2016). *NCLEX-RN® examination: Test plan for the National Council Licensure Examination for Registered Nurses.* Retrieved from https://www.ncsbn.org/RN_Test_Plan_2016_Final.pdf

Snyder, M. (1985). *Independent nursing interventions.* Hoboken, NJ: John Wiley & Sons.

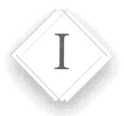

Foundations for Use of Complementary Therapies

Complementary therapies have become widely known and used in Western healthcare, particularly in nursing. According to the National Center for Complementary and Integrative Health (NCCIH), a national survey in the United States documented that 33% of American adults use complementary therapies (National Center for Complementary and Integrative Health [NCCIH], 2016). Use of these therapies occurs also on a global scale. Throughout the text, perspectives from individuals worldwide provide a view on the use of complementary therapies in their respective countries. Not only are complementary therapies used within conventional healthcare, but other systems of care and the healing practices that were initiated a millennium ago are also receiving increasing attention. Expanding the perspectives on therapies used in other health systems will provide nurses with knowledge about therapies that are practiced by people in multiple cultures across the globe and will lead to more personalized quality care.

Chapter 1 provides an overview of the long tradition of use of complementary therapies in nursing and the growing acceptance of their place in healthcare. In accordance with this growing acceptance and integration into healthcare, the National Center for Complementary and Alternative Medicine changed its title to the National Center for Complementary and Integrative Health. The term *integrative health* reflects the blending of complementary therapies and conventional health practices into a healthcare delivery system. With growth in the number of refugees and immigrants and the increase in global travel, it is paramount that healthcare providers be more aware of the great diversity in health practices that exist and secure from patients a thorough assessment of the practices used as some, particularly natural, products may interact with medications being prescribed.

Two therapies—presence (Chapter 2) and therapeutic listening and communication (Chapter 3)—are critical elements in the implementation of any complementary therapies. Many patients and families voice appreciation of a nurse who was "really present when providing care." *Presence* is difficult to define. An old adage goes, "You know it when you see it." The multiple facets of therapeutic listening and communication (Chapter 3), both verbal and nonverbal, are likewise important keys to providing holistic care. Nonverbal communication, including really listening and observing, can assume even greater importance when interacting with people from other cultures in the context of a therapeutic relationship. The knowledge of customs—as basic as whether it is acceptable to shake the hands of the patient and family or touch someone of another gender—is foundational in establishing the kind of therapeutic relationship that is integral to the success of complementary therapies.

Chapter 4 focuses on creating an optimal healing environment. More health facilities are devoting attention to light, color, and other aspects of the environment. Research is beginning to substantiate the impact that the environment has on outcomes of care.

Systems of care (Chapter 5), particularly Tibetan medicine, is a new chapter describing systems and practices that differ significantly from the conventional system of care with which readers are most familiar. Having a basic understanding of other systems will assist nurses in providing care to the growing diversity of cultures found in patient populations. Although it is unlikely that nurses will ever embrace an entire system of nonconventional healthcare, they may identify a practice or therapy from a system that would be useful for them to use for their patients or for self-care.

REFERENCE

National Center for Complementary and Integrative Health. (2016). *NCCIH facts-at-a-glance and mission*. Retrieved from https://nccih.nih.gov/about/ataglance

Evolution and Use of Complementary Therapies and Integrative Healthcare Practices

MARIAH SNYDER AND RUTH LINDQUIST

Complementary and alternative therapies, or as occasionally labeled *unconventional*, have become an integral part of healthcare in the United States and other countries. The term *complementary therapies* is used in this book. The word *complementary* conveys that a procedure is used as an adjunct to Western or conventional therapies. Another term, *alternative*, which is also in the title of this text, indicates a therapy that is used in place of a Western approach to healthcare. Nurses, in their practice, use both types of therapies. For example, nurses may use progressive muscle relaxation with a person with high stress to lower the stress level or a nurse may use progressive muscle relaxation in addition to the medication the patient is receiving to lower the stress level. A term that is receiving increasing use is *integrative healthcare*, which conveys that both biomedical and complementary therapies or other systems of care are part of the offerings at a healthcare facility.

The National Institutes of Health (NIH) has changed the title for the center created to focus on complementary therapies from the National Center for Complementary and Alternative Medicine (NCCAM) to the National Center for Complementary and Integrative Health (NCCIH). What is important to note is that the new title states *integrative health* and eliminates *medicine*. The title also recognizes the increasing use of complementary therapies in healthcare.

DEFINITION AND CLASSIFICATION

Numerous definitions of *complementary therapies* exist. The broad scope of the therapies and the many health professionals and therapists who are involved in delivering them create challenges for finding a definition that captures the breadth of this field. NCCIH defines *complementary health approaches* as the use of practices and products of nonmainstream origin (NCCIH, 2016a). *Integrative health* is the term used when complementary therapies/practices are used in conjunction with mainstream healthcare (NCCIH, 2016a). These definitions convey the inclusion of different therapies in countries in which Western biomedicine predominates, as opposed to countries in which another health system is dominant, such as traditional Chinese medicine (TCM). According to the WHO (2012), a large number of healing practices in developing countries comprise indigenous traditional health practices rather than Western biomedical approaches.

The lack of precision in the definition of *complementary therapies* poses challenges when comparing findings across surveys that have been conducted on the use of complementary procedures. Some surveys have included a large number of complementary practices, whereas others have been limited in scope. For example, in the NCCAM/National Center for Health Statistics Survey (NCCIH, 2017a), adding prayer for health purposes to the analyses increased the percentage of use of complementary therapies from 36% to 62% (National Center for Complementary and Integrative Health, 2017).

The field of complementary therapies is constantly changing as new therapies are identified; a number of these are from other systems of care or used in indigenous cultures. The NCCIH classifies complementary health approaches into two categories: natural products and mind and body practices. Exhibit 1.1 identifies common therapies in each category. In addition, some of the other systems of care are noted. A number of the therapies included in Exhibit 1.1 have been a part of nursing for many years. The NCCIH lists do not include a number of the complementary therapies included in this text, such as presence, active listening, biofeedback, and light therapy. However, these are therapies often used by nurses.

According to a finding from the 2012 National Health Interview Survey (NHIS), natural products are the most widely used complementary therapy. Nearly 18% of American adults used a dietary supplement other than vitamins and minerals. Natural products are widely available. To date, there is little regulation of this area.

The class of mind and body practices encompasses a wide spectrum of practices and ranges from massage and yoga to energy therapies such as healing touch and acupuncture. As can be noted in Exhibit 1.1, chiropractic and osteopathic manipulation are included in the mind and body practice category. Some view chiropractic and osteopathy as specific systems of care. A significant number of the therapies found in the mind and body practices class have been used by nurses for years, whereas others have recently become therapies that a number of nurses incorporate into their nursing care.

The NCCIH classifies "other systems of care" as *other complementary health approaches*. As noted in Exhibit 1.1, this category encompasses a vast array of systems of care, including *practices of traditional healers*. Many times, these systems of care have been used for millennia by indigenous people around the globe. Stephens, Porter, Nettleton, and Willis (2006) noted that many of these systems have very sophisticated ideas of health and well-being that more closely approximate the health definition proposed by the WHO, in which health is more than the absence of disease.

Other methods for classifying complementary therapies exist. One of these is provider-based and nonprovider-based administration. Therapies that are provider based require a health professional or therapist to administer them, whereas therapies that are nonprovider based do not require the presence of a professional. For example, a therapist is required for acupuncture, but one is not necessarily required for acupressure. Herbal preparations and food supplements—the most used groups of complementary therapies—are self-administered. For a number of therapies, once the technique has been taught, a therapist is not needed. Meditation is an example of this type of a self-administered therapy. Nonprovider therapies are less costly than provider-administered therapies.

Globally, as people migrate for economic reasons, wars, drought, or political factors, health professionals are becoming increasingly aware of culture-specific health practices used in other countries. These practices may be carried out by shamans, healers, family members, or the patient. Knowledge about common practices in various ethnic groups assists nurses in providing culturally sensitive and safe care to promote health. A danger that health professionals face is assuming all people from a country or an area of the world engage in the same health practices. For example, Africa is a vast continent, and cultural practices vary significantly across the continent, as do practices across the tribes within a nation. This is also true for Native American tribes, with practices depending on the plants available for healing within given geographical areas.

Exhibit 1.1. NCCIH Classification for Complementary Therapies and Integrative Practices and Examples of Therapies

Natural Products
Therapies use substances found in nature. Examples: herbs (botanicals), vitamins, minerals, dietary supplemented probiotics.

Mind and Body Practices
This category includes a diverse group of therapies: Chiropractic and osteopathic manipulation, massage, meditation, yoga, acupuncture, relaxation techniques, imagery, hypnotherapy, and movement therapies, and tai chi.

Other Complementary Health Approaches
Whole systems of care are built on theory and practice and often evolved apart from and earlier than Western medicine. Each has its own therapies and practices. Examples include TCM, Ayurvedic, traditional healers, naturopathy, and homeopathy.

NCCIH, National Center for Complementary and Integrative Health; TCM, traditional Chinese medicine.
Source: National Center for Complementary and Integrative Health. (2016a). NCCIH facts-at-a glance and mission. Retrieved from https://nccih.nih.gov/about/ataglance

USE OF COMPLEMENTARY THERAPIES

Interest in, and use of, complementary/alternative therapies has remained fairly constant in recent years in the United States, with slightly more than 30% of adults reporting use of complementary therapies (NCCIH, 2016b). Prior to the emergence of health professionals' interest in complementary therapies, many individuals often used these therapies (e.g., prayer, meditation, herbal preparations); however, they did not refer to them as being complementary therapies. Surveys have addressed use by adults in the United States (Clarke, Black, Stussman, Barnes, & Nahin, 2015; Laiyemo, Nunlee-Bland, Lombardo, Adams, & Laiyemo, 2015). Clarke et al. (2015), using the NHIS for 2012, found a slight decrease in reported adult use of complementary therapies from the NHIS 2007 survey: 35% in 2007 to 33.2% in 2012. The percentage of use for children 4 to 17 years was lower than for adults: 11.6% (NCCIH, 2016b). Findings from the NHIS reported a lower use of complementary therapies by Hispanic adults (22%) and non-Hispanic Black adults (19.3%) compared with non-Hispanic White adults (37.9%) (Clarke et al., 2015).

Interest in the use of complementary therapies is a phenomenon found not only in the United States, but also in many other countries. Research on the use of these therapies has been conducted in various countries, including the United Kingdom (Posadzki, Watson, Alotaibi, & Emst, 2013), Germany (Linde, Alscher, Friedrichs, Joos, & Schneider, 2014), Japan (Hori, Mihaylov, Vasconcelos, & McCoubrie, 2008), and Iran (Balouchi, Rahanama, Hastings-Tolsma, Shoja, & Bolaydehyi, 2016). The number of people using complementary therapies varied in these survey reports, but it was 50% or higher, indicating a wide use of these therapies.

Numerous studies have explored the use of complementary therapies in specific health conditions, including cancer (Ben-Arye et al., 2014), asthma (George & Topaz, 2013), neck pain (Brosseau et al., 2012), and arthritis (Hoerster, Butler, Mayer, Finlayson, & Gallo, 2011). The Cochrane Database of Systematic Reviews (2016) contains reviews of the efficacy of numerous complementary therapies in the treatment of specific conditions. In addition to their use for health conditions, complementary therapies are often used to promote a healthy lifestyle. An example would be the use of tai chi to promote flexibility and prevent falls in older adults.

Researchers have attempted to identify characteristics of users of complementary therapies. Nguyen, Davis, Kaptchuk, and Phillips (2011) found that more women than men use these therapies. They also noted that a higher percentage of individuals using complementary therapies have academic degrees compared with a nonuser group. This may relate to economics and the ability to pay out-of-pocket for complementary therapies. These findings were further validated in the NHIS conducted by the National Center for Health Statistics of the Centers for Disease Control and Prevention (CDC) (Barnes, Bloom, & Nahin, 2008). Goetz et al. (2013) compared the use of complementary therapies by people in active military service with the use by civilians. Their findings revealed a much higher use by active military personnel (44.5%) compared with civilians (36%).

Natural products are the most commonly used complementary therapy by both adults and children (NCCIH, 2016a). Exhibit 1.2 displays the 10 most commonly used therapies by adults identified on the 2012 NHIS survey.

Exhibit 1.2. 10 Most Commonly Used Complementary Therapies in Adults in the United States

Natural products	17.7%*
Deep breathing	10.9%
Yoga, tai chi, qigong	10.1%
Chiropractic or osteopathic manipulation	8.4%
Meditation	8.0%
Massage	6.9%
Special diets	3.0%
Homeopathy	2.2%
Progressive relaxation	2.1%
Guided imagery	1.7%

*This listing does not compute to 100% because there were other therapies on the survey that were used by less than 1.7% of those surveyed.

Source: National Center for Complementary and Integrative Health. (2016a). NCCIH facts-at-a glance and mission. Retrieved from https://nccih.nih.gov/about/ataglance

The growing interest in and use of complementary therapies has prompted groups to explore why people elect to use a complementary or integrative health practice. In a report from an international panel looking at the economic factors related to the use of complementary therapies, Coulter, Herman, and Nataraj (2013) noted that complementary and integrative health therapies often target the whole person rather than a specific symptom or disease. This holistic philosophy underlying many of the complementary therapies differs significantly from the dualistic or Cartesian philosophy that for several centuries has permeated Western medicine. Although use of a specific symptom or condition may be the focus of the therapy, often the person who is treated reports a greater sense of harmony or balance. People often seek care from complementary therapists or care at facilities that offer complementary therapies because they want to be treated as a whole person—and not treated as "a heart attack" or "a fractured hip."

The integration of complementary therapies with biomedical therapies is a growing trend in healthcare as the scientific basis for the use of numerous complementary therapies increases. (See Chapter 28 for examples of institutions in which integrative healthcare is provided.) With the growing number of older adults and the increase in chronic health conditions, practices that may be used to manage symptoms and increase quality of life have great appeal.

The personal qualities of a complementary practitioner (whether a nurse, physician, or other therapist) are key in the healing process. Having a practitioner who is caring, which has been integral to the nursing profession through the years, is also a key component in administering complementary therapies. Two aspects of caring administration of complementary therapies—presence and active listening—are covered in subsequent chapters. Both convey caring. Remen (2000), a physician who is involved in cancer care, has stated:

> I know that if I listen attentively to someone, to their essential self, their soul, as it were, I often find that at the deepest, most unconscious level, they can sense the direction of their own healing and wholeness. If I can remain open to that, without expectations of what the someone is supposed to do, how they are supposed to change in order to be better, or even what their wholeness looks like, what can happen is magical. By that I mean that it has a certain coherency or integrity about it, far beyond any way of fixing their situation or easing their pain that I can devise on my own. (p. 90)

The heightened interest in complementary therapies prompted the NIH to establish the Office of Alternative Medicine in 1992, which was elevated to the National Center for Complementary and Alternative Medicine (NCCAM) in 1998. The name was changed to the Center for Complementary and Integrative Health (NCCIH) in 2014. What was significant about the establishment of the center in 1992 was that consumers, rather than health professionals, led the lobbying for its creation.

The mission of the NCCIH is to define, through rigorous scientific investigation, the usefulness and safety of complementary therapies and integrative healthcare and their role in improving health (NCCIH, 2016a). The NCCIH has developed a strategic framework that includes:

- Advancing fundamental science and methods development for complementary therapies and integrative health
- Improving care for hard-to-manage symptoms
- Fostering health promotion and disease prevention

The NCCIH also has two crosscutting objectives:

- Enhancing the complementary and integrative health workforce
- Disseminating objective evidence-based information on complementary and integrative health interventions (NCCIH, 2016a)

The NCCIH's website contains information about complementary therapies, research opportunities, and outcomes of recent surveys.

REIMBURSEMENT AND REGULATION

The costs and cost-effectiveness of complementary therapies are difficult to determine. Thus, scientifically sound investigations on the outcomes of specific interventions are needed. Many of the current studies have used a small sample size and/or have design flaws. Because people may use a complementary therapy to accomplish several outcomes, it becomes a challenge to measure all of these outcomes and to find tools that capture these seemingly diverse goals. Investigating the cost of integrative health poses even greater challenges, but it is important for models to be developed (Pelletier, Herman, Metz, & Nelson, 2010).

Are complementary therapies cost-effective in terms of outcomes of care? Lind, Lafferty, Tyree, and Diehr (2010) examined differences in costs of healthcare for patients with back pain, fibromyalgia, and menopause symptoms who used complementary therapies and for those who did not. They found that those using complementary therapies had overall lower healthcare costs—$1,420 less on average—than those who did not use these therapies. Other researchers reported that individuals with chronic illnesses who used complementary therapies were more likely to report feeling healthier (Nguyen et al., 2011).

With the continuing emphasis on controlling healthcare costs in the United States, studies examining the cost of complementary therapies and integrative healthcare will receive increasing attention. The impact that a therapy has on producing positive outcomes is highly important, but also outcomes such as quality of life and adherence need to be included in investigations. This is especially true in those with multiple chronic illnesses, such as in the aging population.

Some of the challenges relate to the holistic focus of many of the complementary therapies. Does massage relieve knee pain? Does a reduction in pain result in fewer days missed from work? Does the reduction in pain result in a better mood state that has an effect on social interactions? These are only a small number of outcomes that may result from massage reducing knee or other pain. The multitude of possible outcomes poses many challenges for researchers in terms of determining the cost-effectiveness of a specific therapy.

Third-party payers such as insurance companies pay for a limited number of complementary therapies. The therapies most frequently covered are chiropractic medicine, acupuncture, and biofeedback. In some instances, physician referral is required for reimbursement. Patients should consult with their insurer to see if and what complementary therapies may be covered. According to the NHIS 2012 survey, Americans spend $30.2 billion out-of-pocket each year on complementary therapies. This money was divided among health practitioners ($14.7 billion), natural products ($12.8 billion), and other complementary therapy approaches ($2.7 billion) (NCCIH, 2017b). Obviously, people must believe that complementary techniques produce positive results if they continue to personally pay for these aids. Although the amount spent on complementary therapies seems large, it is less than 10% of out-of-pocket payments made by Americans for healthcare (NCCIH, 2017).

Some states, such as Washington, require the inclusion of complementary therapists in private, commercial insurance offerings (Lafferty et al., 2006). Other states have instituted legislation that provides protection for persons using complementary procedures. For example, legislation in Minnesota established the Office of Alternative and Complementary Health Care Practices (Minnesota Department of Health, Health Occupation Program, 2017). This office provides information for consumers, delineates rights for users, and suggests questions to ask a practitioner. An important aim of this office is to provide protection for those seeking care from a nonhealthcare-licensed provider.

Practitioners administering complementary therapies may or may not be licensed health professionals. Concern has been voiced about the preparation of all who administer complementary therapies but particularly about nonhealthcare professionals. Regulation of both healthcare and nonhealthcare professionals is done by states and in some instances at the city level. A number of professional organizations such as the National Board of Chiropractic Examiners, the Healing Touch Program, and the National Holistic Nurses establish standards and administer certification examinations for practitioners in these therapies. Many healthcare facilities have requirements for complementary therapists working in their facility. For example, they may require that practitioners administering healing touch be certified.

Because of the diversity in educational preparation and the lack of state requirements for some complementary therapy practitioners, it is important that the individual seeking a therapist inquire about practitioner/provider experience and background. Also, if concerns exist, the person should contact the Department of Health in his or her state for further information.

CULTURE-RELATED ASPECTS OF COMPLEMENTARY THERAPIES

Human cultures pervade the globe. One's culture lends structure to a shared way of life in health and illness. All cultures have either systems of healthcare or numerous healthcare practices/therapies that are used by the members of that culture. Although some healthcare practices of other cultures have become part of the compendium of complementary therapies, such as yoga, many of these remedies remain unknown to Western healthcare providers. Because of the largest refugee population since World War II, large number of immigrants, migrations of people due to climate changes, and an increase in global travel, knowledge of the healthcare practices of other cultures has become paramount in providing healthcare.

Migration of people brings not only their diseases, but also their healthcare practices. Traditional healers traveling in populations of refugees include midwives, herbalists, shamans, priests or priestesses, bonesetters, and surgeons. There is a great need for healers because 47% of global morbidity is attributable to chronic conditions, with 60% mortality arising from such conditions (Manderson & Smith-Morris, 2010). Quinlan (2011) stated that 85% of traditional remedies are herbal, and more than 70% of the world's population depends on common herbal medicine for their primary care. Beliefs about the cause of a number of chronic conditions point to the type of therapies selected to treat or "cure" that condition. Some individuals may seek care from a sorcerer. Humoral balance is a focus in some cultural systems of care such as TCM (yin/yang) and Latin American medicine (hot/cold). Therapies to promote this balance such as chi in TCM and other systems in Latin American medicine may be used by immigrants from these areas.

Entire systems of healthcare have survived for thousands of years in various regions of the world. With the increasing movement of people either for short periods of time such as for study, business, or vacation or for permanent immigration, aspects of diverse systems of care will be encountered both by those in transit and by healthcare providers in their home country. The impact of Western medicine in most areas of the world is growing. However, individuals will continue to use all or portions of their traditional system of healthcare. These different ways of healing can work well together; however, it is imperative for Western care providers to assess for therapies or practices that may be used so that the patient receives safe care. Because minimal information is known about the outcomes of many of these therapies, close observations are needed to ensure that they are enhancing, not interfering with, biomedical treatment.

Sidebar 1.1 details the use of plant medicines over the centuries in Peru.

SIDEBAR 1.1. THE USE OF MEDICINAL PLANTS IN PERU

Miryam Benites Cerna

I am a nurse and have been working for more than 25 years in rural and urban areas of northern Peru. During this time, I have been able to observe and guide the use of herbs or plants used for medicinal purposes.

There is evidence that ancient Peruvians used plants for therapeutic purposes 6,000 years before Christ. The inhabitants of pre-Inca cultures were keen observers of the environment that surrounded them and, therefore, of the plants that grew in their environment. For thousands of years, the inhabitants of Peru, especially those living in rural areas, have used various plants for medicinal purposes; some were grown in the wild, and others were cultivated especially for this purpose. This cultural practice has not been lost because it has been transmitted orally from one generation to the next. Families and communities are the depositories and practitioners of this ancient wisdom.

In some cases, the whole plant or part of it is used to cure or alleviate pain, and in other cases, infusions are administered to the patient. Some of the disorders that are treated with medicinal plants are trauma to the skeletal system; bacterial, fungal, or viral infections; parasites; and respiratory, digestive, and urinary disorders. They are also used as regulators of the hormonal, reproductive, and even psychic systems.

Here are some examples of well-known and commonly used plants:

- *Cola de caballo* is used as a diuretic to improve kidney function and to heal wounds.
- *Manzanilla* is an infusion of stems, leaves, and flowers used to relieve stomach pains. It is also used as a tranquilizer and for diarrhea in children.
- *Altamisa* involves heating branches and then rubbing them on limb areas affected by rheumatism. Fresh branches are placed under a bed to expel fleas.
- *Cerraja* is a concoction of leaves used to relieve digestive disorders and hepatitis.
- *Supiquegua* or *pedorrera* is an infusion is used for indigestion and stomach gases.
- *Toronjil* is an aromatic plant used as an antispasmodic or as a relaxant and sedative of the nervous system.
- *Panisara* is used to relieve symptoms of a light cold and cough and to strengthen the respiratory system.
- *Matico* is an infusion of leaves taken for flu and coughs. Dried and crushed leaves are used to heal wounds.
- *Llantén* is a concoction prepared from leaves and used to heal wounds. An infusion of the leaves serves as an anti-inflammatory agent.
- *Pie de perro* is an infusion used as an anti-inflammatory for the kidneys.
- *Cedron* is used as an infusion for digestive problems and intestinal gases.

Although nurses may not know exact details of healing traditions in other cultures, it is helpful for them to gain some knowledge about the specific heritage of a patient. With today's technology, key points about the health practices of the culture can be obtained from web sources. When nurses are familiar with the patient's worldview, they can ask patients and family members about specific needs and preferences that are natural parts of the individual's or the family's healing traditions.

Sidebar 1.2 paints a worldview and the healing traditions of a nurse raised in the Middle East.

SIDEBAR 1.2. INTERNATIONAL PERSPECTIVE—PALESTINE

Jehad Adwan

Growing up in a refugee camp in Rafah, on the Gaza Strip, I heard stories from my parents and grandparents about how they treated their sick. My paternal grandfather, Hassan, died long before I was born, but my grandmother, Aisha, lived until I was 15 years old. Hassan was perceived by his village as man of God (*Darwish*). He once predicted, according to the story my father told us many times, that my father (his son, Zaki) would fall and hurt himself or even die while sleeping one hot summer night on the roof—as many people did during summer. He asked his wife, Aisha, to remove the large pottery jars (used to cool water off in the shade) from under the assumed spot where my father would fall. Sure enough, my father fell that night and landed on soft sand rather than on a pottery jar. He was unscathed.

My grandmother inherited the skill of massage from her mother. Massaging the sick has been practiced in Palestine for many generations. My great-grandmother specialized in massage, which she learned from her mother. She incorporated hand skills and locally harvested olive and sesame seed oils with spiritual recitation of healing verses from the Qur'an. This skill is usually kept in families and handed down from mother to daughter or father to son. I still feel her warm hands on my neck and chest as a child whenever I had a cold or sore throat. The warm oil in her hands touching my neck and chest with her firm yet gentle pressure on the troubled spot—combined with her reassuring whisper of the Qur'an verses—were hypnotizing. In a calming voice she would whisper:

> Say, I seek refuge in the Lord of daybreak from the evil of that which He created; from the evil of darkness when it settles; from the evil of the blowers in knots [witchcraft]; and from the evil of an envier when he envies. (Qur'an 113, 1–5)

Envy was often perceived as a cause of illness and misfortune in Palestine. However, as people become more accustomed to Western-style healthcare practices, fewer believe today that envy alone is the source of illness; and it's becoming more accepted that physical and environmental factors cause illness. Traditional healing, however, still exists to a large extent in rural communities

(continued)

that modern clinics and hospitals often cannot reach. You can find traditional healers delivering babies, fixing bones, and prescribing herbal and natural remedies for a variety of minor ailments and diseases. Some of these remedies include hibiscus teas, honey, vinegar, and numerous local herbs such as sage, thyme, and anise.

My older brother, Ra'ed, a superintendent for our hometown school district, is a strong believer in herbal medicine. We used to argue about the efficacy of these herbal remedies—he defended them, whereas I took the side of the Western-style approach of pharmacology. In retrospect, I see where he was coming from. I believe that although not all traditional Palestinian remedies do what they claim, there are elements that I do miss about them. I miss my grandmother's gentle, healing touch on my tiny neck and body as a sick little boy. I miss her comforting voice. If her touch wasn't comforting and healing to me, I don't know what else was.

An example of the importance of knowledge about cultural health practices can be found in Native American traditional healthcare practices. As noted previously, the health professional must not make generalizations about health practices of Native Americans because great variations exist among the more than 500 Native American nations. Traditional healing practices of Native American cultures were often embedded in stories, legends, symbolism, ceremonies and spiritual treatments; these healing traditions have played an important role in the well-being of traditional Native American people (Koithan & Farrell, 2011). Purifying the body is a foundational healing component of health rituals in a number of Native American nations. The basis for cleansing is to rid the person of bad feelings, negative energy, or bad spirits. The individual is cleansed both physically and spiritually (Borden & Coyote, 2012). Cleansing can take a variety of forms such as smudging or sweat lodges. Sage and sweetgrass are commonly used by Great Plains Native Americans for their smudging ceremonies. Borden and Coyote describe a smudging ceremony:

[B]urn the clippings of the herbs [dried], rub your hands in the smoke, and then gather the smoke and bring it into your body—or rub it onto yourself; especially onto any area you feel needs spiritual healing. Keep praying all the while that the unseen powers of the plant will cleanse your spirit. Sometimes, one person will smudge another, or a group of people using hands—or more often a feather—to lightly brush the smoke over the other person(s). (p. 3)

Native American families may wish to use smudging for family members who are hospitalized. It will require creativity on the part of nurses and others to make this possible.

The rights of indigenous peoples to their cultural beliefs and healthcare practices are receiving increasing attention. The United Nations has promulgated a Declaration on the Rights of Indigenous Peoples (UNDRIP; Carrie, Mackey, & Laird, 2015). Although the declaration is not binding for member nations, it behooves healthcare practitioners to become more aware of the practices of peoples who are coming to biomedical facilities for healthcare. It is important for healthcare workers to inquire about the use of healthcare practices and not show repugnance at seemingly "strange" practices. One area in which knowledge is particularly needed is the use of herbal preparations. In many cultures, it is not one herb but a combination of multiple herbal preparations that are used; information on the entirety of all herbs in any potions being taken is needed.

The inclusion of immigrants and indigenous persons in research on complementary therapies and other biomedical research is sorely needed, as is the exploration of the effectiveness of the health practices of indigenous cultures. One area in which research on the practices of indigenous people has been done is in the use of sweat lodges in the treatment of addiction in Native Americans. These practices were found to be effective both with the addiction and in the spiritual well-being of persons (Rowan et al., 2014).

The complementary therapy chapters that follow each detail how the specific therapy is implemented in countries other than the United States. Although similarities across nations and cultures in administration of therapies are noted, cultural differences are recognized in the handling of therapies globally. International sidebars that highlight both cross-cultural similarities and differences are included in most chapters.

IMPLICATIONS FOR NURSING

Although the term *complementary therapies* was not used until recently, numerous therapies and their underlying philosophy have been a part of the nursing profession since its beginnings. In *Notes on Nursing* (1935/1992), Florence Nightingale stressed the importance of creating an environment in which healing could occur and the significance of therapies such as music in the healing process. Complementary therapies today simply provide yet another opportunity for nurses to demonstrate caring for patients.

As noted in the chapters on self-care, education, practice, and research, nursing has embraced complementary practices. Although it is indeed gratifying to see that medicine and other health professions are recognizing the importance of listening and presence in the healing process, nurses need to assert that many of these therapies have been taught in nursing programs and have been practiced by nurses for centuries. Procedures such as meditation, imagery, support groups, music therapy, humor, journaling, reminiscence, caring-based approaches, massage, touch, healing touch, active listening, and presence have been practiced by nurses throughout time.

Complementary therapies are receiving increasing attention within nursing. Journals such as the *Journal of Holistic Nursing* and *Complementary Therapies for Clinical Practice* are devoted almost exclusively to complementary solutions. Many professional journals have devoted entire issues to exploring the use of complementary remedies. Articles inform nurses about complementary therapies and ways that specific procedures can be used with various conditions, including use for the promotion of health.

Because of the increasing use of complementary therapies by patients, it is critical that nurses possess basic knowledge about these therapies. Chang and Chang

(2015) reviewed studies done on nurses' knowledge and attitudes about complementary therapies. Although 66.4% of the participating nurses reported positive attitudes about these therapies, 77.4% did not possess a good understanding of the risks and benefits of complementary therapies. A sizable number of the nurses felt uncomfortable in discussing use of complementary therapies with their patients.

It is not feasible for nurses to know about *all* of the vast number of therapies, but the following are some skills and knowledge nurses should possess:

- Skills in obtaining a comprehensive health history to accurately ascertain patients' use of a broad range of complementary therapies
- Ability to assess the appropriateness and safety of therapies used
- Ability to answer basic questions about the use of complementary techniques
- Knowledge to refer patients to reliable sources of information
- Knowledge to suggest therapies having evidence of benefit for specific conditions
- Knowledge to provide guidelines for identifying competent therapists
- Ability to assist in determining whether insurance will reimburse for a specific therapy
- Knowledge and skills to administer a select number of complementary remedies

Obtaining a complete health history requires that questions about the use of complementary therapies be an integral part of the health history. Many patients may not volunteer information about using complementary procedures unless they are specifically asked; others may be reluctant to share this information unless the practitioner displays an acceptance of complementary techniques. Although facts are needed about all complementary therapies, getting feedback about use of herbal preparations is critical because interactions between certain prescription drugs and certain herbal preparations may pose a threat to health.

The vast number of complementary therapies makes it impossible for nurses to be knowledgeable about all of them, but familiarity with the more common therapies will assist health providers in answering basic questions. Many organizations, professional associations, individuals, and groups have excellent websites that provide information about specific therapies. Caution is needed, however, in accepting information from any website. These are some questions to consider when accessing a website for unbiased and honest information about a complementary therapy:

- What is the purpose of the site?
- What group/organization operates and/or funds the site?
- Who, such as an editorial board, selects the data contained on the site?
- How often is the content updated?
- Is there a way for the user to contact someone if questions arise about site content?

Chapter 30 provides more detailed information for evaluating websites. Also, each chapter provides websites related to that therapy.

CONCLUSION

More and more people not only know about complementary therapies but are using them or considering using them. Thus, it is essential for nurses to increase their knowledge about these therapies, which are often used with Western biomedical treatments. Patients may desire an emphasis on holistic care that underlies many complementary techniques. Holistic practice has permeated nursing for centuries, and incorporating complementary procedures into nursing care carries on this tradition.

REFERENCES

Balouchi, A., Rahanama, M., Hastings-Tolsma, M., Shoja, M., & Bolaydehyi, E. (2016). Knowledge, attitude and use of complementary and integrative health strategies: A preliminary survey of Iranian nurses. *Journal of Integrative Medicine, 14*, 121–127.

Barnes, P. M., Bloom, B., & Nahin, R. L. (2008). *Complementary and alternative medicine use among adults and children: United States, 2007.* (National Health Statistics Report No. 12). Hyattsville, MD: National Center for Health Statistics. Retrieved from https://www.cdc.gov/nchs/data/nhsr/nhsr012.pdf

Ben-Arye, E., Massalha, E., Bar-Sela, G., Silbermann, M., Agbarya, A., Saad, B., ... Schiff, E. (2014). Stepping from traditional to integrative medicine: Perspectives of Israeli-Arab patients on complementary medicine's role in cancer care. *Annals of Oncology, 25*, 476–480.

Borden, A., & Coyote, S. (2012). *The smudging ceremony.* Retrieved from http://www.asunam.com/smudge_ceremony.html

Brosseau, L., Wells, G., Tugwell, P, Casimiro, L, Novikov, M., Loew, L., ... Cohoon, C. (2012). Ottawa panel evidence-based clinical practice guidelines on therapeutic massage for neck pain. *Journal of Bodywork and Movement Therapies, 16*(3), 300–325.

Carrie, H., Mackey, T., & Laird, S. (2015). Integrating traditional indigenous medicine into Western biomedical health systems: A review of Nicaraguan health policies and Miskitu health services. *International Journal for Equity in Health, 1*, 129. doi:10.1186/s12939-015-0260-1

Chang, H., & Chang, H. (2015). A review of nurses' knowledge, attitudes, and ability to communicate the risks and benefits of complementary and alternative medicine. *Journal of Clinical Nursing, 24*, 1466–1478.

Clarke, T., Black, L., Stussman, B., Barnes, P., & Nahin, R. (2015). Trends in the use of complementary health approaches among adults: United States, 2002–2012. *National Health Statistics Reports, 79*, 1–15.

Cochrane Database of Systematic Reviews. (2017). What is Cochrane evidence and how can it help you? Retrieved from www.cochrane.org/what-is-cochrane-evidence

Coulter, I. D., Herman, P. M., & Nataraj, S. (2013). Economic analysis of complementary, alternative, and integrative medicine: Considerations raised by an expert panel. *BMC Complementary and Alternative Medicine, 13*, 191. doi:10.1186/1472-6882-13-191

George, M., & Topaz, M. (2013). A systematic review of complementary and alternative medicine for asthma self-management. *Nursing Clinics of North America, 48*, 53–149.

Goetz, C., Marriott, B. P., Finch, M. D., Bray, R. M., Williams, T. V., Hourani, L. L., ... Jonas, W. B. (2013). Military report more complementary and alternative medicine use than civilians. *Journal of Alternative and Complementary Medicine, 20*, 509–517.

Hoerster, K. D., Butler, D. A., Mayer, J. A., Finlayson, T., & Gallo, L. C. (2011). Use of conventional care and complementary/alternative medicine among U.S. adults with arthritis. *Preventive Medicine, 54*(1), 13–17.

Hori, S., Mihaylov, I., Vasconcelos, J. C., & McCoubrie, M. (2008). Patterns of complementary and alternative medicine use amongst outpatients in Tokyo, Japan. *BMC Complementary and Alternative Medicine, 8*, 14. doi:10.1186/1472-6882-8-14

Koithan, M., & Farrell, C. (2011). Indigenous Native American healing traditions. *Journal for Nurse Practitioners, 6*(6), 477–478. doi:10.1016/j.nurpra.2010.03.016

Lafferty, W., Tyree, P. T., Bellas, A. S., Watts, C., Lind, B., Sherman, K., ... Grembowski, D. E. (2006). Insurance coverage and subsequent utilization of complementary and alternative medical (CAM) providers. *American Journal of Managed Care, 12*, 397–404.

Laiyemo, M., Nunlee-Bland, G., Lombardo, F., Adams, G., & Laiyemo, A. (2015). Characteristics and health perceptions of complementary and alternative medicine users in the United States. *American Journal of the Medical Sciences, 349*, 140–144.

Lind, B. K., Lafferty, W. E., Tyree, P. T., & Diehr, P. K. (2010). Comparison of health care expenditures among insured users and nonusers of complementary and alternative medicine in Washington state: A cost minimization analysis. *Journal of Alternative and Complementary Medicine, 16*, 411–417.

Linde, K., Alscher, A., Friedrichs, C., Joos, S., & Schneider, A. (2014). The use of complementary and alternative therapies in Germany—a systematic review of nationwide surveys. *Forschende Komplementarmedizin, 21*, 111–118.

Manderson, L., & Smith-Morris, C. (2010). *Chronic conditions, fluid states: Chronicity and the anthropology of illness.* New Brunswick, NJ: Rutgers University Press.

Minnesota Department of Health, Health Occupation Program. (2017). *Consumer Guide: Complementary and Alternative Medicine.* Retrieved from http://www.health.state.mn.us/divs/hpsc/hop/ocap/ocapbroc2012.pdf

National Center for Complementary and Integrative Health. (2016a). NCCIH facts-at-a glance and mission. Retrieved from https://nccih.nih.gov/about/ataglance

National Center for Complementary and Integrative Health. (2016b). What complementary and integrative approaches do Americans use? Retrieved from https://nccih.nih.gov/research/statistics/NHIS/2012/key-findings

National Center for Complementary and Integrative Health. (2017a). The use of complementary and alternative medicine in the United States. Retrieved from https://nccih.nih.gov/research/statistics/2007/camsurvey_fs1.htm

National Center for Complementary and Integrative Health. (2017b). Paying for complementary and integrative health approaches. Retrieved from https://nccih.nih.gov/health/finacial

Nguyen, L. T., Davis, R. B., Kaptchuk, T. J., & Phillips, R. S. (2011). Use of complementary and alternative medicine and self-rated health status: Results from a national survey. *Journal of General Internal Medicine, 26*(4), 399–404.

Nightingale, F. (1992). *Notes on nursing.* Philadelphia, PA: Lippincott. (Original work published 1935).

Pelletier, K., Herman, R., Metz, P., & Nelson, C. (2010). Health and medical economics applied to integrative medicine. *Explore: The Journal of Science & Healing, 6*, 86–99.

Posadzki, P., Watson, L. K., Alotaibi, A., & Ernst, E. (2013). Prevalence of use of complementary and alternative medicine (CAM) by patients/consumers in the UK: Systematic review of surveys. *Clinical Medicine, 13*(2), 126–131.

Quinlan, M. (2011). Ethnomedicine. In M. Singer & P. Erickson (Eds.), *A companion to medical anthropology* (pp. 381–404). Ames, IA: Wiley-Blackwell.

Remen, R. N. (2000). *My grandfather's blessings.* New York, NY: Riverhead Books.

Rowan, M., Poole, N., Shea, B., Gone, J. P., Mykota, D., Farag, M., ... Dell, C. (2014). Cultural interventions to treat addictions in indigenous populations: Findings from a scoping study. *Substance Abuse Treatment, Prevention, and Policy, 9*, 34. doi:10.1186/1747-597X-9-34

Stephens, C., Porter, J., Nettleton, C., & Willis, R. (2006). Disappearing, displace, and undervalued: A call to action of indigenous health worldwide. *Lancet, 367*(9527), 2019–2028.

World Health Organization. (2012). *Health of indigenous peoples.* Retrieved from http://www.who.int/mediacentre/factsheets/fs326/en/index.html

Presence

MARIAH SNYDER

Presence is a practice that is used often by health professionals and also by many people in ordinary daily interactions. When the person we are interacting with is looking beyond us or flipping through messages on a smartphone, we know the person is not giving us full attention. We feel a sense of separation and disrespect. The description of presence related by Albom (1997) in *Tuesdays with Morrie* succinctly captures the essential elements of presence. Albom is reporting how Morrie, a man with advanced amyotrophic lateral sclerosis, views presence:

> I believe in being fully present. That means you should be with the person you're with. When I'm talking with you now, Mitch, I try to keep focused only on what is going on between us. I am not thinking about something we said last week. I am not thinking about what's coming up this Friday. I am not thinking about doing another Koppel show, or about medications I'm taking. I am talking to you; I am thinking about you. (pp. 135–136)

Presence plays an integral part in the use of all complementary therapies. Being fully present to the person adds to the effectiveness of the therapy being administered.

DEFINITION

Philosophical views of existentialism helped develop the concept of presence for nursing. Sartre (1943/1984) described awareness of the other as a means toward knowing a person and a way of presence. Sartre coined the term *authentic self* as bringing self to "being with" a person. According Nelms (1996), presence is the heart of nursing practice. Being truly there and being with are core definitions of *presence*.

The connection between philosophy and nursing regarding the concept of presence began to emerge in the 1960s. Vaillot (1962) used the phenomenon of presence to describe therapeutic relationships as crucial to patient care. According to Paterson and Zderad (1976), is the process of being available with the whole of oneself and open to the experience of another through a reciprocal interpersonal encounter. They defined *presence* as an intervention that the nurse uses to establish a relationship with the patient. Presence is an integral component of their theory of humanistic nursing.

Presence implies openness, receptivity, readiness, and availability on the part of the nurse. Many nursing situations require the close proximity of the nurse to another person; however, that in itself does not constitute presence. To be truly present, the nurse conveys an openness to a "person-with-needs" and with an "availability-in-a-helping way" (Paterson & Zderad, 1976). Reciprocity often emerges through this type of interaction.

Benner (1984) coined the verb *presencing* to denote the existential practice of being with a patient. "Presencing" is one of the eight competencies Benner identified as constituting the helping role of the nurse. More recently, McMahon and Christopher (2011) developed a midrange theory of nursing presence in which they identified five variables that characterize presence: individual client characteristics, characteristics of the nurse, shared characteristics within the nurse–patient dyad, the environment, and the intentional decisions of the nurse related to practice.

Kostovich (2012) identified the following as attributes as composing presence: teaching, surveillance, concern, empathy, companionship, educated skillfulness, availability, responsive listening, coordination of care, spiritual enhancement, reassurance, and personalization of care (p. 169). These served as the basis for developing her scale for measuring presence.

Presence may be reciprocal when both parties are connecting and may be meaningful to both the patient and the nurse. Melnechenko (2003) noted, "To be invited to share in another's unfolding health, to be asked to journey with another through the process of moving and choosing, is without doubt an honor and privilege" (p. 24). Hessel (2009), in a concept analysis of presence, noted that presence involves a spiritual connection that is felt when the nurse and the patient share the experience of being together. In presence, the nurse is available to the patient with the wholeness of the unique individual being.

Presence is much more than being physically present. According to Hessel (2009), it requires nurses to completely focus their attention on their patients, including being free of other thoughts and responsibilities to allow for a true connectedness though sharing the human experience (p. 278). Edvardsson and colleagues (2017) used the term *patient-centeredness,* which captures what presence focuses on: the patient. In an editorial in the *Journal of PeriAnesthesia Nursing,* Hooper (2013) states:

> While patients may recognize that the presence of the nurse at the bedside carrying out routine activities such as monitoring vital signs, administering medications, etc. is critical to their safe passage across the surgical continuum, they are most reassured when the nurse is actively, intentionally present and engaged with the patient. (p. 255)

The universality of presence and caring has been documented (Jonsdöttir, Litchfield, & Pharris, 2004). Presence transcends cultures and modes of communication. The Buddhist way of life, through mindfulness, implies one is attentive, aware, and fully present in the moment (Kabat-Zinn, 1990). Even if the nurse and patient are unable to communicate verbally, the patient often perceives the presence of a caring nurse.

SCIENTIFIC BASIS

Conducting research on presence poses many challenges due to its subjective nature. The majority of research has been qualitative. Only recently have scales to measure presence been developed (Kostovich, 2012). The reliability and validity of Kostovich's 25-item Presence of Nursing Scale has been established. Such a scale will assist in validating the importance of presence in the practice of nursing and other professions.

Nurse scientists have described presence as a subconstruct of the broad concept of caring (Nelms, 1996; Watson, 1985). Caring requires the nurse to be keenly attentive to the needs of the patient, the meaning the patient attaches to the illness or problem, and the way that the patient wishes to proceed. The use of presence helps the patient heal, discover others, and find meaning in life.

Research on the expert practice of critical care nurses has demonstrated the importance of presence. Minick (1995) found that connectedness with the patient was important not only as a caring behavior, but also because it assisted the nurse in the early identification of postoperative problems. Therapeutic presence may help nurses be more attentive and detect subtle changes that may not be evident without it. Nurses lacking connectedness were perceived by their patients as detached. Wilkin and Slevin (2004) further validated the importance of the critical care nurse being present to the patient as essential, as were the skills needed to reach unresponsive and intubated patients.

When presence is used as a complementary therapy, consequences or effects occur for the patient, family, and nurse. Easter (2000) reported a decrease in pain for the patient, an increase in satisfaction for the nurse, and improved mental well-being for the nurse through presence. According to Drick (2003), presence creates healing and changes the atmosphere in the nurse–patient relationship. Jonas and Crawford (2004) reported lower, more stable heart rates as a result of healing presence within minutes to hours of the intervention. Tavernier (2006) identified three consequences of presence: (a) relationship, (b) healing, and (c) reward. The importance of presence in care has been recognized and valued as a key nursing intervention. A midrange theory of nursing presence, developed by McMahon and Christopher (2011), identifies presence as integral to the nurse–patient relationship. The nurse must have the ability to recognize the need for presence and be open to the invitation to be present. Further investigation on why and how presence plays a positive and vital role in health outcomes needs to be encouraged.

INTERVENTION

Presence is an intervention used by nurses but requires constant intention due to the often-hectic work situations. Nurses may increase their use of true presence by being there with a patient, practicing journaling and mindfulness meditation, or engaging in purposeful activities such as smiling and centering. These activities enable a person to experience presence and evoke it as an intervention.

Centering

Presence entails conscious attention to the upcoming interaction with the patient. The nurse must be available with the whole self and be open to the personal and care needs of the patient. This process is called *centering*, and it is a meditative state. The nurse takes a short time, sometimes only 10 or 20 seconds, to eliminate distractions, so that the focus can be on the patient. Some people find that taking a deep breath and closing the eyes helps in freeing them of distractions and becoming centered. This may be done outside the room (or other setting) in which the encounter will occur. Centering may also be as simple as the nurse pausing before contact with the patient and repeating the patient's name to help focus attention on that person.

Bartels (2014) discusses the use of "The Pause" for being with a person who has died. The nurse or team takes 45 to 60 seconds to focus on the life of the patient who has died. The concept of "The Pause" could be implemented in situations with unresponsive patients or those with dementia.

Technique

Exhibit 2.1 lists the key component of presence and the skills necessary for practicing it. Sensitivity to others requires the nurse to be an excellent listener and observer. (Therapeutic listening is addressed in Chapter 3.) Good observation skills assist nurses in identifying nuances in expression and communication that may reveal the real concerns of the patient. Presence often means periods of silence in which subtle interchanges occur. Continuing attentiveness on the part of the nurse is a critical aspect of this therapy. Both the nurse and the client experience a sense of union or joining for a moment in time. Focusing on the moment—not the past or the future—is inherent in being present.

Little is known about the length of a therapy session or the times when therapeutic presence should be used. Often, the nurse identifies it intuitively: "It just seems like this patient truly needs me now." Because of the intense nature of the interaction, the length of time the nurse is present to the patient may seem greater even though only 30 seconds or a minute may have passed. Although presence

Exhibit 2.1. Skills for Implementing Presence

Key Component	Skills
Holistic attention to patient	Centering
	Active listening
	Openness to others
	Sensitivity
	Verbal communication that is at the level of the patient
	Use of touch when culturally appropriate
	Nonverbal demonstration of acceptance

Exhibit 2.2. Possible Outcomes of Presence

- Patient feeling comforted and supported
- Patient sensing that whole being is cared for
- Patient level of stress decreased
- Patient feeling less lonely
- Patient having an increased sense of peace and hope
- Patient feeling increased self-worth
- Patient perceiving decreased pain
- Patient feeling motivated and encouraged
- Nurse having an increased sense of who the patient is
- Nurse having increased satisfaction with care

---

is often used with another therapy or treatment, identifying when patients need someone to just be present for a few minutes may be the most effective technique in helping the patient feel cared for.

Measurement of Outcomes

Measuring outcomes of presence interventions involve both the patient and the nurse because of their reciprocal interaction. Comments from the patient about feeling cared for, being able to express concerns, and perceiving understanding are some outcome measures derived from patient satisfaction tools. McMahon and Christopher (2011) reviewed literature on presence and identified potential client outcomes. These are shown in Exhibit 2.2. The correlation between patient satisfaction and person-centered care was shown in study by Edvardsson, Watt, and Pearce (2017). Several of the variables having high correlations were (a) a place where staff seem to have time for patients, (b) a place where staff takes notice of what a patient says, (c) sensitivity toward the patient, and (d) empathy toward or identification with the patient. Incorporating the effects of presence in patient surveys should be considered among the important outcomes indicating a positive health experience and healing. Because of the intangibles that often occur with the use of presence, finding words or indices to measure presence may be challenging.

PRECAUTIONS

The major precaution in the use of presence is to take one's cue from the patient and not force an encounter. A true presence encounter considers the wants and needs of the patient and is not for the nurse's primary benefit. If the nurse is truly centered on the patient and aware of the needs of the patient, the nurse will act in accordance with the wishes and needs of the patient (Paterson & Zderad, 1976).

A negative consequence of presence is that colleagues may be critical of the nurse who spends time "just being" with patients and/or families. Certainly, this should not be a deterrent to the use of presence, but rather a concern that should be discussed and resolved by nursing staff. Finfgeld-Connett (2006) stated that a supportive work environment that starts at the highest administrative level of the facility helps promote the use of presence.

Professional maturity has been identified as a factor having an impact on the use of presence. McMahon and Christopher (2011) noted that novice nurses may be so focused on the skill to be performed that they are unable to detect the subtle signs that the patient requires the intervention of presence.

USES

Presence can be used in any nursing situation. Patients struggling with a new diagnosis, an exacerbation of a condition, or a loss are especially in need of moments of presence. An and Jo (2009) found that a 30-minute nursing-presence intervention reduced stress in older adults in nursing homes. The use of presence is also important with patients in hospice settings.

Presence is especially needed with patients in critical care settings (Wilkin & Slevin, 2004) and emergency departments (Wiman & Wikblad, 2004). Patients and their families often feel lost in high-tech critical care settings. The use of presence helps prevent critical care nurses from being viewed by their patients as emotionally distant and focusing only on machines and technology. Other patient populations in which the use of presence has been documented as significant to care include women with postpartum psychosis (Engqvist, Ferszt, & Nilsson, 2010) and in midwifery practice (Hunter, 2009). Karlou, Papathanassoglou, and Patiraki (2015) explored caring behaviors of cancer patients in Greece.

Although not specific to presence, Tornøc, Danbolt, Kvigne, and Sørlie (2015) detail a mobile hospice nurse model for training care workers in how to meet the spiritual and existential care needs of dying patients. The team demonstrated and worked with staff to decrease the staff workers' fears in interacting with dying patients and to provide the interacting care needed to meet the needs of this group of patients. Some long-term care facilities have a volunteer service for dying residents who do not have a family member to sit with them as they near death. This is "being with," and although the dying person may not give any indication of the presence, holding a hand or touching conveys that the person is not alone.

As healthcare and nursing encompass more technology, including telemedicine, as part of the modes for delivery of care, explorations of virtual presence are needed. Educators using distance teaching have been investigating the impact of the emotional presence of the instructor on learners and the effect this has on learning outcomes. Sandelowski (2002) noted that nurses and people involved in designing technology are interested in creating environments for patients and nurses to produce feelings of interaction that are immediate, intimate, and *real*. The rapidly increasing use of telephones, home monitoring, and other forms of telemedicine challenge nurses to convey attentive care in these settings that includes presence. Nurses can ask themselves, "Am I truly listening, present to the patient who is invisible?" Mastel-Smith, Post, and Lake (2015) entitled their article about online teaching as "Are You There, and Do You Care?" This is a question nurses involved in online care should ask themselves.

CULTURAL APPLICATIONS

Culture is closely interlaced with nationality, race/ethnicity, social class, and even generations and is important in considering the meaning of presence for the patient, family, and nurse. Presence may also hold a special interpretation for the individual based on past experience or family influence. The key is to identify and acknowledge the meaning of presence for the patient and all family members in the relationship. Mitchell (2006) provides an exemplar of presence among young, middle-aged, and older adults. The themes of attentive presence and "being with" in the exemplar are apparent in each of the generations. As described by Mitchell, cultural connection is necessary for bringing meaning to life experience and is emotional and healing.

In addition, each person has a preference for a communication style, which may be influenced by cultural background. In several cultures, using gestures of respect and knowing the person hold high importance in establishing a relationship. In other cultures, too much eye contact may be seen as offensive. Communication and trust are shown to be the largest factors that create connection among Hispanic families (Evans, Coon, & Crogan, 2007). Conversational silence is important in some cultures as a mechanism to becoming present with another person or the environment. Buddhists use silence as a respectful technique for being present and are comfortable with long periods of silence, whereas other cultures may not be. Mindfulness, being in the present moment and aware of everything around oneself, is the Buddhist way of life.

Interacting with patients and families from a culture different than that of the nurse may take more time than the nurse is accustomed to giving in a situation. Patience may be required to give adequate explanations or respond to the tug on one's hand when verbal communication fails. A warm smile and just standing by the bed for a moment convey that a nurse does care and wishes for a better understanding and verbal communication.

In Sidebar 2.1, a nurse from Pakistan relates the use of presence while caring for a patient in her country. It conveys the universality of the use of presence by nurses across the world.

SIDEBAR 2.1. USE OF "PRESENCE IN NURSING" IN PAKISTAN

Naheed Meghani

Pakistan, being a developing country, has fewer resources than many countries. There is a nursing shortage and hence cultural and socioeconomic realities intersect. In Pakistan, when possible, nurses rely on family members or volunteers to be with the patient. In Pakistani culture, there is a family value system, and a family member's illness is regarded as a family matter. The nurses work collaboratively with the family member(s) who stay with the patient, and their presence is comforting and healing to the patient. Nurses' presence is also reassuring to the patients to allay fear and anxiety. Having the familiar face of a family member helps in achieving the goal of promoting comfort and healing. In the event when nurses have too many patients assigned and are pressed for time, they prioritize which patients would benefit most from their presence.

(continued)

One of the examples I remember vividly from my nursing experience was of a patient (a truck driver) who was brought into the hospital after an accident. I found in the patient's chart that some roadside witnesses of the accident brought him to the hospital. He was unconscious and did not have any family members with him. When he regained consciousness and was stable, he was transferred to our unit. This patient was always quiet, disinterested, and staring at the ceiling. He would not finish his meals and sometimes skip them, saying he wasn't hungry. He started refusing his medications, too. I had 30 patients assigned to me, but I prioritized that this particular patient needing my presence. I sat on the chair beside his bed and asked him, while making appropriate eye contact, what he would like to share. He started crying and revealed that he missed his family, who lived in a rural area quite distant and probably were unable to visit. He wasn't sure if they even knew that he had been in an accident. He worried that he would never see them again.

I told him it was all right to cry about not being with his family and offered him some water. I sat by him and told him that as his nurse, I was concerned about his health and well-being and that although it was not possible for his family to visit, perhaps there was a way he could talk to them over the phone or to write them. He told me that they did not have a telephone and although he knew how to read and write, no one at his home knew how to do so. I felt very sad and quite helpless. I asked him if there was anything he would like changed in his surroundings to make him feel better. He asked if we could move his bed by the window so that he can see the tree that reminded him of a tree in the front of his house. I asked permission from another patient, and we switched the bed assignments so the trucker had the bed closer to the window. He was very grateful. I gave him paper and a pen so that he could draw a picture of the tree for his family. I sent that to his family. I also connected him with other patients on the unit and their family members. I reassured him that we were figuring out a way to connect with his family and coordinating the next steps of care. The patient started to connect with other patients and their families. The patient became stable and was discharged home. When he was leaving the unit, he gave me a paper (a thank you note), on which he had drawn a tree and a sun rising. He said, "That tree gave me hope and reminded me of my home. Then I wanted to get better so I could see my family. You helped me see that there was hope."

This was emotionally and spiritually uplifting for me that my attentiveness and presence made a difference in this patient's life. I believe that it is essential to assess, understand, and respond to what is a meaningful presence for a patient from a cultural perspective. Presence is meaningful when the nurse is open to the reciprocal interaction; however, with sensitivity to the knowledge of the culture, any related previous experiences or cues from the patient or family will assist the nurse in these interactions.

FUTURE RESEARCH

Nurses document assessments made and treatments administered, but rarely do they document the use of presence and the outcomes of this therapy. Despite the challenges in identifying and documenting outcomes of presence, current interest in complementary therapies provides an opportunity for nurses to validate the positive outcomes of the use of presence. Areas in which research is needed include the following:

- Although every patient could benefit from presence, what are assessments that would alert nurses to patients who most need the therapy of presence?
- What strategies can be used to teach nursing students and other health professionals ways to implement presence? The article by Tornøc and colleagues (2015) suggest strategies that may be helpful.
- With telemedicine rapidly increasing, how can presence be introduced into these contacts with patients? Is physical presence essential for patients to feel caring and personal interest by nurses?
- As diversity in patient populations increases, what are ways nurses can learn about cultural behaviors in cultures so that presence is practiced in the appropriate manner?

REFERENCES

Albom, M. (1997). *Tuesdays with Morrie*. New York, NY: Doubleday.

An, G., & Jo, K. (2009). The effect of a nursing presence program on reducing stress in older adults in two Korean nursing homes. *Australian Journal of Advanced Nursing, 26*, 79–85.

Bartels, J. (2014). The pause. *Critical Care Nurse, 34*, 74–75.

Benner, P. (1984). *From novice to expert: Excellence and power in clinical nursing practice*. Menlo Park, CA: Addison-Wesley.

Drick, C. A. (2003). Back to basics: The power of presence in nursing care. *Journal of Gynecologic Oncology Nursing, 13*(3), 13–18.

Easter, A. (2000). Construct analysis of four modes of being present. *Journal of Holistic Nursing, 18*, 362–377.

Edvardsson, D., Watt, E., & Pearce, F. (2017). Patient experiences of caring and person-centeredness are associated with perceived nursing care quality. *Journal of Advanced Nursing, 73*, 217–227.

Engqvist, I., Ferszt, G., & Nilsson, K. (2010). Swedish registered nurses' description of presence when caring for women with post-partum psychosis: An interview study. *International Journal of Mental Health Nursing, 19*, 193–196.

Evans, B. C., Coon, D., & Crogan, N. L. (2007). *Personalismo* and breaking barriers: Accessing Hispanic populations for clinical services and research. *Geriatric Nursing, 28*(5), 289–296.

Finfgeld-Connett, D. (2006). Meta-synthesis of presence in nursing. *Journal of Advanced Nursing, 55*, 708–714.

Hessel, J. (2009). Presence in nursing practice: A concept analysis. *Holistic Nursing Practice, 23*, 276–281.

Hooper, V. (2013). The caring presence of nursing: A qualitative focus. *Journal of PeriAnesthesia Nursing, 28*, 255–256.

Hunter, L. (2009). A descriptive study of "being with women" during labor and birth. *Journal of Midwifery & Women's Health, 54*, 111–118.

Jonas, W. B., & Crawford, C. C. (2004). The healing presence: Can it be reliably measured? *Journal of Alternative and Complementary Medicine, 10*, 751–756.

Jonsdóttir, H., Litchfield, M., & Pharris, M. D. (2004). The relational core of nursing practice in partnership. *Journal of Advanced Nursing, 47*, 241–248.

Kabat-Zinn, J. (1990). *Full catastrophe living*. New York, NY: Delacorte.

Karlou, C., Papathanassoglou, E., & Patiraki, E. (2015). Caring behaviors in cancer care in Greece: Comparison of patients', their caregivers', and nurses' perceptions. *European Journal of Oncology Nursing, 19*, 244–250.

Kostovich, C. T. (2012). Development and psychometric assessment of the Presence of Nursing Scale. *Nursing Science Quarterly, 25*, 167–175.

Mastel-Smith, B., Post, J., & Lake, P. (2015). Online teaching: 'Are you there, and do you care?' *Journal of Nursing Education, 54*, 145–151.

McMahon, M., & Christopher, K. (2011). Toward a mid-range theory of nursing presence. *Nursing Forum, 46*(2), 71–82.

Melnechenko, K. (2003). To make a difference: Nursing presence. *Nursing Forum, 38*, 18–24.

Minick, P. (1995). The power of human caring: Early recognition of patient problems. *Scholarly Inquiry for Nursing Practice: An International Journal, 9*, 303–317.

Mitchell, M. (2006). Understanding true presence with elders: A story of joy and sorrow. *Perspectives, 30*(3), 17–19.

Nelms, T. P. (1996). Living a caring presence in nursing: A Heideggerian hermeneutical analysis. *Journal of Advanced Nursing, 24*, 368–374.

Paterson, J. G., & Zderad, L. T. (1976). *Humanistic nursing*. New York, NY: Wiley.

Sandelowski, M. (2002). Visible humans, vanishing bodies, and virtual nursing: Complications of life, presence, place, and identity. *Advances in Nursing Science, 24*, 58–70.

Sartre, J. P. (1943/1984). *Being and nothingness*. New York, NY: Washington Square Press.

Tavernier, S. (2006). An evidence-based conceptual analysis of presence. *Holistic Nursing Practice, 20*, 152–156.

Tornøc, K., Danbolt, L., Kvigne, K., & Sørlie, V. (2015). A mobile hospice nurse teaching team's experience: Training care workers in spiritual and existential care for dying—A qualitative study. *BMC Palliative Care, 14*, 43. doi:10.1186/s12904-015-0042-y

Vaillot, S. M. C. (1962). *Commitment to nursing: A philosophical investigation*. Philadelphia, PA: Lippincott.

Watson, J. (1985). *Nursing: Human science and human care: A theory of nursing*. Norwalk, CT: Appleton-Century-Crofts.

Wilkin, K., & Slevin, E. (2004). The meaning of caring to nurses: An investigation into the nature of caring work in an intensive care unit. *Journal of Clinical Nursing, 13*, 50–59.

Wiman, E., & Wikblad, K. (2004). Caring and uncaring encounters in nursing in an emergency department. *Journal of Clinical Nursing, 13*, 422–429.

Therapeutic Listening

SHIGEAKI WATANUKI, MARY FRAN TRACY, AND RUTH LINDQUIST

Listening is an active and dynamic process of interaction that requires intentional effort to attend to a client's verbal and nonverbal cues. Listening is an integral part and foundation of nurse–client relationships and one of the most effective therapeutic techniques available to nurses. The theoretical underpinnings of listening can be traced back to counseling psychology and psychotherapy. Rogers (1957) used counseling and listening to foster independence and promote growth and development of clients. Rogers also emphasized that empathy, warmth, and genuineness with clients were necessary and sufficient for therapeutic changes to occur. Listening has been identified as a significant component of therapeutic communication with patients and therefore fundamental to a therapeutic relationship between the nurse and the patient (Foy & Timmins, 2004). Listening is also a key to improving health professionals' teamwork effectiveness and patient safety in complex clinical settings (Denham et al., 2008). Listening is foundational in the administration of complementary therapies.

DEFINITION

Many modifiers are used with the word listening—*active, attentive, empathic, therapeutic,* and *holistic.* The choice of modifier seems to depend more on an author's paradigm than on differences in the descriptions of listening (Fredriksson, 1999). Unless active listening was explicitly used by researchers in the articles reviewed in this chapter, the term *therapeutic listening* is used here to focus on the formal, deliberate actions of listening for therapeutic purposes (Lekander, Lehmann, & Lindquist, 1993). *Therapeutic listening* is defined as "an interpersonal, confirmation process involving all the senses in which the therapist attends with empathy to the client's verbal and nonverbal messages to facilitate the understanding, synthesis, and interpretation of the client's situation" (Kemper, 1992, p. 22). Beyond the therapist, this empathetic attending pertains to nurses and to other care providers.

SCIENTIFIC BASIS

Therapeutic listening is a topic of interest and concern to a variety of disciplines. A number of qualitative and quantitative studies provide a scientific basis of intervention effects in relation to process—behavioral changes of providers that foster communication—and outcomes, including improved client satisfaction and other clinical indicators.

Evidence from a neuropsychological experiment using functional brain imaging demonstrates the powerful interpersonal impact of listening (Kawamichi et al., 2015). When the study participants perceived the experience of "being actively listened to," or had positive emotional appraisal of such an interaction and the listener, their brains showed an activated "reward system," as evidenced by neural activation in the ventral striatum and the right anterior insula (Kawamichi et al., 2015). When the participants believed they were being actively listened to, they also expressed increased willingness to cooperate with the listener.

A systematic review of 20 intervention studies that aimed to improve patient–doctor communication revealed the effectiveness of interventions that typically increased patient participation and clarification (Harrington, Noble, & Newman, 2004). Although few improvements in patient satisfaction were found, significant improvements in perceptions of control over health, preferences for an active role in healthcare, adherence to recommendations, and clinical outcomes were achieved. Likewise, preferable client outcomes were found in another study in nursing. A survey of 195 parents of hospitalized pediatric patients demonstrated that healthcare providers' use of immediacy and perceived listening were positively associated with satisfaction, care, and communication (Wanzer, Booth-Butterfield, & Gruber, 2004).

Qualitative studies provide rich understanding of the nature of therapeutic listening and explore the meaning and experience of being listened to in the context of real-world settings. Self-expression opportunities that enable clients to be listened to and understood can promote clients' self-discovery—meaning reconstruction and healing (Sandelowski, 1994). A discourse analysis of 20 nurse–patient pairs at community hospitals, however, indicated insufficient active listening skills on the part of nurses (Barrere, 2007). The study results showed that nurses often missed cues when patients needed them to listen to their concerns or overlooked potential opportunities for health teaching, especially in "asymmetrical" communication patterns (dominance of nurse or patient) compared with "symmetrical" patterns (nurse–patient communication involving active listening).

Conversely, in a qualitative study using unstructured interviews with patients regarding their experiences with nurse communication, McCabe (2004) found that most participants had positive experiences of empathetic communication by nurses. In situations when patients felt this did not occur, they attributed the lack of communication more with the nurses needing to complete tasks and being extremely busy rather than a deficiency in the nurse. McCabe concludes that nurses can communicate well if they approach communication from a patient-centered perspective rather than a task-centered perspective. Based on these findings, one may ask whether listening cues were actually missed in the study by Barrere (2007) because nurses didn't have adequate listening skills or felt they didn't have adequate time to do a listening intervention.

The utility of active listening training has been shown in an experiment with undergraduate students (Bodie, Vickery, Cannava, & Jones, 2015). The undergraduate students were randomly assigned to disclose their upsetting problem to either trained listeners or untrained listeners. The study results showed that active listening behavior promoted a greater emotional improvement of the students; however, active listening did not affect perceived improvement in relational assurance and problem solving of the students (Bodie et al., 2015).

A combination of learning sessions (cognitive interventions), administrative support, and coaching activities (affective and behavioral interventions) enables long-term improvement in communication styles of nurses. A quasi-experimental study was undertaken to test the effectiveness of an integrated communication skills training program for 129 oncology nurses at a hospital in China. Continued significant improvements in overall basic communication skills, self-efficacy, outcome expectancy beliefs, and perceived support in the training group were observed after 1 and 6 months of training intervention. No significant improvements were found in the control group (Liu, Mok, Wong, Xue, & Xu, 2007).

These studies attempted to identify complex relationships among multiple phenomena and variables, including the immediate and long-term effects of training interventions, clinical supervision and support, and cognitive and behavioral changes on the part of nurses. Further systematic studies are needed to enhance knowledge related to intervention effectiveness, especially the link between client characteristics, client satisfaction, and type of interventions. This is particularly important in light of today's healthcare emphasis and reimbursement aligned with patient satisfaction, patient engagement, and symptom management such as alleviation of pain. The Centers for Medicare & Medicaid Services (CMS) views RN–patient communication as one of several critical aspects of patients' hospital experiences (CMS, 2014, 2015). That is why a question regarding RN–patient communication is on the *Hospital Consumer Assessment of Healthcare Providers and Systems (HCAHPS) Survey*, a patient satisfaction survey that all hospitals are required to conduct and publicly report and on which a portion of their reimbursement is based (CMS, 2014, 2015).

INTERVENTION

Therapeutic listening enables clients to better understand their feelings and to experience being understood by another caring person. It has been said that there may be no more fundamental behavior for supporting others in the process of disclosing stress than through active listening (Bodie et al., 2015), and it is thought to be a crucial skill for nurses and healthcare providers (Halpern, 2012). Effective engagement in therapeutic listening requires nurses to be aware of verbal and nonverbal communication that conveys explicit and implicit messages. When verbalized words contradict nonverbal messages, communicators rely more often on nonverbal cues; facial expression, tone of voice, and silence become as important as words in determining the meaning of a message (Kacperek, 1997). Nonverbal communication is inextricably linked to verbal communication and can change, emphasize, or distract from the words that are spoken (Bush, 2001).

Developing Therapeutic Listening Skills

Listening is a skill that needs to be practiced and refined, just like other more tangible nursing skills. In today's healthcare environment with ever-present time pressures, it may be easy to become a "provider" of listening using visible behaviors such as nodding, eye contact, and not monitoring the time, rather than being an empathetic listener who truly engages and actively participates with the discloser (Halpern, 2012). Nurses may view others or be viewed themselves as not being productive when taking the time to act as a listener rather than performing other more visible, tangible nursing interventions. It is important to recognize that it requires practice and education to transform "ordinary" listening skills into "therapeutic" listening. In the process of learning therapeutic listening, the listener may actually learn to do less than more, undoing habitual reactions and interactions (Lee & Prior, 2013). There can be a tendency for nurses to talk more and offer advice rather than to stay in the listening mode as a means for the discloser to guide the problem-solving process (Chan, 2010).

One must learn to be aware of what is occurring when listening: Am I filtering content through my personal lens? What am I doing with my body? Am I having an emotional reaction to what is being said? Am I formulating a response rather than staying engaged in listening? (Lee & Prior, 2013).

There are multiple ways to practice and refine therapeutic listening skills, both in education programs and in clinical practice. In education, use of traditional and contemporary methods, such as role playing and simulations, may be helpful; both of those scenarios developed specifically around therapeutic-listening situations or were embedded within scenarios that are emotionally charged, such as end-of-life conversations after acute physiological events. Scenarios can occur with colleagues, instructors, or actors playing the part of clients. They can also be videotaped or audiotaped and reviewed for learning opportunities. It is also important for instructors and preceptors to both role-model in the clinical setting and provide feedback in observations of the student. The Calgary–Cambridge Referenced Observation Guide may be a helpful tool for instructors to use when educating students in this skill (Kurtz, Silverman, & Draper, 1998; Silverman, Kurtz, & Draper, 1998).

In clinical practice, more experienced colleagues and leaders can also role-model, mentor, and provide feedback in daily interactions as well as more formal conversations with patients and families such as care conferences. Mentors can offer phrases and techniques to improve listening skills. In the mental health setting, clinical supervision is frequently used to formally build skills such as therapeutic listening as a component of developing therapeutic relationships (Chan, 2010).

Guidelines

Listening is an active process, incorporating explicit behaviors, as well as attention to choice of words, quality of voice (pitch, timing, and volume), and full engagement in the process (Burnard, 1997). Therapeutic listening requires a listener to tune in to the client and to use all the senses in analyzing, inferring, and evaluating the stated and underlying meaning of the client's message. As providers feel increasing time pressures, it can be easy to attempt to guide or limit the conversation rather than allowing the patient to fully express concerns. However, to be fully heard without interruption can be viewed as supportive by the patient (Bryant, 2009) and may ultimately strengthen the therapeutic relationship. Therapeutic listening requires concentration and an ability to differentiate between what is actually being said and what one wants or expects to hear. It may be difficult to listen accurately and interpret messages that one finds difficult to relate to or to listen to information that one may not want to hear. When not fully engaged, it can be easy to become distracted or to start formulating a response rather than to stay focused on the message.

Therapeutic listening is both a cognitive and an emotional process (Arnold & Underman Boggs, 2007). Jones and Cutcliffe (2009) state that therapeutic listening requires a critical competency of self-management and resilience in the midst of emotional situations. They state it involves the need to be comfortable with ambiguity and emotional discomfort. Nurses should be prepared with statements to use in response to expression of negative emotions to encourage the speaker to further discuss their feelings (Adams, Cimino, Arnold, & Anderson, 2012). Several components have been identified as being foundational to therapeutic listening:

1. Rephrasing the patient's words and thoughts to ensure clarity and accuracy
2. Reflecting feeling
3. Conveying an understanding of the speaker's perceptions
4. Assumption checking
5. Asking questions and prompting to clarify (Bodie et al., 2015; DeVito, 2006)

These and other techniques for therapeutic listening intervention are presented in Exhibit 3.1.

Therapeutic listening with children can be even more complex because it frequently involves the presence or participation of more parties: nurse, child, parents, and/or other family members. This may take particular skill on the part of the nurse, who attends to both the spoken messages and the nonverbal communication/reactions of two or more people simultaneously. In addition, the nurse must be sensitive to the information and cues of either the child or the caregiver, depending on the child's age and developmental stage.

Adolescents especially may be willing to talk openly with an adult who is not a family member. However, they may respond quickly, abruptly, or defensively to any perceived indications of judgment, indifference, or disrespect on the part of the listener. It is extremely important with adolescents to be fully attentive, allow for complete expression of thoughts, and avoid statements or facial expressions that imply disapproval or that can be misinterpreted.

In addition, with the increased use of technology in everyday healthcare environments (e.g., telehealth, telemedicine, charting at the bedside through electronic health records) it is imperative to consider how the use of technology can either impede or enhance the use of therapeutic listening skills.

A listening technique referred to as *change-oriented reflective listening* targets behavioral change in healthcare providers (Strang, McCambridge, Platts, & Groves, 2004) and has a strong potential for incorporation into the repertoire of nursing interventions. This technique has been adapted from the core principles of motivational interviewing (Rollnick et al., 2002). Change-oriented reflective listening is a brief motivational enhancement intervention that encourages providers'

Exhibit 3.1. Therapeutic Listening Techniques

Active presence: Active presence involves focus on clients to interpret the message that they are trying to convey, on recognition of themes, and on hearing what is left unsaid. Short responses such as "yes" or "uh-huh" with appropriate timing and frequency may promote clients' willingness to talk.

Accepting attitude: Conveying an accepting attitude is assuring and can help clients feel more comfortable about expressing themselves. This can be demonstrated by short affirmative responses or gestures.

Clarifying statements: Clarifying statements and summarizing can help the listener verify message interpretation and create clarity, as well as encourage specificity rather than vague statements to facilitate communication. Rephrasing and reflection can assist the client in self-understanding. Using phrases such as "tell me more about that" and "what was that like?" may be helpful, rather than asking "why," which may elicit a defensive response. Typically statements such as these are used with an introductory phrase that conveys speculation and an attempt to clarify (e.g., it seems that, it appears that, …)

> *Paraphrasing*: The listener repeats what speakers said using their own words to the best of how the listener understood it.
>
> *Reflecting feelings*: The listener references the speaker's statements with an attempt to accurately convey and mirror the feelings underlying the statements, which is different than paraphrasing.
>
> *Assumption checking*: The listener uses short questions to verify accuracy in understanding the speaker's disclosure.

Use of silence: The use of silence can encourage the client to talk, facilitate the nurse's focus on listening rather than the formulation of responses, and reduce the use of leading questions. Sensitivity toward cultural and individual variations in the seconds of silence may be developed by paying detailed attention to the patterns of client communication.

Tone: Tone of voice can express more than words through empathy, judgment, or acceptance. The intensity of the tone should be matched to the message received to avoid minimizing or overemphasizing.

Nonverbal behaviors: Clients relaying sensitive information may be very aware of the listener's body language, which will be viewed as either accepting of the message or closed to it, judgmental, and/or disinterested. Eye contact or nodding are essential to conveying the listener's true interest and attention. Maintaining a conversational distance and judicious use of touch may increase the client's comfort. Cultural and social awareness are important so as to avoid undesired touch.

Environment: Distractions should be eliminated to encourage the therapeutic interchange. Therapeutic listening may require careful planning to provide time for undivided attention or may occur spontaneously. Some clients may feel very comfortable having family present; others may feel inhibited when others are present.

consideration of the quality of primary care and then stimulates their intent to change behavior in the direction desired. This method takes the form of a brief telephone conversation (15–20 minutes), in which reflective listening statements are interspersed with open questions about the issue at hand. A menu of questions with the range of possible areas for discussion is constructed in advance. The technique has been successfully piloted with general practitioners to motivate them to intervene with opiate users and as part of alcohol intervention (McCambridge, Platts, Whooley, & Strang, 2004; Strang et al., 2004).

Communicating with a patient and family in difficult situations necessitates careful and considerate listening skills. Basic communication skills such as the "ask-tell-ask" and "tell me more" principles have been introduced to oncology settings (Back, Arnold, Baile, Tulsky, & Fryer-Edwards, 2005) and end-of-life care in critical care settings (Hollyday & Buonocore, 2015; Shannon, Long-Sutehall, & Coombs, 2011). The first "ask" is used for the provider to assess perceptions and understanding of a patient or family regarding the current situation or issue at hand. This step would help the provider to obtain a basic idea about the patient's or family's level of knowledge or emotional state. The "tell" portion is used for the provider to convey the most pressing needed or desired information to the patient/family. The information should be provided in understandable, brief chunks, kept to no more than three pieces of information at a time. Then the second "ask" is used to check understanding of the patient/family and to answer their additional questions. The "ask-tell-ask" cycle would be repeated until a final "ask" is a summary of agreed-on decisions or plans. "Tell me more" can be used to get back on track when the conversation appears diverted. It also can be used to allow patient/family to share more of their emotions while letting the health provider get past initial reactions and respond in a less defensive or emotional mode (Back et al., 2005; Shannon et al., 2011).

Measurement of Outcomes

Inclusion of multiple measurements, such as self-report, behavioral observation, physiological indicators, and qualitative accounts, provides rich data for the study of therapeutic listening. For example, the Active Listening Observation Scale (ALOS-global) is a validated seven-item behavioral observational scale that measures the general practitioner's attentiveness and acknowledgment of suffering among patients presenting minor ailments (Fassaert, van Dulmen, Schellevis, & Bensing, 2007).

Challenges for outcome measurement may include the isolation of therapeutic listening as an independent variable from other confounding variables. Other challenges may be related to the complexity of the multifaceted phenomenon of therapeutic listening that may necessitate different study designs. Antecedents to interventions, such as clients' characteristics, have to be taken into consideration; likewise, the process-related components of interventions, such as short- and long-term improvements in nurses' knowledge, skills, and attitudes after training and client outcomes, need to be evaluated (Harrington et al., 2004; Kruijver, Kerkstra, Francke, Bensing, & van de Weil, 2000).

Positive changes in psychological variables such as anxiety, depression, hostility, nurse–patient communication, or nursing care satisfaction are potential client outcomes of therapeutic listening. It may also be useful to examine physiological measures (e.g., heart rate, blood pressure, respiratory rate, immunological measures, electroencephalography results) as outcomes of therapeutic interchange. Outcomes may include clinical variables such as patients' response to illness, mood, treatment adherence, disease control, morbidity, and healthcare cost. Boudreau,

Cassell, and Fuks (2009) believe that therapeutic listening can result in multiple outcomes: listening gives patients opportunities to articulate concerns that provide insight into their "personhood"; it can generate data for providers to use in the provision of optimal care, and it may actually assist in healing.

PRECAUTIONS

Therapeutic listening has at its heart the intent to be helpful; however, a few precautions are warranted. Questions that start with the word "why" may take clients out of the context of their experience or feelings and direct them into an intellectual thinking mode or cause defensive responses. Rather, phrases such as "tell me more about that," or "what was that like?" (Shattell & Hogan, 2005, p. 31) may be helpful.

The provider needs to be engaged fully when using therapeutic listening. If the provider is only half-listening, is using selective listening, or is distracted, patients may sense that their concerns are being minimized, or the provider may reach an inaccurate diagnosis. This weakens the therapeutic relationship between patient and provider (Boudreau et al., 2009).

The provider also needs to be aware of the potential negative self-consequences if the caregiver is involved in emotionally charged situations. Clinical supervision may be helpful for the provider in addressing such difficulties (Jones & Cutcliffe, 2009).

Practitioners and clinicians are encouraged to raise positive expectations and cautioned to selectively use active listening skills, especially with patients with minor ailments. When patients were in a good mood state before the consultation, the active listening behavior of general practitioners was observed to correlate with nonadherence of medication regimens. Rather, general practitioners' sensitivity to the emotional state of a patient and provision of clear explanations of the condition and preferable prognosis were observed to correlate with patients' reduced anxiety and better overall health (Fassaert, van Dulmen, Schellevis, van der Jagt, & Bensing, 2008).

Maintaining professional boundaries during therapeutic listening is important; empathy should be demonstrated but within the professional relationship with clients. Referrals for professional counseling may be indicated in cases such as psychiatric crises. Ethical dilemmas may result if the principle of respecting clients' autonomy and confidentiality conflicts with the principle of maintaining professional responsibility and integrity, such as taking action based on sensitive information shared in the therapeutic exchange. Open discussion and negotiation of the use of such sensitive information, within the context of the nurse–client relationship, relies on the trust relationship that has been established such that the trust is retained or even deepened.

USES

Therapeutic listening is an intervention applicable to a virtually unlimited number of care situations. It is beneficial for practitioners to continue listening to a patient throughout the entire visit. Indeed, according to a study of audiotaped office visits, approximately 21% to 39% of patients disclosed

---

Exhibit 3.2. Selected Uses of Listening With Patient Populations or in Care Settings

- Adolescent mental health (Claveirole, 2004)
- Cancer (Back et al., 2005; Liu et al., 2007)
- Culturally diverse populations (Davidhizar, 2004)
- Day surgery (Foy & Timmins, 2004)
- Emergency care (Kristensson & Ekwall, 2008)
- End-of-life care in critical care settings (Shannon et al., 2011)
- Heart failure: To improve self-care (Riegel et al., 2006, 2017)
- Major depressive disorder (Davidson et al., 2015)
- NICU: Mothers' depression management (Segre, Orengo-Aguayo, & Siewert, 2016)
- Older adults (Williams, Kemper, & Hummert, 2004)
- Preschoolers with developmental disabilities (Bazyk, Cimino, Hayes, Goodman, & Farrell, 2010)
- Women with breast cancer (Cohen et al., 2012)
- Young people in foster care (Murphy & Jenkinson, 2012)

---

new and vital information in the closing moments of an appointment (White, Levinson, & Roter, 1994; Rodondi et al., 2009). Soliciting the patient's agenda at least twice during the visit may decrease such situations, also known as "by-the-way" syndrome (Rodondi et al., 2009). Managers in the health-care field may also reap benefits from active listening (Kubota, Mishima, & Nagata, 2004).

Selected patient population–based examples in which the use of listening is described are included in Exhibit 3.2. The Websites section that follows presents websites of national and international professional organizations where online resources for therapeutic listening can be found.

Technology is ever-advancing and becoming increasingly important in ensuring that patients have effective means to communicate and ways to be fully heard and understood. Devices such as Passy–Muir tracheal valves that can allow mechanically ventilated patients to speak, computer programs that can "speak" the patient's electronic input, and laryngeal devices are now more frequently available and expected to promote communication. When alternative methods are being used, nonverbal communication is even more important to observe and monitor.

CULTURAL APPLICATIONS

Sensitivity and awareness of cultural variations in communication styles are vital to intervention effectiveness. Cultural differences in meanings of certain words, styles, and approaches, or in certain nonverbal behaviors such as silence, touch, eye contact, or smile, may adversely affect the effectiveness of therapeutic communication. For example, there may be tendencies for clients from certain cultures to talk loudly, to be direct in conversation, and to come to the point quickly. Clients from other cultures may tend to talk softly, be indirect in their communication, or "talk around" points while emphasizing attitudes and feelings. In some cultures, it is believed that open expression of emotions is unacceptable. Whether in the dominant culture or in nondominant cultures, however, people may simply smile when they do not comprehend. The skills of therapeutic listening are particularly useful in ensuring that communication in such cases is effective.

It is important that nurses explore and understand clients' cultural values and assumptions, as well as their patterns of behavior related to communication, while avoiding stereotyping (Seidel et al., 2011). Awareness of cultural differences is key to therapeutic communication. Sidebars 3.1 through 3.3 illustrate the importance of therapeutic listening in very diverse cultural contexts. Sidebar 3.1 provides an exemplar of the use of therapeutic listening in context of a healthcare setting in Japan. It underscores the challenge of working with an Asian culture wherein elders may hesitate to express concerns and where they may perceive questioning medical providers to be improper or socially unacceptable. Sidebar 3.2 presents the challenge of overcoming barriers of cultural differences in healthcare and the need for establishing trust in the therapeutic relationship through careful listening to achieve mutually desired healthcare outcomes. A final cultural example is provided in Sidebar 3.3, which emphasizes the centrality of family and proposes their inclusion in therapeutic listening surrounding the patients' care.

SIDEBAR 3.1. NURSES' THERAPEUTIC LISTENING SKILLS USED FOR OLDER POSTESOPHAGECTOMY PATIENTS IN TOKYO, JAPAN

Shigeaki Watanuki

Many esophageal cancer patients in Japan undergo thoracoabdominal esophageal surgery. Such patients frequently experience multiple signs and symptoms after surgery for months and sometimes even years due to gastrointestinal (GI) conditions. These conditions may include vocal cord paralysis, esophageal stenosis, or reflux, which may result in coughing, dysphagia, difficulty swallowing, vomiting, weight loss, or reduced physical activity.

Surgeons, due to their limited time and large number of patients, have only a few minutes to listen to postsurgical patients in outpatient departments. Older Japanese patients usually hesitate to ask their primary doctors (surgeons) about their signs and symptoms, changes in daily life, or biopsychosocial concerns. It is as though these elders think they have problems that are "too small" to ask their doctors. Such problems, however, are often very

(continued)

important and may actually be an indication of major complications or GI conditions; reporting them may aid in diagnosis.

Nurses' therapeutic listening skills play a key role in detecting patients' problems. Nurses at this hospital are trained in the "ask-tell-ask" and "tell me more" educational programs. Designated nurses are assigned to the GI surgical outpatient department to see postsurgical patients and to listen to their stories. In addition, nurses are specifically trained to use systematic questions and assessment skills that enhance identifying the patients' GI problems and symptoms. Such questions include general (e.g., fatigue, insomnia), GI-related (e.g., nausea and vomiting, constipation, diarrhea, constipation), and esophagectomy-related symptoms (e.g., dysphagia, reflux, difficulty swallowing, choking, coughing). If the nurses "sense" patients' problems through therapeutic exchange, they continue to explore the type and degree of the patients' problems and the way that the problems affect their daily lives. The nurses listen to the patients' entire experiences of living after esophagectomy while paying attention to any potential signs of hesitation or emotional distress that the patients may not show or state clearly. The nurses are aware that older Japanese patients usually do not want to admit they "have problems or difficulties;" however, they do have problems or difficulties. With nurse reassurance and encouragement, patients may go on: "actually, I am concerned this symptom may be...," or "yeah, I was going to say I have been bothered by this symptom for weeks...."

One day, a nurse saw a patient who complained of nothing special but had eaten sushi the previous evening as a celebration of his 80th birthday—3 months after his esophagectomy. The nurse kept exploring the patient's story, and found that he had continuously experienced a decline in food intake because of an increased difficulty in passing food through his esophagus. The nurse assessed that such a condition might be associated with esophageal stenosis, an indication of a need for balloon or bougie dilation by his surgeon. The nurse immediately reported this to the surgeon. The surgeon examined the patient and, as expected, diagnosed severe esophageal stenosis. This patient's condition might otherwise have been overlooked by nurses and surgeons, if this nurse had not had an outstanding "sense" and effective therapeutic listening skills.

The nurses also provide assurance and positive feedback if the patients are on the right track and are trying to adhere to the expected "healthy behavior." Such behavior includes eating small amounts of food slowly, engaging in regular physical activity, and keeping the upper body elevated while asleep. If patients would benefit from behavioral changes in their daily lives, nurses work with them to find acceptable common ground.

After seeing patients, the nurses convey the clients' critical information or questions to the surgeon if indicated and desired. Otherwise, nurses encourage the patients to relay their concerns to the surgeons or may ask surgeons questions on behalf of patients. The patients and surgeons of this department have reported that the nurses are sensitive to the patients' needs and have noted how helpful nurses are in working together on behalf of the patients. The nurses' outstanding therapeutic listening skills truly enhance the quality of care at the outpatient department of this hospital.

SIDEBAR 3.2. THE ROLE OF COMPLEMENTARY AND ALTERNATIVE THERAPIES IN CARING FOR SOMALI PATIENTS

Nasra Giama

Therapeutic listening as part of therapeutic communication with Somali patients may not only build trust, but also help provide culturally sensitive care. It can help avoid adverse interactions between traditional therapies and those used in Western medicine.

Numerous types of complementary and alternative therapies are used by Somalis, including massage, prayer and spiritual healing, plant-based treatments, and herbs. The most popular herbs are Fenugreek and black seed (oil or seed form), and specialized diets are used to treat certain diseases. For example, natural products may be used to induce diarrhea to cleanse the colon and digestive system (*qaras bixin*); the purpose is to expel sickness-causing pathogens. Traditional healers and spiritual leaders may be called on to use the Qur'an, as well as the teachings from the Prophet, to provide tailored treatment remedies and prayers for sick individuals. Listening to recitations of the Qur'an is calming, healing, and humbling; through the recitations, one may come to appreciate God's (Allah's) blessings and may ask for the higher being to sending healing (Ahmed, 1988).

Trained traditional healers in Somalia may use cutting (blood-letting to remove spoiled blood), burning/cauterization (consistent with the Somali saying, "Disease and fire cannot stay together in the same place"), and cupping (Ahmed, 1988). Traditional healers typically find it difficult to practice in the Western world because of laws prohibiting certain practices. However, Somalis may seek traditional care because it is what they know and how they perceive their illness. They seek it from healers and spiritual leaders whom they trust. Often, these are sought before entry into the more foreign Western healthcare system.

To provide patient-centered, culturally sensitive care to Somali patients, therapeutic listening is important (Guerin, Guerin, Diiriye, Omar, & Yates, 2004). There are important questions to be asked related to complementary and alternative therapies and healing practices, and the nurse should listen carefully and respectfully to the answers. Tips for nurses:

1. Ask patients for their understanding or explanations of the illnesses they are experiencing. What do they think is the cause?
2. Ask what patients have done at home for self-care, or ask about other remedies or healing practices they may have sought and used. Identify through conversation with patients and caregivers what things they do (or have done), in addition to the treatment plan recommended by the healthcare team?
3. Provide a "showing," or demonstration, of any complementary or alternative therapy, if offered to a Somali patient in context of the Western healthcare system. Clearly explain its purpose. A Somali

(continued)

patient may know and have used certain therapies but be unfamiliar with the English terms for them. The nurse can listen carefully to the patient to determine whether the therapy is understood and, if so, whether it is desired.

References

Ahmed, A. (1988.). Somali traditional healers, role and status. *Medicine and Traditional Medicine*, 240–247. Retrieved from http://dspace-roma3.caspur.it/bitstream/2307/1050/5/33_A.%20 M.%20AHMED%20-%20Somali%20traditional%20healers,%20role%20and%20status. pdf;jsessionid=E66E51EF5CAA227F7FA8BC1C378E8DA0

Guerin, B., Guerin, P., Diiriye, R., Omar, R., & Yates, S. (2004). Somali conceptions and expectations concerning mental health: Some guidelines for mental health professionals. *New Zealand Journal of Psychology*, 33(2), 59–67.

SIDEBAR 3.3. THERAPEUTIC COMMUNICATION WITH MEXICAN PATIENTS INCLUDES LISTENING TO FAMILIES

Karim Bauza

First, in providing care to Mexican patients, one must understand the absolute importance of family. Culturally, in Mexico and other Latin American countries, family holds things together. From the perspective of my culture and Mexican/Latina heritage, I know that if something happens to me, I have a strong family support system to rely on. The importance of family extends to medical care contexts. Some nurses would like to care for patients without family present; working with family members in difficult healthcare contexts can be frustrating. Having family in the room or answering their questions may be difficult, but family have expectations and responsibilities to be on top of the care and to help in making decisions for their family member. If I were injured and hospitalized, my whole family would be in the room. Someone would be with me (or desire to be) 100% of the time.

Listening to the family in the hospital is important. If a family member were to be intubated, you would be able to get significant information from family (e.g., patient allergies and personal preferences). In Latina cultures, family is a resource. It would be unusual for family not to be present or not to visit regularly when a family member is hospitalized. Coming from this family-centered culture, it is shocking when I care for non-Latino patients and sometimes family may not be there or visit for days at a time. Family is a great resource that is often underutilized. If I had a family member who was hospitalized, I would want the nurse to make me feel included. I would be listening to how my family member will get better. How could my loved one be more comfortable? How are their holistic needs being met?

(continued)

The difference in knowledge and practice between the large urban tertiary care centers and what is available in small towns or locations in Mexico is significant. There are "medical deserts" in Mexico. There are cultural differences that should be considered. For example, in the Mexican culture, someone with sniffles may take penicillin—penicillin for everything. It is available without prescription. If a patient arrives in the United States from Mexico requiring healthcare, they would have many questions, which may go unasked and unanswered if a therapeutic relationship is not developed through mutual listening. In this process, nurses should try their best to include the family. We learned this in our basic education, but its importance cannot be overemphasized.

So, what would I recommend a nurse do? Listen. Many Mexican or Latina patients may not know why they are taking their prescribed medications; listen to what they think is the purpose of the treatment or medication. Use therapeutic listening skills to build the bridge to get closer to them in a therapeutic relationship to close the gap between what they are thinking about their care and health and what they may need to know to ensure desired therapeutic outcomes. Use listening skills to gather important information about Latina patients' medical and cultural background and understanding of their health or illness. As a nurse, a priority is to understand their expectations of treatment outcomes. To achieve positive healthcare outcomes, it is important to reach common understandings with the patient and family members who may support the patients or provide care. Otherwise, problems with medical adherence to the prescribed drugs, medical treatments, or therapies are likely. Without careful listening for understanding and reaching mutual expectations and goals for care, medical therapies may be doomed to fail. For example, in the case of wound care, it is important that the patient and family have the supplies and understanding of the timing and techniques of dressing changes—otherwise, the wound won't be properly dressed and the patient is likely to return with infection.

Listening needs to occur on both sides in a relationship. It should not only be the nurse or provider saying, "This is my expectation for your treatment and outcome." The nurse may need to be the one who listens first; nurses can model listening and respect. Two-sided listening has an important role in the caregiving relationship. Nurses can listen to hear what the patient and family understands and what they are seeking from care. Only through listening and truly hearing can the nurse know and understand patient and family preferences and demonstrate caring. In this manner, trust is developed, and patients and families can be confident that the nurse and providers have their best interest at heart.

Language Challenges

Interpreter-mediated healthcare encounters can be a challenge for therapeutic interchange. The issue of translation and interpretation in healthcare includes more than the differences in language use. Interpretation should be founded on a word-for-word translation while incorporating nuances and maintaining semantic equivalency of communication. Difficulties in translation and interpretation in healthcare encounters are illustrated, for example, in a study by Flores et al. (2003) of Spanish–English interpretations in pediatric encounters. The study found that there were, on average, 31 errors in medical interpretation per clinical encounter. Most errors were categorized as "omissions" of important information and had potential clinical consequences. Those serious errors were more likely to be committed by nonprofessional interpreters—including nurses, social workers, and siblings—as compared with those committed by hospital interpreters. Use of appropriately trained and experienced interpreters is a necessity for clients who have language barriers.

Another study showed that non–English-speaking family members are at increased risk of receiving less information about the patient's condition, as evidenced by less family conference time and shorter duration and less proportion of clinician speech during a conference (Thornton, Pham, Engelberg, Jackson, & Curtis, 2009). This study also showed that non–English-speaking families receive less reported emotional support from their healthcare providers, including valuing families' input, easing emotional burdens, and actively listening (Thornton et al., 2009). Healthcare professionals' cultural sensitivity and considerations are vital to promoting quality of care for patients/families with language barriers.

FUTURE RESEARCH

Many research questions have potential for exploration in the area of therapeutic listening. Systematic studies are needed to develop a body of knowledge. The study designs will require new paradigms beyond traditional randomized controlled trials for, among other things, ethical and feasibility reasons. Qualitative studies, case reports, or mixed-method designs may be better options for understanding the nature and effects of therapeutic listening. Some potential questions for future research are:

- Can therapeutic listening via telephone or other interactive technology (synchronous or asynchronous) be effective at a distance?
- What are the effects of listening by healthcare providers on patient satisfaction and other outcomes of care?
- Are interventions to enhance listening on the part of healthcare providers cost-effective and legitimate areas on which to focus continuous quality improvement to increase patient safety and quality of care?
- How do multicultural differences manifest in the processes and effectiveness of therapeutic listening?

WEBSITES

- International Communication Association (www.icahdq.org)
- International Listening Association (www.listen.org)
- Communication Institute for Online Scholarship (www.cios.org)
- EACH: International Association for Communication in Health Care (www.each.eu)
- AACH: Academy on Communication in Healthcare (www.achonline.org)

REFERENCES

Adams, K., Cimino, J. E. W., Arnold, R. M., & Anderson, W. G. (2012). Why should I talk about emotion? Communication patterns associated with physician discussion of patient expressions of negative emotion in hospital admission encounters. *Patient Education and Counseling*, *89*(1), 44–50.

Arnold, E. C., & Underman Boggs, K. (2007). *Interpersonal relationships: Professional communication skills for nurses* (5th ed.). London, UK: W. B. Saunders.

Back, A. L., Arnold, R. M., Baile, W. F., Tulsky, J. A., & Fryer-Edwards, K. (2005). Approaching difficult communication tasks in oncology. *CA: A Cancer Journal for Clinicians*, *55*(3), 164–177.

Barrere, C. C. (2007). Discourse analysis of nurse-patient communication in a hospital setting: Implications for staff development. *Journal of Nurses in Staff Development*, *23*, 114–122.

Bazyk, S., Cimino, J., Hayes, K., Goodman, G., & Farrell, P. (2010). The use of therapeutic listening with preschoolers with developmental disabilities: A look at the outcomes. *Journal of Occupational Therapy, Schools, and Early Intervention*, *3*(2), 124–138.

Bodie, G. D., Vickery, A. J., Cannava, K. E., & Jones, S. (2015). The role of "active listening" in informal helping conversations: Impact on perceptions of listener helpfulness, sensitivity, and supportiveness and discloser emotional improvement. *Western Journal of Communication*, *79*(2), 151–173. doi:10.1080/10570314.2014.943429

Boudreau, J. D., Cassell, E., & Fuks, A. (2009). Preparing medical students to become attentive listeners. *Medical Teacher*, *31*, 22–29.

Bryant, L. (2009). The art of active listening. *Practice Nurse*, *37*(6), 49–52.

Burnard, P. (1997). *Effective communication skills for health professionals* (2nd ed.). Cheltenham, UK: Nelson Thornes.

Bush, K. (2001). Do you really listen to patients? *RN*, *64*(3), 35–37.

Centers for Medicare and Medicaid Services. (2014). HCAHPS: Patients' perspectives of care survey. Retrieved from https://www.cms.gov/Medicare/Quality-Initiatives-Patient-Assessment-Instruments/HospitalQualityInits/HospitalHCAHPS.html

Centers for Medicare and Medicaid Services. (2015). HCAHPS fact sheet. Retrieved from http://hospitalcoremeasures.com/pdf/hcahps/HCAHPS_Fact_Sheet_June_2015.pdf

Chan, Z. C. Y. (2010). Supervision of nurses using the five principles on practising nursing. *Journal of Nursing Administration*, *18*, 111–112.

Cohen, M., Anderson, R. C., Jensik, K., Xiang, Q., Pruszynski, J., & Walker, A. P. (2012). Communication between breast cancer patients and their physicians about breast-related body image issues. *Plastic Surgical Nursing*, *32*(3), 101–105.

Claveirole, A. (2004). Listening to young voices: Challenges of research with adolescent mental health service users. *Journal of Psychiatric & Mental Health Nursing*, *11*(3), 253–260.

Davidhizar, R. (2004). Listening—A nursing strategy to transcend culture. *Journal of Practical Nursing*, *54*(2), 22–24.

Davidson, S. K., Harris, M. G., Dowrick, C. F., Wachtler, C. A., Pirkis, J., & Gunn, J. M. (2015). Mental health interventions and future major depression among primary care patients with subthreshold depression. *Journal of Affective Disorders*, *177*, 65–73.

De Vito, J. A. (2006). *The interpersonal communication book* (11th ed.). Needham Heights, MA: Allyn & Bacon.

Denham, C. R., Dingman, J., Foley, M. E., Ford, D., Martins, B., O'Regan, P., & Salamendra, A. (2008). Are you listening … are you really listening? *Journal of Patient Safety*, *4*(3), 148–161.

Fassaert, T., van Dulmen, S., Schellevis, F., & Bensing, J. (2007). Active listening in medical consultations: Development of the Active Listening Observation Scale (ALOS-global). *Patient Education and Counseling*, *68*(3), 258–264.

Fassaert, T., van Dulmen, S., Schellevis, F., van der Jagt, L., & Bensing, J. (2008). Raising positive expectations helps patients with minor ailments: A cross-sectional study. *BMC Family Practice*, *9*, 38. doi:10.1186/1471-2296-9-38

Flores, G., Laws, M. B., Mayo, S. J., Zuckerman, B., Abreu, M., Medina, L., & Hardt, E. J. (2003). Errors in medical interpretation and their potential clinical consequences in pediatric encounters. *Pediatrics*, *111*(1), 6–14.

Foy, C. R., & Timmins, F. (2004). Improving communication in day surgery settings. *Nursing Standard, 19*(7), 37–42.

Fredriksson, L. (1999). Modes of relating in a caring conversation: A research synthesis on presence, touch and listening. *Journal of Advanced Nursing, 30,* 1167–1176.

Halpern, J. (2012, Spring). Attending to clinical wisdom. *Journal of Clinical Ethics, 23*(1), 41–46.

Harrington, J., Noble, L. M., & Newman, S. P. (2004). Improving patients' communication with doctors: A systematic review of intervention studies. *Patient Education and Counseling, 52*(1), 7–16.

Hollyday, S. L., & Buonocore, D. (2015). Breaking bad news and discussing goals of care in the intensive care unit. *AACN Advanced Critical Care, 26*(2), 131–141.

Jones, A. C., & Cutcliffe, J. R. (2009). Listening as a method of addressing psychological distress. *Journal of Nursing Management, 17*(3), 352–358.

Kacperek, L. (1997). Non-verbal communication: The importance of listening. *British Journal of Nursing, 6,* 275–279.

Kawamichi, H., Yoshihara, K., Sasaki, A. T., Sugawara, S. K., Tanabe, H. C., Shinohara, R., ... Sadato, N. (2015). Perceiving active listening activates the reward system and improves the impression of relevant experiences. *Social Neuroscience, 10*(1), 16–26.

Kemper, B. J. (1992). Therapeutic listening: Developing the concept. *Journal of Psychosocial Nursing and Mental Health Services, 30*(7), 21–23.

Kristensson, J., & Ekwall, A. (2008). Psychometric properties of the consumer emergency care satisfaction scale: Tested on persons accompanying patients in emergency department. *Journal of Nursing Care Quality, 23,* 277–282.

Kruijver, I. P., Kerkstra, A., Francke, A. L., Bensing, J. M., & van de Wiel, H. B. (2000). Evaluation of communication training programs in nursing care: A review of the literature. *Patient Education and Counseling, 39,* 129–145.

Kubota, S., Mishima, N., & Nagata, S. (2004). A study of the effects of active listening on listening attitudes of middle managers. *Journal of Occupational Health, 46*(1), 66–67.

Kurtz, S. M., Silverman, J. D., & Draper, J. (1998). *Teaching and learning communication skills in medicine.* Oxford, UK: Radcliffe Medical Press.

Lee, B., & Prior, S. (2013). Developing therapeutic listening. *British Journal of Guidance & Counseling, 41*(2), 91–104.

Lekander, B. J., Lehmann, S., & Lindquist, R. (1993). Therapeutic listening: Key nursing interventions for several nursing diagnoses. *Dimensions of Critical Care Nursing, 12,* 24–30.

Liu, J. E., Mok, E., Wong, T., Xue, L., & Xu, B. (2007). Evaluation of an integrated communication skills training program for nurses in cancer care in Beijing, China. *Nursing Research, 56,* 202–209.

McCabe, C. (2004). Nurse-patient communication: An exploration of patients' experiences. *Issues in Clinical Nursing, 13,* 41–49.

McCambridge, J., Platts, S., Whooley, D., & Strang, J. (2004). Encouraging GP alcohol intervention: Pilot study of change-oriented reflective listening (CORL). *Alcohol & Alcoholism, 39*(2), 146–149.

Murphy, D., & Jenkinson, H. (2012). The mutual benefits of listening to young people in care, with a particular focus on grief and loss: An Irish foster carer's perspective. *Child Care in Practice, 18*(3), 243–253.

Riegel, B., Dickson, V. V., Garcia, L. E., Masterson Creber, R., & Streur, M. (2017). Mechanisms of change in self-care in adults with heart failure receiving a tailored, motivational interviewing intervention. *Patient Education and Counseling, 100,* 283–288.

Riegel, B., Dickson, V. V., Hoke, L., McMahon, J. P., Reis, B. F., & Sayers, S. (2006). A motivational counseling approach to improving heart failure self-care: Mechanisms of effectiveness. *Journal of Cardiovascular Nursing, 21,* 232–241.

Rodondi, P. Y., Maillefer, J., Suardi, F., Rodondi, N., Cornuz, J., & Vannotti, M. (2009). Physician response to "by-the-way" syndrome in primary care. *Journal of General Internal Medicine, 24,* 739–741.

Rogers, C. R. (1957). The necessary and sufficient conditions of therapeutic personality change. *Journal of Consulting Psychology, 21,* 95–103.

Rollnick, S., Allison, J., Ballasiotes, S., Barth, T., Butler, C. C., Rose, G. S., & Rosengren, D. B. (2002). Variations on a theme: Motivational interviewing and its adaptations. In W. R. Miller &

S. Rollnick (Eds.), *Motivational interviewing: Preparing people for change* (2nd ed., pp. 270–283). New York, NY: Guilford Press.

Sandelowski, M. (1994). We are the stories we tell: Narrative knowing in nursing practice. *Journal of Holistic Nursing, 12,* 23–33.

Seidel, H. E., Ball, J. W., Dains, J. E., Flynn, J. A., Solomon, B. S., & Stewart, R. W. (Eds.). (2011). Cultural awareness. In *Mosby's guide to physical examination* (7th ed., pp. 32–45). St. Louis, MO: Mosby.

Segre, L. S., Orengo-Aguayo, R. E., & Siewert, R. C. (2016). Depression management by NICU nurses: Mothers' views. *Clinical Nursing Research, 25,* 273–290.

Shannon, S. E., Long-Sutehall, T., & Coombs, M. (2011). Conversations in end-of-life care: Communication tools for critical care practitioners. *Nursing in Critical Care, 16*(3), 124–130.

Shattell, M., & Hogan, B. (2005). Facilitating communication: How to truly understand what patients mean. *Journal of Psychosocial Nursing and Mental Health Service, 43*(10), 29–32.

Silverman, J. D., Kurtz, S. M., & Draper, J. (1998). *Skills for communicating with patients.* Oxford, UK: Radcliffe Medical Press.

Strang, J., McCambridge, J., Platts, S., & Groves, P. (2004). Engaging the reluctant GP in care of the opiate users. *Family Practice, 21*(2), 150–154.

Thornton, J. D., Pham, K., Engelberg, R. A., Jackson, J. C., & Curtis, J. R. (2009). Families with limited English proficiency receive less information and support in interpreted intensive care unit family conferences. *Critical Care Medicine, 37*(1), 89–95.

Wanzer, M. B., Booth-Butterfield, M., & Gruber, K. (2004). Perceptions of health care providers' communication: Relationships between patient-centered communication and satisfaction. *Health Communication, 16,* 363–384.

White, J., Levinson, W., & Roter, D. (1994). "Oh by the way": The closing moments of the medical visit. *Journal of General Internal Medicine, 9,* 24–28.

Williams, K., Kemper, S., & Hummert, M. L. (2004). Enhancing communication with older adults: Overcoming elderspeak. *Journal of Gerontological Nursing, 30*(10), 17–25.

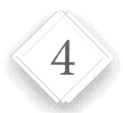

Creating Optimal Healing Environments

MARY JO KREITZER AND TERRI ZBOROWSKY

Nurses have long been leaders in creating optimal healing environments (OHEs). Florence Nightingale, the founder of modern nursing, described the role of the nurse as helping the patient attain the best possible condition so that nature can act and self-healing occur (Dossey, 2000). Nightingale recognized the nurse's role in both caring for the patient and managing the physical environment. She wrote about the importance of natural light, fresh air, noise reduction, and infection control, as well as spirituality, presence, and caring. Her philosophy embodied the notion that people have the innate capacity to heal and as nurses, we create the conditions that support healing within a person. Increasingly, a base of evidence about the creation of OHEs is emerging from many disciplines, including nursing, interior design, architecture, neuroscience, psychoneuroimmunology, and environmental psychology, among others. Just as evidence-based practice informs clinical decision making, evidence-based design impacts the planning and construction of healthcare facilities. Nurses need to be informed about the ways in which the physical environment affects health outcomes so that they can contribute to the design of patient care units and other healthcare facilities that will optimize the health and well-being of patients, their families, and the staff. Nurses are also in a unique position to carry out needed research on the impact of specific design interventions on intended outcomes.

DEFINITION

The word *healing* comes from the Anglo-Saxon word *haelen*, which means "to make whole." Healing environments are designed to promote harmony or balance of mind, body, and spirit; to reduce anxiety and stress; and to be restorative. An OHE model developed by Zborowsky & Kreitzer (2009) and depicted in Figure 4.1 illustrates that an OHE is created through a deep and dynamic interplay among people, place, and process. In this model, "people" includes the caregivers and support team that surround the patient. The characteristics and competencies of the staff and the knowledge, skills, and attitudes that they embody are some of the most critical elements of an OHE. The "place" element focuses on the physical space where care is provided and the geography that surrounds the patient, family, and caregiver. "Place" elements include meeting functional requirements or program needs, access to nature, positive distractions, design elements that help create aesthetics, ambient environment, and ecosystem sustainability (see Exhibit 4.1 for definitions). The "process" element refers to the care processes as well as the leadership processes that support a culture aligned with creating an OHE. Care processes include conventional, integrative, and behavioral interventions.

This model of OHE illustrates that optimally, there is coherence and alignment between the "people—nurses, patients and families," the "processes—caregiving in the context of patient centered care," and in a "place—physical environment" that is designed to maximize positive outcomes for patients, their family, and staff. The reality is that much of care occurs in old, dysfunctional facilities. Even healthcare facilities built 20 years ago lack the available space and mechanical systems to function well today due to changes in building codes, guidelines, and best practice in care models. An inadequate space makes it more difficult to attain a truly healing environment, although the elements of the caregiver and the care provided are even more critical than the physical place or space. Today, there is a better understanding of, and rigorous research that describes ways of choosing, elements of "place" that support and enable an OHE.

The primary emphasis of this volume is on the evidence and clinical applications of complementary and alternative therapies that nurses can use to enhance their practice. This chapter focuses on the physical environment in which care is provided and the ways in which evidence can be used to create environments that contribute to positive health outcomes.

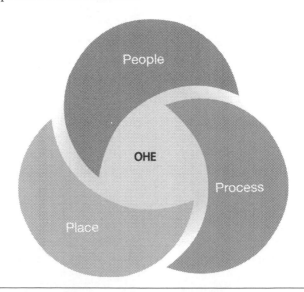

Figure 4.1   People, place, and process: The role of place in creating OHEs. OHEs, optimal healing environments.

Source: Reprinted from Zborowsky, T., & Kreitzer, M. J. (2009). People, place, and process: The role of place in creating optimal healing environments. *Creative Nursing, 15*(4), 186–190.

Exhibit 4.1. OHE "Place" Element Definitions

Meets Functional Requirements: Functional requirements are identified during the programming phase of the design process (see Facility Guidelines Institute [FGI] guidelines for more information: https://www.fgiguidelines.org/wp-content/uploads/2015/08/2001guidelines.pdf). These requirements include patient and staff safety, space for social support, and staff work areas, among others.

   Access to Nature: Includes actual or visual access to natural settings or designed nature settings. Access to daylight.

   Positive Distractions: Includes elements of the design environment that are of a two- or three-dimensional nature (e.g., artwork, water features, fire places).

   Design Elements: Includes the design elements—color, texture, shape, form, and volume—that contribute to the creation of furniture, fabric, and room layout, among other design artifacts.

   Ambient Environment: Includes the design elements of artificial light, sound, odor, and heating, ventilation, and air conditioning (HVAC).

   Supports a Sustainable Ecosystem: Includes the economic, social, and ecological impact of the design elements of the building and impact of any construction.

OHEs, optimal healing environments.

SCIENTIFIC BASIS

A growing body of evidence links the physical environment to health outcomes. According to a review of the research literature on evidence-based healthcare design (Ulrich et al., 2008), over 1,000 rigorous empirical studies link the design of a hospital's physical environment with healthcare outcomes. The studies cover a broad scope, with evidence linking:

- *Single-bed rooms* with reduced hospital-acquired infections, reduced medical errors, reduced patient falls, improved patient sleep, and increased patient satisfaction
- *Decentralized supplies* with increased staff effectiveness
- *Appropriate lighting* with decreased medical errors and decreased staff stress
- *Ceiling lifts* with decreased staff injuries

Although many of the studies focus on topics such as infection control, patient falls, staff productivity, and staff injuries, a growing number of studies focus on other aspects of the environment that contribute to healing.

As described by Malkin (2008), design strategies that focus on creating healing environments have in common the goal of reducing stress and include:

- Connections to nature (e.g., artwork with a nature theme, views to the outside, interior gardens, plants)
- Options that give patients choices and control (e.g., room service menu, choice of music and art, ability to control lighting and temperature)
- Spaces that provide access to social support (e.g., family zones within patient rooms that offer sleeping space, storage, and adequate seating)

- Positive distractions (e.g., music, water features, aviaries, videos of nature, aquariums, sculpture)
- Reductions of environmental stressors such as noise and glare from direct light sources (e.g., carpet, indirect lighting, elimination of overhead paging)

Design Theories and Best Practices Related to Healing Environments and Clinical Applications

Access to Nature

OHE "place" elements include theories that support creating healing spaces in healthcare. For example, biophilia is a theory that supports the concept of access to nature. Biophilia is the inherent human inclination to "affiliate" with natural systems and processes. The concept, originally proposed by eminent biologist Edward O. Wilson (1984), has grown into a broader framework that increasingly is shaping the design of the man-made environment, including hospitals and other healthcare facilities. Biophilic design emphasizes the necessity of maintaining, enhancing, and restoring the beneficial experience of nature and describes attempts to do so through the use of environmental features that embody characteristics of the natural world, such as color, water, sunlight, plants, natural materials, and exterior views and vistas (Kellert, 2008).

The theory of biophilia has been empirically tested in clinical settings. Outcomes measured most often include stress and pain reduction. For example:

- A study of elderly residents in an urban long-term care facility revealed that residents attach considerable importance to having access to window views of outdoor spaces with prominent features such as plants, gardens, and birds (Kearney & Winterbottom, 2005).
- Patients in a dental clinic reported less stress on days when a large nature mural was hung in the waiting room compared with days when there was no nature scene (Heerwagen, 1990).
- In a prospective randomized trial of blood donors, it was found that donors who viewed a wall-mounted television playing a nature videotape had lower blood pressure and pulse rates than subjects who were viewing a television playing either a videotape of urban scenes or game or talk shows (Ulrich, Simons, & Miles, 2003).
- Ulrich, Lunden, and Eltinge (1993) found that patients following heart surgery who viewed photos of trees and water required fewer doses of strong pain medication and reported less anxiety than patients who viewed abstract images or were assigned to a control group with no picture.

There is some evidence that the more engrossing a nature distraction, the greater the potential for pain alleviation. Miller, Hickman, & Lemasters (1992), in a study of burn patients, found that distracting patients during burn dressings by having them view nature scenes on a bedside TV accompanied by music lessened both pain and anxiety. In a randomized prospective trial of patients undergoing bronchoscopy, patients who viewed a ceiling-mounted nature scene and listened to nature sounds reported less pain than patients in the control group who looked at a blank ceiling. Following a review of the literature on the use of virtual reality as adjunct analgesic technique, Wismeijer and Vingerhoets (2005) concluded that "nature exposures" may tend to be more diverting, and hence pain-reducing, if they involve sound as well as visual stimulation and maximize realism and immersion.

Roe and Aspinall (2011) reported on two quasi-experiments that compared the restorative benefits of walking in urban and rural settings in two groups of adults with good and poor mental health. The authors examined two aspects of restoration, mood, and personal project techniques to capture an underexplored aspect of cognitive restoration through reflection on everyday life tasks. Results were consistent with a restorative effect of landscape. The rural walk was advantageous to affective and cognitive restoration in both health groups when compared with an urban walk. However, beneficial change took place to a greater extent in the poor health group. Differential outcomes between health groups were found in the urban setting, which was most advantageous to restoration in the poor mental health group. This study extends restorative environments research by showing that the amount of change and context for restoration can differ among adults with variable mental health.

Emerging research us a multi-method approach to understand the effect nature has on patients. In a case study of 19 subjects living in an assisted living facility, Goto, Park, Tsunetsugu, Herrup, and Miyazaki (2013) found that exposure to organized gardens can affect both the mood and the cardiac physiology of elderly individuals. Among other findings, they revealed that the subjects' heart rates were significantly lower in the Japanese garden than in the other environments studied; measures of subjects' sympathetic function were also significantly lower.

Positive Distractions

Art falls under another of the "place" elements of positive distractions. A number of studies have examined patient preferences for art and the effect of art on stress, recovery, and pain, among other outcomes. Studies have consistently documented that patients prefer nature over other subject matter and that they overwhelmingly prefer realistic art and strongly dislike abstract images (Winston & Cupchik, 1992). Findings such as these, consistent with the theory of biophilia, have led to the use of evidence-based design guidelines in healthcare facilities to guide the selection of art. According to Ulrich and Gilpin (2003), visual art should be unambiguously positive. Recommended subject matter includes waterscapes with calm or nonturbulent water, landscapes with visual depth or openness, nature settings depicted during warmer seasons when vegetation is verdant and flowers are visible, garden scenes, outdoor scenes in sunny conditions, and avoidance of overcast or foreboding weather. Pati and Nanda (2011) used a quasi-experimental design to examine pediatric patients' behavior during five distraction conditions ranging from a slide show to video with music. All distraction conditions were created on one flat-screen plasma TV monitor mounted on a stand in the waiting areas. Data analysis showed that the introduction of distraction conditions was associated with more calm behavior and less fine and gross movement, suggesting significant calming effects associated with the distraction conditions. Data also suggest that positive distraction conditions are significant attention grabbers and could be an important contributor to improving the waiting experience for children in hospitals by improving environmental attractiveness. Nanda, Zhu, and Jansen (2012) conducted a systematic review of neuroscience articles on the emotional states of fear, anxiety, and pain to understand how emotional response is linked to the visual characteristics of an image at the level of brain behavior. Findings indicate there is a paucity of research in this area and a compelling area for future research on the direct impact the imagery of artwork can have on emotional processing centers in the brain.

Nanda, Eisen, Zadeh, and Owen (2010) investigated the impact of different visual art conditions on agitation and anxiety levels of patients by measuring the rate of pro re nata (PRN; as needed) incidents and collecting nurse feedback. Results showed that PRN medication dispensed by nurses for anxiety and agitation was significantly lower on days when a realistic nature image of a landscape was displayed as compared with days when abstract or no art was displayed. The authors concluded that positive distractions, such as visual art depicting restorative nature scenes, could help reduce mental health patients' anxiety and agitation in healthcare settings. It also makes a case that the environment can have a powerful impact on healing in mental health settings. The emergence of simulated nature products has raised the question regarding the effectiveness of these approaches. Pati, Freier, O'Boyle, Amor, and Valipoor (2016) conducted a between-subject experimental design, in which outcomes from five inpatient rooms with sky-composition ceiling fixtures were compared with corresponding outcomes in five identical rooms without the intervention. The experimental group of subjects exhibited shorter times spent in the room, lower diastolic blood pressure, lower acute stress, lower anxiety, decreased pain, better sleep quality, and higher environmental satisfaction. The authors concluded that the salutogenic benefits of photographic sky compositions render them better than traditional ceiling tiles and offer an alternative to other nature interventions.

Ambient Environment

Light is an aspect of the "place" element, the ambient environment. Chronobiology is an interdisciplinary field of inquiry that focuses on biological rhythms. Discoveries in "chronotherapeutics" have documented that time patterning of medications in synchrony with body rhythms can enhance effectiveness and safety. Other studies have focused on the impact of environmental factors such as light and temperature on body rhythms. A significant body of literature has focused on the impact of light on depression. In a study of psychiatric patients, Beauchemin and Hays (1996) found that patients in sunnier rooms stayed an average of 2.6 fewer days than those in sunless rooms. A meta-analysis of 20 randomized controlled trials by Golden et al. (2005) on the impact of light treatment on nonseasonal and seasonal depression quantified the effect of light treatment as equivalent to that of antidepressant pharmacotherapy trials. Light has also been found to be related to patients' perception of pain. In a study (Walch et al., 2005) of post–spinal surgery experiences, patients who were admitted to rooms with greater sunlight intensity reported less pain and stress and took 22% fewer analgesic medications. Results such as these support careful site planning to ensure adequate access to daylight and provide justification for larger windows in patient rooms or the use of bright (but diffused) artificial light in areas where sufficient daylight is inaccessible. Using a pretest/post-test quasi-experimental study in two intensive care units, Shepley, Gerbi, Watson, Imgrund, and Sagha-Zadeh (2012) studied the impact of daylight and window views on patient pain levels, length of stay, staff errors, absenteeism, and vacancy rates. Researchers concluded that high levels of natural light and window views may positively affect staff absenteeism and staff vacancy, whereas factors such as medical errors, patient pain, and length of stay still require additional research. In summary, there is growing evidence that views of nature and light are beneficial for patients as well as staff.

Interestingly, evolving research explores the impact of lighting, both daylight and electrical lighting, on circadian entrainment of the elderly who live with neurocognitive disorders. In a systematic literature review, Joseph, Choi, and Quan (2015) found one multidimensional intervention, which included a daily sunlight exposure of 30 minutes or more, resulted in a significant decrease in daytime sleeping in intervention participants with no change in controls. In addition, there was a modest decrease in the mean duration of nighttime awakenings in intervention participants versus an increase in controls. They noted that although there is inconsistent support for the impact of bright light on direct sleep measures, findings do consistently suggest that bright light treatment may be effective in improving rest–activity rhythms (which results in better sleep at night and greater wakefulness in the daytime) for residents with dementia (Ancoli-Israel et al., 2003; Dowling, Mastick, Hubbard, Luxenberg, & Burr, 2005). Figueiro et al. (2008) conducted a study that incorporated a 24-hour lighting design intervention to meet the physiological needs of older adults in residential care environments (see Exhibit 4.2). Although this study did not find significant difference in sleep quality, nighttime sleep, or daytime awake hours in the small sample of seven assisted living residents, residents overwhelmingly preferred the new lighting conditions and felt they could read better under this condition compared with the old lighting condition. In the discussion section of the review, Joseph et al. (2015) noted that this study is significant because it offered concrete lighting design solutions that can be incorporated within new or existing environments.

Exhibit 4.2. Applied Lighting Interventions

Figueiro et al. (2008) applied the following architectural lighting scheme to improve circadian entrainment and increase architectural legibility for the elderly with dementia:

1. High circadian stimulation during the day and low circadian stimulation during the night
2. Good visual conditions during waking hours
3. Nightlights that provide perceptual cues for navigation and that improve postural stability and control for transitioning from a sitting into a standing position
4. High contrasts between daytime and nighttime light levels
5. Glare-free lighting
6. Shadow-free visual environments

These lighting interventions appear to be applicable to many other settings of care, including home environments.

This area of study—the impact of place on creating OHEs—is growing rapidly. In a 2014 study, Zborowsky analyzed a sample of 67 healthcare design–related research articles from 25 nursing journals to validate the extent to which current topics align with Nightingale's environmental theory. She found that sound and noise ranked high among the dependent variables and sleep among the independent variables (the result of sound and noise). As stated by Nightingale, "Unnecessary noise is the most cruel absence of care which can be inflicted either on sick or well" (Nightingale, 1860, p. 27). Like Nightingale, nurses today are in a strategic position to study and design healing environments that optimize health outcomes for patients, families, and staff.

INTERVENTION

Case Study Applications of OHEs

To illustrate the use of OHEs, we focus here on three exemplars—North Hawaii Community Hospital in Waimea, Hawaii, and two Minnesota facilities, Abbott Northwestern Hospital in Minneapolis and Regions Hospital in St. Paul.

North Hawaii Community Hospital

North Hawaii Community Hospital, an affiliate of the Queens Health Systems, embodies the culture of the community in the way in which it has operationalized the concept of an OHE. The footprint of the hospital was aligned so that the front is oriented to the Kohala Mountain, and the back to the mountain Mauna Kea. Earl Bakken, one of the founders of the hospital, had the vision that the hospital itself would be an "instrument of healing," rather than a "warehouse for sick bodies" (E. Bakken, personal communication, January 2008). All patient rooms are private and have access to views of nature and fresh air through sliding doors that open to the outside. Art in patient's rooms is culturally meaningful and can be changed. Hallways are carpeted and there is minimal overhead paging. Soft music is playing in public spaces. Familiar cultural patterns, textures, and colors are used in wallpapers, carpeting, and furniture coverings. *Ti* plants at all entrances and corners of the building are believed to filter out bad spiritual energy. An interior bamboo garden also offers spiritual protection and represents strength and resilience. All patient rooms have sleep chairs or extra beds for guests to stay over, and there are no limits on the number of visitors or visiting hours. An *ohana* (Hawaiian for "family") room includes a kitchen so that families can prepare special meals. Skylights in halls and windows in the operating rooms were incorporated into the design to enable staff to stay attuned to day/night cycles. In addition to these and many other mechanical, architectural, and engineering adaptations, the hospital embraced a philosophy of blended medicine that encourages the integration of complementary therapies and culturally based healing practices. The vision of North Hawaii Community Hospital is to become the most healing hospital in the world.

Abbott Northwestern Hospital

The design of the Neuroscience/Orthopaedic/Spine Patient Care Center at Abbott Northwestern's new Heart Hospital in Minneapolis, Minnesota, integrates the elements of Abbott Northwestern's Healing Environment Aesthetic Standards, including the principles of feng shui and patient-centered care, while acknowledging the needs of staff. This 128-bed inpatient unit located on two floors of the Heart Hospital was designed to incorporate the latest technology to aid in meeting patient and safety requirements, as well as implement the organization's holistic approach to healing. To accomplish these goals, patient rooms were "zoned" so that the needs of each user of the space would be addressed:

* The *patient zone* provides a view to the outside from every bed; a flower/card shelf; private safes for valuables; art work and care provider information on the footwall; and a small refrigerator for favorite foods.
* The *family zone* incorporates an upholstered bench seat/sleeper, a reading light with private switch, and a data outlet for Internet access.
* The *caregiver zone* includes a bedside work area with a sink, computer, and ceiling-mounted, patient-lift system with a custom track to assist with turning, moving, or toileting a patient.

Other family and patient amenities in the unit include access to a two-story atrium with soothing water walls and a waiting room with a panoramic view of the city, kitchenette, and fireplace. In addition to the bedside computer in each patient room, facilities for staff workflow include decentralized support rooms such as clean utility, soiled utility, nutrition, and medication rooms. A staff-respite area, a private room for staff to use, includes a lounge chair, an ottoman, a phone, and an outside view. Beyond the clinical outcomes, this design provides balance for the psychological, social, and spiritual needs of the staff, the patients, and their families. Ultimately, the new patient care center design aspired to create a unique healthcare environment for this center of excellence at Abbott Northwestern Hospital.

Regions Hospital

A primary objective of a building project at Regions Hospital, a large tertiary care facility located in St. Paul, Minnesota, was to replace shared patient rooms with private patient rooms. To do this, the hospital undertook the largest construction project ever to occur in the city. The new hospital bed tower includes an expansion of the emergency department, replacement of the operating suite, and the addition of 144 private patient rooms. Design principles included an overarching goal to enhance patient safety. To accomplish this goal in the bed tower, many new features were built into the design:

* **Standardization of patient rooms.** First, staff realized that standardization of all the patient rooms was imperative. Although each floor has a different service line, even different acuity levels that range from intensive care to orthopedics, all patient rooms are laid out in the same way.
* **Unique staff access and visibility.** Each patient room has a separate doorway for patients and families as well as one for staff. Staff work areas directly adjacent to the patient room include a view window with an integral blind. Staff share this alcove between two rooms, a design feature particularly important for ICU staff. Patient visibility and ease of access to the patient should enhance patient safety by increasing staff presence.

- **Enhanced family zones.** In addition, family zones in the rooms are gener-
ous, with the intent to encourage family-centered patient care. Families have
the ability to stay overnight in most rooms.
- **Inclusion of acuity-adaptable patient rooms.** Patient rooms on the cardiac
unit were designed to be "acuity adaptable"; that is, they allow patients to stay
in the same room as their acuity level varies. The concept is based on data
suggesting that reduced transfers of patients decreases medical incidents and
errors (Hendrich, Fay, & Sorrels, 2004).
- **Patient access to the toilet.** Finally, as the patient rooms are mirrored,
at least half of patient rooms have direct access to the patient toilet. No
studies to date have been able to document that this is a safer layout for
patients, but with a growing number of patient rooms being designed this
way, Regions provides the perfect setting to study the impact of this layout
on patient safety.

CULTURAL APPLICATIONS AND PRECAUTIONS

The increased diversity of the U.S. population has added a level of complexity
to the design of healthcare environments. As noted by Kopec and Han (2008),
entering a healthcare environment can be frightening and disempowering, particularly when a patient's traditional and spiritual beliefs differ from that of the
dominant culture. Thus, it is becoming increasingly important to carefully weigh
all design decisions that impact the physical environment, including the use of
color and cultural symbols, as well as other visual, auditory, and tactile design
elements.

To Asians, for example, the color red symbolizes good luck whereas the color
white is associated with mourning and death. The color green has positive associations within the Islamic tradition because it is associated with vegetation and
life and is believed to have been the prophet Mohammed's favorite color. Kopec
and Han (2008) have identified a number of ways in which the needs of Muslim
patients might be accommodated. A curtain inside the door, for instance, could
help patients maintain visual privacy and modesty while allowing healthcare providers on rounds to announce their presence, giving patients time to prepare themselves to be seen. Understanding that followers of Islam face the northeast when
they pray could be taken into consideration when orienting the bed and furnishings
in the room. Given the diversity of spiritual, religious, and cultural beliefs and practices, however, it would be nearly impossible—from a design perspective, as well as
practically and financially—to accommodate all the specifics and nuances of every
tradition in the design of healthcare settings. Thus, the goal of design can only be
to strive to express core, universal values while seeking to devise design elements
that can be flexible. Sidebar 4.1, written by a nurse from Liberia, reminds us that
it is not only the physical environment that can enhance healing. It is important
to understand diverse cultural perspectives of healing and healing environments so
that nurses can work to overcome the challenges that these present in the provision
of culturally sensitive, patient-centered care.

Another cultural perspective is presented in Sidebar 4.2. This sidebar emphasizes the healing potential of natural and built environments and the ancient understanding of their potential effects on healing.

SIDEBAR 4.1. HEALING ENVIRONMENTS IN LIBERIA, WEST AFRICA

Maria Tarlue Keita

I am from the Krahn tribe, a small tribe in Liberia, West Africa, which is one of 16 tribes in Liberia. However, I am confident in saying that the healing environment I describe reflects the culture of the Liberian people in general.

When I think of the healing environment in the United States, what comes to mind are the beautiful, well-designed rooms, readily available medications, and high-tech medical devices. The healing environment in my culture consists of four major parts: family presence, food, spirituality, and complementary therapies.

Presence as a Healing Environment

When people from Liberia are in the hospital, it is important for staff to understand the importance of presence. Family and friends come in dozens to visit. However, there are always one or two people who stay in the room at all times to support the sick person. The role of the assigned person(s) is to coordinate the care of the patient between hospital caregiver and the family and to provide direct support such as encouragement and reassurance to the patient. The presence of friends and family reduces anxiety and builds trust with hospital staff. A healing environment is incomplete without the presence of a family member or a friend with the sick.

It is an expectation in my culture that people stay with one who is ill. The role of the family is to help in the care of the sick with activities of daily living, even when in a formal hospital setting.

Food as a Healing Environment

Food is another very important part of the healing environment in my culture. Special foods, such as a pepper soup made with hot spices, are offered to sick people. If solid food is prepared, it is usually anything that can be easily swallowed. *Depa* and *fufu* are like mashed potatoes made from fresh or dried cassava, yams, or plantains. So-called slippery soups are also easy to swallow. Sick people, it is believed, obtain cleansing and nasal decongestion from various soups.

Complementary Therapy as a Part of a Healing Environment

A warm bath with or without herbs is considered to be very therapeutic in my culture and is therefore offered to sick people. A routine daily bath is an expectation. Herbs are often boiled with the bath water and the hot bath is given to the patient.

Spirituality

Providing regular prayers and the presence of religious symbols is an essential part of the healing environment; however, these may come with different levels

(continued)

of spirituality. Many families may believe that without intervention from above, conventional medicine will not bring about healing.

The combination of conventional medicine and a healing environment in the Liberian culture is sometimes a challenge to healthcare providers in the United States. Family involvement in conventional medicine is limited based on how a healing environment is perceived by Liberians. Hospital staff is usually overwhelmed by the presence of many family members in rooms of patients from Liberia or most African cultures.

SIDEBAR 4.2. ANCIENT HEALING ENVIRONMENTS OF GREECE

Ioanna Gryllaki

I have given the topic of the environment's role in healing much consideration. After reflecting on my own most recent experience in the public hospitals of Greece and consulting my resident family members about their experiences, I have come to the conclusion that unfortunately, modern Greece does not have the resources or motivation to use its beautiful landscape to induce healing. The reality of the economic depression in Greece has taken a hit not only on its natural and financial resources, but also on the spirit of the Greek people. In Ancient Greece, the most famous healing temples were the 2,400-year-old Asclepions, which were dedicated to the god of healing, Asclepius (Holloway, 2015). The estimated 320 of these beautiful healing temples acted as hospitals in Ancient Greece, with the most famous temples located in Epidaurus, Cos, and Pergamum (Holloway, 2015). In ancient days, the priests and physicians who oversaw the care provided at the Asclepions embraced a holistic approach to healing that included treatments such as massage and herbal medicines— treatments embedded in the context of soul-uplifting healing environments to optimize the body's power for health and healing. The healers of the day held a view that one's soul needed mending as well as one's body (Holloway, 2015). However, these ancient temples are no longer being funded or used by Greeks. Although this is the stark reality of Greece today, the dormant power of the healing environments within these treasures awaits future reawakening to benefit its people and visitors to this historic land.

Reference

Holloway, A. (2015, October 25). 2,400-year-old healing temple dedicated to Asclepius, god of healing, excavated in Greece. *Ancient Origins*. Retrieved from http://www.ancient-origins.net/news-history-archaeology/2400-year-old-healing-temple-dedicated- asclepius-god-healing-excavated-020587

Nurses can promote the health and well-being by providing simple tips for modifying and enhancing the environment of patients' homes. These simple, yet effective tips are presented in Exhibit 4.3.

Exhibit 4.3. Creating Healing Environments and Enhancing Well-Being: Tips for the Home

- *Open a window.* Allowing fresh air to circulate through your home lets you breathe easier. This also rids the air of pollutants, including harmful chemicals that may accumulate from products, equipment such as air conditioners, and furniture.
- *Bring the outside in.* Studies have demonstrated that exposure to nature can reduce stress levels and improve well-being. Viewing nature from a window or looking at nature-related images can give a sense of retreat throughout the day.
- *Create a quiet, comfortable space* that allows you to escape and reflect. Meditation is an important part of overall well-being and has been shown to increase (hard-to-access) alpha-wave patterns in the brain that have been associated with less stress and anxiety.
- *Use calming colors.* Color can have a wide range of effects on human mood and emotions. Colors with blue undertones have the ability to calm the mind and create a greater sense of relaxation. Light waves corresponding to the color blue are found to have the greatest effect on regulating the circadian rhythms that are directly related to moods.
- *Avoid clutter in the home*; it can create unnecessary stress! Because our brains are constantly categorizing what we see, it is important to keep the space around us organized and free of clutter.
- *Personalize your space* with items, furnishings, and finishes that bring you joy and that have meaning. Personalizing one's space gives one a sense of control and a deeper connection to a space.
- *Have a sense of control* in your home environment. This can include temperature controls, space allocation and organization, noise levels, security, and safety. Most important, your home should function according to the way you live.

Source: Adapted from Angelita Scott, personal communication, April 1, 2013.

FUTURE RESEARCH

More research is needed to understand the impact of design interventions on the environment of care. Future studies need to rigorously examine the many factors that contribute to healing environments and should focus on staff, as well as patient outcomes. Healthcare outcomes for patients may include the reduction of stress, reduced length of stay, decreased incidence of nosocomial infections, reduced pain, improved sleep, increased satisfaction, and reduced number of falls. Outcomes for nursing staff may include decreased injuries, decreased stress, reduced number of sick days taken, and increased effectiveness, productivity, and satisfaction. The OHE framework provides one way to help establish study parameters. As U.S. healthcare facilities construction spending continues to be robust, nurses need to be actively engaged in contributing to the design and evaluation of healing environments that will optimize the health and well-being of patients, family members, and staff.

WEBSITES

The following websites contain additional information on healing environments:

- The Center for Health Design (www.healthdesign.org)
- Earl E. Bakken Center for Spirituality & Healing, University of Minnesota (www.takingcharge.csh.umn.edu/what-is-a-healing-environment) (www.takingcharge.csh.umn.edu/explore-healing-practices/healing-environment) (www.takingcharge.csh.umn.edu/explore-healing-practices/healing-environment/what-impact-does-environment-have-us)

REFERENCES

Ancoli-Israel, S., Gehrman, P., Martin, J. L., Shochat, T., Marler, M., Corey-Bloom, J., & Levi, L. (2003). Increased light exposure consolidates sleep and strengthens circadian rhythms in severe Alzheimer's disease patients. *Behavioral Sleep Medicine, 1*, 22–36.

Beauchemin, K. M., & Hays, P. (1996). Sunny hospital rooms expedite recovery from severe and refractory depressions. *Journal of Affective Disorders, 40*(1–2), 49–51.

Dossey, B. M. (2000). *Florence Nightingale: Mystic, visionary, healer.* Springhouse, PA: Springhouse.

Dowling, G. A., Mastick, J., Hubbard, E. M., Luxenberg, J. S., & Burr, R. L. (2005). Effect of timed bright light treatment for rest-activity disruption in institutionalized patients with Alzheimer's disease. *International Journal of Geriatric Psychiatry, 20*, 738–743.

Figueiro, M., Saldo, E., Rea, M. S., Kubarek, K., Cunningham, J., & Rea, M. S. (2008). Developing architectural lighting designs to improve sleep in older adults. *The Open Sleep Journal, 1*, 40–51.

Golden, R. N., Gaynes, B. N., Ekstrom, R. D., Hamer, R. M., Jacobsen, F. M., Suppes, T., … Nemeroff, C. B. (2005). The efficacy of light therapy in the treatment of mood disorders: A review and meta-analysis of the evidence. *American Journal of Psychiatry, 162*(4), 656–662.

Goto, S., Park, B.-J., Tsunetsugu, Y., Herrup, K., & Miyazaki, Y. (2013). The effect of garden designs on mood and heart output in older adults residing in an assisted living facility. *Health Environments Research & Design Journal, 6*(2), 27–42.

Heerwagen, J. H. (1990). The psychological aspects of windows and window design. In K. H. Anthony, J. Choi, & B. Orland (Eds.), *Proceedings of 21st Annual Conference of the Environmental Design Research Association* (pp. 269–280). Oklahoma City, OK: Environmental Design Research Association.

Hendrich, A., Fay, J., & Sorrells, A. (2004). Effects of acuity-adaptable rooms on flow of patients and delivery of care. *American Journal of Critical Care, 113*(1), 35–45.

Joseph, A., Choi, Y., & Quan, X. (2015). Impact of the physical environment of residential health, care, and support facilities (RHCSF) on staff and residents: A systematic review of the literature. *Environment & Behavior, 48*(10), 1203–1241.

Kearney, A. R., & Winterbottom, D. (2005). Nearby nature and long-term care facility residents: Benefits and design recommendations. *Journal of Housing for the Elderly, 1*(3/4), 7–28.

Kellert, S. R. (2008). Dimensions, elements and attributes of biophilic design. In S. R. Kellert, J. H. Heerwagen, & M. L. Mador (Eds.), *Biophilic design* (pp. 3–20). Hoboken, NJ: John Wiley.

Kopec, D., & Han, L. (2008). Islam and the healthcare environment: Designing patient rooms. *Health Environments Research and Design Journal, 1*(4), 111–121.

Malkin, J. (2008). *A visual reference for evidence-based design.* Concord, CA: The Center for Health Design.

Miller, A. C., Hickman, L. C., & Lemasters, G. K. (1992). A distraction technique for control of burn pain. *Journal of Burn Care and Rehabilitation, 13*(5), 576–580.

Nanda, U., Eisen, S., Zadeh, R., & Owen, D. (2010). Effect of visual art on patient anxiety and agitation in a mental health facility and implications for the business case. *Journal of Psychiatric and Mental Health Nursing, 18*, 386–393.

Nanda, U., Zhu, X., & Jansen, B. H. (2012). Image and emotion: From outcomes to brain behavior. *Health Environments Research & Design Journal, 5*(4), 40–59.

Nightingale, F. (1860). *Notes on nursing: What it is, what it is not.* London, England: Harrison and Sons.

Pati, D., Freier, P., O'Boyle, M., Amor, C., & Valipoor, S. (2016). The impact of simulated nature on patient outcomes: A study of photographic sky compositions. *Health Environments Research & Design Journal, 9*(2), 36–51.

Pati, D., & Nanda, U. (2011). Influence of positive distractions on children in two clinic waiting areas. *Health Environments Research & Design Journal, 4,* 124–140.

Roe, J., & Aspinall, P. (2011). The restorative benefits of walking in urban and rural settings in adults with good and poor mental health. *Health & Place, 17,* 103–113.

Shepley, M. M., Gerbi, R. P., Watson, A. E., Imgrund, S., & Sagha-Zadeh, R. (2012). The impact of daylight and views on ICU patients and staff. *Health Environments Research & Design Journal, 5*(2), 46–60.

Ulrich, R. S., & Gilpin, L. (2003). Healing arts. In S. B. Frampton, L. Gilpin, & P. Charmel (Eds.), *Putting patients first: Designing and practicing patient-centered care* (pp. 117–146). San Francisco, CA: Jossey-Bass.

Ulrich, R. S., Lunden, O. L., & Eltinge, J. L. (1993). Effects of exposure to nature and abstract pictures on patients recovering from heart surgery. [Paper presented at the Thirty-Third Meeting of the Society for Psychophysiological Research.] *Psychophysiology, 30*(Suppl. 1), 7.

Ulrich, R. S., Simons, R. F., & Miles, M. A. (2003). Effects of environmental simulations and television on blood donor stress. *Journal of Architectural & Planning Research, 20*(1), 38–47.

Ulrich, R. S., Siring, C., Zhu, X., Dubose, J., Seo, H., Choi, Y., … Joseph, A. (2008). A review of the research literature on evidence-based healthcare design. *Health Environments Research & Design Journal, 1*(3), 61–125.

Walch, J. M., Rabin, B. S., Day, R., Williams, J. N., Choi, K., & Kang, J. D. (2005). The effect of sunlight on post-operative analgesic medication usage: A prospective study of patients undergoing spinal surgery. *Psychosomatic Medicine, 67,* 156–163.

Wilson, E. O. (1984). *Biophilia: The human bond with other species.* Cambridge, MA: Harvard University Press.

Winston, A. S., & Cupchik, G. C. (1992). The evaluation of high art and popular art by naive and experienced viewers. *Visual Arts Research, 18,* 1–14.

Wismeijer, A. J., & Vingerhoets, J. J. (2005). The use of virtual reality and audiovisual eyeglass systems as adjunct analgesic techniques: A review of the literature. *Annals of Behavioral Medicine, 30*(3), 268–278.

Zborowsky, T. (2014). The legacy of Florence Nightingale's environmental theory: Nursing research focusing on the impact of healthcare environments. *Health Environments Research & Design Journal, 7*(4), 19–34.

Zborowsky, T., & Kreitzer, M. J. (2009). People, place, and process: The role of place in creating optimal healing environments. *Creative Nursing, 15*(4), 186–190.

Systems of Care: Sowa Rigpa—The Tibetan Knowledge of Healing

MIRIAM E. CAMERON

Healthcare systems are burdened by caring for individuals whose chronic disease (lack of ease) often results from unhealthy lifestyle choices. As people become more health conscious, they are looking outside of conventional healthcare for answers to better health. In the United States, more than 30% of adults and approximately 12% of children use complementary and alternative therapies. Complementary therapies are nonmainstream practices that are integrated into conventional care, whereas alternative therapies are nonmainstream practices used in place of conventional healthcare (National Center for Complementary and Integrative Health [NCCIH], 2016).

Too often, complementary and alternative therapies lack scientific evidence. An example is homeopathy, a therapy that developed in Germany at the end of the 18th century. Central tenets of homeopathy are (a) like cures like, which means a disease can be cured by a substance that produces similar symptoms in healthy people, and (b) the law of minimum dose, meaning that the *lower* the dose of medication, the *greater* its effectiveness. In evaluating this therapy, research is needed because little scientific evidence exists to support the use of homeopathy as an effective treatment for any specific condition (NCCIH, 2017b).

Three ancient, yet timely, complementary and alternative therapies are gaining popularity in the United States: traditional Chinese medicine; Ayurveda from India; and *Sowa Rigpa*, Tibet's knowledge of healing, commonly called Tibetan medicine. For thousands of years, these traditions have taught that (a) each person is born with a unique combination of energies and (b) health is balance and disease is imbalance. Chinese medicine describes two principal energies: hot energy (*yang*) and cold energy (*yin*) (NCCIH, 2017c; Earl E. Bakken Center for Spirituality & Healing, University of Minnesota, 2017b). Ayurveda and Tibetan medicine identify three primary energies: movement energy (*loong* in Tibetan, *vata* in Ayurveda), hot energy (*tripa* in Tibetan, *pitta* in Ayurveda), and cold energy (*baekan* in Tibetan, *kapha* in Ayurveda) (Earl E. Bakken Center for Spirituality & Healing, University of Minnesota, 2017b;

Earl E. Bakken Center for Spirituality & Healing, University of Minnesota, 2016; Gonpo, 2015a; NCCIH, 2017a). Although science does not readily adapt to investigating these holistic systems, publications are exploding with studies about the benefits of their interventions (Earl E. Bakken Center for Spirituality & Healing, University of Minnesota, 2017b; Earl E. Bakken Center for Spirituality & Healing, University of Minnesota, 2016; Lindquist, Snyder, & Tracy, 2014).

This chapter explores Tibetan medicine, a complementary therapy with promising scientific evidence pertinent to nursing (Cameron, et al., 2012). Tibetan medicine and nursing share a holistic perspective in considering every individual to have unique, interrelated mental, physical, and spiritual needs. Both disciplines aim to address these needs. Nurses can use Tibetan medicine as self-care and in nursing. Including Tibetan medicine in integrative nursing expands healing options and promotes relationship-based, individualized, quality care (Bauer-Wu, et al., 2014; Earl E. Bakken Center for Spirituality & Healing, University of Minnesota, 2017c).

DEFINITION

History, Philosophy, and Psychology of Tibetan Medicine

The earliest inhabitants of Tibet learned to thrive in the Himalayas, the tallest mountains on earth. Observing wildlife, Tibetans relied on natural resources to heal and sustain them. They practiced *Bon*, Tibet's indigenous shamanism, based on the interrelatedness of mind, body, and natural world. When Buddhism came to Tibet, Tibetan medicine practitioners blended *Bon* and Buddhism with influences from Ayurveda; yoga; and Chinese, Persian, and Greek traditions. In the 8th century, Yuthok Yonten Gonpo, a famous doctor, compiled these teachings into the *Gyueshi*, the fundamental text of Tibetan medicine (Gonpo, 2015a; Gonpo, 2015b).

Today Tibetan medical colleges base their programs on the *Gyueshi*, commentaries, research, experience, and current theories of health and disease. An example is Men-Tsee-Khang (2017) Tibetan Medical Institute in Dharamsala, India. Graduates are called Doctor of Tibetan Medicine. Recently, Tso-Ngon (Qinghai) University Tibetan Medical College in Xining, China (Amdo, Tibet) developed a master's degree and PhD in Tibetan medicine. Faculty created a bachelor's degree in Tibetan medicine nursing. Graduates take the same national licensing exam as other nurses in China.

Tibetan medicine is based on four profound concepts: karma, suffering, healing, and happiness. *Karma* is the universal law of cause and effect: "As one sows, so does one reap." To be healthy and happy, one needs to make choices that create health and happiness. Ethical behavior is essential to avoid the turmoil resulting from unethical actions. Sometimes choices have an immediate, obvious effect, but other times effects are not clear. For example, eating unhealthy food or telling lies may not reap poor consequences immediately but eventually cause suffering and even disease. One needs to develop awareness of both immediate and long-term effects of one's choices (Cameron, 2002; Earl E. Bakken Center for Spirituality & Healing, University of Minnesota. (2016).

Suffering results from interpreting situations negatively. The Sanskrit term for suffering is *dukkha*, meaning "dissatisfaction" (lack of satisfaction). Most of human life is spent trying to avoid suffering and increase pleasure, too often in ways that inadvertently cause suffering. Pain and suffering are not the same (Cameron, 2002; Gonpo, 2015a; Gonpo, 2015b). For example, one experiences pain from a sprained ankle. One also will suffer by angrily asking, "Why do bad things always happen to me?" To avoid suffering, one can say, "I'm glad I didn't break my ankle. My sprained ankle is telling me to slow down, and I'll do it!"

Healing means to reestablish balance and create optimal health. One needs to purify negativity, behave ethically, and develop a healthy mind. A positive, compassionate mindset helps one to make choices that maintain balance. Even on one's deathbed, healing the mind is advisable and possible, although the body is deteriorating (Earl E. Bakken Center for Spirituality & Healing, University of Minnesota, 2016; Men-Tsee-Khang, 2009).

Happiness is the purpose of life! Happiness means lasting peace and well-being resulting from a healthy mind and balanced living. One creates meaning by seeing one's life as part of a bigger, purposeful picture. This includes behaving with integrity according to the highest ethical values. Like a lotus flower growing in mud, one transforms life's "mud" into nourishment to rise and bloom (Cameron, 2002).

Five Elements, Three Energies, Seven Constitutions

Tibetan medicine teaches that energy is the very source of existence. Because everyone is made of energy, everyone is interconnected with everyone else, everything, and the natural world. Energy has five aspects or characteristics, translated as elements. The elements explain qualities and physiological functions that work synergistically to maintain physical, mental, and spiritual health. Everyday terms illustrate the universal, energetic qualities, as described in Exhibit 5.1 (Gonpo, 2015a, Gonpo, 2015b; Men-Tsee-Khang, 2009).

The five elements combine to form three primary energies: *loong, tripa,* and *baekan.* Each of the three energies has divisions and subdivisions, as well as defining characteristics and behavior. Everyone is born with a unique combination of the three primary energies called one's *constitutional nature* or *constitution.* The dominant energy or energies give the name to each constitution (Gonpo, 2015a, Gonpo, 2015b; Gyatso, 2010). Exhibit 5.2 lists the three primary energies, the Tibetan term for each energy, and the element(s) composing each energy. Exhibit 5.3 lists the seven possible constitutions.

Exhibit 5.1. The Five Elements of Tibetan Medicine

- **Earth** is the aspect of energy that produces stability and structure.
- **Water** is the aspect of energy that provides moisture, lubrication, and smoothness.
- **Fire** is the aspect of energy that drives growth, development, metabolism, and digestion.
- **Air** is the aspect of energy that governs movement, including blood and lymph circulation.
- **Space** is the aspect of energy that allows the other four elements to interact and coexist.

Exhibit 5.2. Three Primary Energies, Tibetan Terms, and Five Elements		
Primary Energy	**Tibetan Term**	**Composed of This Element**
Movement	*Loong* (pronounced LOONG)	Air
Heat	*Tripa* (pronounced TEE-pah)	Fire
Cold	*Baekan* (pronounced BA-kun)	Earth, water

Ordinarily, one's inborn constitution does not change. However, the three primary energies can rise, fall, or become disturbed because of multiple variables. Examples are thoughts, food, beverages, stress, weather, environment, other people, lifestyle choices, time of day, and stage in life. To be healthy and happy, one must make choices that keep the current percentages of *loong, tripa*, and *baekan* consistent with their percentages in one's inborn constitution. By learning about one's inborn constitution, one can maintain balance, enhance strengths, and transform weaknesses into assets or at least keep them from becoming obstacles to health (Gonpo, 2015a, Gonpo, 2015b; Gyatso, 2010).

For example, one may be born with about 45% *tripa*, 40% *baekan*, and 15% *loong* (*tripa/baekan* constitution; see Figure 5.1). To be healthy and happy, one must keep the current percentages of the three primary energies at about these inborn percentages. Change in one energy affects the other two energies; increasing *tripa* (hot energy) can decrease *baekan* (cold energy), and vice versa. Imbalance occurs well before physical symptoms of disease appear (Men-Tsee-Khang, 2009).

Regardless of one's inborn constitution, *baekan* rises in the first stage of life to help children grow and develop. *Tripa* rises during the second and third stages of life when adults need heat energy to set and meet goals, work, raise a family, and fulfill other tasks. In the fourth and final stage, *loong* rises so that older adults can become less grounded and more spiritual as they prepare to let go and die (Cameron, 2002; Gonpo, 2015a).

Exhibit 5.3. The Seven Constitutions of Tibetan Medicine

- **Loong:** *Loong* dominates *tripa* and *baekan*.
- **Tripa:** *Tripa* dominates *loong* and *baekan*.
- **Baekan:** *Baekan* dominates *loong* and *tripa*.
- **Loong/tripa** or **tripa/loong:** *Loong* and *tripa* dominate *baekan*.
- **Tripa/baekan** or **baekan/tripa:** *Tripa* and *baekan* dominate *loong*.
- **Loong/baekan** or **baekan/loong:** *Loong* and *baekan* dominate *tripa*.
- **Loong/tripa/baekan:** All three energies are equal, a rare, highly evolved constitution.

15%

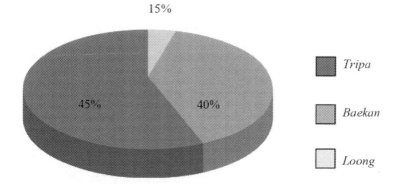

Figure 5.1. Example of a *Tripa/Baekan* Constitution

Relationship Between the Three Primary Energies and Three Mental Poisons

Suffering begins in the mind. Thoughts impact the three primary energies, health, and happiness. For example, happy, compassionate thoughts calm mind and body. Anger raises the heart rate and blood pressure; causes shallow, irregular breathing; and depresses the immune system. When engaging in three categories of afflictive thought patterns, called *mental poisons*, one is likely to make unhealthy lifestyle choices that result in suffering and illness, as listed in Exhibit 5.4 (Cameron, 2002; Gonpo, 2015a).

One's inborn constitution makes one vulnerable to a particular mental poison. For example, a *loong* constitution makes one prone to engaging in greed, attachments, and desire. The likely results are anxiety and other health problems associated with *loong*. In other words, greed causes and results from *loong* imbalance. Likewise, anger causes and results from *tripa* imbalance, and delusion causes and results from *baekan* imbalance (Gonpo, 2015a, Gonpo, 2015b; Gyatso, 2010).

When one energy goes out of balance, the other two energies likely will go out of balance, too. Anxiety and insomnia often begin the process. *Loong* rises too high, which affects *tripa* and *baekan*. Chronic imbalance in all three energies is difficult

Exhibit 5.4. Three Mental Poisons, Three Primary Energies, and Health Problems

Mental Poison	Imbalance in This Primary Energy	Imbalance Can Lead to These Health Problems
Greed, attachments, desire	*Loong*	Anxiety, movement disorders, insomnia, mental illness, addictions
Anger, hostility, aggression	*Tripa*	Inflammations, infections, metabolic/hormonal problems
Delusion, confusion, close-mindedness	*Baekan*	Respiratory disorders, obesity, diabetes

to unravel and can produce complex health problems, such as cancer, cardiovascular disease, and autoimmune disorders. Creating a healthy mind and making good choices is the first essential step toward healing and health (Earl E. Bakken Center for Spirituality & Healing, University of Minnesota, 2016; Men-Tsee-Khang, 2009).

SCIENTIFIC BASIS

For hundreds of years, doctors of Tibetan medicine have conducted evidence-based research. They have documented the results of interventions and prescribed the most effective ones (Bauer-Wu et al., 2014; Gonpo, 2015a, Gonpo 2015b; Gyatso, 2010). Western scientific researchers are validating many of their health claims. Numerous studies have been published about benefits of interventions essential to Tibetan medicine. Recent studies include positive results of Tibetan meditation (Pagliaro et al., 2016), Tibetan art (Baumann, Murphy, & Ganzer, 2015), Tibetan yoga (Milbury et al., 2015; NCCIH, 2017d), breathing techniques, massage, mindfulness, imagery, aromatherapy, music, biofeedback, nutrition, presence, listening, reiki, and being in nature (Earl E. Bakken Center for Spirituality & Healing, University of Minnesota, 2016; Earl E. Bakken Center for Spirituality & Healing, University of Minnesota, 2017b; Lindquist et al., 2014).

Compassion, the essence of Tibetan medicine, is a philosophical stance of kindness based on the understanding that all phenomena are made of the same five elements. So-called compassion fatigue does not result from too much compassion but from codependency, excessive reliance on other people for approval and identity (Gonpo, 2015a). Tibetan medicine teaches a positive relationship among self-compassion, compassion, healing, and health, which numerous studies have confirmed (Zessin, Dickhauser, & Garbade, 2015). Recently, researchers found this relationship in U.S. veterans of the wars in Iraq and Afghanistan (Dahm et al., 2015), interpersonal relations (Kneafsey, Brown, Sein, Chamley, & Parsons, 2016), people with depression (Kotsou & Leys, 2016), individuals experiencing adversity (Lim & DeSteno, 2016), pregnant women's fetal–maternal attachment (Mohamadirizi & Kori, 2016), people with chronic pain (Purdie & Morley, 2015), adolescents (Shepperd, Miller, & Smith, 2015), and altruistic individuals (Weng, Fox, Hessenthaler, Stodola, & Davidson, 2015).

Sinclair et al. (2016) mapped compassion literature in clinical healthcare and found limited empirical understanding of compassion. After reviewing nursing literature, McCaffrey and McConnell (2015) concluded that compassion is a human experience of deep significance to nursing but needs precise understanding. Tibetan medicine offers in-depth understanding of compassion that can benefit the discipline of nursing, individual nurses, and nursing practice. Nurses can use these teachings to treat themselves and others with compassion and be a happy, healing presence (Cameron, 2002).

Scientific research is lacking about Tibetan medicine as a holistic system. Such research is challenging because the physical, mental, and spiritual components of Tibetan medicine work synergistically. Bauer-Wu et al. (2014) found Tibetan medicine as a holistic system to be safe and have positive effects on quality of life, disease regression, and remission in individuals with cancer and blood disorders.

Cameron, et al. (2012) tested and refined two tools based on Tibetan medicine as a holistic system: (a) Constitutional Self-Assessment Tool (CSAT) and (b) Lifestyle Guidelines Tool (LGT). The primary purpose was to provide self-assessment tools for

---

Exhibit 5.5. Instructions for Completing the Constitutional Self-Assessment Tool (CSAT)

- Before completing the tools, learn basic teachings of Tibetan medicine, as in this free, online information (Earl E. Bakken Center for Spirituality & Healing, University of Minnesota, 2016).
- Complete the CSAT in a quiet, reflective environment, without time pressures.
- Do an accurate, honest assessment of who you *really* are, not the person you wish to be.
- Consult with someone who knows you well to help you assess yourself accurately.
- Base your answers on your overall life, not just your current situation.
- Use the CSAT result to complete the LGT and calm *loong*, cool *tripa*, or warm *baekan*.

---

people who don't have access to doctors of Tibetan medicine. The CSAT and LGT had high content validity; the CSAT had moderate criterion validity. When participants followed the instructions in Exhibit 5.5, assessment accuracy (criterion validity) of the CSAT increased. The tools are posted online for anyone to complete for free (Earl E. Bakken Center for Spirituality & Healing, University of Minnesota, 2017a).

Most studies that have been carried out have focused on the medicinal agents used by Tibetan medicine practitioners. Such research is challenging because Tibetan medicinal agents often are composed of 100 or more ingredients to treat symptoms, reverse imbalance, and promote healing (Kalsang, 2016). Studies have been done on rats and in laboratories to identify whether specific ingredients can benefit humans; results are promising. Recent studies showed decreased MCF7 breast cancer cells (Bassa et al., 2016); less neuropathic pain (Fan, Li, Gong, & Wang, 2016); antitumor activity (Choedon, Mathan, & Kumar, 2015; Fan et al., 2015); and lower uric acid (Kou et al., 2016). *Padma 28*, a Tibetan medicinal agent, lessened pain and increased walking distance in individuals with intermittent claudication (Stewart, Morling, & Maxwell, 2016). Because Tibetan medicinal agents are not readily available, this research currently has limited use in nursing.

INTERVENTION

Tibetan medicine has numerous, easy-to-use, free or inexpensive interventions. These are summarized in the earlier exhibits and the descriptions that follow. Nurses can use these interventions for their own self-care and in integrative nursing.

Complete a Constitutional Analysis

The gold standard is to consult with a qualified, experienced Tibetan medicine doctor, called a Tibetan medicine practitioner in the United States. During a consultation, the practitioner asks the client questions, reads the pulses, analyzes the urine, and looks at the tongue. Using this information, the practitioner identifies the client's inborn constitution; energies that are out of balance (if any); methods to bring them back into balance; and supportive lifestyle choices (Bauer-Wu, et al., 2014; Earl E. Bakken Center for Spirituality & Healing, University of Minnesota, 2016; Men-Tsee-Khang, 2009).

Because few people have access to such a practitioner, nurses can complete, and encourage clients to complete, the CSAT and LGT, the first published, research-based self-assessment tools about Tibetan medicine (Cameron et al., 2012). The CSAT and LGT can be completed anonymously, for free, 24/7, at https://www.csh.umn.edu/education/focus-areas/tibetan-medicine/assessment-and-guidelines-tools (Earl E. Bakken Center for Spirituality & Healing, University of Minnesota, 2017a).

Create a Healthy Body

The CSAT identifies one's current dominant energy, which may not be the same as the dominant energy in one's inborn constitution if imbalance exists. Using the CSAT result, follow that LGT column to calm *loong*, cool *tripa*, or warm *baekan*. If, for example, one's CSAT result is *tripa*, do what is listed in the *tripa* column to cool *tripa*. Doing the CSAT and LGT periodically can teach one to balance the primary energies, heal symptoms, and reverse the source of imbalance (Earl E. Bakken Center for Spirituality & Healing, University of Minnesota, 2017a; Cameron et al., 2012).

As stated in the LGT, one can create balance by ingesting foods and beverages opposite to one's current dominant energy. When one is stressed out and *loong* is high, eat warm, nutritious soup to reduce *loong*. On a hot day when *tripa* is high, one can eat cool foods like salads. During a cold winter when *baekan* rises, one can eat warm, spicy foods. Exhibit 5.6 summarizes how to behave in a way opposite to the energy that is out of balance. Conversely, if any of the three energies falls too low, one can use the LGT to engage in behaviors that increase this energy (Earl E. Bakken Center for Spirituality & Healing, University of Minnesota, 2017a).

Heal the Three Mental Poisons

Exhibit 5.7 lists meditations and actions to heal negativity (Cameron, 2002; Gyatso, 2010).

Exhibit 5.6. Bring the Three Primary Energies Into Balance With Opposite Behavior

Energy Out of Balance	Behaviors to Treat Imbalance
Loong (movement energy)	Calm *loong* by doing what is warm, grounded, and calming. For example, listen quietly to calming music.
Tripa (hot energy)	Cool *tripa* by doing what is dry and cool. For example, avoid vigorous exercise on a hot day.
Baekan (cold energy)	Warm *baekan* by doing what is dry and warm. For example, wear warm clothes on a cool day; exercise vigorously.

Exhibit 5.7. Heal the Three Mental Poisons			
Mental Poison	**Imbalance**	**Meditate on**	**Action**
Greed, attachments, desire	*Loong*	Impermanence: Continuous change	Behave with generosity, loving kindness, acceptance.
Anger, hostility, aggression	*Tripa*	Compassion: Yearn for everyone to be free of suffering	Relieve suffering by asking, "What can I do to help?"
Delusion, confusion, close-mindedness	*Baekan*	Wisdom: Wake up and see things as they *really* are	Develop mindfulness of the present moment.

Create a Healthy Mind

The focus in creating a healthy mind is on mindfully making lifestyle choices that lead to happiness, rather than suffering. Tibetan medicine integrates ethics, spirituality, and healing. A healthy mind results from creation of an ethical, spiritual life in which one can flourish. One thrives by practicing the qualities of happiness: love, compassion, wisdom, kindness, honesty, contentment, integrity, forgiveness, joy, peace, tolerance, meaning, altruism, humility, equanimity, responsibility, and patience (Cameron, 2002; Gonpo, 2015a, Gonpo, 2015b; Gyatso, 2010).

Meditation is a powerful intervention to create a happy mind and optimal health. As numerous studies have found, meditation opens the heart, promotes compassion, and enhances the immune system (Earl E. Bakken Center for Spirituality & Healing, University of Minnesota, 2017b). During meditation, the mind may seem like a jumping monkey, leaping from thought to thought. Tibetan meditation tames the monkey-mind (Earl E. Bakken Center for Spirituality & Healing, University of Minnesota, 2016).

In Tibetan medicine, the purpose of meditation is to become familiar with the mind. This process involves bringing unconscious and subconscious thoughts into the conscious mind to heal negativity. Many options exist: One can meditate while sitting, walking, lying down, dancing, or listening to calm music. Exercising first may promote quiet during sitting meditation. Ideally, one develops a meditative perspective all the time (Cameron, 2002).

Specific strategies include the following:

- Start with a 2-minute meditation on the breath every hour or two (Exhibit 5.8).
- Do Tonglen meditation to fill the heart with compassion and purify the mind and body (Exhibit 5.9).
- Do Loving-Kindness meditation to enhance the immune system (Exhibit 5.10).

Exhibit 5.8. Two-Minute Meditation on Your Breath

- Make yourself comfortable sitting, standing, walking, or lying down.
- Straighten your back, relax your body, breathe deeply, and focus on your breath.
- Engage in circular breathing: Breathe slowly, deeply, and evenly through your nose, from your abdomen, with your in-breath the same length as your out-breath, and no break in-between.
- When your attention moves away from your breath, bring it back to your breath.

Exhibit 5.9. Tonglen Meditation: "Breathe in suffering and breathe out compassion"

- Make yourself comfortable sitting, standing, walking, or lying down.
- Straighten your back, relax your body, breathe deeply, and focus on your breath.
- Engage in circular breathing: Breathe slowly, deeply, and evenly through your nose, from your abdomen, with your in-breath the same length as your out-breath, and no break in-between.
- *Do Tonglen for yourself:* As you breathe in, let all negativity in your mind and body come to the surface. On your out-breath, breathe out these toxins completely and fill yourself with compassion.
- *Do Tonglen for someone you love:* Breathe in your loved one's suffering and breathe out compassion to the person. Open your heart to your loved one.
- *Do Tonglen for someone about whom you feel neutral (clerk in a store, etc.):* Breathe in the person's suffering, and breath out compassion to the person. Open your heart to this individual.
- *Do Tonglen for someone you dislike:* Breathe in the person's suffering and breathe out compassion to this individual. Open your heart to the person and let go of any negativity.
- *Do Tonglen for the world:* Breathe in the suffering of the world, and breathe out compassion to the world. Open your heart to everyone's suffering and let go of any negativity.
- *Purification:* Visualize the suffering you breathed in as black smoke in your heart's center, and breathe it out completely. Fill your heart with compassion for yourself, everyone, and everything.

Exhibit 5.10. Loving-Kindness Meditation

- Make yourself comfortable sitting, standing, walking, or lying down.
- Straighten your back, relax your body, breathe deeply, and focus on your breath.
- Engage in circular breathing: Breathe slowly, deeply, and evenly through your nose, from your abdomen, with your in-breath the same length as your out-breath, and no break in-between.

(continued)

● When you are deeply relaxed and focused, say these words with an altruistic intention:
   ▪ May I be well; may all beings be well.
   ▪ May I be happy; may all beings be happy.
   ▪ May I be peaceful; may all beings be peaceful.
   ▪ May I be loved; may all beings be loved.

These meditations use circular breathing. Engaging in circular breathing all the time, not just during meditation, brings in life-force (*prana* in Sanskrit), oxygenates cells, and releases toxins. Nurses can do the meditations and teach them to clients. Meditating before treatments and surgery calms both mind and body (Earl E. Bakken Center for Spirituality & Healing, University of Minnesota, 2016).

Prepare for a Good Death

Death is not separate from life, but part of life. According to Tibetan medicine, one dies like one lives. To die well, one must live well. Negativity that is not healed during life likely will cause disturbance while dying. By creating a healthy mind, one can face death with acceptance, peace, and even joy (Cameron, 2002; Gonpo, 2015a, Gonpo, 2015b).

Effectiveness

Nurses can determine the effectiveness of these interventions by asking themselves and clients if they feel better than before using them. Conventional care can be an excellent option when Western pharmaceuticals, technology, and surgery are needed to treat acute illness. Tibetan medicine can be effective to create a healthy mind, live a healthy life, heal or manage chronic disease, and die peacefully. The two approaches can complement each other; for example, a client who is undergoing conventional treatment for cancer could use Tibetan medicine to heal from chemotherapy and radiation (Bauer-Wu et al., 2014; Earl E. Bakken Center for Spirituality & Healing, University of Minnesota, 2016).

Even beginners can use Tibetan medicine to decrease stress, anxiety, and headaches, and to improve digestion and sleep. However, most health problems develop over time; Tibetan medicine may not alleviate them right away. Serious imbalance may require careful, long-term rebalancing. Tibetan medicine advocates gradual change. Optimal benefits occur from systematic use (Cameron, 2002; Gyatso, 2010).

PRECAUTIONS

Precautions are advisable when using Tibetan medicine or any other healing system (Earl E. Bakken Center for Spirituality & Healing, University of Minnesota, 2016). Exhibit 5.11 lists precautions to ensure coordinated, safe care.

Take precautions before consulting with Tibetan medicine practitioners. Because the practice of Tibetan medicine is not yet widespread in the United States, standardization, accreditation, and licensure have not yet been established. Some

---

Exhibit 5.11. Precautions When Using Tibetan Medicine

- *Do not* use Tibetan medicine to replace effective conventional care or as a reason to postpone seeing conventional health professionals about health problems.
- Learn as much as you can about your inborn constitution and your health problems.
- Carefully select qualified professionals you trust, but listen to your internal wisdom.
- Advocate for yourself, rather than just accepting what health professionals tell you.
- Explain to your health professionals how you manage your health and medications you take.

---

people lacking credentials claim to practice Tibetan medicine. Be sure to consult only with practitioners who have graduated from a legitimate Tibetan medical college, such as Men-Tsee-Khang (2017).

In the United States, Tibetan medicine practitioners must follow state laws regulating unlicensed practitioners of complementary and alternative healthcare. For example, Chapter 146A of the Minnesota Statutes (2017) states that unlicensed practitioners cannot call themselves a doctor; refer to clients as patients; and use treatments, such as acupuncture, covered by other licensing boards. They must give each client a detailed bill of rights about their qualifications and the client's rights and responsibilities.

If Tibetan medicine practitioners prescribe Tibetan medicinal agents, precautions are needed. Most such medicines are composites of herbs picked in the Himalayan Mountains (Kalsang, 2016). These Tibetan herbal preparations work slowly and have few, if any, side effects. In the United States, Tibetan medicinal agents are categorized as dietary supplements regulated by the U.S. Food and Drug Administration (FDA). In general, regulations are less stringent than for Western pharmaceuticals.

A few Tibetan medicines contain minerals and poisonous plants to detoxify the body and stimulate healing (Ma et al., 2015). In two studies, Tibetan medicines containing detoxified mercury did not lead to mercury in participants' blood (Sallon et al., 2006; Sallon et al., 2017). Until more testing is done, Tibetan medicinal agents containing minerals and poisonous plants should be avoided. Additionally, use of Tibetan medicines together with Western pharmaceuticals should be avoided, as they may interact and be unsafe. Women who are pregnant or nursing, and parents who want to use Tibetan medicinal agents for children, should first consult with qualified health professionals.

USES

Nurses can use Tibetan medicine as self-care and as part of integrative nursing. Sidebar 5.1 explains how one registered nurse uses Tibetan medicine in her personal life and her nursing practice.

FUTURE RESEARCH

Published scientific studies about Tibetan medicine generally report positive results, but much more research is needed. Tibetan medicine's holistic philosophy

SIDEBAR 5.1. A TIBETAN NURSE INTEGRATES NURSING AND TIBETAN MEDICINE

Tashi Lhamo

My parents grew up in Tibet and moved to India, where I was born. Because I wanted to help others, I entered the Tibetan medicine program at Men-Tsee-Khang Tibetan Medical Institute in Dharamsala, India. I graduated as a Doctor of Tibetan Medicine and worked with senior doctors. After immigrating to the United States in 2002, I went to college and studied nursing. Now I am a staff nurse on a busy medical–surgical unit of a large metropolitan hospital. Tibetan medicine is essential to my nursing practice.

Tibetan medicine teaches that the purpose of life is to be happy. Everyone is born with a unique combination of three principal energies: *loong* (movement), *tripa* (hot), and *baekan* (cold). What we think, eat, drink, and do can cause them to rise, fall, or become disturbed. Health is balance and disease is imbalance. To be happy and healthy, we need to make lifestyle choices that keep the current percentages of these energies consistent with our inborn constitution. By using Tibetan medicine as self-care, we become aware of how our thoughts and behaviors affect our body, mind, health, and happiness.

Tibetan medicine helps me to give quality nursing care by understanding my clients on the level of their three principal energies. I view each client as unique and encourage the person to make healthy choices, let go of negativity, and create optimal health. Tibetan medicine teaches me to be mindful of my surroundings and treat each client with compassion, loving kindness, empathetic joy, and equanimity. Also, Tibetan medicine reminds me to practice self-compassion and nurture myself to be healthy physically, mentally, and spiritually. Medical–surgical nursing can be very stressful. Stressed-out nurses will benefit by using Tibetan medicine as self-care and in integrative nursing.

and psychology pose challenges for conducting Western scientific research. The profound interventions affect mind and body in ways that may not be reproducible and quantifiable. New qualitative methods may be needed.

Well-designed studies can test Tibetan medicine's theories about the three primary energies, the seven constitutions, and the relationship between energy imbalance and health problems. Other research questions are:

- How does Tibetan medicine as a holistic approach affect mental health, immunity, longevity, happiness, chronic illness, regeneration, and preparation for death?
- What are relationships between each of the seven constitutions and measurements of anxiety, insomnia, anger, depression, addictions, compassion, biological markers, and specific illnesses?
- How can nurses and clients be taught to use Tibetan medicine for self-care?
- How can nurses effectively integrate Tibetan medicine into nursing care?
- How can nurses be encouraged to practice self-compassion, as taught by Tibetan medicine?

In summary, Tibetan medicine shows promise as a complementary and alternative therapy in nursing. Both disciplines promote mindfulness, self-understanding, and healthy lifestyle choices. Nurses who use Tibetan medicine as self-care and integrate Tibetan medicine into nursing practice enhance healing and health. More people making healthy lifestyle choices based on Tibetan medicine and other promising holistic therapies benefit themselves, healthcare systems, and society.

REFERENCES

Bassa, L. M., Jacobs, C., Gregory, K., Henchey, E., Ser-Dolansky, J., & Schneider, S. S. (2016). *Rhodiola crenulata*. *Phytomedicine, 23*(1), 87–94.

Bauer-Wu, S., Lhundup, T., Tidwell, T., Lhadon, T., Ozawa-de Silva, C., Dolma, J., et al. (2014). Tibetan medicine for cancer. *Integrative Cancer Therapies, 13*(6), 502-512.

Baumann, S. L., Murphy, D. C., & Ganzer, C. A. (2015). A study of graduate nursing students' reflections on the art of Tibetan medicine. *Nursing Science Quarterly, 28*(2), 156–161.

Cameron, M. E. (2002). *Karma & happiness: Tibetan odyssey in ethics, spirituality, & healing.* New York, NY: Roman & Littlefield.

Cameron, M. E., Torkelson, C., Haddow, S., Namdul, T., Prasek, A., & Gross, C. R. (2012). Tibetan medicine and integrative health. *Explore: The Journal of Science and Healing, 8*(3), 158–171.

Choedon, T., Mathan, G., & Kumar, V. (2015). The traditional Tibetan medicine Yukyung Karne. *BMC Complementary and Alternative Medicine, 15*, 182.

Dahm, K. A., Meyer, E. C., Neff, K. D., Kimbrel, N. A., Gulliver, S. B., & Morissette, S. B. (2015). Mindfulness, self-compassion, posttraumatic stress disorder symptoms, and functional disability in U.S. Iraq and Afghanistan war veterans. *Journal of Traumatic Stress, 28*(5), 460–464.

Earl E. Bakken Center for Spirituality & Healing, University of Minnesota. (2017a). *Constitutional Self-Assessment Tool and Lifestyle Guidelines Tool.* Retrieved from https://www.csh.umn.edu/education/focus-areas/tibetan-medicine/assessment-and-guidelines-tools

Earl E. Bakken Center for Spirituality & Healing, University of Minnesota. (2017b). *Learning modules for healthcare professionals.* Retrieved from https://www.csh.umn.edu/education/online-learning-modules-resources/online-learning-modules.

Earl E. Bakken Center for Spirituality & Healing, University of Minnesota. (2017c). *Integrative nursing.* Retrieved from https://www.csh.umn.edu/education/focus-areas/integrative-nursing/principles-integrative-nursing

Earl E. Bakken Center for Spirituality & Healing, University of Minnesota. (2016). *Tibetan medicine.* Retrieved from https://www.takingcharge.csh.umn.edu/explore-healing-practices/tibetan-medicine

Fan, H., Li, T., Gong, N., & Wang, Y. (2016). Shanzhiside methylester, the principle effective iridoid glycoside from the analgesic herb *Lamiophlomis rotata*, reduces neuropathic pain by stimulating spinal microglial beta-endorphin expression. *Neuropharmacology, 101*, 98-109.

Fan, J., Wang, Y., Wang, X., Wang, P., Tang, W., Yuan, W., et al. (2015). The antitumor activity of *Meconopsis horridula Hook. Cellular Physiology & Biochemistry, 37*(3), 1055–1065.

Gonpo, Y. Y. (2015a). *Root Tantra and Explanatory Tantra (Gyueshi)* (T. Paljor, P. Wangdu, & S. Dolma, Trans.). Dharamsala, India: Men-Tsee-Khang.

Gonpo, Y. Y. (2015b). *Subsequent Tantra* (T. Paljor, Trans.). Dharamsala, India: Men-Tsee-Khang.

Gyatso, D. S. (2010). *Mirror of beryl* (G. Kilty, Trans.). Boston, MA: Wisdom Publications.

Kalsang, T. (2016). *Cultivation and conservation of endangered medicinal plants: Tibetan medicinal plants for health.* Dharamsala, India: Men-Tsee-Khang.

Kneafsey, R., Brown, S., Sein, K., Chamley, C., & Parsons, J. (2016). A qualitative study of key stakeholders' perspectives on compassion in healthcare. *Journal of Clinical Nursing, 25*, 70–79.

Kotsou, I., & Leys, C. (2016). Self-compassion scale (SCS): Psychometric properties of the French translation and its relations with psychological well-being, affect and depression. *PLOS ONE, 11*(4), e0152880. doi:10.1371/journal.pone.0152880

Kou, Y., Li, Y., Ma, H., Li, W., Li, R., & Dang, Z. (2016). Uric acid lowering effect of Tibetan Medicine *RuPeng15*. *Journal of Traditional Chinese Medicine*, *36*(2), 205–210.

Lim, D., & DeSteno, D. (2016). Suffering and compassion: The links among adverse life experiences, empathy, compassion, and prosocial behavior. *Emotion*, *16*(2), 175–182.

Lindquist, R., Snyder, M., & Tracy, M. F. (2014). *Complementary & alternative therapies in nursing* (7th ed.). New York, NY: Springer Publishing.

Ma, L., Gu, R., Tang, L., Chen, Z. E., Di, R., & Long, C. (2015). Important poisonous plants in Tibetan ethnomedicine. *Toxins*, *7*(1), 138–155.

McCaffrey, G., & McConnell, S. (2015). Compassion. *Journal of Clinical Nursing*, *24*(19–20), 3006–3015.

Men-Tsee-Khang. (2009). *Fundamentals of Tibetan medicine*. Dharamsala, India: Author.

Men-Tsee-Khang. (2017). *Men-Tsee-Khang, 1916-2017*. Retrieved from http://men-tsee-khang.org/

Milbury, K., Chaoul, A., Engle, R., Liao, Z., Yang, C., Carmack, C., et al. (2015). Couple-based Tibetan yoga program for lung cancer patients and their caregivers. *Psychooncology*, *24*, 117–120.

Minnesota Statutes. (2017). *Chapter 146A*. Complementary and alternative health care practices. Retrieved from https://www.revisor.mn.gov/statutes/?id=146A

Mohamadirizi, S., & Kordi, M. (2016). The relationship between multi-dimensional self-compassion and fetal-maternal attachment in prenatal period in referred women to Mashhad Health Center. *Journal of Education and Health Promotion*, *5*, 21.

National Center for Complementary and Integrative Health. (2017a). *Ayurvedic medicine*. Retrieved from https://nccih.nih.gov/health/ayurveda

National Center for Complementary and Integrative Health. (2017b). *Homeopathy*. Retrieved from https://nccih.nih.gov/health/homeopathy

National Center for Complementary and Integrative Health. (2017c). *Traditional Chinese medicine*. Retrieved from https://nccih.nih.gov/health/chinesemed

National Center for Complementary and Integrative Health. (2017d). *Yoga*. Retrieved from https://nccih.nih.gov/health/yoga

National Center for Complementary and Integrative Health. (2016). *Complementary, alternative, or integrative health: What's in a name?* Retrieved from https://nccih.nih.gov/health/integrative-health

Pagliaro, G., Pandolfi, P., Collina, N., Frezza, G., Brandes, A., Galli, M., et al. (2016). A randomized controlled trial of tong len meditation practice in cancer patients: Evaluation of a distant psychological healing effect. *Explore: The Journal of Science & Healing*, *12*(1), 42-49.

Purdie, F., & Morley, S. (2015). Self-compassion, pain, breaking social contract. *Pain*, *156*(11), 2354–2363.

Sallon, S., Namdul, T., Dolma, S., Dorjee, P., Dolma, D., Sadutshang, T., et al. (2006). Mercury in traditional Tibetan medicine: panacea or problem? *Human & Experimental Toxicology*, *25* (7), 405-412.

Sallon, S., Dory, Y., Barghouthy, Y., Tamdin, T., Sangmo, R., Tashi, J., et al. (2017). Is mercury in Tibetan Medicine toxic? Clinical, neurocognitive and biochemical results of an initial cross-sectional study. *Experimental Biology & Medicine*, *242*, 316-332.

Shepperd, J. A., Miller, W. A., & Smith, C. T. (2015). Religiousness and aggression in adolescents. *Aggressive Behavior*, *41*(6), 608–621.

Sinclair, S., Norris, J. M., McConnell, S. J., Chochinov, H. M., Hack, T. F., Hagen, N. A., et al. (2016). Compassion: a scoping review of the healthcare literature. *BMC Palliative Care*, *15*, 6.

Stewart, M., Morling, J. R., & Maxwell, H. (2016). Padma 28 for intermittent claudication. *Cochrane Database of Systematic Reviews*, *3*, 007371. doi:10.1002/14651858.CD007371.pub3

Weng, H. Y., Fox, A. S., Hessenthaler, H. C., Stodola, D. E., & Davidson, R. J. (2015). The role of compassion in altruistic helping and punishment behavior. *PLOS ONE*, *10*(12), e0143794. doi:10.1371/journal.pone.0143794

Zessin, U., Dickhauser, O., & Garbade, S. (2015). Relationship between self-compassion and well-being: A meta-analysis. *Applied Psychology, Health, and Well-being*, *7*(3), 340–364.

Mind–Body–Spirit Therapies

Mind and body practices are one of the two major categories that the National Center for Complementary and Integrative Health (NCCIH) has designated for complementary therapies. According to the NCCIH, "Mind and body practices include a large and diverse group of procedures or techniques administered or taught by a trained practitioner or teacher" (NCCIH, 2016). Deep breathing, yoga, and tai chi are among the most popular mind and body practices according to the 2012 National Health Interview Survey (NHIS; Clarke, Black, Stussman, Barnes, & Nahin, 2015).

Although the NCCIH has reduced the number of categories for complementary and integrative health practices to two major classes (natural products, and mind and body practices), the editors of this text have elected to use the classification categories of previous editions. Thus, a number of the therapies NCCIH include in mind and body practices we have placed in the categories of manipulative and body-based therapies, and energy therapies.

Because the philosophy of nursing is holistic, "spirit" was added to the title for this section. Not only does the mind affect the body and the body the mind, but the spiritual aspect also has an impact on a person's overall functioning. Nursing has moved away from the Cartesian philosophy in which the body and mind (and spirit) were seen as functioning independently of each other. Cartesian philosophy has for centuries dominated Western medicine. Refuting this dichotomy can be seen in the impact that a severe headache has on one's ability to think, to move, and to pray.

A growing body of research on imagery (Chapter 6) exists. Imagery is one of the therapies that can be taught to patients without a practitioner. Many CDs, DVDs, and smartphone apps for guided imagery exist. Dentists were perhaps the first practitioners to make use of music intervention (Chapter 7) for distraction and relaxation during procedures. Research on music in fields such as with patients with dementia is offering encouraging results. Ancient Greek philosophers wrote about the healing effects of humor (Chapter 8). It was not until Norman Cousins in the 1970s reported on his personal use of humor in the treatment of his health problems that humor assumed a more recognized role as a complementary therapy.

The body of supporting research for therapies in this section is increasing, particularly for therapies such as yoga (Chapter 9) and meditation (Chapter 11). The body of research existing for biofeedback (Chapter 10) also continues to increase, particularly its use with multiple health care problems. Much of the research for these three therapies has been done by non-nurse researchers, but the findings provide direction to nurses in selecting and implementing therapies.

Journaling (Chapter 12) and storytelling (Chapter 13) are therapies in which less formal research has been conducted. It is interesting to contrast these two therapies—with journaling being more accepted by people whose culture has a written history—while storytelling has a greater appeal to oral cultures. Research on animal-assisted therapies (Chapter 14) is increasing. Animal-assisted therapy has found a niche in care centers and living facilities for elders, hospitals, and other settings. Although many think of dogs and cats as the animals used in animal-assisted therapy, horses, dolphins, fish, birds, and other creatures are also used.

Of particular help in determining the impact of mind–body–spirit therapies on physical, mental, and spiritual well-being has been the development of instruments not only to measure the outcomes of specific therapies, but also to demonstrate the areas of the brain that might be involved. A growing number of researchers are also examining holistic effects of these therapies on outcomes such as resilience, satisfaction with care, and improvement of quality of life. However, as could be said for many complementary therapies, more research needs to be done, especially with populations for whom specific therapies hold promise.

Many of the therapies in this category such as imagery, music, prayer, humor, journaling, and meditation have been and continue to be a part of nursing's armamentarium of interventions. A number of therapies in this group, such as yoga and journaling, are commonly used by nurses in their self-care.

The integration of mind–body–spirit is an integral part of many healing practices in many non-Western and indigenous health care systems. The spirit realm characterizes many healing practices in Native American tribes/nations. Thus, nurses need to be attentive to therapies that are not discussed in this section of the book but are an integral part of the health care of people from other cultures who may be receiving care in Western health care facilities.

REFERENCES

Clarke, T., Black, L., Stussman, B., Barnes, P., & Nahin, R. (2015, February 10). Trends in the use of complementary health approaches among adults: United States, 2002-2012. *National Health Statistics Reports, 79*, 1–16.

National Center for Complementary and Integrative Health. (2016). *NCCIH facts-at-a-glance and mission*. Retrieved from https://nccih.nih.gov/about/ataglance

Imagery

MAURA FITZGERALD AND MARY LANGEVIN

Imagery is a mind–body intervention that uses the power of the imagination to bring about change in physical, emotional, or spiritual dimensions. Throughout our daily lives, we constantly see images, feel sensations, and register impressions. A picture of lemonade makes our mouths water; a song makes us happy or sad; a smell takes us back to a past moment. Images evoke physical and emotional responses and help us understand the meaning of events.

Imagery is commonly used in healthcare—most often in the form of guided imagery, clinical hypnosis, or self-hypnosis. In the mid-1950s, the American Medical Association and the American Psychiatric Association recognized hypnosis as a therapeutic tool. Nurses, physicians, psychologists, and others use it with adults and children for the treatment of acute and chronic illness, relief of symptoms, and enhancement of wellness. Imagery is a hallmark of stress-management programs and has become a standard therapy for alleviating anxiety, promoting relaxation, improving coping and functional status, gaining psychological insight, and even making progress on a chosen spiritual path.

DEFINITION

Imagery is the formation of a mental representation of an object, place, event, or situation that is perceived through the senses. It is a cognitive behavioral strategy that uses the individual's own imagination and mental processing and can be practiced as an independent activity or guided by a professional. Imagery uses all the senses—visual, aural, tactile, olfactory, proprioceptive, and kinesthetic. Although imagery is often referred to as *visualization*, it includes imagining through any sense and is not just being able to see something in the mind's eye.

Van Kuiken (2004) describes four types of guided imagery: pleasant, physiologically focused, mental rehearsal or reframing, and receptive imagery. While inducing imagery, the individual often imagines seeing, hearing, smelling, tasting, and/or touching something in the image. The image used can be active or passive (playing volleyball vs. lying on the beach). Although for many participants physical and mental relaxation tend to facilitate imagery, this is not necessary—particularly for children, who often do not need to be in a relaxed state. Imagery may be receptive or active. In receptive imagery, the individual pays attention to an area of the body or a symptom and mentally explores thoughts or feelings that arise. In active imagery, the individual evokes thoughts or ideas. Active imagery can be outcome or end-state oriented, in which the individual envisions a goal, such as being healthy and well; or it can be process oriented, in which the mechanism of the desired effect is imagined, such as envisioning a strong immune system fighting a viral infection or tumor.

Imagery and clinical hypnosis are closely related. Clinical hypnosis is a strategy in which a professional guides the participant into an altered state of deep relaxation, and suggestions for changes in subjective experience and alterations in perception are made. Both hypnosis and guided imagery incorporate the use of relaxation techniques, such as diaphragmatic breathing or progressive muscle relaxation, to help the participant focus the attention. In hypnosis, this is referred to as an *induction*. Guided imagery is often used within the context of hypnosis to further deepen the state of relaxation, and in both techniques, suggestions for positive growth, change, or improvement are often made. Because of the close association between these two processes, selected studies on hypnosis are discussed in this chapter.

SCIENTIFIC BASIS

Imagery can be understood as an activity that generates physiologic and somatic responses. It is based on the cognitive process known as *mental imagery*, which is a central element of cognition that operates when mental representations are created in the absence of sensory input. Functional MRI (fMRI) has demonstrated that the mental construction of an image activates the same neural pathways and central nervous system structures that are engaged when an individual is using one or more of the senses (Djordjevic, Zatorre, Petrides, Boyle, & Jones-Gotaman, 2005; D. J. Kraemer, Macrae, Green, & Kelley, 2005). For example, if an individual is imagining hearing a sound, the brain structures associated with hearing become activated. Mental rehearsal of movements activates motor areas and can be incorporated into stroke rehabilitation and sports-improvement programs (Braun, Beurskens, Borm, Schack, & Wade, 2006; Schuster et al., 2011).

Andrasik and Rime (2007) postulated that cognitive tasks, such as mental imagery, can be conceptualized as neuromodulators. *Neuromodulation* is generally defined as the interaction between the nervous system and electrical or pharmacological agents that block or disrupt the perception of pain. By distraction, imagery alters processing in the central, peripheral, and autonomic nervous systems. The perception of a symptom such as pain or nausea is reduced or eliminated.

A key mechanism by which imagery modifies disease and reduces symptoms is thought to be by reducing the stress response, which is triggered when a situation or event (perceived or real) threatens physical or emotional well-being or when the demands of the situation exceed available resources. It activates complex interactions between the neuroendocrine system and the immune system. Emotional responses to situations trigger the limbic system and signal physiologic changes in the peripheral and autonomic nervous systems, resulting in the characteristic fight-or-flight stress response. Over time, chronic stress results in adrenal and immune suppression and may be most harmful to cellular immune function, impairing the ability to ward off viruses and tumor cells (Pert, Dreher, & Ruff, 1998).

The complexity of the human response to stress is best understood through psychoneuroimmunology (PNI), an interdisciplinary field of study that explains the mechanisms by which the brain and body communicate through cellular interactions. Early work was based on rat-model research by Robert Ader and Nicholas Cohen, which confirmed that the immune system could be conditioned by expectations and beliefs (Ader & Cohen, 1981; Ader, Felten, & Cohen, 1991; Fleshner & Laudenslager, 2004). Subsequent research focused on the mechanisms of brain and body communication through cellular interactions, and identified receptors for neuropeptides, neurohormones, and cytokines that reside on neural and immune cells and induce biochemical changes when activated by neurotransmitters.

A cascade of signaling events in response to perceived or actual stress results in the release of hormones from the hypothalamus, pituitary gland, adrenal medulla, adrenal cortex, and peripheral sympathetic nerve terminals. Psychosocial and physical stressors have the potential to upregulate this hypothalamic–pituitary–adrenal (HPA) axis. Chronic hyperactivation of the HPA axis and sympathetic nervous system with the associated increased levels of cortisol and catecholamines can deregulate immune function, whereas moderate levels of circulating cortisol may enhance immune function (Langley, Fonseca, & Iphofen, 2006). Cytokines are secreted by cells participating in the immune response and act as messengers between the immune system and the brain (McCance & Huether, 2002). They also function as neurotransmitters, crossing the blood–brain barrier and affecting sensory neurons. Through these channels, cytokines induce symptoms of fever, increased sensitivity to pain, anorexia, and fatigue, which are adaptive responses that may facilitate recovery and healing (Langley et al., 2006). These interactions between the brain and the immune system are bidirectional, and changes in one system influence the others. The stress response can therefore enhance or suppress optimal immunity (Fleshner & Laudenslager, 2004).

Although immune responses to emotional states are extremely complex, acute stress activates cardiac sympathetic activity and increases plasma catecholamines and natural killer (NK) cell activity, whereas chronic stress (inescapable or unpredictable stress) is associated with suppression of NK cells and interleukin-1-beta and other proinflammatory cytokines (Glaser et al., 2001). These effects appear to be mediated by the influence of stress hormones on T helper components (Th1 and Th2; Segerstrom, 2010). Imagery, by inducing deep relaxation and reprocessing of stressful triggers, interrupts or alters the stress response and supports the immune system. In a review of guided-imagery studies examining immune system function, Trakhtenberg (2008) concluded that there is evidence to support a relationship between the immune system and stress or relaxation.

The degree of response to stress varies according to many factors, including the nature of the stressor, its magnitude and duration, and a person's degree of control over it (Costa-Pinto & Palermo-Neto, 2010). Individuals who have strong physiological responses to everyday stressors have high stress reactivity and are at greater risk for disease susceptibility, even when coping, performance, and perceived stress are comparable. One of the goals of imagery is to reduce stress reactivity by reframing stressful situations from negative responses of fear and anxiety to positive images of healing and well-being (Kosslyn, Ganis, & Thompson, 2001). Donaldson (2000) proposed that thoughts produce physiological responses and activate appropriate neurons. Using imagery to increase emotional awareness and restructure the meaning of a remembered situation by changing negative responses to positive images and meaning alters the physiological response and improves outcomes.

INTERVENTION

Techniques and Guidelines

Imagery has been used extensively in children, adolescents, and adults. Children as young as 4 years old, who have language skills adequate for understanding suggestions, can benefit from imagery (Kohen & Olness, 2011). Young children often are better at imagery because of the natural, active use of their imaginations. Imagery may be practiced independently, with a coach or teacher, or with a DVD, CD, or smartphone app. The most effective imagery intervention is one that is specific to individuals' personalities, their preferences for relaxation and specific settings, their age or developmental stage, and the desired outcomes. The steps of a general imagery session are outlined in Exhibit 6.1.

Exhibit 6.1. General Guided-Imagery Technique

1. Achieving a relaxed state
   a. Find a comfortable sitting or reclining position.
   b. Uncross any extremities.
   c. Close your eyes or focus on one spot or object in the room.
   d. Focus on breathing with your abdominal muscles—being aware of the breath as it enters through your nose and leaves through your mouth. With your next breath let the exhalation be longer and notice how the inhalation that follows is deeper. And as you notice that, let your body become even more relaxed. Continue to breathe deeply; if it is comfortable, gradually let the exhalation become twice as long as the inhalation.
   e. If your thoughts roam, bring your mind back to thinking about your breathing and your relaxed body.
2. Specific suggestions for imagery
   a. Picture a place you enjoy and where you feel good.
   b. Notice what you see, hear, taste, smell, and feel.
   c. Let yourself enjoy being in this place.
   d. Imagine yourself the way you want to be (describe the desired goal specifically).
   e. Imagine what steps you will need to take to be the way you want to be.
   f. Practice these steps now—in this place where you feel good.
   g. What is the first thing you are doing to help you be the way you want to be?
   h. What will you do next?
   i. When you reach your goal of the way you want to be, notice how you feel.
3. Summarizing process and reinforce practice
   a. Remember that you can return to this place, this feeling, and this way of being anytime you want.

(continued)

> **b.** Allow yourself to feel this way again by focusing on your breathing, relaxing, and imagining yourself in your special place.
> **c.** Come back to this place and envision yourself the way you want to be every day.
> **4.** Returning to present
>   **a.** Be aware again of the favorite place.
>   **b.** Bring your focus back to your breathing.
>   **c.** Become aware of the room you are in (drawing attention to the temperature, sounds, or lights).
>   **d.** Let yourself feel relaxed and refreshed and be ready to resume your activities.
>   **e.** Open your eyes when you are ready.

Imagery sessions for adults and adolescents are usually 10 to 30 minutes in length, whereas most children tolerate 5 to 15 minutes. The session typically begins with a relaxation exercise that enables the participant to focus or "center." A technique that works well both for children and adults is engaging in slow and expansive breathing, which facilitates relaxation as the breath moves lower into the chest and the diaphragm, while the abdominal muscles begin to be used more than the upper chest muscles. Other techniques include progressive muscle relaxation or focusing on a word or object. Some children may use their bodies to demonstrate or respond to their image. Although most participants close their eyes, some, especially young children, will prefer to keep their eyes open.

Once the participant is in a relaxed or "altered" state, the practitioner suggests an image of a relaxing, peaceful, or comforting place or introduces an image suggested by the client. Scenes commonly used to induce relaxation include watching a sunset or clouds, sitting on a warm beach or by a fire, or floating through water or space. Some participants, particularly young children, may prefer active images that involve motion, such as flying or playing a sport. The scene used is one that the client finds relaxing or engaging. It is often introduced as a favorite place. Huth, Van Kuiken, and Broome (2006) interviewed children who were participants in a guided-imagery research study, to determine the content of their imagery. The children reported their favorite images as the park, swimming at a beach, amusement parks, and vacationing. They also visualized a variety of familiar places, such as sports events and places that included pets and other animals.

Although mental relaxation is often accompanied by muscle relaxation, this is not always a goal. Participants of any age, but particularly preschool and school-age children, may imagine in an active state. For example, a group of 9- to 12-year-old boys with sickle cell disease were being taught guided imagery as a pain-control technique. When asked what special place they would like to go to, they requested a trip to a local amusement park and a ride on the roller coaster. During the imagery, many of them were physically and vocally active, swaying from side to side and moving their arms up and down. At the end of the visualization, they all reported feeling like they had been in the park (absorption) and gave examples of things they felt, saw, heard, or smelled.

For directed imagery, the practitioner guides the imagery, using positive suggestions to alleviate specific symptoms or conditions (outcome or end-state imagery) or to rehearse or walk through an event (process imagery). Images do not need to be anatomically correct or vivid. Symbolic images may be the most powerful healing images because they are drawn from individual beliefs, culture, and meaning. A cancer patient might imagine sweeping cancer cells away or an individual with pain might imagine a pain-control center with a dial to turn the pain down.

The ability to use guided imagery is related to the individual's hypnotic ability or the ability to enter an altered state of consciousness and to become involved or absorbed in the imagery (Kwekkeboom, Wanta, & Bumpus, 2008). Studies have demonstrated that responsiveness to hypnosis increases through early childhood, peaking somewhere between ages 7 and 14 and then leveling off into adolescence and adulthood. However, clinicians have argued that in clinical settings, in which techniques are adjusted to the child's development, preschool children and younger can be quite responsive to hypnosis (Kohen & Olness, 2011).

Some individuals have naturally high hypnotic abilities; they recall pictures more accurately, generate more complex images, have higher dream-recall frequency in the waking state, and make fewer eye movements in imagery than poor visualizers. However, most individuals can use imagery if the experience is adjusted to their needs and preferences (Carli, Cavallaro, & Santarcangelo, 2007; Olness, 2008). Recognizing individual, cultural, and developmental preferences for settings, situations, and preference for either relaxation or stimulation can improve the effectiveness of the imagery and reduce time and frustration with learning it. Practicing imagery oneself is extremely helpful in guiding others.

Measurement of Outcomes

Evaluating and measuring outcomes are important in determining the effectiveness and value of imagery in clinical practice. The clinical outcomes of imagery are related to the context in which it is used and include physical signs of relaxation; lower levels of anxiety and depression; alteration in symptoms; improved functional performance or quality of life; a sense of meaning, purpose, and/or competency; and positive changes in attitude or behavior. Health services benefits may include reduced costs, morbidity, and length of hospital stay.

The outcomes measured should reflect the client's situation and the conceptual framework providing the rationale for the use of imagery. If imagery is used to facilitate rehabilitation or performance, outcomes would include functional measures such as improved gait or ability to perform a specific task. If imagery is used to control symptoms in clients undergoing chemotherapy for cancer, expected outcomes might include reduced nausea, vomiting, and fatigue; enhanced body image; positive mood states; and improved quality of life. When imagery is used to reduce the stress response and promote relaxation, outcomes may include increased oxygen saturation levels, lower blood pressure and heart rate, warmer extremities, reduced muscle tension, greater alpha waves on electroencephalography, and lower anxiety.

Factors that may influence imagery's success include dose (e.g., duration and frequency of session), client characteristics, and condition being treated. Great variability exists in how frequently imagery is recommended. In an attempt to quantify this effect, Van Kuiken (2004) conducted a meta-analysis of 16 published studies going back to 1996. Although the final sample of 10 studies was too small for statistical analysis, Van Kuiken concluded that imagery practice for up to 18 weeks increases the effectiveness of the intervention. A minimum dose was not determined and further study is needed to explore a dose relationship with outcomes. To help with standardization of imagery interventions and generalizability, documentation should include a detailed description of the specific interventions used, outcomes affected by the imagery, and factors influencing effectiveness.

Individual differences such as imaging ability, outcome expectancy, preferred coping style, relationship with the imagery practitioner, and disease state may all affect the outcome of an imagery experience. In a crossover-design pilot study comparing progressive muscle relaxation therapy (PMRT) and imagery to a control, the combined intervention groups demonstrated improved pain control (Kwekkeboom, Wanta, & Bumpus, 2008). However, the individual responder analysis revealed that subjects did not respond equally to each therapy and that only half of participants had reduced pain from each intervention. Imagery sessions were more likely to have positive results when participants had greater imaging ability, positive outcome expectancy, and fewer symptoms. A study of 323 adult medical patients who received six interactive guided-imagery sessions with a focus on gaining insight and self-awareness demonstrated that participants' ability to engage in the guided-imagery process and the relationship with the practitioner were strong influences on outcome (Scherwitz, McHenry, & Herrero, 2005).

One of the most difficult determinations to make is whether the outcomes are the result solely of imagery or of a combination of factors. Learning and practicing imagery often change other health-related behaviors, such as getting more sleep, eating a healthier diet, stopping smoking, or exercising regularly. The therapist's presence, attention, and compassion also may constitute an intervention independent of the imagery process.

Technology

Technology can be used to make imagery more accessible and available. This can take the form of telemedicine sessions (Freeman et al., 2015), technology tools such as biofeedback to enhance imagery sessions and skill development (Yijing, Xiaoping, Fang, Xiaolu, & Bin, 2015), CDs or videos, smartphone apps that provide imagery sessions or reminders (Hansen, 2015; Meinlschmidt et al., 2016), and online training for healthcare providers (Kemper & Khirallah, 2015; Rao & Kemper, 2017). Freeman et al. (2015) demonstrated a successful telemedicine delivery of imagery-based behavioral interventions to community groups of breast cancer survivors, achieving improvement outcomes. This is a promising technology for rural areas where clients need to travel long distances for services or for clients who have difficulty with transportation. The advent of the smartphone has opened a range of options, including applications that provide background sounds to enhance an imagery session (nature sounds or music), audio of various types of guided-imagery and relaxation sessions, and reminders to do a relaxation or imagery technique. Studies have demonstrated the feasibility of providing audio relaxation using smartphone technology (Hansen, 2015) and using smartphones to send a hyperlink for access to a cognitive intervention the participant can do at a convenient time (Meinlschmidt et al., 2016).

PRECAUTIONS

Imagery is generally a safe intervention, as noted in a systematic review of guided imagery for cancer, in which there were no reports of adverse events or side effects

(Roffe, Schmidt, & Ernst, 2005). However, occasionally a participant reacts negatively to relaxation or to the imagery. Subjects may experience anxiety, particularly when using imagery to reduce stress. Huth, Broome, and Good (2004) reported that two children became distressed during guided-imagery practice sessions; hence, the authors encourage prescreening. Some individuals have anecdotally reported increased discomfort, airway constriction, or difficulty breathing when they focus on diaphragmatic breathing. This is most likely to occur if the participant is experiencing a symptom such as abdominal pain or dyspnea. Using another centering method, such as focusing on an object in the room or repeating a mantra, can reduce this distressing response and still induce relaxation. Some participants may report feeling out of control or "spacey" when deeply relaxed. The guide can help participants become more grounded by focusing on an image such as a tree with strong roots or doing a more alert relaxation such as having the client keep eyes open and focus on an object. Participants may report dizziness that is often related to mild hyperventilation and can be relieved by encouraging them to breathe slower and less deeply.

The expertise and training of the nurse should guide judgment in using imagery to achieve outcomes in practice. Imagery techniques can be easily applied to managing symptoms (e.g., pain, nausea, vomiting) and facilitating relaxation, sleep, or anxiety reduction (see Sidebar 6.1). Advanced techniques often associated with hypnosis—such as age regression and management of depression, anxiety, or post-traumatic stress disorder—require further training.

SIDEBAR 6.1. USE OF GUIDED IMAGERY IN A PEDIATRIC ONCOLOGY CLINIC

Elizabeth McDonough, United States

A young 8-year-old girl with sickle cell anemia came to our clinic needing a transfusion. She was familiar with our clinic and the staff. She was sitting in the bed with the head up. When I began talking of the need to place intravenous access, the girl became very frightened and started climbing up the back of the bed and crying. We did not have topical numbing cream available at that time.

I suggested the girl come back to sitting in the bed and began to talk with her about ways she could help her body and mind relax. I helped her calm with breathing techniques, which helped some. I asked her if there was a place she would like to go to in her mind. She was agreeable to try this and wanted to imagine she was at school because she liked school. Her parents were present throughout the process.

My guiding script involved bringing her to the classroom, encouraging her to "smell the smells of the room; listen to the sounds of your classmates and the noise of the room; see the desks where your classmates are sitting; what projects are you doing?" I repeated this image several times as she became quiet, her eyes closed and breathing calmly.

I proceeded to get my IV supplies ready and inserted the needle as she rested calmly. She did not move her arm as I inserted the needle and taped it into place. The family and child were pleased with the process.

USES

Imagery has been used therapeutically in a variety of conditions and populations (see Exhibit 6.2). Pain and cancer are two conditions in which imagery has been helpful both in adults and in children.

Exhibit 6.2. Conditions for Which Imagery Has Been Tested

Clinical Condition	Selected Sources
In children and adolescents	
Abdominal pain	Ball, Shapiro, Monheim, and Weydert (2003); Cotton et al. (2010); Galili, Shaoul, and Mogilner (2009); Gottsegen (2011); Gulewitsch, Müller, Hautzinger, and Schlarb (2013); Vlieger, Blink, Tromp, and Benninga (2008); Weydert et al. (2006)
Cancer	Richardson, Smith, McCall, and Pilkington (2006); Tsitsi, Charalambous, Papastavrou, and Raftopoulos (2017)
Headache	Fichtel and Larsson (2004)
Hospice care	Russell, Smart, and House (2007)
Pain	Culbert, Friedrichsdorf, and Kuttner (2008); Kline et al. (2010); Wood and Bioy (2008)
Perioperative symptom management (pain, nausea, anxiety, behavioral disorders)	Calipel, Lucas-Polomeni, Wodey, and Ecoffey (2005); Kuttner (2012); Mackenzie and Frawley (2007); Polkki, Pietila, Vehvilainen-Julkunen, Laukkala, and Kiviluoma (2008)
Post-traumatic stress disorder	Gordon, Staples, Blyta, Bytyqi, and Wilson (2008)
Pregnancy and stress	Flynn, Jones, and Ausderau (2016)
Procedural pain	Alexander (2012); Cyna, Tomkins, Maddock, and Barker (2007); Forsner, Norström, Nordyke, Ivarsson, and Lindh (2014); Nilsson, Forsner, Finnström, and Mörelius (2015); Uman, Chambers, McGrath, and Kisely (2008)
Psychiatry	Anbar (2008)
Sickle cell anemia	C. Dobson (2015); C. E. Dobson and Byrne (2014)
Spinal fusion	Charette et al. (2015)
In adults	
Asthma	Lahmann et al. (2009)
Autoimmune disorders	Collins and Dunn (2005); Torem (2007)

(continued)

Clinical Condition	Selected Sources
Cancer treatment—physical and emotional side effects	Charalambous, Giannakopoulou, Bozas, and Paikousis (2015); Chen, Wang, Yang, and Chung (2015); Leon-Pizarro et al. (2007); Roffe et al. (2005)
Depression	Chou and Lin (2006)
Fibromyalgia	Menzies and Kim (2008); Menzies, Lyon, Elswick, McCain, and Gray (2014); Menzies, Taylor, and Bourguignon (2006); Onieva-Zafra, Garcia, and del Valle (2015); Verkaik et al. (2014); Zech, Hansen, Bernardy, and Häuser (2017)
Health and well-being (including stress management)	Beck, Hansen, and Gold (2015); Boehm and Tse (2013); Cardeña, Svensson, and Hejdström (2013); Greene and Greene (2012); Kraemer, Luberto, O'Bryan, Mysinger, and Corton (2016); Watanabe, Fukuda, Hara, Maeda, and Ohira (2006)
Immune response in breast cancer	Lengacher et al. (2008); Nunes et al. (2007)
Medical conditions (general)	Elkins, Johnson, Fisher, and Sliwinski (2013); Kwekkeboom and Bratzke (2016); Peerdeman et al. (2015); Scherwitz et al. (2005); Spiva et al. (2015)
Osteoarthritis	Baird and Sands (2006); Giacobbi et al. (2015)
Pain—abdominal	Boltin et al. (2015); Lindfors et al. (2012); Mizrahi et al. (2012); Palsson and van Tilburg (2015)
Pain—cancer	Kwekkeboom, Wanta, and Bumpus (2008); Kwekkeboom, Hau, Wanta, and Bumpus (2008)
Pain—chronic	Carrico, Peters, and Diokno (2008); Lewandowski, Good, and Draucker (2005); Posadzki, Lewandowski, Terry, Ernst, and Stearns (2012); Proctor, Murphy, Pattison, Suckling, and Farquhar (2008); Turk, Swanson, and Tunks (2008)
Pain—phantom limb	Beaumont, Mercier, Michon, Malouin, and Jackson (2011); Brunelli et al. (2015); MacIver, Lloyd, Kelly, Roberts, and Nurmikko (2008)
Pain—procedural	Alam et al. (2016); Armstrong, Dixon, May, and Patricolo (2014); Flory, Salazar, and Lang (2007); Shenefelt (2013)
Perioperative	Draucker, Jacobson, Umberger, Myerscough, and Sanata (2015); Jacobson et al. (2016); Nelson et al. (2013); Sears, Bolton, and Bell (2013)

(continued)

Clinical Condition	Selected Sources
Pregnancy	Chuang, Liu, Chen, and Lin (2015); DiPietro, Costigan, Nelson, Gurewitsch, and Laudenslager (2008); Jallo, Cozens, Smith, and Simpson (2013); Jallo, Ruiz, Elswick, and French (2014)
Rehabilitation	Braun, Wade, and Beurskens (2011); Dunsky, Dickstein, Marcovitz, Levy, and Deutsch (2008); Hovington and Brouwer (2010); Kim, Oh, Kim, and Choi (2011)
Sleep	Casida et al. (2012); Krakow and Zadra (2006); Lam et al. (2015); Loft and Cameron (2013); Schaffer et al. (2013)
Sports medicine	Driediger, Hall, and Callow (2006); Schuster et al. (2011)

Pain

Pain is a uniquely subjective experience, and proper management depends on individualizing interventions that recognize determinants affecting the pain response. Age, temperament, gender, ethnicity, and stage of development are all considerations when developing a pain-management plan (Gerik, 2005; Young, 2005). Whether pain is from illness, side effects of treatment, injury, or physical stress on the body, emotional factors contribute to pain perception, and mind–body interventions such as imagery can help make pain more manageable (Reed, 2007). Stress, anxiety, and fatigue decrease the threshold for pain, making the perceived pain more intense. Imagery can break this cycle of pain–tension–anxiety–pain. Relaxation with imagery decreases pain directly by reducing muscle tension and related spasms and indirectly by lowering anxiety and improving sleep. Imagery also is a distraction strategy; vivid, detailed images using all senses tend to work well for pain control. In addition, cognitive reappraisal/restructuring used with imagery can increase a sense of control over the ability to reframe the meaning of pain.

There is a considerable body of research examining the efficacy of guided imagery as a therapy to treat pain in adults. Studies have explored the effectiveness of guided imagery in treating cancer pain (Kwekkeboom, Wanta, & Bumpus, 2008), dysmenorrhea (Proctor et al., 2008), orthopedic pain (Charette et al., 2015; Draucker et al., 2015; Jacobson et al., 2016), interstitial cystitis (Carrico et al., 2008), and fibromyalgia (FM; Menzies et al., 2006; Menzies & Kim, 2008). Results have been variable but favorable enough to indicate that guided imagery might help relieve some forms of pain, especially when used as an adjunct to standard care measures. Subjects report positive and negative experience with guided-imagery interventions. Subjects who find guided imagery useful describe it as enjoyable, relaxing, or interesting, whereas subjects who reported negative experiences describe it as unrealistic or annoying (Draucker et al., 2015). Subjects have reported increased sense of self-efficacy (Menzies et al., 2014).

There are many causes of chronic pain, but whatever the underlying etiology, it is generally challenging and costly to treat and has an impact on many aspects of an individual's life. Analgesic therapy often falls short of achieving adequate pain relief, and successful management frequently depends on the use of cognitive behavioral techniques such as imagery (Turk et al., 2008). Two conditions leading to chronic pain in adults are osteoarthritis and FM. In a randomized trial of 28 women with osteoarthritis, participants received either standard care or a 12-week program of guided imagery with relaxation (Baird & Sands, 2006). In the intervention group, scores of health-related quality of life improved. Analysis noted that improvement in scores was not completely explained by improved mobility and pain reduction and that the guided-imagery and relaxation intervention might have had a positive effect on social and emotional functioning.

FM is a condition of chronic widespread pain accompanied by fatigue, disturbed sleep, stiffness, and depression (Menzies & Kim, 2008). The etiology of FM is unknown; however, recent studies have identified abnormal sensory and pain processing as a factor (Verkaik et al., 2014). Guided imagery and hypnosis have both been studied for pain and symptom management in FM, and Menzies and colleagues have done a series of investigations on the effect of guided imagery on FM symptoms (Menzies et al., 2006; Menzies & Kim, 2008; Menzies et al., 2014). In a randomized control trial of 72 female subjects with FM, subjects were randomized into usual care or usual care plus guided imagery (Menzies et al., 2014). The intervention group received CDs with a 20-minute guided-imagery audiotrack and were instructed to use them daily and compared with a usual-care control group. There was improvement in self-efficacy for managing other symptoms, perceived stress and levels of fatigue, pain severity, and depression in the intervention group. There was no difference in biomarkers (C-reactive protein, cytokine). Onieva-Zafra et al. (2015) found improvement in pain relief in a guided-imagery group over a control group; however, Verkaik et al. (2014) found no differences in pain, self-efficacy, or functional status between groups. Two systematic reviews endorse the use of guided imagery for FM but note that the evidence is not of high quality and that studies use a variety of techniques, treatment types (audiotapes, group sessions), number of sessions, and outcomes measured, making it difficult to compare studies (Meeus et al., 2015; Zech et al., 2016).

In spite of the many advances made in the treatment of pediatric pain, the American Academy of Pediatrics and the American Pain Society (2001) reported that children's pain continues to be inadequately assessed and managed. They recommended a multimodal approach to pain management to include both pharmacological and nonpharmacological interventions. Mind–body therapies, including guided imagery, are noted to be safe and effective for children and adolescents (American Academy of Pediatrics Section on Integrative Medicine, 2016).

There are adverse short-term and long-term effects of inadequate pain management in children, including hypoxemia, immobility, altered pulmonary function, post-traumatic stress, and adverse psychological and behavioral patterns (Grunau, Oberlander, & Whitfield, 2001). Distraction imagery is particularly helpful in getting a child through a medical procedure with a safe and effective level of sedation/analgesia and as little movement as possible (Butler, Symons, Henderson, Shortliffe, & Spiegel, 2005). Suggestions to breathe deeply and to relax or be comfortable are combined with vivid images of a favorite place or pleasant experience that draw the attention away from the pain. It is best to introduce the child to breathing techniques and explore favorite images prior to the procedure. However, in critical or emergency situations, imagery has been successfully used without prework (Kohen, 2000). In a randomized study of 44 children from 4 to 15 years of age undergoing voiding cystourethrography, children who were taught self-hypnotic visual imagery before the procedure were compared with controls who received routine care. Results indicated benefits for the intervention group in the form of parental perception of decreased trauma, decreased observational ratings of distress, increased ease of procedure by physician report, and decreased time to complete the procedure (Butler et al., 2005). In a systemic review of controlled trials of interventions for needle-related procedural pain and distress distraction, combined cognitive behavioral interventions and hypnosis showed the most promise (Uman et al., 2008); however, two studies using imagery for venipuncture and vaccination in older children (11–12 years old) found no difference between imagery and standard care groups (Forsner et al., 2014; Nilsson et al., 2015).

Chronic pain in childhood can be challenging to treat and has significant impact on the child's quality of life and engagement in school and social activities. Common chronic pain conditions in childhood are musculoskeletal pain, headaches, and abdominal pain (American Pain Society, 2012). Weydert et al. (2006) assessed the efficacy of imagery and relaxation on abdominal pain. In a randomized trial, a guided-imagery group was compared with a control group taught breathing exercises only. The imagery group had significantly fewer days with pain at 1 and 2 months. In addition, children in the imagery group had fewer than four pain episodes a month and did not miss any activities because of pain. No adverse effects were reported. Another study assigned children with functional abdominal pain and irritable bowel syndrome (and their parents) to a hypnotherapeutic behavioral treatment or wait-list control. The intervention consisted of group sessions in which the participants learned about stress and were taught hypnotic techniques (relaxation, imagery, and suggestions directed at increased wellness and managing pain). Children in the treatment group reported significantly greater reduction in pain scores and pain-related disability (Gulewitsch et al., 2013).

Huth et al. (2004) examined the use of guided imagery as an adjunct to routine analgesics for postoperative tonsillectomy and/or adenoidectomy pain. Significantly less pain was found in the treatment group 1 to 4 hours after surgery but not at 22 to 24 hours after surgery. Children in the imagery group had 28% less sensory pain, 10% less anxiety, and 8% less affective pain than children in the control group. A correlation between state of anxiety and sensory pain was high at both points, and there were no differences in analgesic use between groups. The researchers reported two adverse events in which children became distressed during practice sessions.

Cancer Treatment

Imagery interventions in oncology have focused on physiological and psychological responses to cancer treatment. Guided-imagery research over the past few years has developed to include more randomized clinical trials and larger sample sizes. Areas that have been researched are efficacy in management of symptoms (e.g., pain, nausea), influence on surgical outcomes, improvement in quality of life, and changes in immunity (Roffe et al., 2005). Roffe et al., in a systematic literature search that spanned three decades, uncovered 103 articles investigating guided imagery in cancer care. Of these, 27 were case studies, 56 combined imagery with another treatment (e.g., PMRT, music therapy, hypnosis), 12 were uncontrolled trials, and two were nonrandomized. The authors reviewed in detail six randomized control trials. The collective data suggested that guided imagery is most beneficial on psychosocial and quality-of-life indicators. No effects were found on physical symptoms, which may be partially explained by a paucity of distressing symptoms in the subjects. When guided imagery was compared with other relaxation strategies, all study arms did better than the control, indicating that other relaxation strategies are also beneficial or that there is significant overlap among strategies.

Patients receiving chemotherapy often experience side effects that affect their quality of life. These side effects are often experienced in a cluster that includes nausea, vomiting, fatigue, anxiety, and depression. Studies of imagery have focused on reduction of these symptoms. In clinical cancer care, relaxation strategies such as PMRT are often paired with imagery. This combination has been investigated in a number of studies. In a randomized controlled trial of 60 women undergoing chemotherapy treatment for breast cancer, guided imagery was paired with PMRT to determine their effect on nausea, vomiting, and quality of life (Yoo, Ahn, Kim, Kim, & Han, 2005). Patients in the intervention group demonstrated improvement in anticipatory nausea, postchemotherapy nausea, and quality of life. Positive treatment effects on quality of life were present at 3 and 6 months post-therapy. Similarly, Leon-Pizarro et al. (2007) conducted a randomized controlled trial of 66 gynecologic and breast cancer patients who were undergoing brachytherapy. The intervention group had a 10-minute training period in relaxation and guided imagery and an individualized cassette for home use; the control group received standard care. The treatment group had statistically significant reductions in anxiety, depression, and body discomfort. A study by Charalambous et al. (2016) explored the effectiveness of guided imagery combined with PMRT on this cluster of side effects in a randomized control trial. Patients in the intervention group experienced less fatigue, better quality of life, and less nausea and vomiting. There was also more depression in the control group compared to the intervention group.

Guided imagery is a recognized intervention for women receiving treatment for breast cancer. Serra et al. (2012) studied the effect of a guided-imagery intervention during radiation therapy. A convenience sample of 61 women received a guided-imagery session in the radiation oncology setting immediately before their radiation treatment. Physiological and psychological measurements were evaluated. There was a statistically significant improvement in pulse rate, respiratory rate, and blood pressure between the first and second sessions. There was also a rise in skin temperature, indicating increased peripheral blood flow and decreased sympathetic response. The guided-imagery intervention was determined to be helpful by 86% of the participants.

Quality of life for breast cancer survivors is of concern, especially for women with limited access to psychosocial interventions. A recent study by Freeman et al. (2015), conducted in Alaska, compared in-person group sessions, telemedicine delivery group sessions, and a wait-list as a control group. The intervention group sessions included education on mind–body connections, including mental imagery and sensory experiences. Both the in-person group and the telemedicine group experienced significant changes in cognitive function, sleep disturbance, and quality of life. This research invites new methods for delivering guided-imagery interventions for women with breast cancer who have limited abilities to attend in-person sessions.

A randomized controlled trial conducted in Cyprus in 2015 included subjects with breast cancer and prostate cancer. A total of 236 patients were randomized to receive either a combined guided-imagery and PMRT intervention, which included both supervised and unsupervised sessions, or standard care with computer-based education about their specific cancer. Measurement included anxiety and depression scales and saliva biomarkers. Results included significant decreases in anxiety and depression scores in the intervention group (Charalambous et al., 2015).

In pediatric oncology, the focus of research has largely been on procedural pain and on the use of hypnosis. A review of seven randomized controlled trials and one nonrandomized controlled clinical trial (Richardson et al., 2006) reported reductions in pain and anxiety for hypnosis in pediatric oncology patients undergoing procedures (e.g., bone marrow aspiration, lumbar puncture, venipuncture). Both this review and a previous one (Wild & Espie, 2004) cited methodological limitations, including small, underpowered samples; lack of reporting on the method of randomization; concealment of allocation and/or blinding; lack of information on standard care; and wide variation in procedures used.

Childhood malignancy has a profound effect on the whole family, including parents. A randomized control trial by Tsitsi et al. (2017) explored guided imagery combined with PMRT as an intervention during their child's treatment aimed at reducing parental anxiety and improving mood. Several measurement tools were used. The results supported a statistically significant decrease in tension in the intervention group. Parents in the intervention group also were less sad and had decreased anxiety compared with the control group.

The role of imagery in improving cancer outcomes has been studied for more than two decades. It continues to be difficult to identify the significance of imagery in long-term cancer survival when so many related factors must be considered. Sahler, Hunter, and Liesveld (2003) showed reduced time to engraftment in 23 patients undergoing bone marrow transplant. A common explanation for how imagery may improve cancer outcomes is postulated through increasing cellular immune function. Some studies have demonstrated increases in NK cytotoxicity (Gruzelier, 2002; Lengacher et al., 2008) and NK cell numbers (Bakke, Purtzer, & Newton, 2002), whereas others have found no differences in NK numbers and cytotoxicity (Nunes et al., 2007). Despite inconclusive effects on cancer outcome, imagery interventions have consistently improved coping responses and psychological states in patients with cancer, suggesting that imagery may mediate PNI outcomes in breast and other cancers (Walker, 2004). Further study is needed to determine the clinical significance of immunological effects.

Guided imagery has been identified on the National Institutes of Health, National Center for Complementary and Integrative Health website as one of the 10 most frequently used integrative therapies for cancer (see Figure 6.1). The improved quality of the studies suggests that there is good evidence for guided imagery as an intervention for cancer patients. The Society for Integrative Oncology published a clinical practice guideline for the use of integrative therapies as supportive care for breast cancer patients and reported that guided imagery can be considered for improving quality of life for breast cancer patients (Greenlee et al., 2014).

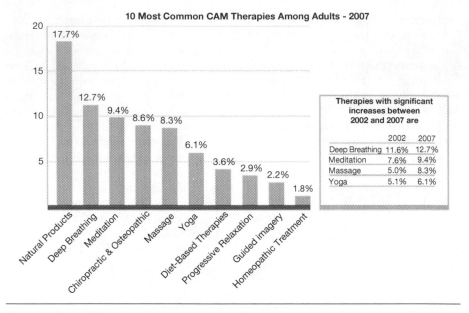

Figure 6.1.   Ten most common CAM therapies among adults, 2007.

CAM, complementary and alternative medicine.

Source: Barnes PM, Bloom B, Nahin R. *CDC National Health Statistics Report* #12. Complementary and Alternative Medicine Use Among Adults and Children; United States, 2007. December 2008.

CULTURAL APPLICATIONS

Modern-day imagery owes it roots to the use of imagery in traditional healing. Achtenberg (1985) described imaging as "the world's oldest and greatest healing resource" (p. 3) and noted that the use of imagery is foundational to the shamanic healing found in many healing traditions. Shamanic healing is a centuries-old practice in which imagery is used within an ecstatic or altered state to access the patient's subconscious mind and belief system (Reed, 2007). This opens communication among mind, body, and spirit to cure, alleviate suffering, and facilitate spiritual transformation. Epstein et al. (2004) noted that in spiritual life, experiences are images reflecting us back to ourselves.

The interest in imagery as part of a therapeutic treatment plan is found globally (see Sidebar 6.2). In addition to the many studies from the United States, research on the use and effectiveness of imagery is prevalent in many other countries: Canada (Beaumont et al., 2011; Kuttner, 2012), Spain (Leon-Pizarro et al., 2007), Brazil (Nunes et al., 2007), Korea (Kim et al., 2011; Yoo et al., 2005), and Japan (Watanabe, Fukuda, Hara, Maeda, & Ohira, 2006; Watanabe, Fukuda, & Shirakawa, 2005). In fact, many of the newer studies, including multiple randomized clinical trials, come from colleagues in other countries.

International research on guided imagery is growing as cancer incidence is increasing worldwide. Nurses are at the forefront of this research, seeking new, effective interventions to mitigate the side effects of treatment (see Sidebar 6.3). Breast cancer incidence rates are increasing globally. A nursing research study in Taiwan evaluated the effects of cancer treatment on women with breast cancer.

The researchers found that guided imagery paired with relaxation had a positive effect on mediating the side effects of anxiety and depression (Chen et al., 2015). In Iran, breast cancer in the most common cancer found in women. A group of nurse researchers studied guided imagery for chemotherapy-induced nausea and vomiting (CINV), one of the most distressing side effects of chemotherapy. If not adequately controlled, it can lead to many other serious side effects such as weight loss, malnutrition, social isolation, depression, insomnia, and dehydration. The intervention was delivered at clinic appointments, and the participants also listened to a guided-imagery CD at home. Guided imagery as an intervention reduced the severity and frequency of CINV (Hosseini, Tirgari, Forouzi, & Janhani, 2016).

SIDEBAR 6.2. USING IMAGERY ONLINE: NEW ZEALAND

Theresa Fleming and Matthew Shepherd

New Zealand or—in the words of the indigenous Maori people—Aotearoa, includes Maori, as well as Pacific, Asian, New Zealand European, and other peoples. Our team set out to develop a computerized therapy to help extend the reach of psychological therapies to teenagers with unmet needs, particularly untreated depression and anxiety. We focused on computerized therapies because face-to-face services are limited, sometimes costly, inconvenient, or not preferred by adolescents. Computerized, or online, therapies have been tested and shown to be effective; however, often these have high dropout rates, many are very text heavy, and may not reflect the interests of diverse peoples.

Over several years we worked with young people, therapists, learning technologists, researchers, and game developers to develop and test a computer program called SPARX (smart, positive, active, realistic, x factor) thoughts. This was shown to be effective in a large randomized controlled trial and is now freely available in New Zealand, funded through the Ministry of Health (https://www.fmhs.auckland.ac.nz/assets/fmhs/faculty/ABOUT/newsandevents/docs/SPARX%20Fact%20sheet.pdf).

SPARX uses cognitive behavioral therapy techniques, storytelling, and metaphor- and play-based learning. These strategies were selected based on evidence and on appeal to Maori and other youth. The program has seven levels or modules that young people can do on their own or with support. SPARX uses both explicit instructional learning and play-based, first-person experiential learning. Each level begins with "the guide," a virtual therapist who welcomes the user, explains what the session is about, and discusses how it relates to real life (instructional learning). The users then go into a game world, where they complete quests and challenges to "right the balance" and reduce negativity in the game world. In general, this is exploratory, play-based learning in the context of a rich visual environment. There is an overarching narrative, and metaphors are often used. At the end of each level, users come back to the guide, who invites them to reflect and develop strategies to use skills from the game in real life. For example, in the volcano province, users must negotiate with angry fire spirits and lift blocks from volcanic vents to prevent explosions. When they return to the guide, they consider what causes them to explode with anger and how to deal with these challenges in real life. In another example, users release the "Bird of Hope" from a chest where it has been trapped.

(continued)

From there, the Bird of Hope follows them and helps them throughout the game; again, this is explicitly linked to how one develops and maintains hope in real life.

The imagery in SPARX was created with input from youth, as well as cultural, learning, and computer game experts. The team included Maori and non-Maori health researchers, clinicians, and youth. The computer game company that developed the software was Maori-led, and cultural experts ensured that the content was appropriate and powerful. Evaluations have shown SPARX to be effective among young people seeking help for depression. There were no differences in its effectiveness between Maori and non-Maori or between males and females. This is exciting because many therapeutic interventions are more appealing to girls and/or majority-culture persons, which may inadvertently increase disparities. Youth feedback has highlighted that the imagery and narrative helped increase the appeal of SPARX and made it easy to understand, remember, and use new skills:

> "The Bird of Hope is encouraging, it's like having someone next to you, by your side, it will be in my memory."
> "I learnt from the game. It was interesting and fun, you do learn from game stuff."
> "It felt personal, you know, like he [the guide] was talking to you, like you got to know him."

Thyroid cancer incidence is also increasing worldwide. In Korea, thyroid cancer is the most common cancer. A group of nurse researchers observed significant stress in patients who were receiving radioactive iodine treatments post-thyroidectomy. They provided guided-imagery CDs to the intervention group and had them view the CD daily for 4 weeks. The control group received standard education about radioactive iodine therapy. There were significant decreases in stress and fatigue in the intervention group (Lee, Kim, & Yu, 2013).

Cultures are broadly categorized as tending toward either individualism or collectivism. La Roche, Batista, and D'Angelo (2010) investigated guided-imagery scripts to determine their level of idiocentrism versus allocentrism. Idiocentrism is the tendency to define oneself in isolation from others and would be found in individualistic societies; allocentrism is the tendency to define oneself in relation to others and would be seen in cultures valuing collectivism. The authors reviewed 123 guided-imagery scripts and found that they tended to be more idiocentric. This may indicate that guided imagery scripts may need to be adapted depending on the user's cultural ethnicity.

When directing a guided-imagery experience, the practitioner should be aware of individual preferences and use images that are understandable and acceptable to the participant. As a rule, the most powerful and meaningful image is one that the participant creates rather than one that is supplied by the guide. Participants are more likely to choose images that are congruent with their cultural, spiritual, and personal beliefs. The guide or therapist is there to help them use those images.

FUTURE RESEARCH

Despite documented relationships between the mind and the body, there continues to be a lack of high-quality intervention trials testing the effectiveness of guided imagery and other mind–body interventions. Although the body of evidence is

SIDEBAR 6.3. COMPARISON OF THE USE OF GUIDED IMAGERY VERSUS MINDFUL ATTENTION WITH CHILDREN IN THAILAND WITH CANCER

Kesanee Boonyawatanangkool

In Thailand, as elsewhere, children with a life-threatening illness such as cancer experience multiple types of distress. These can range from disease symptoms, procedures, and treatments to the psychological discomfort of living with a potentially terminal illness. Indeed, there are numerous challenges inherent to the provision of holistic nursing care to these children throughout their illness trajectory. Guided imagery is an independent nursing intervention that uses psychoneuroimmunological principles to help manage distress symptoms such as pain, anxiety, and fear by directing attention away from difficult events. Conversely, mindfulness involves devoting attention to one's experience in an accepting and nonjudgmental way; however, the effect of this instruction on distress symptoms—including pain and other outcomes—is unknown.

The objective we addressed in our clinical work was to examine whether mindful attention could help children focus on pain, anxiety, or fear without increasing their distress symptoms or decreasing their symptom tolerance. In this clinical evaluation, we compared the effects of mindful attention to a well-established intervention for reduction of difficult symptoms (i.e., guided imagery/self-hypnosis)—an intervention that is designed to take attention away from uncomfortable events.

Anxiety and fear were monitored in children ($n = 58$) 5 to 18 years of age who were hospitalized and receiving chemotherapy. Each child attended and completed a session of guided imagery. Participants then received either mindful attention or guided-imagery instructions designed to direct attention to focus on or away from their pain, anxiety, and fear, respectively.

Our clinical evaluation revealed that children who received the mindful attention instructions demonstrated more awareness of the physical sensations of pain, anxiety, and fear—including thoughts about those sensations—without decreasing tolerance levels. Some of them said, "I am now feeling better; can you help me do this again please?" (e.g., a 14-year-old boy with palliation of rhabdomyosarcoma pain). There were no interactions observed between baseline characteristics of the children and the specific intervention used to address their symptoms.

Based on our clinical observations, we concluded that mindful (trance) attention—compared with guided imagery—was successful in helping the children focus attention on experiences of pain, anxiety, and fear without increased pain intensity or decreased symptom tolerance.

These conclusions were based solely on the clinical experience in my practice setting in Thailand. Factors that we know to be important to the implementation of either intervention with children include the children's knowledge, their developmental stage, trust and rapport, gender and age, pain and other uncomfortable experiences, coping strategies, disease status, religious and

(continued)

cultural beliefs, and family background. Both interventions appeared to be beneficial in reducing distress in children and included shared strategies such as eye-fixation techniques, deep breaths, and progressive muscle relaxation through guided instruction.

growing, with many reports of clinical efficacy, more scientifically rigorous research testing outcomes are needed. For example, Richardson et al. (2006) concluded that there is sufficient evidence for the efficacy of hypnosis to manage procedural pain in pediatric oncology but noted a number of methodological limitations. Small sample sizes, lack of standardized control groups, and inadequate reporting of research methods limit the generalizability of the findings of many imagery studies.

Key questions remain to be answered regarding specific physiological responses to imagery, the influence of imagery on clinical outcomes and quality of life, and the effect of individual factors. As a low-cost, noninvasive intervention, imagery has the potential to be effective in reducing symptoms and distress across several conditions. Questions to be pursued include:

- What is the role of imagery in maintaining health and wellness? Should imagery be a component of preventive medicine? Over time, can imagery reduce stress, improve coping, enhance well-being, create healthier lifestyles, and reduce illness in individuals?
- What is the effect of imagery on clinical outcomes relevant to quality-of-life and health/illness states and does it have an impact on cost effectiveness and quality of care?
- What is the relationship between imagery and other relaxation strategies? Are they more effective when paired or should they be used alone?
- Does the type of imagery produce different outcomes? What imagery protocols or processes are most appropriate in specific conditions (use of recording/app or session with a practitioner; duration and number of sessions)?
- Is it possible to predict the usefulness of an imagery intervention in specific individuals? Are there certain characteristics of individuals that determine their ability to respond to imagery and produce desired outcomes? Are there certain individuals or conditions for which imagery should not be recommended?
- What are the long-term effects of imagery?
- What is the role of practitioner characteristics (type of training, practitioner style, number of different practitioners) in outcomes?

WEBSITES

The following websites contain additional information on guided imagery:

- Academy for Guided Imagery (2017). Workshops and resources (www.acadgi.com)
- American Holistic Nurses Association (2017) (www.ahna.org)

- American Society of Clinical Hypnosis (2017). Certification, workshops, and resources (www.asch.net)
- Association for Music and Imagery (2017). Bonny method of guided imagery and music therapy (www.ami-bonnymethod.org)
- Imagery International (2017) (www.imageryinternational.org)
- National Center for Complementary and Integrative Health Practices (2017). Relaxation techniques for health (https://nccih.nih.gov/health/stress/relaxation.htm)
- National Pediatric Hypnosis Training Institute (2017). Training in pediatric hypnosis (www.nphti.net)

REFERENCES

Achtenberg, J. (1985). *Imagery in healing: Shamanism and modern medicine.* Boston, MA: Shambhala.

Ader, R., & Cohen, N. (1981). Conditioned immunopharmacologic responses. In R. Ader (Ed.), *Psychoneuroimmunology* (pp. 281–319). New York, NY: Academic Press.

Ader, R., Felten, D. L., & Cohen, N. (1991). *Psychoneuroimmunology* (2nd ed.). San Diego, CA: Academic Press.

Alam, M., Roongpisuthipong, W., Kim, N., Goyal, A., Swary, J. H., Brindise, R.T., ... Yoo, S. (2016). Utility of recorded guided imagery and relaxing music in reducing patient pain and anxiety, and surgeon anxiety, during cutaneous surgical procedures: A single-blinded randomized and controlled trial. *Journal* of the American Academy Dermatology, 75, 585–589.

Alexander, M. (2012). Managing patient stress in pediatric radiology. *Radiologic Technology,* 83(6), 549–560.

American Academy of Pediatrics Section on Integrative Medicine. (2016). Mind-body therapies in children and youth. *Pediatrics,* 138(3), e20161896. doi:10.1542/peds.2016-1896

American Pain Society. (2012). *Assessment and management of children with chronic pain: A position statement from the American Pain Society.* Retrieved from http://americanpainsociety.org/uploads/get-Involved/pediatric-chronic-pain-statement.pdf

Anbar, R. D. (2008). Subconscious guided therapy with hypnosis. *American Journal of Clinical Hypnosis, 50*(4), 323–334.

Andrasik, F., & Rime, C. (2007). Can behavioural therapy influence neuromodulation? *Neurological Sciences, 28*(Suppl. 2), S124–S129.

Armstrong, K., Dixon, S., May, S., & Patricolo, G. E. (2014). Anxiety reduction in patients undergoing cardiac catheterization following massage and guided imagery. *Complementary Therapies in Clinical Practice, 20*(2014), 334–338.

Baird, C. L., & Sands, L. (2006). Effect of guided imagery with relaxation on health-related quality of life in older women with osteoarthritis. *Research in Nursing and Health,* 29, 442–451.

Bakke, A. C., Purtzer, M. Z., & Newton, P. (2002). The effect of hypnotic-guided imagery on psychological well-being and immune function in patients with prior breast cancer. *Journal of Psychosomatic Research, 53*(6), 1131–1137.

Ball, T. M., Shapiro, D. E., Monheim, C. J., & Weydert, J. A. (2003). A pilot study of the use of guided imagery for the treatment of recurrent abdominal pain in children. *Clinical Pediatrics,* 42(6), 527–532.

Beaumont, G., Mercier, C., Michon P. E., Malouin, F., & Jackson, P. L. (2011). Decreasing phantom limb pain through observation of action and imagery: A case series. *Pain Medicine, 12,* 289–299.

Beck, B. D., Hansen, A. M., & Gold, C. (2015). Coping with work-related stress through guided imagery and music (GIM): Randomized controlled trial. *Journal of Music Therapy, 52*(3), 323–352.

Boehm, L. B. & Tse, A. M. (2013). Application of guided imagery to facilitate the transition of new graduate registered nurses. *Journal of Continuing Education in Nursing, 44*(3), 113–119.

Boltin, D., Sahar, N., Gil, E., Aizic, S., Hod, K., Levi-Drummer, R., ... Dickman, R. (2015). Gut-directed guided affective imagery as an adjunct to dietary modification in irritable bowel syndrome. *Journal of Health Psychology, 20*(6), 712–720.

Braun, S. M., Beurskens, A. J., Borm, P. J., Schack, T., & Wade, D. T. (2006). The effects of mental practice in stroke rehabilitation: A systematic review. *Archives of Physical Medicine and Rehabilitation, 87,* 842–852.

Braun, S. M., Wade, D. T., & Beurskens, A. J. (2011). Use of movement imagery in neurorehabilitation: Researching effects of a complex intervention. *International Journal of Rehabilitation Research, 34,* 203–208.

Brunelli, S., Giovanni, M., Iosa, M., Ciotti, C., De Giorgi, R., Foti, C., ... Traballesi, M. (2015). Efficacy of progressive muscle relaxation, mental imagery, and phantom exercise training on phantom limb: a randomized control trial. *Archives of Physical Medicine and Rehabilitation, 96,* 181–187.

Butler, L. D., Symons, B. K., Henderson, S. L., Shortliffe, L. D., & Spiegel, D. (2005). Hypnosis reduces distress and duration of an invasive medical procedure for children. *Pediatrics, 115*(1), e77–e85.

Calipel, S., Lucas-Polomeni, M. M., Wodey, E., & Ecoffey, C. (2005). Premedication in children: Hypnosis versus midazolam. *Pediatric Anesthesia, 15,* 275–281.

Cardeña, E., Svensson, C., & Hejdström, F. (2013). Hypnotic tape intervention ameliorates stress: A randomized control study. *International Journal of Clinical and Experimental Hypnosis, 61*(2), 125–145.

Carli, G., Cavallaro, F. I., & Santarcangelo, E. L. (2007). Hypnotizability and imagery modality preference: Do highs and lows live in the same world? *Contemporary Hypnosis, 24*(2), 64–75.

Carrico, D. J., Peters, K. M., & Diokno, A. C. (2008). Guided imagery for women with interstitial cystitis: Results of a prospective, randomized controlled pilot study. *Journal of Alternative and Complementary Medicine, 14*(1), 53–60.

Casida, J. M., Yaremchuk, K. L., Shpakoff, L., Marrocco, A., Babicz, G., & Yarandi, H. (2012). The effects of guided imagery on sleep and inflammatory response in cardiac surgery: A pilot randomized controlled trial. *Journal of Cardiovascular Surgery, 53,* 1–11.

Charalambous, A., Giannakopoulou, M., Bozas, E., & Paikousis, L. (2015). A randomized controlled trial for the effectiveness of progressive muscle relaxation and guided imagery as anxiety reducing interventions in breast and prostate cancer patients undergoing chemotherapy. *Evidenced-Based Complementary and Alternative Medicine, 2015,* 270876. doi:10.1155/2015/270876

Charalambous, A., Giannakopoulou, M., Bozas, E., Marcou, T., Kitslos, P., & Paikousis, L. (2016). Guided imagery and progressive muscle relaxation as a cluster of symptoms management intervention in patients receiving chemotherapy: A randomized control trial. *PLOS ONE, 11*(6). doi:10.1371/journal.pone.0156911

Charette, S., Fiola, J. L., Charest, M. C., Villeneuve, E., Théroux, J., Joncas, J., ... Le May, S. (2015). Guided imagery for adolescent post-spinal fusion pain management: A pilot study. *Pain Management Nursing, 16*(3), 211–220.

Chen, S., Wang, H., Yang, H., & Chung, U. (2015). Effect of relaxation and guided imagery on the physical and psychological symptoms of breast cancer patients undergoing chemotherapy. *Iran Red Crescent Medical Journal, 17*(11), 1–8.

Chou, M. H., & Lin, M. F. (2006). Exploring the listening experiences during guided imagery and music therapy of outpatients with depression. *Journal of Nursing Research, 14*(2), 93–102.

Chuang, L. L., Liu, S. C., Chen, Y. H., & Lin, L. C. (2015). Predictors of adherence to relaxation guided imagery during pregnancy in women with preterm labor. *Journal of Alternative and Complementary Medicine, 21*(9), 563–568.

Collins, M. P., & Dunn, L. F. (2005). The effects of meditation and visual imagery on an immune system disorder: Dermatomyositis. *Journal of Alternative and Complementary Medicine, 11*(2), 275–284.

Committee on Psychosocial Aspects of Children and Family Health, Task Force on Pain in Infants, Children and Adolescents. (2001). The assessment and management of acute pain in infants, children and adolescents. *Pediatrics, 108*(3), 793–797.

Costa-Pinto, F., & Palermo-Neto, J. (2010). Neuroimmune interactions in stress. *NeuroImmunoModulation, 17,* 196–199.

Cotton, S., Roberts, Y. H., Tsevat, J., Britto, M., Succop, P., McGrady, M. E., & Yi, M. S. (2010). Mind-body complementary alternative medicine use and quality of life in adolescents with inflammatory bowel disease. *Inflammatory Bowel Disease, 16*(3), 501–506.

Culbert, T., Friedrichsdorf, S., & Kuttner, L. (2008). Mind-body skills for children in pain. In H. Breivik, W. I. Campbell, & M. K. Nicholas (Eds.), *Clinical pain management: Practice and procedures* (2nd ed., pp. 478–495). London, England: Hodder Arnold.

Cyna, A. M., Tomkins, D., Maddock, T., & Barker, D. (2007). Brief hypnosis of severe needle phobia using switch-wire imagery in a 5-year-old. *Pediatric Anesthesia, 17,* 800–804.

DiPietro, J. A., Costigan, K. A., Nelson, P., Gurewitsch, E. D., & Laudenslager, M. L. (2008). Fetal responses to induced maternal relaxation during pregnancy. *Biological Psychology, 77,* 11–19.

Djordjevic, J., Zatorre, R. J., Petrides, M., Boyle, J. A., & Jones-Gotaman, M. (2005). Functional neuroimaging of odor imagery. *Neuroimage, 24*(3), 791–801.

Dobson, C. (2015). Outcome results of self-efficacy in children with sickle disease pain who were trained to use guided imagery. *Applied Nursing Research, 28,* 384–390.

Dobson, C. E., & Byrne, M. W. (2014). Using guided imagery to manage pain in young children with sickle cell disease. *American Journal of Nursing, 114*(4), 27–36.

Donaldson, V. W. (2000). A clinical study of visualization on depressed white blood cells in medical patients. *Applied Psychophysiology and Biofeedback, 25*(2), 230–235.

Draucker, C. B., Jacobson, A. F, Umberger, W. A., Myerscough, R. P., & Sanata, J. D. (2015). Acceptability of a guided imagery intervention for persons undergoing a total knee replacement. *Orthopedic Nursing, 34*(6), 356–364.

Driediger, M., Hall, C., & Callow, N. (2006). Imagery use by injured athletes: A qualitative analysis. *Journal of Sports Sciences, 24*(3), 261–271.

Dunsky, A., Dickstein, R., Marcovitz, E., Levy, S., & Deutsch, J. (2008). Home-based motor imagery training for gait rehabilitation of people with chronic poststroke hemiparesis. *Archives in Physical Medicine and Rehabilitation, 89,* 1580–1588.

Elkins, G., Johnson, A., Fisher, W., & Sliwinski, J. (2013). A pilot investigation of guided self-hypnosis in the treatment of hot flashes among postmenopausal women. *International Journal of Clinical and Experimental Hypnosis, 61*(3), 342–350.

Epstein, G. N., Halper, J. P., Barrett, E. A., Birdsal, C., McGee, M., Baron, K. P., ... Lowenstein, S. (2004). A pilot study of mind–body changes in adults with asthma who practice mental imagery. *Alternative Therapies, 10*(4), 66–71.

Fichtel, A., & Larsson, B. (2004). Relaxation treatment administered by school nurses to adolescents with recurrent headaches. *Headache, 44,* 545–554.

Fleshner, M., & Laudenslager, M. L. (2004). Psychoneuroimmunology: Then and now. *Behavioral and Cognitive Neuroscience Reviews, 3*(2), 114–130.

Flory, N., Salazar, G. M. M., & Lang, E. V. (2007). Hypnosis for acute distress management during medical procedures. *International Journal of Clinical and Experimental Hypnosis, 55*(3), 303–317.

Flynn, T. A., Jones, B. A., & Ausderau, K. K. (2016). Guided imagery and stress in pregnant adolescents. *American Journal of Occupational Therapy, 70*(5), 700522002 1–7.

Forsner, M., Norström, F., Nordyke, K., Ivarsson, A., & Lindh, V. (2014). Relaxation and guided imagery used with 12-year-olds during venipuncture in a school-based screening study. *Journal of Child Health Care, 18*(3), 241–252.

Freeman, L., White, R., Ratcliff, M., Sutton, S., Stewart, M., Palmer, J., ... Cohen, L. (2015). A randomized trial comparing live and telemedicine delivery of an imagery-based behavioral intervention to breast cancer survivors: Reducing symptoms and barriers to care. *Psycho-Oncology, 24*(8). 1–16.

Galili, O., Shaoul, R., & Mogilner, J. (2009). Treatment of chronic recurrent abdominal pain: Laparoscopy or hypnosis? *Journal of Laparoendoscopic and Advanced Surgical Techniques, 19*(1), 93–96.

Gerik, S. M. (2005). Pain management in children: Developmental considerations and mind–body therapies. *Southern Medical Journal, 98*(3), 295–301.

Giacobbi, P. R., Stabler, M., Stewart, J., Jaeschke, A., Siebert, J. L., & Kelly, G. A. (2015). *Pain Management Nursing, 16*(5), 792–803.

Glaser, R., MacCallum, R. C., Laskowski, B. F., Malarkey, W. B., Sheridan, J. F., & Kiecolt-Glaser, J. K. (2001). Evidence for a shift in the Th-1 to Th-2 cytokine response associated with chronic stress and aging. *Journal of Gerontology. A: Biological Science and Medical Science*, *56*(8), M477–M482.

Gordon, J. S., Staples, J. K., Blyta, A., Bytyqi, M., & Wilson, A. (2008). Treatment of posttraumatic stress disorder in postwar Kosovar adolescents using mind–body skills groups: A randomized controlled trial. *Journal of Clinical Psychiatry*, *69*(9), 1469–1476.

Gottsegen, D. (2011). Hypnosis for functional abdominal pain. *American Journal of Clinical Hypnosis*, *54*, 56–69.

Greene, C., & Greene, B. A. (2012, May–June). Efficacy of guided imagery to reduce stress via the internet: A pilot study. *Holistic Nursing Practice*, *26*(3), 150–163.

Greenlee, H., Baineaves, L., Carlson, L. E., Cohen, M., Deng, G., Hershman, D., … Tripathy, D. (2014). Clinical practice guidelines on the use of integrative therapies as supportive care in patients treated for breast cancer. *Journal of the National Institute Monographs*, *50*, 346–357.

Grunau, R. E., Oberlander, T. F., & Whitfield, M. F. (2001). Demographic and therapeutic determinants of pain reactivity in very low birth weight neonates at 32 weeks postconception age. *Pediatrics*, *107*, 105–117.

Gruzelier, J. H. (2002). A review of the impact of hypnosis, relaxation, guided imagery and individual differences on aspects of immunity and health. *Stress*, *5*(2), 147–163.

Gulewitsch, M. D., Müller, J., Hautzinger, M., & Schlarb, A. A. (2013). Brief hypnotherapeutic-behavioral intervention for functional abdominal pain and irritable bowel syndrome in childhood: A randomized controlled trial. *European Journal of Pediatrics*, *172*, 1043–1051.

Hansen, M. M. (2015). A feasibility pilot study on the use of complementary therapies delivered via mobile technologies on Icelandic surgical patient's reports of anxiety, pain, and self-efficacy in healing. *Complementary and Alternative Medicine*. *15*, 92–104.

Hosseini, M., Tirgari, B., Forouzi, M. A., & Janhani, Y. (2016, November). Guided imagery effects on chemotherapy induced nausea and vomiting in Iranian breast cancer patients. *Complementary Therapies in Clinical Practice*, *25*, 8–12. doi:10.1016/j.ctcp.2016.07.002

Hovington, C. L., & Brouwer, B. (2010). Guided motor imagery in healthy adults and stroke: Does strategy matter? *Neurorehabilitation and Neural Repair*, *24*, 851–856.

Huth, M. M., Broome, M. E., & Good, M. (2004). Imagery reduces children's postoperative pain. *Pain*, *110*(1–2), 439–448.

Huth, M. M., Van Kuiken, D. M., & Broome, M. E. (2006). Playing in the park: What school age children tell us about imagery. *Journal of Pediatric Nursing*, *21*(2), 115–125.

Jacobson, A. F., Umberger, W. A. Palmieri, P. A., Alexander, T. S., Myerscough, R. P., Draucker, C. B., … Kirschbaum, C. (2016). Guided imagery for total knee replacement: A randomized, placebo-controlled pilot study. *Journal of Alternative and Complementary Medicine*, *22*(7), 563–575.

Jallo, N., Cozens, R., Smith, M. W., & Simpson, R. I. (2013). Effects of a guided imagery intervention on stress in hospitalized pregnant women: A pilot study. *Holistic Nursing Practice*, *27*(3), 129–139.

Jallo, N., Ruiz, J., Elswick, R. K. Jr., & French, E. (2014). Guided imagery for stress and symptom management in pregnant African American women. *Evidence-Based Complementary and Alternative Medicine*, *2014*, 840923. doi:10.1155/2014/840923

Kemper, K. J., & Khirallah, M. (2015). Acute effects of online mind-body skills training on resilience, mindfulness, and empathy. *Journal of Evidence Based Complementary and Alternative Medicine*, *20*(4), 247–253.

Kim, J. S., Oh, D. W., Kim, S. Y., & Choi, J. D. (2011). Visual and kinesthetic locomotor imagery training integrated with auditory step rhythm for walking performance of patients with chronic stroke. *Clinical Rehabilitation*, *25*, 134–145.

Kline, W. H., Turnbull, A., Labruna, V. E., Haufler, L., DeVivio, S., & Ciminera, P. (2010). Enhancing pain management in the PICU by teaching guided mental imagery: A quality-improvement project. *Journal of Pediatric Psychology*, *35*(1), 25–31.

Kohen, D. (2000, June). *Integrating hypnosis into practice*. Paper presented at the Introductory Workshop in Clinical Hypnosis. St. Paul: University of Minnesota and the Minnesota Society of Clinical Hypnosis.

Kohen, D., & Olness, K. (2011). *Hypnosis and hypnotherapy with children* (4th ed.). New York, NY: Routledge.

Kosslyn, S. M., Ganis, G., & Thompson, W. (2001). Neural foundations of imagery. *Nature Reviews, 2*, 635–642.

Kraemer, D. J., Macrae, C. N., Green, A. E., & Kelley, W. M. (2005). Musical imagery: Sound of silence activates auditory cortex. *Nature, 434*(7030), 158.

Kraemer, K. M., Luberto, C. M., O'Bryan, E. M., Mysinger, E., & Cotton, S. (2016). Mind-body skills training to improve distress tolerance in medical students: A pilot study. *Teaching and Learning in Medicine, 28*(2), 219–228.

Krakow, B., & Zadra, A. (2006). Clinical management of chronic nightmares: Imagery rehearsal therapy. *Behavioral Sleep Medicine, 4*(1), 45–70.

Kuttner, L. (2012). Pediatric hypnosis: pre-, peri-, and post-anesthesia. *Pediatric Anesthesia, 22*, 573–577.

Kwekkeboom, K. L., & Bratzke, L. C. (2016). A systematic review of relaxation, meditation, and guided imagery strategies for symptom management in heart failure. *Journal of Cardiovascular Nursing, 31*(5), 457–468.

Kwekkeboom, K. L., Hau, H., Wanta, B., & Bumpus, M. (2008). Patients' perceptions of the effectiveness of guided imagery and progressive muscle relaxation interventions used for cancer pain. *Complementary Therapies in Clinical Practice, 14*, 185–194.

Kwekkeboom, K. L., Wanta, B., & Bumpus, M. (2008). Individual difference variables and the effects of progressive muscle relaxation and analgesic imagery interventions on cancer pain. *Journal of Pain and Symptom Management, 36*(6), 604–615.

Lahmann, C., Nickel, M., Schuster, T. Sauer, N., Ronel, J., Noll-Hussong, M., ... Loew, T. (2009). Functional relaxation and guided imagery as complementary therapy in asthma: A randomized controlled clinical trial. *Psychotherapy and Psychosomatics, 78*(4), 233–239.

Lam, T., Chung, K. F., Yeung, W., Yu, B. Y., Yung, K. P., & Ng, T. H. (2015). Hypnotherapy for insomnia: A systematic review and meta-analysis of randomized controlled trials. *Complementary Therapies in Medicine, 23*, 719–732.

Langley, P., Fonseca, J., & Iphofen, R. (2006). Psychoneuroimmunology and health from a nursing perspective. *British Journal of Nursing, 15*(29), 1126–1129.

La Roche, M. J., Batista, C., & D'Angelo, E. (2010). A content analyses of guided imagery scripts: A strategy for the development of cultural adaptations. *Journal of Clinical Psychology, 67*(1), 45–57.

Lee, M. H., Kim, D., & Yu, H. S. (2013). The effect of guided imagery on stress and fatigue in patients with thyroid cancer undergoing radioactive iodine therapy. *Evidence-Based Complementary and Alternative Medicine, 2013*, 130324. doi:10.1155/2013/130324

Lengacher, C. A., Bennett, M. P., Gonzalez, L., Gilvary, D., Cox, C. E., Cantor, A., ... Djeu, J. (2008). Immune responses to guided imagery during breast cancer treatment. *Biological Research in Nursing, 9*(3), 205–214.

Leon-Pizarro, C., Gich, I., Barthe, E., Rovirosa, A., Farrus, B., Casa, F., ... Arcusa, A. (2007). A randomized trial of the effect of training in relaxation and guided imagery techniques in improving psychological and quality-of-life indices for gynecologic and breast brachytherapy patients. *Psycho-Oncology, 16*, 971–979.

Lewandowski, W., Good, M., & Draucker, C. B. (2005). Changes in the meaning of pain with the use of guided imagery. *Pain Management Nursing, 6*(2), 58–67.

Lindfors, P., Unge, P., Arvidsson, P., Nyhlin, H., Björnsson, E., Abrahamsson, H., & Simrén, M. (2012). Effects of gut-directed hypnotherapy on IBS in different clinical settings: Results from two randomized, controlled trials. *American Journal of Gastroenterology, 107*, 276–285.

Loft, M. H., & Cameron, L. D. (2013). Using mental imagery to deliver self-regulation techniques to improve sleep behaviors. *Annals of Behavioral Medicine, 46*, 260–272.

MacIver, K., Lloyd, D. M., Kelly, S., Roberts, N., & Nurmikko, T. (2008). Phantom limb pain, cortical reorganization and the therapeutic effect of mental imagery. *Brain, 131*, 2181–2191.

Mackenzie, A., & Frawley, G, P. (2007). Preoperative hypnotherapy in the management of a child with anticipatory nausea and vomiting. *Anesthesia and Intensive Care, 35*, 784–787.

McCance, K. L., & Huether, S. E. (2002). *Pathophysiology: The biologic basis for disease in adults and children* (4th ed.). St. Louis, MO: Mosby.

Meeus, M., Nijs, J., Vanderheiden, T., Baert, I., Descheemaeker, F., & Struyf, F. (2015). The effect of relaxation therapy on autonomic functioning, in patients with chronic fatigue syndrome or fibromyalgia: A systematic review. *Clinical Rehabilitation, 29*(3) 221–233.

Meinlschmidt, G., Lee, J. H., Stalujanis, E., Belardi, A., Oh, M., Jung, E. K., … Tegethoff, M. (2016). Smartphone-based psychotherapeutic micro-interventions to improve mood in a real-world setting. *Frontiers in Psychology, 7,* 1112. doi:10.3389/fpsyg.2016.01112

Menzies, V., & Kim, S. (2008). Relaxation and guided imagery in Hispanic persons diagnosed with fibromyalgia: A pilot study. *Family and Community Health, 31*(3), 204–212.

Menzies, V., Lyon, E. E., Elswick, R. K., McCain, N. L., & Gray, D. P. (2014). Effects of guided imagery on biobehavioral factors in women with fibromyalgia. *Journal of Behavioral Medicine, 37*(1), 70–80.

Menzies, V., Taylor, A. G., & Bourguignon, C. (2006). Effects of guided imagery on outcomes of pain, functional status, and self-efficacy in persons diagnosed with fibromyalgia. *Journal of Alternative and Complementary Medicine, 12*(1), 12–30.

Mizrahi, M. C., Reicher-Atir, R., Levy, S., Haramati, S., Wengrower, D., Israeli, E., & Goldin, E. (2012). Effects of guided imagery with relaxation training on anxiety and quality of life among patients with inflammatory bowel disease. *Psychology and Health, 27*(12), 1463–1479.

Nelson, E. A., Dowsey, M. M., Knowles S. R., Castle, D. J., Salzberg, M. R., Monshat, K., … Choong, P. F. (2013). Systematic review of the efficacy of pre-surgical mind-body based therapies on post-operative outcome measures. *Complementary Therapies in Medicine, 21,* 697–711.

Nilsson, S., Forsner, M., Finnström, B., & Mörelius, E. (2015). Relaxation and guided imagery do not reduce stress, pain, and unpleasantness for 11 to 12 year-old girls during vaccinations. *ACTA Paediatrica, 104,* 724–729.

Nunes, D. F. T., Rodriguez, A. L., Hoffman, F. S., Luz, C., Filho, A., Muller, M. C., & Bauer, M. E. (2007). Relaxation and guided imagery program in patients with breast cancer undergoing radiotherapy is not associated with neuroimmunomodulatory effects. *Journal of Psychosomatic Research, 63,* 647–655.

Olness, K. (2008). Helping children and adults with hypnosis and biofeedback. *Cleveland Clinic Journal of Medicine, 75*(Suppl. 2), S39–S43.

Onieva-Zafra, M. D., Garcia, L. H., & del Valle, M. G. (2015, January–February). Effectiveness of guided imagery relaxation on levels of pain and depression in patients diagnosed with fibromyalgia. *Holistic Nursing Practice, 29,* 13–21.

Palsson, O. S., & van Tilburg, M. (2015). Hypnosis and guided imagery treatment for gastrointestinal disorders: Experience with scripted protocols developed at the University of North Carolina. *American Journal of Clinical Hypnosis, 58*(1), 5–21.

Peerdeman, K. J., van Laarhoven, A. I. M., Donders, A. R. T., Hopman, M. T. E., Peters, M. L., & Evers, A. W. M. (2015). Inducing expectations for health: Effects of verbal suggestion and imagery on pain, itch, and fatigue as indicators of physical sensitivity. *PLOS ONE, 10*(10), e0139563. doi:10.1371/journal.pone.0139563

Pert, C. B., Dreher, H. E., & Ruff, M. R. (1998). The psychosomatic network: Foundations of mind–body medicine. *Alternative Therapies in Health and Medicine, 4*(4), 30–41.

Polkki, T., Pietila, A. M., Vehvilainen-Julkunen, K., Laukkala, H., & Kiviluoma, K. (2008). Imagery-induced relaxation in children's postoperative pain relief: A randomized pilot study. *Journal of Pediatric Nursing, 23*(3), 217–224.

Posadzki, P., Lewandowski, W., Terry, R., Ernst, E., & Stearns, A. (2012). Guided imagery for non-musculoskeletal pain: A systematic review of randomized clinical trials. *Journal of Pain and Symptom Management, 44*(1), 95–104.

Proctor, M. L., Murphy, P. A., Pattison, H. M., Suckling, J., & Farquhar, C. M. (2008). Behavioural interventions for primary and secondary dysmenorrhoea (review). *Cochrane Database of Systematic Reviews, 4,* 1–24.

Rao, N., & Kemper, K. J. (2017). The feasibility and effectiveness of online guided imagery training for health professionals. *Journal of Evidence-Based Complementary & Alternative Medicine, 22*(1), 54–58.

Reed, T. (2007). Imagery in the clinical setting: A tool for healing. *Nursing Clinics of North America, 42,* 261–277.

Richardson, J., Smith, J. E., McCall, G., & Pilkington, K. (2006). Hypnosis for procedure-related pain and distress in pediatric cancer patients: A systematic review of effectiveness and methodology related to hypnosis interventions. *Journal of Pain and Symptom Management, 31*(1), 70–84.

Roffe, L., Schmidt, K., & Ernst, E. (2005). A systematic review of guided imagery as an adjuvant cancer therapy. *Psycho-Oncology, 14*, 607–617.

Russell, C., Smart, S., & House, D. (2007). Guided imagery and distraction therapy in paediatric hospice care. *Paediatric Nursing, 19*(2), 24–25.

Sahler, O. L., Hunter, B. C., & Liesveld, J. L. (2003). The effect of using music therapy with relaxation imagery in the management of patients undergoing bone marrow transplantation: A pilot feasibility study. *Alternative Therapies in Health and Medicine, 9*(6), 70–74.

Schaffer, L., Jallo, N., Howland, L., James, K., Glaser, D., & Arnell, K. (2013). Guided imagery: An innovative approach to improving maternal sleep quality. *Journal of Perinatal and Neonatal Nursing, 27*(2), 151–159.

Scherwitz, L. W., McHenry, P., & Herrero, R. (2005). Interactive guided imagery therapy with medical patients: Predictors of health outcomes. *Journal of Alternative and Complementary Medicine, 11*(1), 69–83.

Schuster, C., Hilfiker, R., Amft, O., Scheidhauer, A., Andrews, B., Butler, J., ... Ettlin, T. (2011). Best practice for motor imagery: A systematic literature review on motor imagery training elements in five different disciplines. *BMC Medicine, 9*, 75. Retrieved from http://www.biomedcentral.com/1741-7015/9/75

Sears, S. R., Bolton, S., & Bell, K. (2013). Evaluation of "Steps to Surgical Success" (STEPS): A holistic peripoerative medicine program to manage pain and anxiety related to surgery. *Holistic Nursing Practice, 27*(6), 349–357.

Segerstrom, S. (2010). Resources, stress, and immunity: An ecological perspective on human psychoneuroimmunology. *Annals of Behavioral Medicine, 40*, 114–125.

Serra, D., Parris, C. R., Carper, E., Homel, P., Fleishman, S. B., Harrison, L. B., & Chadha, M. (2012). Outcomes of guided imagery in patients receiving radiation therapy for breast cancer. *Clinical Journal of Oncology Nursing, 16*(6), 617–623.

Shenefelt, P. D. (2013). Anxiety reduction using hypnotic induction and self-guided imagery for relaxation during dermatologic procedures. *International Journal of Clinical and Experimental Hypnosis, 61*(3), 305–318.

Spiva, L., Hart, P. L., Gallagher, E., McVay, F., Garcia, M., & Malley, K., ... Smith, N. (2015). The effects of guided imagery on patients being weaned from mechanical ventilation. *Evidence-Based Complementary and Alternative Medicine, 2015*, 802865. doi:10.1155/2015/802865

Torem, M. S. (2007). Mind-body hypnotic imagery in the treatment of auto-immune disorders. *American Journal of Clinical Hypnosis, 50*(2), 157–170.

Trakhtenberg, E. C. (2008). The effects of guided imagery on the immune system: A critical review. *International Journal of Neuroscience, 118*, 839–855.

Tsitsi, T., Charalambous, A., Papastavrou, E., & Raftopoulos, V. (2017). Effectiveness of a relaxation intervention (progressive muscle relaxation and guided imagery) to reduce anxiety and improve mood of parents of hospitalized children with malignancies: A controlled trial in the Republic of Cyprus and Greece. *European Journal of Oncology Nursing, 26*, 9–18. doi:10.1016/j.ejon.2016.10.007

Turk, D. C., Swanson, K. S., & Tunks, E. R. (2008). Psychological approaches in the treatment of chronic pain patients—when pills, scalpels and needles are not enough. *Canadian Journal of Psychiatry, 53*(4), 213–223.

Uman, L. S., Chambers, C. T., McGrath, P. J., & Kisely, S. (2008). A systematic review of randomized controlled trials examining psychological interventions for needle-related procedural pain and distress in children and adolescents: An abbreviated Cochrane Review. *Journal of Pediatric Psychology, 33*(8), 842–854.

Van Kuiken, D. (2004). A meta-analysis of the effect of guided imagery practice on outcomes. *Journal of Holistic Nursing, 22*(2), 164–179.

Verkaik, R., Busch, M., Koeneman, T., Van Den Berg, R., Spreeuwenberg, P., & Francke, A. L. (2014). Guided imagery in people with fibromyalgia: A randomized controlled trial of effects on pain, functional status and self-efficacy. *Journal of Health Psychology, 19*(5), 678–688.

Vlieger, A. M., Blink, M., Tromp, E., & Benninga, M. (2008). Use of complementary and alternative medicine by pediatric patients with functional and organic gastrointestinal diseases: Results from a multicenter survey. *Pediatrics, 122*, e446–e451. Retrieved from http://www.pediatrics.org/cgi/content/full/122/2/e446

Walker, L. G. (2004). Hypnotherapeutic insights and interventions: A cancer odyssey. *Contemporary Hypnosis, 21*(1), 35–45.

Watanabe, E., Fukuda, S., Hara, H., Maeda, Y., & Ohira, H. (2006). Differences in relaxation by means of guided imagery in a healthy community sample. *Alternative Therapies, 12*(2), 60–66.

Watanabe, E., Fukuda, S., & Shirakawa, T. (2005). Effects among healthy subjects of the duration of regularly practicing a guided imagery program. *BMC Complementary and Alternative Medicine, 5*(21), 1–8.

Weydert, J. A., Shapiro, D. E., Acra, S. A., Monheim, C. J., Chambers, A. S., & Ball, T. M. (2006). Evaluation of guided imagery as treatment for recurrent abdominal pain in children: A randomized controlled trial. *BMC Pediatrics, 6*(29), 1–10.

Wild, M. R., & Espie, C. A. (2004). The efficacy of hypnosis in the reduction of procedural pain and distress in pediatric oncology: A systematic review. *Developmental and Behavioral Pediatrics, 25*(3), 207–213.

Wood, C., & Bioy, A. (2008). Hypnosis and pain in children. *Journal of Pain and Symptom Management, 35*(4), 437–446.

Yijing, Z., Xiaoping, D., Fang, L., Xiaolu, J., & Bin, W. (2015). The effects of guided imagery on heart rate variability in simulated spaceflight emergency tasks performers. *BioMed Research International, 2015*, 687020. doi:10.1155/2015/687020

Yoo, H. J, Ahn, S. H, Kim, S. B., Kim, W. K., & Han, O. S. (2005). Efficacy of progressive muscle relaxation training and guided imagery in reducing chemotherapy side effects in patients with breast cancer and in improving their quality of life. *Supportive Care in Cancer, 13*, 826–833.

Young, K. D. (2005). Pediatric procedural pain. *Annals of Emergency Medicine, 45*(2), 160–171.

Zech, N., Hansen, E., Bernardy, K., & Häuser, W. (2017). Efficacy, acceptability and safety of guided imagery/hypnosis in fibromyalgia—A systematic review and meta-analysis of randomized controlled trials. *European Journal of Pain, 21*, 217–227.

Music Intervention

LINDA L. CHLAN AND ANNIE HEIDERSCHEIT

Music has been used throughout history as a treatment modality (Haas & Brandes, 2009). From the time of the ancient Egyptians, the power of music to affect health has been noted (Davis, Gfeller, & Thaut, 2008). Nursing pioneer Florence Nightingale recognized the healing power of music (1860/1969). Today, nurses can use music in a variety of settings to benefit patients and clients.

DEFINITION

The *American Heritage Dictionary of the English Language,* fifth edition (2016) defines *music* as "the art of arranging sounds in time so as to provide a continuous, unified and evocative composition, as through melody, harmony, rhythm, and timbre." *The Oxford Dictionary of Music* (Rutherford, Kennedy, & Kennedy, 2013) identifies several elements that serve as the building blocks of music.

- **Rhythm** is the timing in music and is a phenomenon that is universal to all music. Rhythm includes tempo, beat, meter, and the duration of tones. It is what provides the movement in music. Rhythm influences motor skills and activates muscles. Slow rhythms can invoke a sense of peace and calm. Strong and intense rhythms can foster a sense or feelings of energy or power.
- **Melody** is the movement of pitches and tones in time. Melody is the relationship between the pitches. The movement and frequency of these pitches impacts our experience. Frequency and pitch are produced by the number of vibrations of a sound—the highness or lowness of a musical tone, noted by the letters A, B, C, D, E, F, and G. Higher pitches have more rapid vibrations that tend to act as stimulants, whereas lower pitches have slower vibrations that can bring about relaxation. Melody is often the element in music a listener follows that can serve to engage or distract the mind.
- **Harmony** is related to melody in that it is the sound produced when pitches are played or sung simultaneously. Harmony communicates a sense of relationship, how the notes connect or relate to one another. Harmony often conveys the emotions in music. When harmony is consonant or pleasing

in sound, there is a feeling of calm connection. Harmony that is dissonant creates a sense of tension, conflict, and unpleasantness. It is important to note that cultural norms determine what a listener deems enjoyable and pleasant. Different cultures use different tonal systems.

- **Timbre** is the characteristic sound of the instrument playing the music or of the voice singing. The construction, shape, materials, and technique of the player impact timbre of an instrument. The timbre of a voice is impacted by the body and the technique of the vocalist. The psychological significance of timbre includes associations with feelings, memories, and events.
- **Form** is the structure or design of music. It can be considered the container within which music is organized. For example, symphonies follow a form of four movements, whereas in a song, there are lyrics and a chorus. The organization in form provides a sense of comfort and predictability.
- **Dynamics** in music are the changes in sound intensity or volume. Dynamics range from loudness to softness. The intensity in dynamics can impact our experience with music. Softer or quieter music can create a sense of calm, closeness, and intimacy; louder music can create a feeling of energy and power.

Music therapists are well versed in using and implementing the healing elements of music to meet the specific and individualized needs of patients. In the United States and around the world, music therapists are employed in a wide variety of healthcare settings and facilities (American Music Therapy Association, 2014; World Federation of Music Therapy, 2014). Although music therapists are specifically trained to use music in various therapeutic ways, there are many situations in which nurses can implement music intervention into a patient's plan of care. So as not to confuse the practice of music therapy (facilitated by a board-certified music therapist) with the use of music from a nursing perspective, the term *music intervention* is used in this chapter.

SCIENTIFIC BASIS

Music is a complex auditory stimulus that affects the physiological, psychological, and spiritual dimensions of human beings (Bruscia, 2014). Individual responses to music can be influenced by personal preferences, experiences, demographic characteristics, the environment, education, and cultural factors (Heiderscheit, 2013). Processing of musical stimuli by the brain's auditory cortex includes musical perception, recognition, and emotion (Okumura et al., 2014). Musical factors such as melody, chords, and consonance, activate the brain bilaterally (Okumura et al., 2014). Listening to music that is perceived to be personally pleasurable can elicit an emotional response that is thought to be associated with dopamine activity in the brain's mesolimbic reward system (Salimpoor, Benovoy, Larcher, Dagher, & Zatorre, 2011).

Entrainment, a physics principle, is a process whereby two objects vibrating at similar frequencies tend to cause mutual sympathetic resonance, resulting in their vibrating at the same frequency (Dissanayake, 2009). Entrainment also refers to the synchronization of body rhythms to an external rhythm (Bruscia, 2014; Crowe, 2004; Hodges & Sebald, 2011). Music and physiological processes (including heartbeat, blood pressure, brain waves, body temperature, digestion, and adrenal hormones) involve rhythms and vibrations that occur in a regular, periodic manner and consist of oscillations (Crowe, 2004). The rhythm and tempo of music can be used to synchronize or entrain body rhythms (e.g., heart rate and respiratory pattern), with resultant changes in physiological states. Certain properties of music (less than 80 beats per minute with fluid, regular rhythm) can be used to promote relaxation by causing body rhythms to slow down or entrain with the slower beat and regular, repetitive rhythm (Bradt, Dileo, & Grocke, 2010; Davies et al., 2016; Pelletier, 2004; Robb, Nichols, Rutan, Bishop, & Parker, 1995).

Likewise, music can decrease anxiety by occupying attention channels in the brain with meaningful, distractive auditory stimuli (Heiderscheit, 2013). Music intervention provides a patient with a familiar, comforting stimulus that can evoke pleasurable sensations while focusing the individual's attention onto the music (distraction) instead of on stressful thoughts (Nilsson, 2009a), pain, discomfort, or other environmental stimuli (Heiderscheit, 2013).

INTERVENTION

Determining a patient's music preferences through assessment is essential; among the tools developed for this purpose is an assessment instrument by Chlan and Heiderscheit (2009) that elicits information on how frequently music is listened to; the type of music selections, artists, groups, and genres preferred; and the individual's reasons for listening to music. For some people, the purpose of listening to music may be to relax, whereas others may prefer music that distracts, stimulates, and invigorates. After assessment data have been gathered, appropriate techniques with specific music can then be devised and implemented (Heiderscheit, Breckenridge, Chlan, & Savik, 2014; Heiderscheit, Chlan, & Donley, 2011).

Techniques

The use of music for intervention can take many forms, such as (passive) listening to selected compact discs (CDs) or individual music downloads from the Internet, as well as actively singing or drumming. A number of factors should be kept in mind when considering the specific technique: the type of music and personal preferences, active music making versus passive listening, individual versus group involvement, length of time involved with the music, and desired outcomes. Two of the more commonly used music-intervention techniques are discussed here: individual listening and group music making.

Individual Music Listening

Providing the means for patients to listen to music is the intervention technique most frequently implemented by nurses. CDs or MP3 downloads from a reputable Internet source (such as www.MyMusicInc.com or iTunes) make it easy to provide music intervention for patients in a wide range of healthcare settings. Portable CD/MP3 players are relatively inexpensive; they are small and can be used in even the most crowded confines, such as critical care units. CD/MP3 players have superior sound clarity and track seeking that enables immediate selection of a desired piece of music. Tablet devices can be used to provide a menu of music choices. Comfortable headphones allow patients private listening that does not disturb others. Equipment selected for music intervention should be easy for patients to use with minimal effort or with assistance. Small MP3 players or tablet devices are more expensive than CD/MP3 players and should be reserved for patients with intact dexterity and sufficient visual acuity to operate these units.

Nurses can encourage patients and their family members to bring in their own music from home to use while hospitalized. Patients may already have their own preferred music available via a mobile device or digital tablet. With only a very modest outlay of money, a nursing unit can establish a music library containing a wide variety of selections to suit various musical preferences. The Public Radio Music Source (www.prms.org) offers diverse music for purchase. It is also easy to individualize CDs or MP3 files to accommodate the preferences of each patient. Attention to copyright laws is necessary when reproducing CDs or downloading music from Internet sites (for guidance refer to www.copyright.gov).

Although various musical genres are available on the radio or Internet radio (e.g., Pandora), commercial messages and talking are deterrents to using these sources for music intervention. Likewise, one cannot control the quality of the radio signal reception or the specific music selections.

Group Music Making

Music can be used for patient groups as a powerful integrating force. Music creates and fosters connection and interrelationships among the members, as well as between the listener and the music (MacDonald, Kreutz, & Mitchell, 2012). One method of group music making is drumming, a form of rhythmic auditory stimulation. Drumming has been found to reduce post-traumatic stress disorder (PTSD) symptoms in a small group of soldiers, both by serving as an outlet for rage and for regaining a sense of control (Bensimon, Amir, & Wolf, 2008). Drumming circles can induce relaxation by entraining theta and alpha brain waves, leading to altered states of consciousness by activation of the limbic brain region with the lower brain (Winkelman, 2003) and by increasing natural killer (NK) cell activity (Bittman et al., 2001; Wachi et al., 2007). Group drumming has been used effectively to reduce burnout and improve mood in nursing students (Bittman et al., 2004), decrease employee burnout and improve mood states of staff working in long-term-care settings (Bittman, Bruhn, Stevens, Westengard, & Umbach, 2003), foster creativity and body movement in long-term-care residents (Bittman et al., 2004), decrease agitation (Choi, Lee, Cheong, & Lee, 2009), enhance recovery from a variety of chemical addictions (Winkelman, 2003), and reduce PTSD symptoms and depression (Carr et al., 2012).

Before implementing this type of group music making, nurses should consult with experts trained in the use of group drumming. The American Music Therapy Association website (www.musictherapy.org) can provide assistance in locating a music therapist for consultation. Interested nurses can visit the HealthRhythms website at Remo.com to locate an endorsed HealthRhythms facilitator in a specific area or to learn more about HealthRhythms training. HealthRhythms is a group-drumming protocol developed by Remo, Inc.; training is offered throughout the United States each year. Furthermore, diversity in the preferences, interests, and abilities of individuals in a group or the difficulties of securing an appropriate site for a group session may necessitate handling music on an individual basis; group sessions also require more planning than individual sessions.

Types of Music for Intervention

Careful attention to the selection of the music contributes to its therapeutic effect. For example, music to induce relaxation has a consistent and steady rhythm (less than 80 beats per minute); melody that is smooth, flowing, and predictable, with a small range of interval dynamics; and harmonic structure that is consonant and pleasing, with instrumentation that the individual enjoys (Ghetti, 2012; Grocke & Wigram, 2007). It is important to note that past experiences can influence one's response to music and that music can elicit a powerful emotional response or reaction at times.

Older adults may enjoy patriotic and popular songs from an earlier era (often music from their late teens to early twenties) or hymns with slower tempos played with familiar instruments (Moore, Staum, & Brotons, 1992). Religious music may be preferred and welcomed by those unable to attend spiritual services and for whom faith is important.

New Age or contemporary music may be preferred by some people. This kind of music differs from traditional music and is characterized by tension and release that may not be appropriate for relaxation because of the novelty of the stimulus and the absence of the usual forms found in more conventional music. Music perceived as unfamiliar causes an orienting response that may undermine goals for intervention (Maranto, 1993). A patient's music preference is of primary importance with consideration for the unique preferences that exist from one patient to another (Heiderscheit, 2013).

Guidelines

Music intervention for the purpose of relaxation uses music as a pleasant stimulus to block out sensations of anxiety, fear, and tension and to divert attention from unpleasant thoughts (Thaut, 1990). A minimum of 20 minutes of music is necessary for inducing relaxation. Some form of diversion exercise, such as deep breathing, is also required prior to initiating music intervention (Guzzetta, 1995). Guidelines for the use of music intervention are provided in Exhibit 7.1 and discussed here.

Although the definition of relaxing music may vary by individual, factors affecting response to music include musical preferences, familiarity of selections, and cultural background. Relaxing music should have a tempo at or below a resting heart rate (less than 80 beats per minute); predictable dynamics; a fluid melodic movement; pleasing harmonies; regular rhythm without sudden changes; and tonal qualities that include strings, flute, piano, or specially synthesized music (Ghetti, 2012; Robb et al., 1995). One of the most widely used classical music selections for relaxation is Pachelbel's Canon in D Major, which is frequently included in commercially available diversion CDs. In the last several years, many music companies have been producing recordings specifically packaged as music for relaxation. There is a wide array of recordings available in various genres and styles that can also include various instrumentation and environmental sounds. Exhibit 7.1 outlines the basic steps for handling music intervention for promoting relaxation.

Exhibit 7.1. Guidelines for Music Intervention for Relaxation

1. Ascertain that patient has adequate hearing.
2. Ascertain patient's like/dislike for music.
3. Assess music preferences and previous experience with music for relaxation.
4. Provide a choice of relaxing selections; assist with CD/MP3/tablet selections as needed.
5. Determine agreed-on goals for music intervention with patient.
6. Complete all nursing care prior to intervention; allow for a minimum of 20 minutes of uninterrupted listening time.
7. Gather equipment (CD or MP3 player, tablet device, CDs, headphones, fresh batteries) and ensure all are in good working order.
8. Test volume and comfort of volume level with patient prior to intervention.
9. Assist patient to a comfortable position as needed; ensure call-light is within easy reach and assist patient with equipment as needed.
10. Enhance environment as needed (e.g., draw blinds, close door, and turn off lights).
11. Post a "Do Not Disturb" sign to minimize unnecessary interruptions.
12. Encourage and provide patient with opportunities to practice relaxation with music.
13. Document patient responses to music intervention.
14. Discuss feelings of patient after using music intervention. Identify whether patient encountered any challenges or problems with the equipment.
15. Revise intervention plan and goal(s) as needed.

Initiating music intervention without first assessing a person's likes and dislikes may produce deleterious effects. Because of music's effect on the limbic system, it can bring about intense emotional responses. Use of portable players with headphones may be inappropriate or prohibited for patients in psychiatric settings, who may use the equipment cords for self-harm.

CD, compact disc.

Measurement of Outcomes

The outcome indices for evaluating the effectiveness of music intervention vary, depending on the purpose for which the music is used. Results may be physiological and/or psychological alterations and include a decrease in anxiety or stress arousal, promotion of relaxation, increase in social interaction, reduction in the need for medications, and increase in overall well-being. The nurse should carefully consider the goals of intervention and select outcome measurements and appropriate instruments accordingly.

PRECAUTIONS

It is imperative that music preferences be assessed prior to initiating a music-listening intervention. Everyone has "musical memories," and listening to a piece of music can bring up negative emotions that can be detrimental to an individual's well-being and also negatively impact the goals of intervention.

Likewise, using music for diversion in patients with tenuous or unstable cardiovascular status should be done with extreme caution. Patients should be closely monitored for any untoward cardiovascular responses.

Age-Related Implications or Adjustments Needed for Optimal Implementation

Older adults may require additional precautions prior to using music for therapeutic purposes. For instance, volume and bass may need to be adjusted to match hearing acuity. Headphones are ideal for masking background noise that can interfere with hearing acuity. Careful selection of equipment for music-listening interventions requires special attention to dexterity and/or vision impairments. Diminishing dexterity or vision may impact the frequency or use of individual music listening.

USES

Music has been tested as a therapeutic intervention with many different patient populations; most of the nursing literature focuses on individualized music listening. Exhibit 7.2 shows the patient populations and the numerous therapeutic purposes that music has served. Two frequent uses are highlighted here.

Exhibit 7.2. Uses of Music Intervention

Orientation/Minimizing Disruptive Behaviors
- Older adults (Cooke, Moyle, Shum, Harrison, & Murfield, 2010; Hicks-Moore, 2005; Thomas & Smith, 2009)

Decreasing Anxiety
- Patients awaiting dental treatment (Thoma et al., 2015)
- Surgical patients (Johnson, Raymond, & Goss, 2012; Kain, Sevarino, Alexander, Pincus, & Mayes, 2000; Lee, Henderson, & Shum, 2004; Yung, Chui-Kam, French, & Chan, 2002)
- Cancer patients (Clark et al., 2006; Ferrer, 2007)
- Patients undergoing endoscopy procedures (Wang et al., 2014)
- Patients with end-stage renal disease on maintenance hemodialysis (Kim, Evangelista, & Park, 2015)
- Patients undergoing flexible sigmoidoscopy (Chlan, Evans, Greenleaf, & Walker, 2000; Lee et al., 2002)
- Ventilator-dependent patients in an ICU (Almerud & Peterson, 2003; Chlan, 1998; Chlan et al., 2013; Davis & Jones, 2012; Heiderscheit et al., 2011; Wong, Lopez-Nahas, & Molassiotis, 2001)

Pain Management
- Individuals with acute pain (Dunn, 2004; Good et al., 2001; Huang, Good, & Zauszniewski, 2010; Koelsch et al., 2011; Laurion & Fetzer, 2003; Shertzer & Keck, 2001)

(continued)

- Chronic pain management (Guetin et al., 2012)
- Nursing care procedures/pediatrics (Whitehead-Pleaux, Zebrowski, Baryza, & Sheridan, 2007)
- Interventional radiological procedures—decrease in pain and sedation (Kulkarni, Johnson, Kettles, & Kasthuri, 2012)

Stress Reduction and Relaxation
- NICU patients (Kemper, Martin, Block, Shoaf, & Woods, 2004); nursing students (Bittman et al., 2004)
- Mechanically ventilated ICU patients (Conrad et al., 2007)
- Hospitalized psychiatric patients (Yang et al., 2012)
- Sleep enhancement for medical intensive care unit patients (Su et al., 2013)

Stimulation
- Cognitive recovery and mood poststroke (Sarkamo et al., 2008)
- Sleep disturbances in college students (Harmat, Takacs, & Bodizs, 2008)
- Head injury (Formisano et al., 2001)

Distraction
- Adjunct to spinal or general anesthesia (Lepage, Drolet, Girard, Grenier, & DeGagne, 2001; Nilsson, Rawal, Unesthahl, Zetterberg, & Unosson, 2001)
- Bone marrow biopsy and aspiration (Shabanloei, Golchin, Esfani, Dolatkhah, & Rasoulian 2010)
- Burn care (Fratianne et al., 2001; Prensner, Yowler, Smith, Steele, & Fratianne, 2001)
- Groin hemostasis with C-clamp application after percutaneous coronary intervention (Chan et al., 2006)
- Hemodialysis-associated pain and anxiety (Lin, Lu, Chen, & Chang, 2012; Pothoulaki et al., 2008)
- Cardiac laboratory environmental enhancement (Thorgaard, Henriksen, Pedersbaek, & Thomsen, 2003)
- Radiation therapy (Clark et al., 2006)

Mood management
- Managing negative or depressive mood states (Heiderscheit & Madson, 2015)

Decreasing Anxiety and Stress

One of the strongest effects of music is anxiety reduction (Chlan et al., 2013; Pelletier, 2004). Music can enhance the immediate environment, provide a diversion, and lessen the impact of potentially disturbing sounds for (Heiderscheit, 2013) patients experiencing a variety of endoscopic procedures (Wang et al., 2014) and surgical procedures (Ebneshahidi & Mohseni, 2008; Ghetti, 2012; Nilsson, 2009b). The effect of music intervention on the stress response has been documented in cardiac surgery patients (Yung et al., 2002) and in ventilator-dependent ICU patients (Almerud & Peterson, 2003; Chlan, 1998; Chlan et al., 2013; Conrad et al., 2007; Heiderscheit et al., 2011; Wong et al., 2001). Empowering ICU patients receiving mechanical ventilatory support to self-manage anxiety levels with their preferred relaxing music results in the need for less intense sedative medication regimens (Chlan et al., 2013). Music can be an efficient intervention for enriching the NICU environment and reducing stress (Kemper et al., 2004) with improvements such as enhanced oxygenation during suctioning (Chou, Wang, Chen, & Pay, 2003) and increased feeding rates (Standley, 2003). Listening to specially composed sedating piano music has been found to induce relaxation and promote sleep in a small sample of patients in a medical ICU (Su et al., 2013).

Distraction

Music is an effective adjunctive intervention for creating distraction, particularly for procedures that induce untoward symptoms and distress, such as pain and anxiety with hemodialysis (Kim et al., 2015; Lin et al., 2012; Pothoulaki et al., 2008) and in patients undergoing endoscopy (Wang et al., 2014). Music listening can effectively distract anticipatory anxiety while awaiting a dental hygiene procedure (Thoma et al., 2015). It has been found to be an adept diversional adjunct in the care of individuals with burns (Formisano et al., 2001; Prensner et al., 2001), in the management of nausea and pain intensity after bone marrow transplantation (Sahler, Hunter, & Liesveld, 2003), in people undergoing regular hemodialysis (Pothoulaki et al., 2008), and for reduction in the amount of sedation required for adults during colonoscopy (Lee et al., 2002; Smolen, Topp, & Singer, 2002).

How to Locate a Music Therapist for Consult or Collaboration

Given the importance of music-preference assessment and knowledge of the physiological and psychological influences of music on the individual listener, it may be appropriate for a nurse to consult or collaborate with a professional music therapist prior to instituting music-listening interventions. One source that nurses can access to locate a music therapist in the United States is:

American Music Therapy Association
8455 Colesville Road, Suite 1000
Silver Spring, MD 20910
www.musictherapy.org
(301) 589-3300

To locate a music therapist internationally, the World Federation of Music Therapy can be accessed at www.musictherapyworld.net.

CULTURAL APPLICATIONS

Although music may indeed be considered a universal phenomenon, there is no universal language to music. Various cultures structure music differently from what is usual to the average Western listener. For example, music from Eastern cultures contains very different tone structures and timbre, which can be foreign to the Western listener. Likewise, individuals from a non-Western culture may find the classical music of Mozart or Beethoven foreign sounding and irritating. These structural differences in what various cultures consider music are crucial to consider when implementing music-listening interventions.

Across five pain-intervention studies, Caucasians preferred orchestral music, African Americans favored jazz, and Taiwanese enjoyed harp music (Good et al., 2000). However, other investigators have found that minority older adults tend to prefer music that is familiar to their own cultural background rather than Western music (Lai, 2004). These disparate findings highlight the need for careful music-preference assessment prior to intervention. It is imperative to keep in mind that music intervention should never be used in place of pharmacological therapy for the management of acute pain. Music can, however, serve as an adjunctive intervention for pain management.

There is interest in music for clinical applications around the world, and researchers in the context of their clinical settings are exploring the benefits of music to address patient conditions that they encounter. Sidebar 7.1 provides a theoretical and clinical example of music therapy in India.

SIDEBAR 7.1. MUSIC THERAPY AS A SALUTOGENIC APPROACH INTO MEDICAL CARE: INDIAN PERSPECTIVES

Sumathy Sundar

Setting the Scene

In India, music therapy has been introduced into regular medical care. This innovation allows a shift from the pathogenic approach (focusing on factors causing diseases) to a salutogenic approach (focusing on factors influencing health; Sundar, 2016). This is supported by a steady surge of empirical evidence in understanding the mechanisms underlying the therapeutic effects of music. On one hand, the scientific aspect of music therapy is understood in a universal music therapy language. On the other hand, the "field of play" (Kenny, 2013) in music therapy is explained and understood in terms of the indigenous cultural practices and healing traditions with the use of the unique microtonal Indian music. There are both strengths and challenges in integrating these two paradoxes of science and traditions in music therapy practice in India.

Hospital-Based Clinical Practice

The "field of play" for music therapy in India is a beautiful reconciliation of science and tradition.

Although the scientific aspects of understanding the benefits of music and the therapeutic processes remain in the global framework, traditional healing practices are scientifically validated wherever possible in understanding the benefits of music therapy applications. This is the most challenging part because traditional healing practices are inherent not so much with words but by the "feeling in one's body, heart, and soul," as well as one's belief in these practices. It is important to recognize that these practices require validation.

(continued)

Relevant musicological and spiritual theories are also integrated in practice and research. A few popular healing applications used in the Indian music therapy "field of play" are *Raga Cikitsa*, Ayurveda, and Time Theory of *Ragas*. As there is increasing evidence suggesting the role of emotional factors in diseases, the beneficial effects of different *ragas* (*Raga Cikitsa*) are explained by eliciting positive emotions in the listener. These emotional responses to music can be explained by several mechanisms such as (a) brain stem reflexes, (b) rhythmic entrainment, (c) evaluative conditioning, (d) contagion, (e) visual imagery, (f) episodic memory, and (g) musical expectancy (Juslin, Liljestrom, Vastfjall, & Lundqvist, 2010). Time Theory of *Ragas* is another interesting concept in Indian classical music in that each *raga* is assigned a specific time of the day/night for performing/listening. It is believed that effects of a *raga* are best produced when it is performed or listened to during the specific time period assigned to it. This perspective can be tested by integrating concepts of the Time Theory of *Ragas* and the chronobiological Ayurvedic concepts of assigning the bio-logical energies of *Vata, Pitta*, and *Kapha* humors in different 24-hour-day time zones according to their active and inactive functional states (Sundar, Durai, & Parmar, 2016).

In India, music therapists work in many hospital clinical departments, including pediatrics, nephrology, obstetrics and gynecology, respiratory med-icine, cardiology, oncology, dermatology, surgery, and psychiatry. Likewise, music therapists work in the areas of procedural support (both diagnostic and interventional), pain management, neurological rehabilitation, and community settings serving psychiatric and transgender individuals, older adults, and chil-dren with special needs in outreach programs. Some common referral areas for music therapy include preprocedural anxiety, pain perception, sleep qual-ity, clinical depression, quality of life, emotional regulation, attention, behav-ioral disorders, and communication issues. Music therapists also work with pregnant women to help them through a healthy pregnancy and delivery of a healthy baby through a traditional *Garbh-Sanskar* (learning in the womb) pro-gram and to reduce their delivery anxiety.

Conclusion

Music therapy practice in India is strongly influenced by its cultural practices and musical traditions. Efforts are being made by music therapist researchers to explore, evaluate, understand, apply, and integrate concepts of Indian music healing traditions into current music therapy practice.

References

Juslin, P., Liljestrom, S., Vastfjall, D., & Lundqvist, L. (2010). How does music evoke emotions? Exploring underlying mechanisms. In P. Juslin & J. Sloboda (Eds.), *Handbook of music and emotion: Theory research, applications* (pp. 605–642). Oxford, UK: Oxford University Press.

Kenny, C. (2013). Music therapy theory: Yearning for beautiful ideas. *Voices Resources*. Retrieved from http://testvoices.uib.no/community/?q=fortnightly-columns/2001-music-therapy-theory-yearning-beautiful-ideas

(*continued*)

Sundar, S. (2016). Can interdisciplinary collaborative research result in newer under-
standings towards therapeutic effects of music? [Editorial]. *Annals of Sri Balaji
Vidyapeeth*, 5(2), 6.
Sundar, S., Durai, P., & Parmar, P. (2016). Indian classical music as receptive music
therapy improves *tridoshic* balance and major depression in a pregnant woman.
International Journal of Ayurveda and Pharma Research, 4(9), 8–11.

FUTURE RESEARCH

Although the evidence base is increasing, the following are areas in which research
is needed to further build the science of music intervention:

- Meta-analyses have been published on the consistent effects of music
  intervention on preoperative anxiety (Bradt, Dileo, & Shim, 2013; Dileo,
  Bradt, & Murphy, 2008), anxiety reduction in critically ill patients receiving
  mechanical ventilatory support (Bradt & Dileo, 2014; Bradt et al., 2010),
  coronary heart disease patients (Bradt, Dileo, & Potvin, 2013), and oncology
  patients (Bradt, Dileo, Magill, & Teague, 2016). Whereas music consistently
  induces favorable outcomes, pooled effect sizes can be small. Common limitations are the inconsistent use of instruments to measure phenomena, such
  as anxiety, and lack of multisite clinical trials with a well-described music-
  intervention protocol. Additional investigation is needed that builds on the
  findings of these meta-analyses through the consistent use of instruments
  to measure important clinical outcomes and the conduct of multisite clinical trials. One source for obtaining valid and reliable instruments to measure a variety of health outcomes is from the Patient-Reported Outcomes
  Measurement Information System (PROMIS) (www.healthmeasures.net/
  explore-measurement-systems/promis)
- Additional exploration into the management of symptom clusters would
  enhance the scientific base of music intervention. For example, patients with
  cancer typically experience nausea, vomiting, distress, and fatigue with treatments. Can the implementation of carefully selected music and its delivery
  improve a constellation of symptoms? Can cancer patients be taught symptom management through the self-initiation of tailored or preferred music?
- Cost and cost savings are significant issues in healthcare today. Little is
  known about the potential cost savings that could be realized with music
  intervention. Study is needed to determine whether music is a cost-effective or
  cost-neutral intervention and, if cost-effective, in which patient-care or symp-
  tom-management settings this is so.
- Much of the nursing review focuses on immediate or short-term effects of
  music intervention. It is not known whether music can be effective for managing symptoms and distress in those with chronic conditions or if it can
  improve their quality of life. Appropriate longitudinal research designs are
  needed to answer these questions.
- There is a paucity of explorations as to the appropriate or optimal timing
  for the delivery of music intervention to enhance effectiveness—and for
  which specific patient populations or symptoms. Likewise, there are scant

suggestions for the frequency of implementation music intervention and for specific symptoms.

- There is limited research on the impact of music intervention on patient satisfaction or on the patient's overall experience. Patient satisfaction with music intervention is an important outcome and quality indicator in a variety of healthcare settings. Appropriate measures and instruments are needed to capture quality data, which requires further research.
- There is an urgent need for the utilization of innovative research designs and more rapid integration of music listening into clinical practice. Music listening has been documented to be a safe nonpharmacological intervention that holds great benefit in numerous patient populations. Dissemination and implementation of music listening interventions into clinical settings is needed to ensure rapid uptake of these research findings into clinical practice in a more expedient manner. Furthermore, patients and family members can be included in the design to promote a more patient-centered approach to music-listening interventions.

Although an intervention study itself is labor intensive, there is a need for additional investigation on music intervention. The knowledge base about music intervention for promotion of patient health and well-being can be expanded through high-quality research and by dissemination of those findings in a timely manner. To further build a strong body of knowledge surrounding the implementation and outcomes of music intervention, the authors of this chapter recommend an interdisciplinary approach: nurses and music therapists conducting collaborative research. From quality evidence, music-intervention implementation guidelines can then be integrated into patient care.

REFERENCES

Almerud, S., & Peterson, K. (2003). Music therapy—A complementary treatment for mechanically ventilated intensive care patients. *International Critical Care Nursing, 19*(1), 21–30.

American Heritage Dictionary of the English Language (4th ed.). (2016). Boston, MA: Houghton Mifflin Harcourt.

American Music Therapy Association. (2014). *AMTA member and workforce analysis.* Silver Spring, MD: Author.

Bensimon, M., Amir, D., & Wolf, Y. (2008). Drumming through trauma: Music therapy with post-traumatic soldiers. *Arts in Psychotherapy, 35*(1), 34–48.

Bittman, B., Berk, L., Felten, D., Westengard, J., Simonton, O., Pappas, J., & Ninehouser, M. (2001). Composite effects of group drumming music therapy on modulation of neuroendocrine-immune parameters of normal subjects. *Alternative Therapy Health Medicine, 7,* 38–47.

Bittman, B., Bruhn, K., Stevens, C., Westengard, J., & Umbach, P. (2003). Recreational music-making: A cost effective group interdisciplinary strategy of reducing burnout and improving mood states in long-term care workers. *Advances in Mind-Body Medicine, 19*(3/4), 4–15.

Bittman, B. B., Snyder, C., Bruhn, K. T., Liebfreid, F., Stevens, C. K., Westengard, J., & Umbach, P. O. (2004). Recreational music-making: An integrative group intervention for reducing burnout and improving mood states in first-year associate degree nursing students: Insights and economic impact. *International Journal of Nursing Education Scholarship, 1,* Article 12.

Bradt, J., & Dileo C. (2014). Music interventions for mechanically ventilated patients. *Cochrane Database of Systematic Reviews,* (12), CD006902. doi:10.1002/14651858.CD006902.pub3

Bradt, J., Dileo, C., & Grocke, D. (2010). Music interventions for mechanically ventilated patients. *Cochrane Database of Systematic Reviews,* (12), CD006902. doi:10.1002/14651858.CD006902.pub2

Bradt, J., Dileo, C., Magill, L., & Teague, A. (2016). Music interventions for improving psychological and physical outcomes in cancer patients. *Cochrane Database of Systematic Reviews*, (8), CD006911. doi:10.1002/14651858.CD006911.pub3

Bradt, J., Dileo, C., & Potvin, N. (2013). Music for stress and anxiety reduction in coronary heart disease patients. *Cochrane Database of Systematic Reviews*, (12), CD006577. doi:10.1002/14651858.CD006577.pub3

Bradt, J., Dileo, C., & Shim, M. (2013). Music interventions for preoperative anxiety. *Cochrane Database of Systematic Reviews*, (6), CD006908. doi:10.1002/14651858.CD006908.pub2

Bruscia, K. (2014). *Defining music therapy* (3rd ed.). University Park, IL: Barcelona Publishers.

Carr, C., d'Ardenne, P., Sloboda, A., Scott, C., Wang, D., & Priebe, S. (2012). Group music therapy for patients with persistent post-traumatic stress disorder: An exploratory randomized controlled trial with mixed methods evaluation. *Psychology and Psychotherapy: Theory, Research and Practice*, *85*(2), 179–202.

Chan, M. F., Wong, O. C., Chan, H. L., Fong, M. C., Lai, S. Y., Lo, C. W., … Leung, S. K. (2006). Effects of music on patients undergoing C-clamp procedure after percutaneous coronary interventions. *Journal of Advanced Nursing*, *53*(6), 669–679.

Chlan, L. (1998). Effectiveness of a music therapy intervention on relaxation and anxiety for patients receiving ventilatory assistance. *Heart & Lung*, *27*(3), 169–176.

Chlan, L., Evans, D., Greenleaf, M., & Walker, J. (2000). Effects of a single music therapy intervention on anxiety, discomfort, satisfaction, and compliance with screening guidelines in outpatients undergoing screening flexible sigmoidoscopy. *Gastroenterology Nursing*, *23*(4), 148–156.

Chlan, L., & Heiderscheit, A. (2009). A tool for music preference assessment in critically ill patients receiving mechanical ventilatory support: An interdisciplinary approach. *Music Therapy Perspectives*, *27*(1), 42–47.

Chlan, L., Weinert, C., Heiderscheit, A., Tracy, M. F., Skaar, D., Guttormson, J., & Savik, K. (2013). Effects of patient directed music intervention on anxiety and sedative exposure in critically ill patients receiving mechanical ventilatory support. *Journal of the American Medical Association*, *309*(22). doi:10.1001/jama.2013.5670

Choi, A., Lee, M., Cheong, K., & Lee, J. (2009). Effects of group music intervention on behavioral and psychological symptoms in patients with dementia: A pilot controlled trial. *International Journal of Neuroscience*, *119*(4), 471–481.

Chou, L., Wang, R., Chen, S., & Pay, L. (2003). Effects of music therapy on oxygen saturation in premature infants receiving endotracheal suctioning. *Journal of Nursing Research*, *11*(3), 209–215.

Clark, M., Isaacks-Donton, G., Wells, N., Redlin-Frazier, S., Eck, C., Hepworth, J. T., & Chakravarthy, B. (2006). Use of preferred music to reduce emotional distress and symptom activity during radiation therapy. *Journal of Music Therapy*, *43*(3), 247–265.

Conrad, C., Niess, H., Jauch, K. W., Bruns, C., Hartl, W., & Welker, L. (2007). Overture for growth hormone: Requiem for interleukin-6? *Critical Care Medicine*, *35*(12), 2709–2713.

Cooke, M. L., Moyle, W., Shum, D. H., Harrison, S. D., & Murfield, J. E. (2010). A randomized controlled trial exploring the effect of music on agitated behaviours and anxiety in older people with dementia. *Aging & Mental Health*, *14*(8), 905–916.

Crowe, B. (2004). *Music and soul making: Toward a new theory of music therapy*. Oxford, UK: Scarecrow Press.

Davies, R., Baker, F., Tamplin, J., Bajo, E., Bolger, K., Sheers, N., & Berlowitz, D. (2016). Music-assisted relaxation during transition to non-invasive ventilation in people with motor neuron disease: A qualitative case series. *British Journal of Music Therapy*, *30*(2), 74–82.

Davis, T., & Jones, P. (2012). Music therapy: Decreasing anxiety in the ventilated patient: A review of the literature. *Dimensions of Critical Care Nursing*, *31*(3), 159–166.

Davis, W., Gfeller, K., & Thaut, M. (2008). *An introduction to music therapy: Theory and practice*. New York, NY: McGraw-Hill.

Dileo, C., Bradt, J., & Murphy, K. (2008) Music for preoperative anxiety (Protocol). *Cochrane Database of Systematic Reviews*, (1), CD006908. doi:10.1002/14651858.CD006908

Dissanayake, W. (2009). Bodies swayed to music: The temporal arts as integral to ceremonial ritual. In S. Malcok & C. Trevarthen (Eds.), *Communicative musicality: Exploring the basis of human companionship* (pp. 17–30). Oxford, UK: Oxford University Press.

Dunn, K. (2004). Music and the reduction of post-operative pain. *Nursing Standard, 18*(36), 33–39.

Ebneshahidi, A., & Mohseni, M. (2008). The effect of patient-selected music on early postoperative pain, anxiety, and hemodynamic profile in cesarean section surgery. *Journal of Alternative and Complementary Medicine, 14*(7), 827–831.

Ferrer, A. (2007). The effect of live music on decreasing anxiety in patients undergoing chemotherapy treatment. *Journal of Music Therapy, 44*(3), 242–255.

Formisano, R., Vinicola, V., Penta, F., Matteis, M., Brunelli, S., & Weckel, J. (2001). Active music therapy in the rehabilitation of severe brain injured patients during coma recovery. *Annali Dell Instituto Superiore di Sanitá, 37*(4), 627–630.

Fratianne, R., Prensner, J., Huston, M., Super, D., Yowler, C., & Standley, J. (2001). The effect of music-based imagery and musical alternate engagement on the burn debridement process. *Journal of Burn Care & Rehabilitation, 22*(1), 47–53.

Ghetti, C. (2012). Music therapy as procedural support for invasive medical procedures: Toward the development of music therapy theory. *Nordic Journal of Music Therapy, 21*(1), 3–35.

Good, M., Picot, B., Salem, S., Chin, C., Picot, S., & Lane, D. (2000). Cultural differences in music chosen for pain relief. *Journal of Holistic Nursing, 18*(3), 245–260.

Good, M., Stanton-Hicks, M., Grass, J., Anderson, G. C., Lai, H., Roykulcahroen, V., ... Adler, P. A. (2001). Relaxation and music to reduce postsurgical pain. *Journal of Advanced Nursing, 33*(2), 208–215.

Grocke, D., & Wigram, T. (2007). *Receptive methods in music therapy: Techniques and clinical applications for music therapy clinicians, educators and students.* London, UK: Jessica Kingsley.

Guetin, S., Ginies, P., Siou, D. K., Picot, M. C., Pommie, C., Guldner, E., ... Touchon, J. (2012). The effects of music intervention in the management of chronic pain: A single-blind, randomized, controlled trial. *Clinical Journal of Pain, 28*(4), 329–337.

Guzzetta, C. (1995). Music therapy: Hearing the melody of the soul. In B. Dossey, L. Keegan, C. Guzzetta, & L. Kolkmeier (Eds.), *Holistic nursing* (pp. 670–698). Gaithersburg, MD: Aspen.

Haas, R., & Brandes, V. (Eds.). (2009). *Music that works: Contributions of biology, neurophysiology, psychology, sociology, medicine and musicology.* New York, NY: Springer Wien.

Harmat, L., Takacs, J., & Bodizs, R. (2008). Music improves sleep quality in students. *Journal of Advanced Nursing, 62*(3), 327–335.

Heiderscheit, A. (2013). Music therapy in surgical and procedural support for adult medical patients. In J. Allen (Ed.), *Guidelines for music therapy with adult medical patients* (pp. 17–34). Gilsum, NH: Barcelona Publishers.

Heiderscheit, A., Breckenridge, S., Chlan, L., & Savik, K. (2014). Music preferences of mechanically ventilated patients participating in a randomized controlled trial. *Music and Medicine, 6*(2), 29–38.

Heiderscheit, A., Chlan, L., & Donley, K. (2011). Instituting a music listening intervention for critically ill patients receiving mechanical ventilation: Exemplars from two patient cases. *Music and Medicine, 3*(4), 239–245.

Heiderscheit, A., & Madson, A. (2015). Use of the iso principle as a central method in mood management: A music psychotherapy clinical case study. *Music Therapy Perspectives, 33*(1), 45–52.

Hicks-Moore, S. (2005). Relaxing music at mealtime in nursing homes. *Journal of Gerontological Nursing, 31*(12), 26–32.

Hodges, D., & Sebald, D. (2011). *Music in the human experience: An introduction to music psychology.* New York, NY: Routledge.

Huang, S., Good, M., & Zauszniewski, J. (2010). The effectiveness of music in relieving pain in cancer patients: A randomized controlled trial. *International Journal of Nursing Studies, 47*(11), 1354–1362.

Johnson, B., Raymond, S., & Goss, J. (2012). Perioperative music or headsets to decrease anxiety. *Journal of Perianesthesia Nursing, 27*(3), 146–154.

Kain, Z., Sevarino, F., Alexander, G., Pincus, S., & Mayes, L. (2000). Preoperative anxiety and post-operative pain in women undergoing hysterectomy: A repeated-measures design. *Journal of Psychosomatic Research, 49*, 417–422.

Kemper, K., Martin, K., Block, S., Shoaf, R., & Woods, C. (2004). Attitudes and expectations about music therapy for premature infants among staff in the neonatal intensive care unit. *Alternative Therapies in Health & Medicine, 10*(2), 50–54.

Kim, Y., Evangelista, L., & Park, Y. G. (2015). Anxiolytic effects of music interventions in patients receiving incenter hemodialysis: A systematic review and meta-analysis. *Nephrology Nursing Journal, 42*(4), 339–347.

Koelsch, S., Fuermetz, J., Sack, U., Bauer, K., Hohenadel, M., Wiegel, M., & Heinke, W. (2011). Effects of music listening on cortisol levels and propofol consumption during spinal anesthesia. *Frontiers in Psychology, 2*, 58. doi:10.3389/fpsyg.2011.00058

Kulkarni, S., Johnson, P. C., Kettles, S., & Kasthuri, R. S. (2012). Music during interventional radiological procedures, effect on sedation, pain and anxiety: A randomized controlled trial. *British Journal of Radiology, 85*(10), 1059–1063.

Lai, H. L. (2004). Music preference and relaxation in Taiwanese elderly people. *Geriatric Nursing, 25*(5), 286–291.

Laurion, S., & Fetzer, S. J. (2003). The effect of two nursing interventions on the postoperative outcomes of gynecologic laparoscopic patients. *Journal of Perianesthesia Nursing, 18*(4), 254–261.

Lee, D., Henderson, A., & Shum, D. (2004). The effect of music on preprocedure anxiety in Hong Kong Chinese day patients. *Journal of Clinical Nursing, 13*, 297–303.

Lee, D. W. H., Chan, K., Poon, C., Ko, C., Cha, K., Sin, K., & Chan, A. C. W. (2002). Relaxation music decreases the dose of patient-controlled sedation during colonoscopy: A prospective randomized controlled trial. *Gastrointestinal Endoscopy, 55*(1), 33–36.

Lepage, C., Drolet, P., Girard, M., Grenier, Y., & DeGagne, R. (2001). Music decreases sedative requirements during spinal anesthesia. *Anesthesia and Analgesia, 93*, 912–916.

Lin, Y. J., Lu, K. C., Chen, C., & Chang, C. C. (2012). The effects of music as therapy on the overall well-being of elderly patients on maintenance hemodialysis. *Biological Research for Nursing, 14*(3), 277–285.

MacDonald, R., Kreutz, G., & Mitchell, L. (2012). *Music, health, and wellbeing.* New York, NY: Oxford University Press.

Maranto, C. (1993). Applications of music in medicine. In M. Heal & T. Wigram (Eds.), *Music therapy in health and education* (pp. 153–174). London, UK: Jessica Kingsley.

Moore, R., Staum, M., & Brotons, M. (1992). Music preferences of the elderly: Repertoire, vocal ranges, tempos, and accompaniments for singing. *Journal of Music Therapy, 29*(4), 236–252.

Nightingale, F. (1969). *Notes on nursing.* New York, NY: Dover. (Original work published 1860.)

Nilsson, U. (2009a). The effect of music intervention in stress response to cardiac surgery in a randomized clinical trial. *Heart & Lung, 38*(3), 201–207.

Nilsson, U. (2009b). Soothing music can increase oxytocin levels during bed rest after open-heart surgery: A randomized control trial. *Journal of Clinical Nursing, 8*, 2153–2161.

Nilsson, U., Rawal, N., Unesthahl, L., Zetterberg, C., & Unosson, M. (2001). Improved recovery after music and therapeutic suggestions during general anesthesia: A double-blind randomized controlled trial. *Acta Anesthesiologica Scandinavica, 45*, 812–817.

Okumura, Y., Asano, Y., Takenaka, S., Fukuyama., S., Yonezawa, S., Kasuya, Y., & Shinoda, J. (2014). Brain activation by music in patients in a vegetative or minimally conscious state following diffuse brain injury. *Brain Injury, 28*(7), 944–950.

Pelletier, C. (2004). The effect of music on decreasing arousal due to stress: A meta-analysis. *Journal of Music Therapy, 41*, 192–214.

Pothoulaki, R., MacDonald, P., Flowers, E., Stamataki, V., Filiopoulos, D., Stamatiadis, D., & Stathakis, C. (2008). An investigation of the effects of music on anxiety and pain perception in patients undergoing haemodialysis treatment. *Journal of Health Psychology, 13*(7), 912–920.

Prensner, J. D., Yowler, C. J., Smith, L. F., Steele, A. L., & Fratianne, R. B. (2001). Music therapy for assistance with pain and anxiety management in burn treatment. *Journal of Burn Care & Rehabilitation, 22*(1), 83–88.

Public Radio Music Source. (2018). Public Radio market. Retrieved from www.prms.org

Robb, S., Nichols, R., Rutan, R., Bishop, B., & Parker, J. (1995). The effects of music-assisted relaxation on preoperative anxiety. *Journal of Music Therapy, 32*(1), 3–12.

Rutherford, T., Kennedy, M., & Kennedy, J. (2013). *The Oxford dictionary of music* (6th ed.). Oxford, UK. Oxford University Press.

Sahler, O., Hunter, B., & Liesveld, J. (2003). The effect of using music therapy with relaxation imagery in the management of patients undergoing bone marrow transplantation: A pilot feasibility study. *Alternative Therapies in Health and Medicine, 9*(6), 70–74.

Salimpoor, V., Benovoy, M., Larcher, K., Dagher, A., & Zatorre, R. (2011). Anatomically distinct dopamine release during anticipation and experience of peak emotion to music. *Nature Neuroscience, 14*(2), 257–262.

Sarkamo, T., Tervaniemi, M., Laitinen, S., Forsblom, A., Soinila, S., Mikkonene, M., ... Hietanen, M. (2008). Music listening enhances cognitive recovery and mood after middle cerebral artery stroke. *Brain, 131*, 866–876.

Shabanloei, R., Golchin, M., Esfani, A., Dolatkhah, R., & Rasoulian, M. (2010). Effects of music therapy on pain and anxiety in patients undergoing bone marrow biopsy and aspiration. *Association of Operating Room Nurses Journal, 91*(6), 746–751.

Shertzer, K., & Keck, J. (2001). Music and the PACU environment. *Journal of Perianesthesia Nursing, 16*(2), 90–102.

Smolen, D., Topp, R., & Singer, L. (2002). The effect of self-selected music during colonoscopy on anxiety, heart rate and blood pressure. *Applied Nursing Research, 16*(2), 126–130.

Standley, J. M. (2003). The effect of music-reinforced nonnutritive sucking on feeding rate of premature infants. *Journal of Pediatric Nursing, 18*(3), 169–173.

Su, C. P., Lai, H. L., Chang, E. T., Yiin, L. M., Perng, S. J., & Chen, P. W. (2013). A randomized controlled trial of the effects of listening to non-commercial music on quality of nocturnal sleep and relaxation indices in patients in medical intensive care unit. *Journal of Advanced Nursing, 69*(6), 1377–1389.

Thaut, M. H. (1990). Physiological and motor responses to music stimuli. In R. F. Unkefer (Ed.), *Music therapy in the treatment of adults with mental disorders: Theoretical bases and clinical interventions* (pp. 33–49). New York, NY: Schirmer Books.

Thoma, M., Zemp, M., Kreienbuhl, L., Hofer, D., Schmidlin, P., Attin, T., ... Nater, U. (2015). Effects of music listening on pre-treatment anxiety and stress levels in a dental hygiene recall population. *International Journal of Behavioral Medicine, 22*, 498 505.

Thomas, D., & Smith, M. (2009). The effect of music on caloric consumption among nursing home residents with dementia of the Alzheimer's type. *Activities, Adaptation & Aging, 33*, 1–16.

Thorgaard, B., Henriksen, B., Pedersbaek, G., & Thomsen, I. (2003). Specially selected music in the cardiac laboratory—An important tool for improvement of the well-being of patients. *European Journal of Cardiovascular Nursing, 3*(1), 21–26.

Wachi, M., Koyama, M., Utsuyama, M., Bittman, B., Kitagawa, M., & Hirokawa, K. (2007). Recreational music-making modulates natural killer cell activity, cytokines, and mood states in corporate employees. *Medical Science Monitor, 13*(2), 57–70.

Wang, M., Zhang, L., Zhang, Y., Zhang, Y., Xu, X. D., & Zhang, Y. C. (2014). Effect of music in endoscopy procedures: Systematic review and meta-analysis of randomized controlled trials. *Pain Medicine, 15*, 1786-1974.

Whitehead-Pleaux, A., Zebrowski, N., Baryza, M., & Sheridan, R. (2007). Exploring the effects of music therapy on pediatric pain: Phase 1. *Journal of Music Therapy, 34*(3), 217–241.

Winkelman, M. (2003). Complementary therapy for addiction: "Drumming out drugs." *American Journal of Public Health, 93*(4), 647–651.

Wong, H., Lopez Nahas, V., & Molassiotis, A. (2001). Effects of music therapy on anxiety in ventilator-dependent patients. *Heart & Lung, 30*(5), 376–387.

World Federation of Music Therapy. (2014). WFMT strategic plan. Retrieved from http://www.wfmt.info/resource-centers/publication-center/wfmt-documents

Yang, C. Y., Chen, C. H., Chu, H., Chen, W. C., Lee, T. Y., Chen, S. G., & Chou, K. R. (2012). The effect of music therapy on hospitalized psychiatric patients' anxiety, finger temperature, and electroencephalography: A randomized clinical trial. *Biological Research for Nursing, 14*(2), 197–206.

Yung, P., Chui-Kam, S., French, P., & Chan, T. (2002). A controlled trial of music and preoperative anxiety in Chinese men undergoing transurethral resection of the prostate. *Journal of Advanced Nursing, 39*(4), 352–359.

8

Humor

SHIRLEY K. TROUT

There seems to be a nearly universal consensus that humor and laughter are good for humans and that good humor promotes good health. The phrase "laughter is the best medicine" has been tossed about as proven as the sun rising in the east each morning. But is it? And if laughter *should be* the best medicine, does that mean therapeutic humor would be, as well? Does the medicine help just the body, or could laughter—and perhaps humor—help the whole person in other ways? The fact is, there is very little conclusive evidence that definitively demonstrates that either laughter or humor can improve physical health.

Despite the existence of only limited research that supports the use of humor as a healing modality, many professions have an interest in its role in maintaining and promoting health and healing. Interestingly, it was Norman Cousins's personal story, an anecdote in research terms, that launched today's interest in humor and laughter as a viable therapy for healing (Cousins, 1979). His intriguing experience with using laughter to overcome illness helped initiate today's emerging interdisciplinary fields of psychoneuroimmunology and, somewhat less directly, positive psychology. There is a growing body of evidence that validates humor as an appropriate complementary therapy.

DEFINITION

Too often, the two related yet far different terms *laughter* and *humor* are used interchangeably as though they are one and the same. Even authors of peer-reviewed publications are sometimes guilty of this error. To use the two terms interchangeably reflects a common lack of serious consideration of either and completely ignores specifics within each. For example, when referring to laughter, do authors mean mirthful laughter or nonemotional laughter? Referring to humor, is it comedy, wit, or mirth? Regarding therapeutic humor, is it the study about coping humor, sense of humor, or types of humor? In general, are researchers asking the right questions and using rigor in their study design and analyses?

Humor

Although the term *humor* has never been definitively defined by experts, it is clearly distinct from the personality-based consideration of sense of humor (Svebak, Kristoffersen, & Aasarod, 2006). Any definition of humor must be developed from a particular theory, such as superiority/disparagement, arousal, incongruity–resolution, or reversal, each of which has its respective body of theory-development literature. The definition of *humor* selected for this chapter is based on the incongruity theory. *Humor* is defined as "simply one element of the comic—as are wit, fun, nonsense, sarcasm, ridicule, satire, or irony—and basically denotes a smiling attitude toward life and its imperfections: an understanding of the incongruities of existence" (Ruch, 1998, p. 6).

Therapeutic Humor

When defining *therapeutic humor*, it helps to make clear what it is *not*. Therapeutic humor is not laughter, which is a physiological phenomenon (although laughter almost always becomes a part of the consideration of humor). It is not comedy, which has a singular purpose of making people laugh. Humor may be used to poke fun *at* the illness or some other element of the health condition or environment, *not* used to poke fun at an individual. Humor helps people laugh *with* each other.

Psychotherapist Steve Sultanoff clarifies the key difference between, for example, comedy-club humor and therapeutic humor: "The purposeful intention of using therapeutic humor as a complementary therapy must clearly be *for the benefit of the client or patient* [emphasis added] and not for the therapist's [i.e., nurse's] personal gratification or merely for pleasure" (Steve Sultanoff, personal communication, December 4, 2012). Therapeutic humor has been defined as "any intervention that promotes health and wellness by stimulating a playful discovery, expression, or appreciation of the absurdity or incongruity of life's situations. This intervention may enhance health or be used as a complementary treatment of illness to facilitate healing or coping, whether physical, emotional, cognitive, social, or spiritual" (Association for Applied and Therapeutic Humor [AATH], 2000).

SCIENTIFIC BASIS

To put the evidence into perspective, it is important to understand some of the history of today's interest in therapeutic humor and laughter. In 1963, psychiatric researcher Dr. William Fry published a small book titled, *Sweet Madness: A Study of Humor*, in which he organized his personal thoughts about humor's relationship to mental health. This theoretical publication and its author were mostly confined to the academic community. Sixteen years later, in 1979, *Saturday Review* editor Norman Cousins (1915–1990) introduced to popular culture his award-winning book *Anatomy of an Illness as Perceived by the Patient*. In this work, Cousins recounts his personal journey of forcing a debilitating and painful illness, ankylosing spondylitis, into remission by using a self-prescribed (with his physician's approval) regimen of mirthful laughter and megadoses of vitamin C. His thought for trying this was: If negative thinking can make you ill (validated by research by that time), then could positive thinking make you well? Interestingly, Mr. Cousins's book is credited with launching today's growing interest in humor and laughter as complementary therapies in healthcare.

The International Society for Humor Studies (ISHS; www.hnu.edu/ishs) is a scholarly organization specifically dedicated to furthering the study and understanding of humor in a wide range of disciplines, including therapeutic humor–related areas. This community of scholars has helped aggregate and strengthen research efforts within this emerging field. As with all professional development, nurses are encouraged to examine original research to evaluate the studies, their strengths, and potential applicability. More important, the ISHS provides connections with an international community of scholars informing the conversations around therapeutic humor.

In general, it is agreed that humor is fundamentally a social phenomenon. However, because it involves cognitive processing, it is available to individuals in isolation as well. Some of the most compelling qualitative examples of humor's value as a coping mechanism for individuals, as well as groups, are revealed by those who have experienced captivity. Lipman's compilation of interviews with Holocaust survivors serves as a powerful testimony as to how valuable humor may be to human survival. Lipman (1991) noted that "during the Holocaust, religion and humor served a like—though not identical—purpose" (p. 11). He concluded that "the former [religion] oriented one's thoughts to a better existence in the next world, the latter [humor] pointed to emotional salvation in this one" (p. 11).

Within the realm of social interaction, researchers have worked to understand how humor is used to incorporate, embrace, and even celebrate the contradictions, incongruities, and ambiguities inherent in interpersonal relationships (Mulkay, 1988). Within this sphere, Martin (2007) cautions that more study is required before the full extent of the interpersonal, cognitive, mental health, coping, and other psychological impacts of humor can be fully understood.

One finding has scientific attention and some preliminary empirical support: Even the mere *anticipation* of a humorous or laughter event triggers a positive impact on a variety of biological (serum catecholamines and cortisol) health indicators (L. S. Berk, Tan, & Berk, 2008). In addition, there appears to be a secret weapon available to nurses that may, one day, undergird the connection between therapeutic humor and the effectiveness of nursing care: *Get the patient to smile!* The more pleasant (mirthful) the emotion accompanying the smile, the greater the positive responses. Researchers do not yet fully understand everything about why and how this works, but even simply moving one's facial muscles into a smiling position appears to improve stress- and mood-related indicators, similar to what happens in anticipation of a joyful event. In one revealing study, subjects who simply held a pencil in their mouths to stimulate the facial muscles used in smiling rated cartoons as funnier and reported greater increases in positive mood (compared with subjects who held the pen in a way that inhibited such muscle contractions; Strack, Martin, & Stepper, 1988).

Selected Evidence

In a review of recent health-related literature, numerous articles were found in which the authors touted the benefits of humor-related interventions and programs or presented studies that described its physiological effects. No recent systematic reviews of randomized controlled trials of humor-related therapies were identified. Earlier narrative reviews generally confirm the findings of the studies included in the present review, that some laughter and humor therapies accrued health benefits without ill effects/contraindications (McCreaddie & Wiggins, 2008; Mora-Ripoll, 2011). Studies examined effects of humor-related interventions, such as laughter yoga, clowning, humor groups, and humorous videos. In general, the studies identified were small (many pilot or feasibility studies), with weak (e.g., quasiexperimental or nonblinded) designs. It is difficult to synthesize the available studies in the literature because there is a significant range in the interventions studied, and even when there were common intervention modalities, the studies' used protocols varied (e.g., timing, frequency, other ways that the modality was operationalized). Furthermore, the studies were conducted in a very wide range of populations (e.g., children, elderly) and settings (e.g., palliative care, cancer care, and behavioral health treatment settings; hospitals; long-term care), and they targeted different outcomes.

Despite the shortcomings of the available evidence base, interest in the potential health benefits of humor, laughter, and positive mood continues. Selected studies published in 2014 or after illustrate the scientific interest in the health effects of a wide variety of humor-related interventions in a broad array of practice settings and populations of patients with a variety of conditions (see Table 8.1). It is clear that humor and humor-related interventions are likely to engender ongoing interest among scientists and healthcare providers because of their intuitive, inherent appeal and the perceived benefits to patients and families.

Martin (2007) concludes that "of all the health benefits claimed for humor and laughter, the most consistent research support has been found for the hypothesized analgesic effects" (p. 331). He goes on to say. "Although humor may not produce all the health benefits that have been claimed, at least it is not likely to be harmful and it can enhance people's enjoyment if not the duration of their lives" (p. 331).

As is understandably the case with studying a phenomenon as complex as humor, one can certainly find arguments against virtually every finding published. Table 8.2 provides some of the significant findings related to therapeutic humor, along with at least one citation related to a finding that is representative of the body of research examining and exploring the respective conclusions. The citations included were selected to include one or more of the key scholars involved in this area of study.

INTERVENTION

Therapeutic humor is as much of an art as it is a science. Therefore, with practice, study, and self-reflection, individuals can find their own personal rhythm and style for how, when, and with whom to engage in this complementary therapy. Humor that is genuinely therapeutic requires a caring heart, keen attention to detail, considerate timing, and creativity. What works for one person may not work for another; a one-size-fits-all formula may never exist. Furthermore, humor does not always work, regardless of how well intentioned the nurse who uses it. In time, however, one gets better by being willing to learn from past experiences, being open to feedback, and striving to improve practice.

Humor typically works because of an incongruence that surprises the receiver. Few people enter a healthcare setting focused on anything but the health concern that brought them there. This provides ample opportunities to shift the wit of patients and their families. The comedic gap that is associated with incongruities may be used in many situations.

Table 8.1 Selected Recent Studies Illustrating Humor-Related Interventions and Outcomes

Authors (Date)	Type of Humor Intervention	Population/Condition Groups; (Sample Size = N)	Selected Outcomes/Effects
Ben-Pazi (2017)	Clown-care	Children with cerebral palsy having injections ($N = 45$) randomized to clown or standard care	Pain during injections was reduced with clown-care, even when crossed over into standard care group.
Felluga et al. (2016)	Clowntherapy	Children in emergency room ($N = 40$) randomized to clown group or control group	Anxiety, but not pain, were reduced.
Meiri, Ankri, Hamad-Saied, Konopnicki, and Pillar (2016)	"Clowning"	Children age 2–10 years having blood drawn, randomly assigned to clowning, local anesthetic, or control ($N = 100$)	Duration of crying was lower in clown group compared with control; parental perception of child anxiety and beneficial effects were superior with clown group.
Cai, Yu, Rong, and Zhong (2014)	Humor skill training intervention	Adults ($N = 30$) with schizophrenia; randomized to humor skill training or control group (handwork)	Sense of humor and rehabilitative outcomes were improved in the humor group in the rehabilitative stage.
Kim et al. (2015)	Laughter therapy	Adults undergoing cancer radiation ($N = 62$) randomized into laughter therapy or wait-list control	The laughter therapy group reported greater mood disturbance reduction, greater decrease in mood disturbance, and greater self-esteem.
Ghodsbin, Ahmadi, Jahanbin, and Shrif (2015)	Laughter therapy	Senior citizens at community center ($N = 72$) randomly assigned to laughter therapy or control	Seniors having laughter therapy improved in reported general health, somatic symptoms, insomnia, anxiety, and measures of health.

(continued)

Table 8.1 Selected Recent Studies Illustrating Humor-Related Interventions and Outcomes (*continued*)

Authors (Date)	Type of Humor Intervention	Population/Condition Groups; (Sample Size = *N*)	Selected Outcomes/Effects
Sim (2015)	Program of humor intervention	School-age children with chronic diseases—atopic dermatitis and type 1 diabetes (*N* = 33), were divided into humor intervention or control.	The humor group had significant decreases in behavior problems and increased resilience scores relative to the control group.
Wellenzohn, Proyer, and Ruch (2016)	Five humor-based online positive psychology interventions	Adults (*N* = 632) participated in a placebo-controlled study of five 1-week humor-based activities.	Happiness was enhanced; there was short-term reduction of depression.
Bains et al. (2015)	Humorous videos	Older adults (*N* = 50): one healthy group, one group with type 2 diabetes, and a control group	There were positive improvements in learning ability and short-term memory and decreases in cortisol for humor groups only before and after videos.
Kuru and Kublay (2016)	Laughter therapy	Residents from two nursing homes (*N* = 65): one intervention and one control home	General and subscale scores of health-related quality of life as measured by the Short-Form Health Survey improved significantly in residents receiving laughter therapy.

Table 8.2 Humor and Laughter Research Relevant to Therapeutic Humor

Empirical Facts	Selected Citations	Comments, Including Outcome Measures
Smiling (Duchenne smile) is virtually universally interpreted as a *positive* communication indicating cheerfulness or playful emotions. This smile has been the only positive emotion facial expression to be interpreted with such universal consistency, although several *negative* emotions have been recognized across cultures.	Ekman and Friesen (1978)	Marked the creation of the FACS, which has been used extensively in a wide range of research and continues to demonstrate significant reliability.
Humor appreciation and comprehension evolve from physical to cognitive over one's developmental years.	McGhee (1979)	A foundational humor piece to explore humor's impact on the mind and body. More recently, McGhee is designing research-based applications of humor (see www.laughterremedy.com)
The Duchenne (enjoyment) smile has been shown to be even more responsible for increasing pain tolerance than actual laughing.	Zweyer, Velker, and Ruch (2004)	Enjoyment that was expressed facially was found to be the mediator between perceiving a humorous film and the change in pain perception.
Sense of humor tends to moderate one's reaction to stress or self-reported level of stress, and humor types appear to be related, although results are inconclusive at this time.	Martin and Dobbin (1988)	Many interesting, albeit not absolutely conclusive, findings are emerging related to humor type and a range of psychological outcomes, such as coping and pain tolerance.
Mirthful laughter has been shown to increase HDL cholesterol and decrease LDL immediately, and in one study, improved conditions remained at 4 months follow-up. The *anticipation* of a laughter event has demonstrated similar results in a growing number of studies.	L. S. Berk, Tan, and Berk (2008); L. S. Berk, Tan, and Tan (2008); Mahony, Burroughs, and Hieatt (2001)	Patients in the laughter groups had lower EP and NEP levels by 2 months; increased HDL cholesterol; decreased TNF-alpha, IFN-gamma, IL-6, and CRP levels by 4 months; and a lower incidence of MI (1/10) than the control group (3/10).

(continued)

Table 8.2 Humor and Laughter Research Relevant to Therapeutic Humor (*continued*)

Empirical Facts	Selected Citations	Comments, Including Outcome Measures
		The authors concluded that addition of mirthful laughter may be an effective CV preventive adjunct in diabetes mellitus and metabolic syndrome care. Effects may contribute to lower MI occurrence.
		Note: The *anticipation* of a pleasant (laughter) event resulted in changes at least as strong as and consistent with the laughter event itself, suggesting that the benefits of therapeutic humor may extend beyond humor or laughter per se.
A complex relationship exists between behavior associated with emotion and the human CV system.	Miller and Fry (2009)	Dr. Fry continues to contribute to the science of humor.
The positive emotion elicited by humor appears to be closely related to the pleasurable feelings associated with other agreeable, emotionally rewarding activities, including ingestion of mood-altering drugs (heroin or alcohol), eating, sexual activity, enjoyable music, or video games.	Schultz (2002)	Much remains to be understood about how the brain processes complexities of humor. This research has introduced intriguing findings.
Humor and creativity are closely related in that they both involve a switch of perspective or a new way of seeing things, most convincingly through the positive emotion of mirth.	Isen (2003)	Positive emotional states, including mirth, affect various cognitive processes such as memory, judgment, risk-taking, and decision making.

CRP, C-reactive protein; CV, cardiovascular; EP, epinephrine; FACS, Facial Action Coding System; HDL, high-density lipoprotein; IFN-gamma, interferon-gamma; IL-6, interleukin-6; LDL, low-density lipoprotein; MI, myocardial infarction; NEP, norepinephrine; TNF-alpha, tumor necrosis factor-alpha.

Incongruity

Although many forms of humor exist, incongruity of some sort is considered an essential element of humor (Martin, 2007). The term *incongruity* is familiar in discussions of both humor and comedy, especially regarding the word's definition of being incompatible. That is, when two realities lack harmony or are incompatible with each other, it creates a juxtaposition that can lead to humor, a chuckle, or even a hardy belly laugh. In comedy, incongruity is the key to creating jokes that resonate with an audience and result in laughter. Comedy writers consider the gap between the *reality* (real or perceived) and the *ideal* state (real or perceived). In this gap or space, jokes reside.

Using humor involves a cognitive shift in perspective that allows one to distance oneself from the immediate threat of a problem situation (R. A. Berk, 2001). Indeed, humor and wit may make tolerable the intolerable; in humor, one can speak the unspeakable that one suffers. In healthcare, incongruity and the space that is ripe for humor lie between the present reality for the person or family and the illness condition or even the healthcare institution itself. By laughing at the gap that exists, several socioemotional and cognitive things happen. The *elephant in the room* is acknowledged by making some element of the ideal become the butt of the joke. This reduces the emotion (e.g., fear, anger) created by the perceived size of the gap, which leads to creative thoughts about alternative ways to see, think, or feel. This shift reduces the amount of power given to the *perception* of the ideal, which switches, at least, the cognitive or emotional power to the individual, so there can be movement toward solutions that can actually reduce the size of the gap, even if only emotionally.

Technique

It may be as subtle as a smile and a quick glance that assures the other you caught what he just did or said or as overt as donning a red nose or Spock ears. Several intervention starter ideas are provided in Table 8.3. The ideas presented are merely starting suggestions. Personal preferences and skill levels determine what eventually gets added to each nurse's humor toolbox.

Table 8.3   Simple Therapeutic Humor—Starter Ideas

Brief Descriptions	Comments
Set your heart to focus on others	An "other" focus is always the place to begin.
View humorous videos	Much humor and laughter research compares data between subjects who have and have not viewed funny videos. Funny videos positively affect people in many physiological and emotional ways.
Read and listen to funny material	Internet sites have boosted volume and access to a wide array of fun resources. Old standards written or recorded by funny authors—including Erma Bombeck, Dave Barry, and Steve Allen—can also be used.

(continued)

Table 8.3 Simple Therapeutic Humor—Starter Ideas (*continued*)

Brief Descriptions	Comments
Take time to do something fun	It is beneficial if the nurse considers: When was the last time I did something fun just because it would be fun to do?
Share something funny with another person	Humor is a seed that, when sown, might grow to be even funnier next time it appears.
Lead or join a Laughter Club	Visit www.worldlaughtertour.com for details.
Create your own personal humor collection	Find small items that can fit into your pocket. Red noses can be a staple because they are small and inexpensive; clean ones may be used and new ones given away. Puppets can be great and come in a wide range of types, sizes, and characters.
Dress up your uniform and/or accessories	Paint a smiley face on your stethoscope; embroider or draw a silly name onto your uniform pocket; have a certain pair of scrubs that you have patients sign at a certain milestone.
Hold silly parades	These are fun, especially if census is low and you are aware of every patient's ability to enjoy it.
Create a list of caring clowns	Call on them for special as well as ordinary days. A number of websites can help you get connected. Search "caring clowns" on the Internet.
Keep an eye out for the perfect time	Remember the element of surprise. If a humor intervention becomes too predictable, it loses some of its effectiveness. Just be aware of situations. When you see an opportunity, *take it*; use humor while the timing is right.
Think in terms of…	…fill in the blanks. Explore all six senses (sight, hearing, touch, smell, taste, and *humor*) as you consider these starter ideas: rhyming words, nonsensical explanations, facial expressions, made-up (or not) songs, physical incongruities such as entering a room walking backward rather than forward, repetition and overexaggeration (until they get it that you're joking), balloons or other soft-tossing items. The list is endless once your imagination is engaged.
Be open to their leads	Does your patient tell jokes? Then laugh at the punch line and come up with your own in response (that day or the next). The principle is that when they give you the lead, *respond*.

Numerous resources are available for developing one's humor intervention potential. Search the Internet for resources that can help you with your particular area of interest, such as cancer or aging. Selected sources that are readily available and provide direct access to reliable researchers and practitioners, including pioneers in the field, are listed in Exhibit 8.1.

Guidelines

Regardless of the technique, the primary considerations when applying therapeutic humor should be:

- *Have your heart right.* Focus on the needs of the patient and family members. Keep *their* best interests at the center of your decisions.
- *Tune your senses.* Be keen to patients' present situation or condition so the humor initiated is appropriate, at least to the extent you are able to assess the environment.
- *Be quick to accept their invitation.* While attending to the patient's and/ or the family's needs, pay close attention so that, when they initiate or plant a humorous seed, you can respond and give the moment real life. One of the truly genius benefits of therapeutic humor is the planting

---

Exhibit 8.1. Selected Humor Resources

- **Human and Nursing I: Impact of Humor and Laughter on Physical Health** is an online course created by one of the first contemporary humor researchers, Paul McGhee (www.corexcel.com/courses4/humor.nursing.part1.title.htm)
- **Association for Applied and Therapeutic Humor (AATH)** conferences explore therapeutic humor in a range of disciplines (e.g., health, education, business, and leadership). These conferences are relevant to professionals in applied fields and include many how-to sessions:(www.aath.org/humor-academy)
- **International Society for Humor Studies (ISHS)** is an organization to join to interact with and be informed by the leading researchers in the field. The international and multidisciplinary nature of this organization helps deepen one's scholarly understanding of humor theories, how humor and comedy work, and how deeply humor exists in and impacts the human condition (www.hnu.edu/ishs).
- **Journal of Nursing Jocularity (JNJ)** is a site developed by Karyn Buxman to blog humor-in-nursing stories, to read other nurses' stories, and review occasional educational articles (www.journalofnursingjocularity.karynbuxman.com).
- **World Laughter Tour, Inc.** This organization provides certification for Certified Laughter Leaders, and academic credit from Columbus State Community College, Columbus, Ohio.

of the seed for an eventual twist or in the way some simple element from a collective past emerges in a different context, this time as humor. Accepting a patient's or family's invitation to "lighten up" serves at least two purposes. First, it helps you pass their test to see whether you are there for the patient or for the illness (or the hospital's rules, the head nurse, the end of your shift, and so on). It is a subtle difference, but humor can help assure the patient and family that your presence is for *their* well-being. Second, it communicates to them that you not only have a sense of humor, but also that it is available to be shared. In other words, you 're not just a competent nurse, you're fun as well (and competent, fun nurses make it easier to trust).

Beyond the three core guidelines, the nurse should maintain eye contact. This is important so that effectiveness can be gauged. Keep eye contact long enough for the recipient to *get it*—that the humor gesture just shared was from a caring place in the heart. This is where the therapy demonstrates itself as an art form. The style of famous comedians, such as Jerry Seinfeld, Steve Martin, or Roseanne Barr, can be studied. When they expect a laugh that hasn't come yet, the comic just stares at the audience or into the camera until the audience gets it and laughs. In much the same way, eye contact, even if subtle, sends a powerful message and confirms that the application of humor was received as intended.

Measurement of Outcomes

Measurements can be made that are appropriate to the patient's condition and consistent with the intent or goal for which the intervention was delivered—measurements appropriate to judge the outcome for which therapeutic humor was used. For example, if the intent of the use of therapeutic humor was to reduce stress, a measure of perceived stress could be used such as the Perceived Stress Scale (Cohen, 2012). If therapeutic humor is used to promote comfort (or pain reduction) or positive emotions (or relief of negative emotions), self-report scales of comfort, pain relief, or emotions/mood may be used. These include a visual analog scale for pain, or the Profile of Mood States™ (Heuchert & McNair, 2013) for moods. A number of biophysiological measures could also be used (e.g., blood pressure or heart rate). In conducting research, a number of serum measures that have been used by investigators are described in Table 8.2. The timing of measurement may be immediately on completion of the intervention or at a later time, keeping in mind that the benefits of therapeutic humor may extend beyond humor or laughter.

If the humor attempt does not appear to be working, be prepared to shift quickly and gauge what adjustments need to be made. Some logical first steps include:

- Soften your approach
- Acknowledge that you recognize your attempt at humor wasn't the right call at that moment
- Offer an apology and return to the patient's medical needs

If a patient or family does not respond to an initial humor attempt, this does not necessarily mean humor will never be appropriate with these individuals. Such a determination only can be made once the nurse has spent more time with the client, and after the nurse has had the opportunity to develop a trusting relationship, and greater understanding of the client's and family's condition and circumstances.

PRECAUTIONS

As with any procedural intervention, nurses using therapeutic humor must remain sensitive to the reaction and receptivity of the patient and family members. The nurse must know the health condition of the client and what is appropriate. Other than with an asthmatic patient or another compromised pulmonary condition such as chronic obstructive pulmonary disease (COPD)—or with a few other conditions such as those affecting the cardiovascular system, or a person with fresh stitches or fractured ribs—therapeutic humor carries little risk for serious adverse health impacts. It is possible that the nurse's well-intended use of therapeutic humor may not always be well received. Although this may undermine relationship-building efforts, no lasting physical harm is done; the relationship can be built and nourished in other ways over time. Six caveats are identified:

- Although humor itself is not physically dangerous, nurses should use care if extended, mirthful laughter is initiated with patients with pulmonary (Lebowitz, Suh, Diaz, & Emery, 2011) or heart conditions. Because laughter is a physiological process that involves the entire pulmonary and cardiovascular systems, care must be taken so humor interventions do not stimulate considerable, sustained laughter unless authorized and under careful monitoring. Brutsche et al. (2008) found similar results to Lebowitz et al. (2011), but also found that smiling induced by a humor intervention was able to reduce hyperinflation in patients with severe COPD. Their work suggests that smiling-derived breathing techniques may complement pursed-lips breathing. When providing nursing care to these patients, be confident that the smile, chuckle, and emotional boosts from a humor intervention can provide considerable benefit; however, be cautious when a patient begins to laugh exuberantly.
- Some unknown considerations when interacting with new patients involve their personal history with humor, sense of humor, or humor style. One woman shared that when her brother broke his arm, the entire family was doubled over with laughter—even as they reached the hospital. Emergency department staff had trouble identifying whom to treat amid the hysteria of the family interaction. The woman clarified that it was the family's typical [unusual] response to when a family member gets hurt. Indeed, some families laugh hysterically at and with each other, even during stressful times; others become serious and believe being ill or injured is no laughing matter. Paying close attention to the cues they provide (verbal and nonverbal, including items they carry with them or post nearby) and spending time with patients and their families will help you pick up the clues you need to make the correct decisions most of the time.

- As with all humor attempts early in a nurse–patient relationship, if the patient fails to chuckle as a result, it's not a full picture of the patient's receptivity to or capacity for humor; however, it can provide a starting point for further assessments as your engagement with this client continues. *Start slowly.* As your relationship with the patient matures, humor can be developed in the context of the therapeutic relationship.
- Beware of the potential for a clash of the humor styles. High-humor nurses should be careful to read their patients or other audience carefully so low-humor patients are not disenfranchised by someone who is overly "chipper" or attempting humor too soon.
- Watch the noise. Because most healthcare environments need to remain quiet out of respect for other patients (Maser, 2012), the nurse should use caution to engage techniques that, most predictably, results in a volume appropriate for the setting.
- In general, the results of a therapeutic humor intervention are easiest to predict when shared among people with a somewhat similar culture and ethnicity. In these situations, people tend to share values, beliefs, and norms that help them understand and contribute to shared humor. In essence, the language is familiar enough that everyone understands how to interpret the words or actions. When interacting with people of other cultures, it is also important to remember another law of comedy that, again, can be explained by using the gap described earlier. Individuals in a lesser position, whether real or perceived (e.g., social, economic, political, hierarchical), may laugh at or make fun of people or situations that they perceive to be above them, but they may not make fun *downward*. For example, a high-income (real or perceived), 45-year-old White male is fair game for most of the world, but such men may *not*, publicly, make fun of people of lower condition—determined by the receiver's perception (e.g., lower income, different race, poorer health, noticeably older or younger). Such a politically incorrect attempt at humor hurts and is sure to erase the opportunity to build a trusting relationship, possibly for a long time. People of higher status within any given interaction are free to make fun of themselves or their situation, but they may not make fun of a person or the condition of one of a less-fortunate status. Similarly, professionals should avoid the three most sensitive subjects—politics, religion, and race—when attempting humor. These are sure to serve a contrary purpose every time.

USES

Given these caveats, when used correctly, humor can be offered as a signal to a patient that "you and I are on the same plane." Elaine Tagliareni, RN, chief program officer with the National League for Nursing, has studied the concept of *other* and ways that individuality and personhood are intimately tied to relationships. "Relationships with others involve an ethic of caring and responsibility, vulnerability, and being touched in a unique way, all elements that are at the very core of the nursing experience" (Tagliareni, 2008, p. 322). Regarding the use of humor: if you consider the other person as "different," then you would not attempt the humor because you would assume the recipient would not understand it enough to respond appropriately. Attempts at humor, well used, communicate a sense that, "We may be different in some ways, but not so many that we cannot share a smile together." In any new relationship, it is wise to use this complementary therapy with some extra care; however, therapeutic humor holds considerable power to bridge gaps and build relationships, even among people of differing ethnic backgrounds, cultures, and ages.

Therapeutic Humor With Children

Regardless of age, humor provides important social and emotional functions in children. Joking and laughing about taboo topics and things that make them anxious help children manage negative emotions—especially in unfamiliar and threatening environments, as is often the case involving healthcare.

Just as children have cognitive and physical stages of development, they also have developmental stages in understanding and applying humor—from physical to cognitive. In general, infants understand touch signals (snuggles that make them giggle, playful tickling); toddlers respond with glee to physical humor ranging from peek-a-boo to pratfalls. Preschoolers and early elementary–age children love more cognitive types of humor, such as rhyming, knock-knock jokes, and nonsense. Middle-school–age children are progressively more capable of creating, recognizing, and appreciating incongruity. This age range is also very rigid regarding rules, especially when they see others breaking them. Nurses are wise to make up rules, some general and others personal, for patients in this age range. Young boys age 9 and older generally respond to "disgusting" body humor, but nurses need to take some cues from the parents before encouraging this type of humor. It may be an effective way to build a relationship with patients of this age.

Early in their interaction with people, children typically give cues as to whether or not they have coping humor strategies that can help moderate the stress of a hospital visit or medical procedure. Children get somewhat the same benefits from coping humor as adults, such as stress reduction, pain tolerance, and relationship building, but their coping techniques tend to be fairly specific. Those with available coping skills ask questions and seek information; use problem-focused methods (e.g., behavioral distraction); or engage in positive self-talk. They tend to not dwell on negative emotions or use catastrophic thinking (Goodenough & Ford, 2005).

Some typical humor interventions with children include hospital clowns, humor carts, clown noses and other props, puppets, funny age-appropriate videos, finger play, funny sounds, funny names for a medical device or the doctor, and creation of alternative reality stories. The list is limited only to one's imagination. Whereas an initial humor intervention with lower-humor children may not be as successful as those with a higher sense of humor, it can work.

When engaging a child in therapeutic humor, the nurse should be sure to watch both the reaction of the child and that of the parents. If parents are indicating any concern, provide a wink or other signal so that they understand you are doing this deliberately and that you need them to follow your lead to the end of the ruse or whatever method you are using. If the parent does not respond, shift quickly, respecting the cue that your approach is not fitting or welcomed at this time. Humor with children can result in loud reactive outbursts that may need to be toned down to appropriate noise levels for the environment.

Use of Therapeutic Humor With Older Adults

Older adults also deserve some special considerations when applying humor to strengthen the healing environment. Obviously, because laughter is a physiological activity, respect should be given to the patient's skeletal, cardiovascular, and pulmonary limitations. However, because humor works so well as a social bonding agent, it can be an especially effective intervention when matched with the physical, cognitive, and emotional needs of the patient—such as depression or lack of appetite.

People older than age 65 make up about 13% of the population of the United States and in 2010 were the fastest growing segment of the U.S. population (U.S. Census Bureau, 2010). Humor appreciation has been shown to diminish beyond age 65; however, causes may result from conditions as diverse as hearing loss, deteriorating mental capacity, or dementia or may be because the icons from their earlier days are unknown by the younger generations, thus creating the absence of cultural cohesion—the infamous generation gap.

Patients from this population or their families help others to understand their physical reasons for needing services, but they may not think to provide clues about their cognitive, social, or emotional condition that can help the nurse determine how best to aid with their original health concern.

Nursing education typically provides considerable attention to the physical care needs of the aging person, including how to manage those with declining cognition and deteriorating skeletal–muscular conditions. Little, if any, attention is given to an important self-perception that therapeutic humor can overcome in an instant—their feelings of invisibility (Bunkers, 2001). Spontaneous humor calls for keen attention to detail. By picking up on or initiating humor with older patients, the nurse says to them, "I notice you, you are 'normal' to me, and I care about your well-being—physical and emotional." In short, humor provides the opportunity to connect as real people.

Well-placed humor can be used as an effective initial assessment that can impact the ability to engage older patients fully in care that optimizes their health. The easiest assessment occurs when the patient or family initiates the humor. In this case, the nurse should respond and appreciate the ease with which the family is setting up a positive interaction. As a professional assessment, their humor initiation also provides an indication of this patient's cognitive capacity and social well-being, at least as an initial indicator.

If the humor is not patient-initiated, the nurse continues with nursing procedures, staying ever-aware of the first opportunity to test the waters for an appropriate, well-timed humor *test*. A simple test for cognition could be a silly incongruity joke such as, *Q: Where do you take a sick boat? A: To a dock.* As with all humor attempts early in a nurse–patient relationship, a lack of a chuckle is not a full picture of the client's cognitive capabilities or overall sense of humor, but it can provide a starting point for understanding and knowing this person. Beyond the covert assessment value, an older patient may especially appreciate the humor intervention simply because it can stimulate further conversation, allow the other to be heard, and communicates an extra measure of caring.

At the very least, older patients look forward to seeing the nurse again. In this way, you not only assure these patients of their visibility, tell them that they are important, and indicate that they are deserving of the best care possible, you also share that little secret weapon for the benefit of their health—you got them to smile. In this smile, you improved the well-being of their minds and bodies.

Use of Therapeutic Humor as Part of Self-Care

Therapeutic humor is not only for the benefit of patients. Given the intense, highly unpredictable, and ever-changing environment of today's healthcare settings, nurses can use humor for personal benefits as well. Nurses are encouraged to make and find humor resources that suit their personal tastes. As has been repeated throughout this chapter, even the anticipation of humorous activities can help relieve stress. By using humor to help balance one's own well-being, one becomes more understanding of how therapeutic humor can benefit others.

Therapeutic humor helps reassure the ill and ailing that they are people, first. It enhances a nurse's ability to connect with patients quickly and in ways not yet fully understood. However, therapeutic humor is gaining ground as one of the therapies nurses can call on as a caring professional. Even as empirical evidence continues to reveal the strengths and limitations of this intriguing human phenomenon, nurses are encouraged to build their knowledge and skills so that therapeutic humor can be accountably and artfully applied as a responsible complementary therapy.

CULTURAL APPLICATIONS

Although humor within populations is a universal social phenomenon, it is also culturally specific, based on that group's own set of values, beliefs, and norms. Verbal humor requires knowledge of words' meanings—an obvious barrier across cultural lines. For humor to work therapeutically requires an understanding of the culture's interpretation of nonverbal cues, as well as the culture's relationship with humor, healthcare, and illness. Complicating the impact further is the patient's biophysical, psychological, and spiritual states of being at that moment (Pasquali, 1990). Therapeutic humor in care situations that involve non–English-speaking patients and clients from foreign countries requires extra consideration. Although humor may work well as a healing modality in one cultural context, one cannot be assured that it will work the same way in another.

Use of Therapeutic Humor With East Asian Populations

The teaching of cultural competence with regard to the use of humor in nursing practice may vary across different educational programs within and between countries. In one preliminary study of cultural differences in therapeutic humor in nursing education (Chiang-Hanisko, Adamle, & Chiang, 2009), investigators explored the linkage between nursing theory and practice among three nursing education programs, two in the United States and one in Taiwan. This study found that the Taiwanese faculty members teach more classroom theory and concepts about therapeutic humor than the U.S.-based faculty, but that they observe and practice less therapeutic humor in clinical settings.

Zen Buddhism authority D. T. Suzuki (1971) suggests that humor is prominent in the Zen tradition. Clasquin (2001) adds that Buddhism embraces incongruity-based humor because humor helps transcend the "absurdity of the human condition" and life's incongruities by bringing Buddhists "down to earth" (p. 113). Regardless of whether Buddhism supports the principles of therapeutic humor or whether nursing educators in East Asian countries teach it, for a variety of reasons, nurses may find it difficult to use therapeutic humor techniques in many healthcare settings.

For example, despite including therapeutic humor in the didactic instruction, the Taiwanese participants in the cited study indicated they practice therapeutic humor less, out of respect for the "reverence of illness" that pervades their culture (Chiang-Hanisko et al., 2009). This reverence is founded in Confucianism, which, as early as the second century BCE, purported that illness may be seen as a failure to meet the obligations of filial piety. Chinese philosopher Chu His (960–1279 CE) wrote that "when a parent is ill, the son should look upset; he should neither amuse himself. ... Only after his parent had recovered may he resume his normal way of life" (Ebrey, 1991, p. 28). Chiang-Hanisko et al. (2009) conclude that, when serving Taiwanese patients and their families, "Nurses and caregivers are expected to view hospital and clinical settings as places to uphold the cultural value of reverence of illness. This outlook must be considered before attempting to use therapeutic humor" (p. 57).

Universality of Smiling and Laughter

Sauter, Eisner, Ekman, and Scott (2010) examined the interpretation of vocalizations of emotional cues between Americans and Namibian villagers. They found that a number of negative emotions have vocalizations recognized by both cultures, but only one type of positive vocalization—laughter—was recognized by both groups. Laughter has been interpreted as a playful communication signaling joy in this and most other similar types of studies. This finding is especially meaningful when placed alongside the decades of work on facial display recognition across cultures in which the Duchenne smile is repeatedly recognized as a visual signal of amusement or joy (Elfenbein & Ambady, 2002). With the reassurance that smiling and laughter are universal languages indicating positive emotions, nurses can feel quite confident that humor is, in fact, an appropriate complementary therapy. As a rule, however, nurses should begin initial humor interactions with new patients from other cultures with respectful caution. Efforts to gain understanding of a patient's culture, and their cultural use and perspectives related to humor, can be helpful in guiding the insertion of humor into a therapeutic relationship. Cultural reflections about Ethiopian humor from the perspective of an Ethiopian student nurse are included in Sidebar 8.1.

FUTURE RESEARCH

Little definitive research exists to support the use of humor as a complementary therapy. However, many professions have an interest in humor and its effects, and multidisciplinary traditions may shape the questions asked. The truth of any social science can be revealed more deeply when informed from both empirical, quantitative research—founded in experimentation (Western principles)—*and* inquiry-based, qualitative research—founded in exploring the lived experience and personal stories (Eastern principles) (Creswell, 2013). Therapeutic humor,

SIDEBAR 8.1. THERAPEUTIC HUMOR: PERSPECTIVES FROM BALE-ROBE OROMIA, ETHIOPIA, AFRICA

Salahadin Abda

In Ethiopian culture, humor plays a part in the healing process, and it also has a very important function in our society. We use it a lot. Humor can be expressed in so many ways, and there are some sensitivities and expressions of humor that may be unique to our cultures, but there are so many universal aspects. Humor needs to be appropriate and its use depends on how close people are in their relationship; it can warm relationships and bring people even closer together. It is used socially, in the context of health and illness, in normal processes of life such as aging, and in times surrounding death.

In Ethiopia, we don't have medical care like in Western culture. Our medical treatments are mostly based on cultural medication such as spices or other natural things. In the United States, when one looks for wisdom and healing, we approach it from a Western perspective, and we turn to evidence and the "scientific knowledge" we have about the disease or medical issue. In Ethiopia, the general understanding of health and illness is different; those who are ill benefit significantly from the care they have from the people surrounding them. In the Western framework, we understand stroke as being a blood clot to the brain. In Ethiopia, individuals likely don't have that understanding—they would call it something different and view if from a spiritual framework rather than a physiological one. Spirituality is about connection with the people and the way they talk; it is not something measurable. Even when there is paralysis, prayer and communication are important. The human "connectivity" eases the suffering. How we perceive and how we tear affect how we feel: Our thoughts can magnify our pain or ease the suffering. In Western healthcare settings, in caring for an elder Ethiopian, the Ethiopian family is helpful—children are especially helpful because the elderly person trusts the children. This is important to bridge the huge gap that exists in understanding the pathophysiology of disease and illness, a cultural gap that may otherwise be hard to breach.

Humor may be used in relationships as people connect, as when an elder loses a bodily function (e.g., hearing loss). Humor may help ease the pain and sense of loss. Family and friends may say, "God is coming for you—and taking you little by little!" So, the person may respond by feeling more at ease. It is understandable and acceptable for God to take them little by little. It may ease the sense of loss. It is put into a perspective of, "this is natural, and acceptable; this how it is and how that happens."

Ethiopian people of the same age can say anything to one another based on connectedness and knowledge of intent. Perhaps one exception is to joke about beliefs—and don't joke about spirituality. In my culture, I would not joke about my grandmother's spiritual beliefs. This may not only offend her, but would also cause her to fear for me for such a serious offense. This is understandable. One needs to have a belief or life is senseless.

(continued)

Humor has helped me a lot to communicate. I have learned to develop strong relationships with patients and staff. I grew up in Ethiopia, but I have been in the United States for well over a decade. To some extent, I have adjusted the way that I interact and the way in which I use humor. I adjust my use of it according to the person I am interacting with. First, I need to know them; I need to get some sense of them and their response in preliminary communication. I must know the person who I interact with well. I know that I have been effective with my use of humor in the building of meaningful therapeutic relationships. For example, a patient who had received a heart transplant returned after 2 years—he had some blood-related problem, and couldn't (or wouldn't) eat. He saw me and remembered me; I could make him eat. We ordered his next meal together. The other caregivers were amazed that he ate, saying, "What did you do!" With a warm smile in the context of our relationship, I had shared my belief that, "There is a reason we are here—we pass on and leave behind what is for the next generation and then we go." In the West, we may believe too much about medication. Nutrition is essential; you cannot heal or recover without it. I shared with him, "If you don't eat, you shrink" [and die]. Eating is the only way you can walk away from this hospital."

In working with individuals of the Ethiopian culture, the foundation is a good connection through establishment of a good relationship. Humor can help build and strengthen that. It is something any good nurse can do, and it has endless forms and possibilities in the process of building trust and helping people understand that they are not alone; it can help them be accepting of losses that are a part of life.

especially in nursing, is a field ripe for mixed methods because it affects, and is affected by, physiological, socioemotional, psychological, intellectual, and even spiritual considerations specific to health and healing.

Indeed, much remains to be discovered about the impact of therapeutic humor on human health and ways to use it effectively with people with specific mental and physical health conditions. Future research should use validated scales (Ruch & Deckers, 1993; Svebak, 1974; Thorson & Powell, 1991) so that the evidence base for intervention can be strengthened. Building on or using well-constructed theoretical foundations can also help increase empirical knowledge about the effects of humor on human health. For example, the promising work within the frameworks of two other emerging interdisciplinary fields—positive psychology and caring nursing practices—may go far toward advancing knowledge in the area. Jean Watson's (1988) caring theory identifies the patient, rather than the technology, as the focus of practice; this offers considerable possibilities for understanding how therapeutic humor can contribute to caring nursing practices. There is a need to connect these to fields of study: "Like caring, therapeutic humor is part of the 'dance' of making a personal connection with a patient. When you can get them to smile, you have some hope of making more of that personal touch" (Dr. Jan Boller, personal communication, December 3, 2012). This sentiment is especially poignant in light of the power of the smile, a virtually universal expression of positive affect. Selected areas in which nursing research is needed include the following:

- How may humor be used to build bridges of communication and understanding in the therapeutic relationships in healthcare when patients and providers speak different languages or when they are from different cultures?

* What are the best ways to operationalize humor to promote comfort, health, and healing in the context of different patient situations and circumstances, such as coping with chronic health conditions (e.g., emphysema) or undergoing difficult therapies (e.g., chemotherapy)?
* What biopsychosocial and behavioral outcomes should be selected as standard measures in humor research so that more robust comparisons across studies can be made?

REFERENCES

Association for Applied and Therapeutic Humor. (2000). What is therapeutic humor? Retrieved from http://www.aath.org/general-information

Bains, G. S., Berk, L. S., Lohman, E., Daher, N., Petrofsky, J., Schwab, E., & Deshpande, P. (2015). Humors effect on short-term memory in healthy and diabetic older adults. *Alternative Therapies in Health and Medicine, 21*(3), 16–25.

Ben-Pazi, H., Cohen, A., Kroyzer, N., Lotem-Ophir, R., Shvili, Y., Winter, G., ... Pollak, Y. (2017). Clown-care reduces pain in children with cerebral palsy undergoing recurrent botulinum toxin injections—A quasi-randomized controlled crossover study. *PLOS ONE, 12*(4), e0175028. doi:10.1371/journal.pone.0175028

Berk, L. S., Tan, I., & Tan, S. (2008). Mirthful laughter, as adjunct therapy in diabetic care, attenuates catecholamines, inflammatory cytokines, C-RP, and myocardial infarction occurrence. *FASEB Journal, 22* (Meeting Abstract Supplement), 1226.2.

Berk, L. S., Tan, S. A., & Berk, D. (2008). Cortisol and catecholamine stress hormone decrease is associated with the behavior of perceptual anticipation of mirthful laughter. *FASEB Journal, 22*(Meeting Abstract Supplement), 946.11.

Berk, R. A. (2001). The active ingredients in humor: Psychophysiological benefits and risks for older adults. *Educational Gerontology, 27,* 323–339

Brutsche, M. H., Grossman, P., Muller, R. E., Wiegand, J., Pello, B., Baty, F., & Ruch, W. (2008). Impact of laughter on air trapping in severe chronic obstructive lung disease. *International Journal of Chronic Obstructive Pulmonary Disorders, 3*(1), 185–192.

Bunkers, S. S. (2001). Becoming invisible: Elder as teacher. *Nursing Science Quarterly, 14*(2), 115–119.

Cai, C., Yu, L., Rong, L., & Zhong, H. (2014). Effectiveness of humor intervention for patients with schizophrenia: A randomized controlled trial. *Journal of Psychiatric Research, 59,* 174–178.

Chiang-Hanisko, L., Adamle, K., & Chiang, L. (2009). Cultural difference in therapeutic humor in nursing education. *Journal of Nursing Research, 17*(1), 52–61.

Clasquin, M. (2001). Real Buddhas don't laugh: Attitudes towards humor and laughter in ancient India and China. *Social Identities, 7*(1), 97–116.

Cohen, S. (2012). Dr. Cohen's scales: Perceived stress scale (PSS). Retrieved from http://www.psy.cmu.edu/~scohen/scales.html

Cousins, N. (1979). *Anatomy of an illness as perceived by the patient.* New York, NY: Norton.

Creswell, J. W. (2013). *Research design: Qualitative, quantitative and mixed methods approaches.* Thousand Oaks, CA: Sage.

Ebrey, P. B. (1991). *Chu Hsi's family rituals.* Princeton, NJ: Princeton University Press.

Ekman, P., & Friesen, W. V. (1978). *Facial action coding system (FACS).* Palo Alto, CA: Consulting Psychologists Press.

Elfenbein, H. A., & Ambady, N. (2002). On the universality and cultural specificity of emotion recognition: A meta-analysis. *Psychological Bulletin, 128,* 203–235.

Felluga, M., Rabach, I., Minute, M., Montico, M., Giorgi, R., Lonciari, I., ... Barbi, E. (2016). A quasi randomized-controlled trial to evaluate the effectiveness of clowntherapy on children's anxiety and pain levels in emergency department. *European Journal of Pediatrics, 175*(5), 465–450.

Fry, W. (1963). *Sweet madness: A study of humor.* Palo Alto, CA: Pacific Books.

Ghodsbin, F., Ahmadi, S., Jahanbin, I, & Shrif, F. (2015). The effects of laughter therapy on general health of elderly people referring to Jahandidegan community center in Shiraz, Iran, 2014: A randomized controlled trial. *International Journal of Community Based Nurse Midwifery, 3*(1), 31–38.

Goodenough, B., & Ford, J. (2005). Self-reported use of humor by hospitalized pre-adolescent children to cope with pain-related distress from a medical intervention. *Humor, 18*(3), 279–298.

Heuchert, J. P., & McNair, D. M. (2013). *Profile of mood states*^{TM} (2nd ed.). North Tonawanda, NY: Multi-Health Systems, Inc. Retrieved from http://www.mhs.com/product.aspx?gr=cli&prod=poms2&id=resources

Isen, A.M. (2003). Positive affect as a source of human strength. In L. G. Aspinwall & U. M. Staudinger (Eds.), *A psychology of human strengths: Fundamental questions and future directions for a positive psychology* (pp. 179–195). Washington, DC: American Psychological Association.

Kim, S. H., Kook, J. R., Kwon, M., Son, M. H., Ahn, S. D., & Kim, Y. H. (2015). The effects of laughter therapy on mood state and self-esteem in cancer patients undergoing radiation therapy: A randomized controlled trial. *Journal of Alternative and Complementary Medicine, 21*(4), 217–222.

Kuru, N., & Kublay, G. (2016). The effect of laughter therapy on the quality of life of nursing home residents. *Journal of Clinical Nursing, 26*(21–22), 3354–3362. doi:10.1111/jocn.13687

Lebowitz, K. R., Suh, S., Diaz, P. T., & Emery, C. F. (2011). Effects of humor and laughter on psychological functioning, quality of life, health status, and pulmonary functioning among patients with chronic obstructive pulmonary disease: A preliminary investigation. *Heart and Lung, 40*(4), 310–319.

Lipman, S. (1991). *Laughter in hell: The use of humor during the Holocaust.* North Vale, NJ: Jason Aronson.

Mahony, D. L., Burroughs, W. J., & Hieatt, A. C. (2001). The effects of laughter on discomfort thresholds: Does expectation become reality? *Journal of General Psychology, 128*(2), 217–222.

Martin, R. A. (2007). *The psychology of humor: An integrative approach.* Burlington, MA: Elsevier.

Martin, R. A., & Dobbin, J. P. (1988). Sense of humor, hassles, and immunoglobulin-A: Evidence for a stress-moderating effect of humor. *International Journal of Psychiatry in Medicine, 18,* 93–105.

Maser, S. E. (2012). *Nursing, noise, and norms: Why Nightingale is still right.* Healing HealthCare Systems. Retrieved from http://www.healinghealth.com

McCreaddie, M., & Wiggins, S. (2008). The purpose and function of humour in health, health care and nursing: A narrative review. *Journal of Advanced Nursing, 61,* 584–595.

McGhee, P. (1979). *Humor: Its origin and development.* San Francisco, CA: Freeman.

Meiri, N., Ankri, A., Hamad-Saied, M., Konopnicki, M., & Pillar, G. (2016). The effect of medical clowning on reducing pain, crying, and anxiety in children aged 2-10 years old undergoing venous blood drawing—A randomized controlled study. *European Journal of Pediatrics, 175*(3), 373–379.

Miller, M., & Fry, W. F. (2009). The effect of mirthful laughter on the human cardiovascular system. *Medical Hypotheses, 73*(5), 636–639.

Mora-Ripoll, R. (2011). Potential health benefits of simulated laughter: A narrative review of the literature and recommendations for future research. *Complementary Therapies in Medicine, 19,* 170–177.

Mulkay, M. (1988). *On humor: Its nature and its place in modern society.* New York, NY: Basil Blackwell.

Pasquali, E. A. (1990). Learning to laugh: Humor as therapy. *Journal of Psychosocial Nursing and Mental Health Services, 28*(3), 31–35.

Ruch, W. (Ed.). (1998). *The sense of humor: Explorations of a personality characteristic.* New York, NY: Mouton de Gruyter.

Ruch, W., & Deckers, L. (1993). Do extraverts "like to laugh"? An analysis of the Situational Humor Response Questionnaire (SHRQ). *European Journal of Personality, 7*(4), 211–220.

Sauter, D. D., Eisner, F., Ekman, P., & Scott, S. K. (2010). Cross-cultural recognition of basic emotions through non-verbal emotional vocalizations. *Proceedings of the National Academy of Sciences, 107*(6), 2408–2412. doi:10.1073/pnas.0908239106

Schultz, W. (2002). Getting formal with dopamine and reward. *Neuron, 36*(2), 241–263.

Sim, I. O. (2015). Humor intervention program for children with chronic diseases. *Applied Nursing Research, 28*(4), 404–412.

Strack, F., Martin, L. L., & Stepper, S. (1988). Inhibiting and facilitating conditions of the human smile: A nonobtrusive test of the facial feedback hypothesis. *Journal of Abnormal & Social Psychology, 54*(5), 278–281.

Suzuki, D. T. (1971). *Sengai: The Zen master.* Greenwich, CT: New York Graphic Society.

Svebak, S. (1974). Revised questionnaire on the sense of humor. *Scandinavian Journal of Psychology, 15,* 328–331.

Svebak, S., Kristoffersen, B., & Aasarod, K. (2006). Sense of humor and survival among a county cohort of patients with end-stage renal failure: A two-year prospective study. *International Journal of Psychiatry in Medicine, 36*(3), 269–281.

Tagliareni, M. E. (2008). More like me than different: Reflections on the notion of other. *Nursing Education Perspectives, 29*(6), 322.

Thorson, J. A., & Powell, F. C. (1991). Measurement of sense of humor. *Psychological Reports, 69,* 691–702.

U.S. Census Bureau. (2010). The older population: 2010. Retrieved from http://www.census.gov/prod/cen2010/briefs/c2010br-09.pdf

Watson, J. (1988). *Nursing: Human science and human care. A theory of nursing.* Burlington, MA: Jones & Bartlett.

Wellenzohn, S., Proyer, R. T., & Willibald, R. (2016). Humor-based online positive psychology interventions: A randomized placebo-controlled long-term trial. *The Journal of Positive Psychology, 11*(6), 584–594.

Zweyer, K., Vollcer, B., & Ruch, W. (2004). Do cheerfulness, exhilaration, and humor production moderate pain tolerance? *Humor, 17*(1/2), 85–119.

9

Yoga

MIRIAM E. CAMERON AND CORJENA K. CHEUNG

Anyone can benefit from yoga, regardless of health, beliefs, age, or culture. The systematic practice of yoga heals body and mind. Yoga's do-it-yourself prescription for stress management and well-being, if done properly, has little or no side effects and does not require expensive medications, treatments, or equipment. Millions of people around the world do yoga for fitness and relaxation; however, yoga has a much deeper dimension (Ravishankar, 2016).

Yoga is an ethical, spiritual way of life designed to transform consciousness, as yogis for centuries have advocated and Western researchers are discovering. Yoga teaches that self-centeredness underlies suffering and most disease (lack of ease). Yoga practitioners who let go of ego come to realize that they are linked to every being, the environment, and larger forces in the universe. Grateful for this vast interconnectedness, they reach out to relieve suffering (Ravishankar, 2016).

This chapter explores how nurses can use yoga as an effective therapy for self-care and as a part of integrative nursing (Earl E. Bakken Center for Spirituality & Healing, University of Minnesota, 2017a). Systematic practice of yoga will help nurses distinguish between conventional, constantly changing reality and ultimate reality, allowing their true nature to shine through. Nurses' inner wisdom will flow spontaneously through all the cells of the body, promoting optimal health, peace, and joy (Ravishankar, 2016).

DEFINITION

Yoga is an ancient art, philosophy, and science that originated in India. *Yoga* means "to yoke or unite the mind, body, and universe." According to tradition, two millennia ago Patanjali, a sage in India, systematized yoga into the *Yoga Sutra*. The book consists of 196 precise, concise statements called *sutras*. This unique blend of theoretical knowledge and practical application is the foundational textbook for all schools of yoga (Ravishankar, 2016).

In the *Yoga Sutra*, Patanjali analyzed how we know what we know and why we suffer. He explained that the primary purpose of consciousness is to see things as they *really* are and to make choices that bring about freedom from suffering.

Through yoga, we can rein in our tendency to seek happiness through external phenomena. By turning inward and developing mindfulness of our true nature, Patanjali wrote, we can come to understand how to develop wisdom and happiness. By becoming still inside, we can abide in this deep, absorptive knowing (Hawley, 2011; Ravishankar, 2016).

Patanjali described yoga as consisting of eight interconnected limbs, or aspects of the whole. He visualized the limbs as branches of a tree. Doing all eight limbs simultaneously leads to higher stages of ethics, spirituality, and healing. The first five limbs still the mind and body in preparation for the last three limbs. The eight limbs, their Sanskrit names, and definitions are listed in Exhibit 9.1 (Ravishankar, 2016).

The *Bagavad Gita* (Hawley, 2011), another ancient, sacred text from India, described eight kinds of yoga and their focus, as listed in Exhibit 9.2.

Hatha Yoga and Yoga Therapy

Hatha yoga has become popular around the world. This kind of yoga consists primarily of physical postures, breathing techniques, and relaxation (Muktibodhananda, 2016). Although Hatha yoga focuses on body, the classes can open the door to the deeper ethical, spiritual dimension of yoga. Hatha yoga styles include Himalayan Tradition, Tibetan Yoga, Iyengar, Ashtanga, Viniyoga, Sivananda, Kripalu, and Kundalini (Earl E. Bakken Center for Spirituality & Healing, University of Minnesota, 2017b).

The Yoga Alliance (2017). developed standards for Hatha yoga teachers and schools. A Registered Yoga Teacher (RYT) is a credential earned by Hatha yoga teachers whose training and teaching experience meet the Yoga Alliance Registry Standards. A Registered Yoga School (RYS) is a credential given to schools with a Hatha yoga teachers' training program taught by qualified faculty and a curriculum that meets the Yoga Alliance standards.

Exhibit 9.1. The Eight Limbs of Yoga in Patanjali's *Yoga Sutra*

1. Ethical behavior (*yama*)—nonharming, truthfulness, nonstealing, responsible sexuality, and nonacquisitiveness
2. Personal behavior (*niyama*)—purity, commitment, contentment, self-study, and surrender to the whole; *niyama* includes *sattvic* (pure) mind, food, beverages, air, and environment
3. Posture (*asana*)—physical poses that stretch, condition, and massage the body
4. Breath expansion (*pranayama*)—refinement of the breath to expand *prana* (life force) and get rid of toxins
5. Sensory inhibition (*pratyahara*)—temporary withdrawal of the senses from the external environment to the inner self (e.g., by closing the eyes and looking inward)
6. Concentration (*dharana*)—locking attention on the breath, mantra, image, or something else
7. Meditation (*dhyana*)—increasingly sustained attention, leading to a profound state of peace and awareness
8. Integration (*samadhi*)—a transcendent state of oneness, wisdom, and ecstasy

---

Exhibit 9.2.   Kinds of Yoga and Their Focus, as Described in the
Bagavad Gita

- *Kundalini yoga:* energy
- *Jnana yoga:* knowledge
- *Mantra yoga:* recitation of sacred syllables
- *Tantra yoga:* technique
- *Bhakti yoga:* devotion
- *Karma yoga:* action, good deeds
- *Raja yoga:* control of mind and body through the Eight Limbs of Patanjali
- *Hatha yoga:* willpower to do physical exercises and expand the breath

---

Numerous studies have found yoga to be therapeutic for individuals (Cameron, 2014; National Center for Complementary and Integrative Health [NCCIH], 2017). Yoga therapy takes therapeutic yoga to a higher, more professional level. The International Association of Yoga Therapists (2017) defines *yoga therapy* as the process of empowering individuals to progress toward improved awareness, health, and well-being through the application of yoga teachings and practices. Goals of yoga therapy include eliminating, reducing, and/or managing symptoms that cause suffering; improving function; preventing occurrence or recurrence of underlying causes of illness; and increasing health and well-being.

The practice of yoga therapy requires specialized education and skill development. Yoga therapy is taught together with Ayurveda, a traditional healing system from India (Earl E. Bakken Center for Spirituality & Healing, University of Minnesota (2016a) and Tibetan medicine, a similar traditional healing system from Tibet (Cameron et al., 2012; Earl E. Bakken Center for Spirituality & Healing, University of Minnesota, 2016b). The International Association of Yoga Therapists (2017) certifies yoga therapists and accredits yoga therapy schools. Moreover, the organization is in the process of developing national examinations and licensing for yoga therapists

Most yoga education takes place in community centers with variable quality. Yoga is evolving from a trade into a profession based on yoga's time-tested philosophy and scientific evidence. To ensure safe, knowledgeable practice, yoga education is moving from community centers to academia with more rigorous standards about ethics, anatomy, physiology, and evidence-based practice. Now students can take academic courses to be Hatha yoga teachers. Graduate students can earn a master's degree in yoga therapy. University faculty and PhD students conduct yoga research. Teaching yoga and conducting yoga research in academia promote standardization, professionalism, and evolution of yoga. Increasingly, nursing undergraduates and graduate students are taking these academic courses to become Hatha yoga teachers and yoga therapists while completing nursing degrees (Cameron, 2014; Earl E. Bakken Center for Spirituality & Healing, University of Minnesota, 2017c).

SCIENTIFIC BASIS

Yoga is based on ancient observations, principles, and theories of the mind–body connection. For thousands of years, yogis have passed down this precise knowledge from one generation to the next (Ravishankar, 2016). Western researchers are validating many of these health claims (Noggle, Steiner, Minami, & Khalsa, 2012). Studies have found that yoga generally is a safe, therapeutic intervention that treats symptoms and/or prevents their onset and recurrence ((Earl E. Bakken Center for Spirituality & Healing, University of Minnesota, 2017b; NCCIH, 2017). After reviewing a variety of studies, Boehm and colleagues concluded that yoga produced considerable health benefits (Boehm, Ostermann, Milazzo, & Bussing, 2012).

Yoga improved immunity (Morgan, Irwin, Chung & Wang, 2014). Poor body alignment and improper breathing are major factors in health problems. Yoga had a positive effect on joint disorders (Cramer, Lauche, Haller & Dobos, 2013). Moreover, yoga decreased fatigue and improved physical fitness, balance, strength, flexibility, body alignment, and use of extremities (Galantino et al., 2012). Yoga therapy was an effective sole or additional intervention for patients with depression (Pascoe & Bauer, 2015) and anxiety (Li & Goldsmith, 2014). Okonta (2012) reviewed 10 randomized controlled trials, quasiexperimental studies, and pilot studies; yoga therapy modulated the physiological system of the body, including the heart rate, and reduced blood pressure, blood glucose levels, cholesterol levels, and body weight.

INTERVENTION

Technique

Each of Patanjali's eight limbs is a potential nursing intervention for children, adults, elders, pregnant women, people with disabilities or illnesses, and individuals who are dying (Cameron, 2014; Earl E. Bakken Center for Spirituality & Healing, University of Minnesota, 2017b). For example, some individuals need encouragement to behave with nonviolence and compassion toward the self and others (Limb 1). Nurses can promote cleanliness, nutrition, and self-discipline (Limb 2; Okonta, 2012; Ravishankar, 2016).

Nurses can suggest yoga poses (Limb 3) and breathing techniques (Limb 4) for relaxation and harmony. Exhibit 9.3 explains how to do Corpse Pose and relax deeply. Exhibit 9.4 lists steps for doing Alternate Nostril Breathing to harmonize mind and body. Doing Corpse Pose and Alternate Nostril Breathing can reduce stress before treatments and surgery.

Exhibit 9.3.   Corpse Pose (*Savasana*; Yoga Limb 3)

- Lie on your back with your arms relaxed near your sides; palms up; and head, trunk, and legs straight. If you are uncomfortable, put a pillow or blanket under your head and/or knees.
- Close your eyes, relax, and let your body sink.
- Breathe in a circular manner: slowly, evenly, deeply through your nostrils, from your abdomen, with your in-breath the same length as your out-breath, and no break in between.
- When you are ready, open your eyes, bend your knees, turn to your right, and get up.

Corpse Pose promotes deep relaxation and can decrease hypertension, anxiety, insomnia, stress, and fatigue (Earl E. Bakken Center for Spirituality & Healing, University of Minnesota, 2017b).

Exhibit 9.4. Alternate Nostril Breathing (*Nadi Shodhana*; Yoga Limb 4)

- Sit comfortably with a straight back.
- Breathe in a circular manner: slowly, evenly, deeply through your nostrils, from your abdomen, with your in-breath the same length as your out-breath, and no break in between.
- Place your right thumb on your right nostril, your ring finger on your left nostril, and inhale through both nostrils.
- Use your thumb to close your right nostril; exhale slowly through your left nostril, and then inhale slowly through your left nostril.
- Use your ring finger to close your left nostril; exhale slowly through your right nostril, and then inhale slowly through your right nostril.
- This sequence constitutes one round; repeat for five more rounds.

This *pranayama* technique promotes balance, gives each side of the body equal time, and strengthens the breath in the weaker nostril (Earl E. Bakken Center for Spirituality & Healing, University of Minnesota, 2017b).

Exhibit 9.5. Withdrawal of Senses, Concentration, Meditation (Limbs 5-8)

- Lie in Corpse Pose or sit comfortably with a straight back in a chair or on a meditation cushion; close your eyes, relax, and look inward.
- Breathe in a circular manner: slowly, evenly, deeply through your nostrils, from your abdomen, with your in-breath the same length as your out-breath, and no break in between.
- Focus on your breath.
- As you inhale through your nose, silently count "one." Exhale. On the next in-breath, count, "two," and so on.
- When your mind wanders away, bring it back to your breath and start with one again.
- At 10, go back to one again.
- When you are deeply relaxed and focused, open up to your inner experience; simply observe and let go of whatever arises, without attachment, judgment, or direction.

Withdrawal of the senses, concentration, meditation, and integration promote deep relaxation, healing, balance, replenishment, focus, and development of insight and joy (Earl E. Bakken Center for Spirituality & Healing, University of Minnesota, 2017b).

Nurses can help clients let go of external stimuli to relax and to sleep (Limb 5). Learning to concentrate and meditate can create meaning in suffering and motivation to develop optimal health (Limb 6 and Limb 7). Through a moment of integration or *samadhi*, individuals can experience oneness and joy, even when seriously ill and dying (Limb 8). Exhibit 9.5 explains a breathing exercise to apply Limbs 5 to 8. Meditating on the breath for even 2 minutes can help transform anger and confusion into compassion and clear thinking.

Guidelines

The best way to learn yoga is to do it. Yoga publications, videos, online postings, and modules describe guidelines for beginning through advanced levels (NCCIH, 2017. Some individuals use these resources to learn yoga on their own. Other people benefit from yoga classes and individual instruction. Qualified, experienced teachers can assist nurses to do yoga themselves and to use yoga as a nursing intervention (Earl E. Bakken Center for Spirituality & Healing, University of Minnesota, 2017b).

Effectiveness

Nurses can determine the effectiveness of yoga by asking themselves and clients how they feel after doing it. Most health problems develop over time, and yoga may not alleviate them immediately. Minor health issues may improve quickly, but serious problems may require sustained, patient practice. Yoga advocates gradual change. Optimal benefits occur from systematic practice. Short-term outcomes, however—including a more relaxed attitude, decreased anxiety, optimism, improved balance, improved sleep, and increased musculoskeletal flexibility—are notable. Faithful practice can produce long-term outcomes of better physical, spiritual, and mental health (Cameron, 2014; Ravishankar, 2016).

PRECAUTIONS

Injuries may result from doing yoga poses and breathing techniques in a harmful manner. Examples are straining to do postures, competing with someone, doing postures and breathing techniques right after eating, breathing stale air in a yoga studio, and doing poses fast in a hot environment (Broad, 2012). Yoga discourages anything unnatural, competitive, or hurtful. To avoid injury, nurses can encourage gentleness, mindfulness, self-compassion, and moderation. Although teachers and other aids can be helpful, individuals must listen to their inner wisdom (Earl E. Bakken Center for Spirituality & Healing, University of Minnesota, 2017b). Exhibit 9.6 lists more precautions (NCCIH, 2017).

Exhibit 9.6. Precautions Involving Yoga

- Do not use yoga to replace conventional care or to postpone seeing a health professional.
- If you have a health problem, talk with your health professionals before starting yoga.
- Carefully select the style of yoga; for example, hot yoga may not be good for you.
- Carefully select a practitioner who can help you modify yoga so that you practice safely.
- Give your health professionals a full picture of your health, including your yoga practice.

Currently, Hatha yoga teachers and yoga therapists are not licensed in the United States. Some states, such as Minnesota, passed statutes that regulate unlicensed practitioners of complementary and alternative therapies (Office of the Revisor of Statutes, 2017). Nurses who integrate yoga into their nursing practice must adhere to the higher requirements of their state boards of nursing. Before selecting yoga teachers or yoga therapists, nurses are best off finding out their education, credentialing, and experience. Ideally, hatha yoga teachers have RYT credentials (Yoga Alliance, 2017) and yoga therapists are certified by the International Association of Yoga Therapists (2017).

USES

Yoga is a good fit with nursing because both disciplines treat the whole person. By doing yoga and using yoga as a nursing intervention, nurses will promote nonreactivity of the mind and inner calmness that embraces, rather than denies, challenging circumstances (Cameron, 2014; Earl E. Bakken Center for Spirituality & Healing, 2017a). Exhibit 9.7 lists recent studies about benefits of yoga.

CULTURAL APPLICATIONS

All over the world, people adapt yoga to their culture and values (Earl E. Bakken Center for Spirituality & Healing, 2017b). Yoga is integral to many traditional healing systems such as Ayurveda and Tibetan medicine. These ancient, holistic traditions teach the importance of creating a healthy body and mind to live a yogic life (Earl E. Bakken Center for Spirituality & Healing, 2016a; Cameron et al., 2012). In Sidebar 9.1, Corjena Cheung, a Chinese nurse, describes yoga in Hong Kong.

Exhibit 9.7. Recent Studies About Benefits of Yoga for Individuals With Health Issues

Asthma: Yang et al. (2016)
Cancer: Derry et al. (2015)
Cardiovascular function: Hartley et al. (2014); Mayor (2014)
Cognition and quality of life: Lee, Moon, and Kim (2014)
Diabetes: Chimkode, Kumaran, Kanhere, and Shivanna (2015)
Elders' mobility and fear of falling: Nick, Petramfar, Ghodsbin, Keshavarzi, and Jahanbin (2016)
Intellectual disabilities: Balasubramaniam, Telles, and Doraiswamy (2013)
Low back pain: Cramer et al., (2013)
Osteoarthritis: Cheung, Park, and Wyman (2016)
Neurological, mental, and psychiatric disorders: Roland (2014)
Pain: Hernández, Suero, Barros, González-Mora, and Rubia (2016)
Physical inactivity: Grabara (2016)
Restless legs syndrome: Yoshihara, Hiramoto, Oka, Kubo, and Sudo (2014)
Smoking cessation: Dai and Sharma (2014)
Stress and inflammation: Bower et al. (2014)
Well-being: Hagen and Nayar (2014)

SIDEBAR 9.1. USE OF YOGA IN HONG KONG

Corjena K. Cheung

Yoga has become a fitness trend in Hong Kong. In the 1950s, yogis from India taught small groups of residents in Hong Kong. Graduates who became yoga teachers taught in local community centers. In the late 1990s, Westerners brought different yoga styles to Hong Kong. Starting in 2002, mega yoga studios, operating under fitness centers, became very popular.

Hong Kong, having received yoga from India and the West, has to find its own interpretation of yoga. Because of the glamour and focus on bodily beauty, yoga has a quick-fix appeal. About 90% of yoga students are women, most of whom turn to yoga for weight loss. Yoga is not popular with older adults; they prefer tai chi and qigong, which originated in China.

Although an ancient philosophy and practice from India, yoga in Hong Kong has an added twist from the West. Most residents do yoga as a system of physical exercise. As in the United State, yoga teachers complain that yoga in Hong Kong has become commercial, fixated on the body, and lacking in spirituality. Many residents do not understand the true meaning of yoga, which is to enhance physical, mental, emotional, and spiritual health. The power of yoga has been limited to improving body image and bringing about physical change.

The deeper dimension of yoga needs to be explored in Hong Kong. Some yoga teachers argue that yoga has undergone hundreds of years of research by ancient yoga practitioners, who observed the effects on their students. In recent years, a growing number of well-designed studies have affirmed the health benefits of yoga. Researchers have found that the practice of yoga is safe, useful, and cost-effective for a wide range of people. Ideally, yoga in Hong Kong, as in many modern cities, will evolve from a form of physical exercise to a commonly used, healthy way of life.

FUTURE RESEARCH

More research is needed to understand yoga and the ways that systematic yoga practice can benefit the discipline of nursing, individual nurses, and clients. Research studies about yoga generally report positive effects. The results of each study may be influenced by the participants' characteristics (age, gender, health status, and diagnosis), study entry criteria, type and duration of the yoga intervention, compliance, attrition, and related factors. Because yoga is a relatively new field of research, most studies are pilot studies with small sample sizes, short study periods, methodological flaws, inadequate control groups, and other limitations. The lack of standardized practices and the variety of yoga styles complicate applicability of the findings (Büssing, Khalsa, Michalsen, Sherman, & Telles, 2012; Earl E. Bakken Center for Spirituality & Healing, 2017b; Li & Goldsmith, 2014).

Yoga's holistic, integrated approach poses challenges for conducting scientific research. Yoga practices affect body and mind in a manner that may not be reproducible and quantifiable. Teasing out specific aspects of yoga is difficult and may not produce statistically significant results. Even so, the NCCIH (2017) is funding many yoga studies with promising results.

Nursing would benefit from well-designed studies that address these research questions:

- Which yoga practices are therapeutic for people with which health issues?
- How can nurses and clients be encouraged to use yoga as self-care?
- What are effective strategies for teaching nurses to use yoga as part of integrative nursing?
- Why do yoga injuries occur and what can be done to prevent them?
- What are ways for nurses to collaborate with hatha yoga teachers and yoga therapists?

New qualitative methodologies may be needed to study yoga as a holistic healing system. Investigating the deeper dimension of yoga, rather than focusing on postures, will enrich the findings. Additional research will encourage nurses to use yoga for self-care and integrate yoga into nursing practice.

REFERENCES

Balasubramaniam, M., Telles, S., & Doraiswamy, P. M. (2013). Yoga on our minds: A systematic review of yoga for neuropsychiatric disorders. *Frontiers in Psychiatry*, *3*(117), 1–16.

Boehm, K., Ostermann, T., Milazzo, S., & Bussing, A. (2012). Effects of yoga interventions on fatigue: A meta-analysis. *Evidence-Based Complementary & Alternative Medicine*, *2012*, 124703. doi:10.115/2012/124703

Bower, J. E., Greendale, G., Crosswell, A. D., Garet, D., Sternlieb, B., Ganz, P. A., ... Cole, S. W. (2014). Yoga reduces inflammatory signaling in fatigued breast cancer survivors: A randomized controlled trial. *Psychoneuroendocrinology*, *43*, 20–29.

Broad, W. (2012). *The science of yoga: Risks and rewards*. New York, NY: Simon & Schuster.

Büssing, A., Khalsa, S. B. S., Michalsen, A., Sherman, K. J., & Telles, S. (2012). Yoga as a therapeutic intervention. *Evidence-Based Complementary & Alternative Medicine*, 2012, 174291. doi:10.1155/2012/174291

Cameron, M. E. (2014). *Integrative Nursing: Yoga and Research*. Seoul, S. Korea: The Research Institute of Nursing Science, College of Nursing, Seoul National University.

Cameron, M. E., Torkelson, C., Haddow, S., Namdul, T., Prasek, A., & Gross, C. R. (2012). Tibetan medicine and integrative health: Validity testing and refinement of the constitutional self-assessment tool and lifestyle guidelines tool. *Explore: The Journal of Science and Healing*, *8*(3), 158–171.

Cheung, C., Park, J., & Wyman, J. F. (2016). Effects of yoga on symptoms, physical function, and psychosocial outcomes in adults with osteoarthritis: A focused review. *American Journal of Physical Medicine and Rehabilitation*, *95*(2), 139–151.

Chimkode, S. M., Kumaran, S. D., Kanhere, V. V., & Shivanna, R. (2015). Effect of yoga on blood glucose levels in patients with type 2 diabetes mellitus. *Journal of Clinical and Diagnostic Research*, *9*(4), CC01–CC03.

Cramer, H., Lauche, R., Haller, H., & Dobos, G. (2013). A systematic review and meta-analysis of yoga for low back pain. *Clinical Journal of Pain*, *29*(5), 450–460.

Dai, C. L., & Sharma, M. (2014). Between inhale and exhale: Yoga as an intervention in smoking cessation. *Journal of Evidence-Based Complementary & Alternative Medicine*, *19*(2), 144–149.

Derry, H. M., Jaremka, L. M., Bennett, J. M., Peng, J., Andridge, R., Shapiro, C., et al. (2015). Yoga and self-reported cognitive problems in breast cancer survivors: A randomized controlled trial. *Psycho-Oncology*, *24*(8), 958–966.

Earl E. Bakken Center for Spirituality & Healing, University of Minnesota. (2017a). *Integrative nursing.* Retrieved from https://www.csh.umn.edu/education/focus-areas/integrative-nursing

Earl E. Bakken Center for Spirituality & Healing, University of Minnesota. (2017b). *Yoga.* Retrieved from https://www.csh.umn.edu/education/online-learning-modules-resources/online-learning-modules

Earl E. Bakken Center for Spirituality & Healing, University of Minnesota. (2017c). Y*oga and Tibetan medicine.* Retrieved from http://www.csh.umn.edu/education/focus-areas/yoga-tibetan-medicine.

Earl E. Bakken Center for Spirituality & Healing, University of Minnesota. (2016a). *Ayurveda.* Retrieved from https://www.takingcharge.csh.umn.edu/explore-healing-practices/ayurvedic-medicine

Earl E. Bakken Center for Spirituality and Healing, University of Minnesota. (2016b). *Tibetan medicine.* Retrieved from https://www.takingcharge.csh.umn.edu/explore-healing-practices/tibetan-medicine

Galantino, M. L., Green, L., Decesari, J. A., Mackain, N. A., Rinaldi, S. M., Stevens, M. E., et al. (2012). Safety and feasibility of modified chair-yoga on functional outcome among elderly at risk for falls. *International Journal of Yoga, 5*(2), 146–150.

Grabara, M. (2016). Could hatha yoga be a health-related physical activity? *Biomedical Human Kinetics, 8*(1), 10–16.

Hagen, I., & Nayar, U. S. (2014). Yoga for children and young people's mental health and well-being: Research review and reflections on the mental health potentials of yoga. *Frontiers in Psychiatry, 5,* 35. doi:10.3389/fpsyt.2014.00035

Hartley, L., Dyakova, M., Holmes, J., Clarke, A., Lee, M. S., Ernst, E., & Rees, K. (2014). Yoga for the primary prevention of cardiovascular disease. *Cochrane Database of Systematic Review, 13,* CD010072. doi:10.1002/14651858.CD010072.pub2

Hawley, J. (2011). *The* Bhagavad Gita*: A walkthrough for Westerners.* Novato, CA: New World Library.

Hernández, S. E., Suero, J., Barros, A., González-Mora, J. L., & Rubia, K. (2016). Increased grey matter associated with long-term Sahaja yoga meditation: A voxel-based morphometry study. *PLOS ONE, 11*(3), e0150757. doi:10.1371/journal.pone.0150757

International Association of Yoga Therapists. (2017). *Bridging yoga and health care.* Retrieved from http://www.iayt.org/

Lee, M., Moon, W., & Kim, J. (2014). Effect of yoga on pain, brain-derived neurotrophic factor, and serotonin in premenopausal women with chronic low back pain. *Evidence-Based Complementary & Alternative Medicine, 2014,* 203173. doi:10.1155/2014/203173

Li, A. W. & Goldsmith, C. W. (2014). The effects of yoga on anxiety and stress. *Alternative Medicine Review, 17*(1), 21–35.

Mayor, S. (2014). Yoga reduces cardiovascular risk as much as walking or cycling, study shows. *British Medical Journal, 349,* g7713. doi:10.1136/bmj.g7713

Morgan, N., Irwin, M. R., Chung, M., & Wang, C. (2014). The effects of mind-body therapies on the immune system: Meta-analysis. *PLOS ONE, 9*(7), e100903. doi:10.1371/journal.pone.0100903

Muktibodhananda, S. (2016). *Hatha Yoga Pradipika.* Bihar, India: Yoga Publications Trust.

National Center for Complementary and Integrative Health. (2017). *Yoga.* Retrieved from https://nccih.nih.gov/health/yoga

Nick, N., Petramfar, P., Ghodsbin, F., Keshavarzi, S., & Jahanbin, I. (2016). The effect of yoga on balance and fear of falling in older adults. *Physical Medicine & Rehabilitation, 8*(2), 145–151.

Noggle, J. J., Steiner, N. J., Minami, T., & Khalsa, S. B. (2012). Benefits of yoga for psychosocial well-being in a US high school curriculum: A preliminary randomized controlled trial. *Journal of Developmental & Behavioral Pediatrics, 33*(3), 193–201.

Office of the Revisor of Statutes. (2017). *Chapter 146A. Complementary and alternative health care practices.* Retrieved from https://www.revisor.mn.gov/statutes/?id=146A

Okonta, N. R. (2012). Does yoga therapy reduce blood pressure in patients with hypertension? *Holistic Nursing Practice, 26*(3), 137–141.

Pascoe, M. C., & Bauer, I. E. (2015). A systematic review of randomised control trials on the effects of yoga on stress measures and mood. *Journal of Psychiatric Research,* 68, 270–282.

Ravishankar, S. S. (2016). *Patanjali Yoga Sutras.* Bangalore, India: Sri Sri Publications Trust, India.

Roland, K. P. (2014). Applications of yoga in Parkinson's disease: A systematic literature review. *Parkinsonism and Restless Legs Syndrome, 4,* 1–8.

Yang, Z. Y., Zhong, H. B., Mao, C., Yuan, J. Q., Huang, Y. F., Wu, X. Y., et al. (2016). Yoga for asthma. *São Paulo Medical Journal = Revista paulista de medicina, 134,* 368.

Yoshihara, K., Hiramoto, T., Oka, T., Kubo, C., & Sudo, N. (2014). Effect of 12 weeks of yoga training on the somatization, psychological symptoms, and stress-related biomarkers of healthy women. *BioPsychoSocial Medicine, 8*(1). doi:10.1186/1751-0759-8-1

Yoga Alliance. (2017). *Serving the yoga community.* Retrieved from https://www.yogaalliance.org

Biofeedback

MARION GOOD AND JACLENE A. ZAUSZNIEWSKI

Biofeedback is a technique that teaches people how to gain more control of involuntary bodily functions. Electronic sensors applied to the body allow a person to become more aware (feedback) of processes in his or her body (bio). Many different types of healthcare professionals rely on biofeedback to help their patients cope with a variety of conditions such as chronic pain, regain movement in paralyzed muscles, and learn to relax. Patients who suffer from migraine headaches, high blood pressure, and incontinence are just a few examples of those who can benefit from biofeedback therapy. This chapter provides an overview of biofeedback, its scientific basis, health conditions in which it is useful, and a technique that can be used by nurses trained in its practice.

DEFINITION

Biofeedback is based on holistic self-care perspectives in which (a) the mind and body are not separated and (b) people can learn ways to improve their health and performance. Biofeedback therapists use instruments and teach self-regulation strategies to help individuals increase voluntary control over their internal physiological and mental processes. Biofeedback instruments measure physiological activity such as muscle tension, skin temperature, cardiac activity, and brainwaves and then provide immediate and real-time feedback to the people in the form of visual and/or auditory signals that increase their awareness of internal processes. The biofeedback therapist then teaches individuals to change these signals and to take a more active role in maintaining the health of their minds and bodies. The holistic and self-care philosophies underlying biofeedback and its focus on helping subjects gain more control over personal functioning make the intervention an appropriate one for nurses to use. Over time, a person can learn to maintain these changes without continued use of a feedback instrument (Association for Applied Psychophysiology and Biofeedback [AAPB], 2016).

SCIENTIFIC BASIS

Biofeedback has been around longer and has a wider array of uses than one might think. The following data provide the basis for the use of biofeedback:

- Biofeedback originated from research in the fields of psychophysiology, learning theory, and behavioral theory. It has been used by nurses for decades and is consistent with self-care nursing theories.
- For centuries, it was believed that responses such as heart rate were beyond the individual's control. In the 1960s, scientists found that the autonomic nervous system (ANS) had an afferent, as well as a motor, system, and control of ANS functioning was possible with instrumentation and conditioning.
- For years, many researchers have used electromyograph (EMG) feedback of muscle tension to measure states of relaxation, anxiety, and muscular strength.
- Heart rate variability (HRV) biofeedback was first studied by Soviet scientists in the 1980s. HRV is the amount of fluctuation from the mean heart rate. It represents the interaction between the sympathetic and the parasympathetic systems and specifically targets ANS reactivity. HRV biofeedback is based on the premise that slowed breathing increases HRV amplitude, strengthens baroreflexes, and improves ANS functioning (McKee, 2008). HRV biofeedback is easy to learn and can be used with inexpensive, user-friendly devices, some of which can be used independently in the home.
- Neurofeedback uses EEG feedback to show people their actual patterns in cortical functioning. It also makes use of the brain's ability to change and can train the brain to function better (Neurodevelopment Center Inc., 2016).

The model for biofeedback is a skills-acquisition model in which individuals determine the relationship between ANS functioning and their voluntary muscle or cognitive/affective activities. They learn skills to control these activities, which are then reinforced by a visual and/or auditory display on the biofeedback instrument. The display informs the person whether control has been achieved, reinforcing learning. The following are conditions in which biofeedback has been used:

- Behavioral strategies, such as relaxation or muscle strengthening, are often part of biofeedback treatment to modify physiological activity.
- Biofeedback with relaxation strategies can be used to control autonomic responses that affect brain waves, peripheral vascular activity, heart rate, blood glucose, and skin conductance.
- Biofeedback combined with exercise can strengthen muscles weakened by conditions such as chronic pulmonary disease, knee surgery, or age.

INTERVENTION

Nurses are the ideal professionals to provide biofeedback because of their knowledge of physiology, psychology, and health and illness states. However, to use biofeedback they need to acquire special information, skills, and equipment. It is recommended that information be gained from classes and workshops available in many locations in the United States, a few other countries, and online. Nurses using biofeedback should become certified by the Biofeedback Certification International Alliance (BCIA, www.bcia.org), which offers certifications in general biofeedback, neurofeedback, and pelvic muscle dysfunction biofeedback. People in the following countries have received BCIA certificates: Australia, Austria, Brazil, Canada, China, Egypt, El Salvador, Germany, Greece, Ireland, Israel, Jamaica, Japan, Mexico, the Netherlands, Poland, Republic of Korea, Republic of Singapore, Slovakia, South Africa, Taiwan, Turkey, the United Kingdom, the United States, and Venezuela. The AAPB (www.aapb.org) is also an excellent resource for information.

For professionals in Europe, North and South America, Asia, and Africa, the Biofeedback Foundation of Europe (BFE) sponsors education, training, and research activities in biofeedback. On their website (www.bfe.org), BFE lists these opportunities in the form of conferences, workshops, Internet courses, courseware, and other materials. Both AAPB and BFE recommend the book *Biofeedback Mastery—An Experiential Teaching and Self-Training Manual*, which can be used for teaching and self-directed learning (Peper, Tylova, Gibney, Harvey, & Combatalade, 2009).

Another organization, Biofeedback Resources International (BRI; www.biofeedbackinternational.com), offers self-directed online courses that meet the didactic requirements for BCIA certification and offers software, books, and CDs of biofeedback treatment programs for anxiety, addiction, anger, and pain. Face-to-face training programs with hands-on training and mentoring, however, are strongly recommended. Biofeedback equipment for sale can also be found on the AAPB and the BRI websites.

The International Society for Neurofeedback and Research (ISNR) is a nonprofit member organization for health professionals, researchers, educators, and other individuals who are interested in the promotion of self-regulation of brain activity for healthier functioning. The major mission of the Society is "to promote excellence in clinical practice, educational applications, and research in applied neuroscience in order to better understand and enhance brain function" (https://www.isnr.org.) Although it is based in McLean, Virginia, Society members gather from around the globe for their annual scientific meetings.

Technique

A biofeedback unit consists of a sensor that monitors the patient's physiological activity and a transducer that converts what is measured into an electronic visual or auditory display. Frequently measured physiological parameters include muscle depolarization, which is monitored by electromyelogram (EMG) and peripheral temperature.

Biofeedback provides information about changes in a physiological parameter when behavioral treatments such as relaxation or strengthening exercises are used for a health problem. For example, a relaxation tape helps patients relax the muscles, and the EMG biofeedback instrument informs the learner of progress (i.e., reduced tension in the muscles). Temperature feedback is also used with relaxation treatments. As muscles relax, circulation improves, and the fingers and toes become warmer. When exercises are used to strengthen perineal muscles in preventing urinary incontinence in women, success in contracting the correct muscles may be monitored by a pressure sensor inserted into the vagina. In health conditions exacerbated by stress, biofeedback is often combined with stress-management counseling.

Biofeedback is most frequently used in an office or clinic setting. Both the behavioral and feedback aspects of the therapy should be explained to patients. The length and number of sessions depends on the condition being treated. If the patient has not achieved mastery or control of a function by the end of an agreed-on number of sessions, the reasons and the need for further sessions should be discussed.

The first session is devoted to assessing the patient, choosing the appropriate mode of feedback, discussing the roles of the nurse and the patient, and obtaining baseline measurements. Measuring several parameters helps in getting valid baseline data. Because success is determined by changes from baseline, it is essential that these are accurate and reflect the true status of the parameter being used. The first session is longer than subsequent ones, perhaps lasting 1 to 2 hours. Behavioral exercises are provided.

The therapist plays a key role in the success of biofeedback. It is helpful for the nurse to have advanced training in relaxation, imagery, and stress management counseling. Because practice of the behavioral techniques is vital, the nurse who succeeds in motivating patients to practice at home is most likely to have patients who exceed their goals.

The final sessions focus on integration of the learning into the person's life. The patient is connected to the machine but does not receive feedback while practicing the technique; the nurse monitors the degree of control achieved. Descriptions of stressful situations are provided, and the person is asked to practice the procedure as if in those situations. Final measurements are taken. Follow-up sessions at 1 month and 6 months are advocated.

Guidelines for Biofeedback-Assisted Relaxation

A protocol for using biofeedback with cognitive behavioral interventions for relaxation and stress management is found in Exhibit 10.1. This technique could be used for hypertension, anxiety, asthma, headache, or pain because muscle relaxation improves these conditions. The protocol should be tailored to the patient, condition, and type of feedback.

Various types of relaxation exercises, such as autogenic phases or systematic relaxation, may be used. To increase patient awareness of the relaxed state versus the state of tension, progressive muscle relaxation with alternate contraction and relaxation may be helpful. Imagery may relax patients by distracting the mind and reducing negative or stressful thoughts. Hypnosis and self-hypnosis also produce an alternative state of mind. Soft music relaxes and distracts and may be used with relaxation or imagery.

It is important to keep the requirements for home practice simple, interesting, and meaningful. For example, boredom with the same relaxation instructions, failure to find a convenient time to practice, and lack of noticeable improvements may decrease adherence to home practice. Changing to a new relaxation technique can revive interest. To integrate new skills into daily life, patients can progress to minirelaxation and use of cues (thoughts, positions, or activities) to signal relaxation. Using a qualitative design, Zauszniewski examined six parameters

Exhibit 10.1. Biofeedback Protocol

1. **Before first session**
   - Determine health problem for which biofeedback treatment is sought.
   - Ask for physician's name so that care can be coordinated. Give information on location, time commitment, and cost.
   - Request a 2-week patient log with medications and the frequency and severity of the health problem (e.g., number, intensity, and time of headaches).
   - Answer questions.

2. **First session**
   - Interview patient for a health history; include the specific health condition.
   - Assess abilities for carrying out current medical regimen and behavioral intervention. Assess cultural preferences for behavioral treatments.
   - Discuss rationale for biofeedback, type of feedback, and behavioral intervention.
   - Explain that the role of the nurse is to provide ten 50-minute sessions once a week, using the biofeedback instrument to supply physiological information.
   - Explain that the patient is the major factor in the successful use of biofeedback and that it is important to continue to keep a log of the health problem, including home practice sessions. The patient should consult the physician if other health problems occur.
   - Explain the procedure. If using frontalis muscle tension EMG feedback, apply three sensors to the forehead after cleaning the skin with soap and water and applying gel. Set the biofeedback machine and operate according to instructions.
   - Obtain baseline EMG readings of frontalis muscle tension for 5 minutes while the patient sits quietly with closed eyes.
   - Instruct the patient to practice taped relaxation instructions for 20 minutes while the EMG sensors are on the forehead. Ask the patient to watch the biofeedback display for information on the decreasing level of muscle tension.
   - Review the 2-week record of the health problem and set mutual goals.
   - Give an electronic sound file of the type the patient would like containing instructions for practicing relaxation at home. Provide a log to record practice and responses. Discuss timing, frequency, length, and setting for practice.
   - Discuss self-care for any possible side effects to the behavioral intervention.

3. **Subsequent sessions**
   - Open the session with a 20-minute review of the health-problem log, stressors, and ways used for coping in the past week; provide counseling for adaptive coping.
   - Apply sensors and earphones and let the patient practice relaxation for 20 minutes while watching the display. Quietly leave the room after the patient masters the technique.
   - Vary relaxation techniques to maintain interest and increase skill.
   - Give instructions for incremental integration of relaxation into daily life. For example, add 30-second minirelaxation exercises for busy times of the day (e.g., touch thumbs to middle fingers, close eyes, and feel relaxation spreading through the body).

4. **Final session**
   - Conduct the session as described; obtain final EMG readings.
   - Discuss a plan for ongoing practice and stress management after treatment ends.

Exhibit 10.2. Parameters Used for Feedback to Patients

Airway resistance	Gastric pH
Blood pressure	Heart rate
Blood volume	Heart rate variability
Bowel sounds	Peripheral skin temperature
EEG neurofeedback	Pneumography
EMG muscle feedback	Tidal volume
Forced expiratory volume	Tracheal noise
Galvanic skin response	Vagal nerve stimulation

for evaluating self-management interventions: necessity, acceptability, feasibility, safety, fidelity, and effectiveness. In women experiencing caregiver stress, she used HRV biofeedback training. This is an important examination of the biofeedback recipient's perspective of factors that are necessary for ongoing self-care practice (Zauszniewski, Musil, Herbell, & Givens, 2017).

Although some patients have multiple symptoms that all require treatment, training should address only one symptom at a time. Other symptoms can be treated sequentially after mastery of the first is attained. The patient can decide which symptom will be treated first.

Measurement of Outcomes

Feedback parameters that reflect mastery of the behavioral intervention are found in Exhibit 10.2. Frequently used mastery parameters include heart rate, muscle tension, peripheral temperature, blood pressure, HRV, and EEG neurofeedback. For learning purposes, it is important that the nurse be clear about (a) mastery parameters that consist of ongoing feedback to the patient and (b) outcome parameters that reflect the desired health improvement. For example, temperature feedback is used in peripheral vascular problems, but healthcare outcomes may result in fewer episodes of painful vasoconstriction. Both EMG feedback and temperature feedback are learning modalities used in those with diabetes mellitus, tension headache, and chronic pain. Outcomes may include decreased glycosylated hemoglobin, fewer and/or less severe headaches, cessation of urinary incontinence, and relief of pain.

PRECAUTIONS

Biofeedback should be used cautiously, if at all, in patients with depression psychosis, seizures, and hyperactive conditions. Those with rigid personalities may be unwilling to change their mode of functioning. The nurse should consider that negative reactions may be related to relaxation rather than to biofeedback. Relaxation-related reactions may be avoided by means of patient education and the type of relaxation used (Schwartz & Andrisik, 2003).

Biofeedback-assisted relaxation is expected to lower blood pressure and heart and respiratory rates. Excessive decreases should be avoided in patients with cardiac conditions, hemodynamic instability, or multiple illnesses.

Use of relaxation therapies may also reduce the amount of medication needed to control diabetes mellitus, hypertension, and asthma. This should be discussed with patients and physicians, and responses to therapy should be carefully monitored. For example, in individuals with diabetes, there is the potential for hypoglycemic reactions if patient education is not provided or if adjustments in insulin or diet are not made. Patients should be taught to manage hypoglycemia and blood glucose. The nurse should keep simple carbohydrates, glucagon, and a blood glucose monitor in the office and have the expertise to administer them. Home practice can be timed to avoid low blood glucose (McGrady & Bailey, 2005).

Nurses should therefore consider the person, the health problem, any known adverse reactions to the behavioral intervention used, and negative reactions to the biofeedback itself. For example, perineal muscle strengthening exercises for stress incontinence carry the risk of "accidents" during the muscle strengthening process, which can be compensated for with padding; however, pharyngeal muscle exercises for dysphasia following stroke carry the more serious risk of aspiration as strength is slowly regained. Finally, although there are generally few side effects to using biofeedback with relaxation or exercises to improve function, ineffectiveness is always possible. Nurses should be cautioned to consider the risks of using a mild intervention with variable effectiveness and to also assess for age and culture-related acceptability and effectiveness as the patient tries both biofeedback and the nonpharmacological treatment. On the other hand, the nurse and patient should consider the learning benefits of using nondrug methods and receiving biological feedback on the patient's efforts to improve body functioning.

Electric shock is a potential hazard when any electrical equipment is used. Dangerous levels of current flow may arise from equipment malfunction or operator error. Zauszniewski et al. (2017) studied the perceived safety of a HRV biofeedback intervention from the perspective of caregivers who were the biofeedback recipients. In the case of electricity, objective evaluation of safety is highly important. The AAPB publishes a list of companies whose products have met their safety code.

Although biofeedback is noninvasive, cost-effective, and very promising in the treatment of many conditions, it is not a miracle intervention. It requires that the therapist be knowledgeable about the health problem, intervention, and medication effects, with a sincere interest in patient outcome. It requires the patient to contribute time, attention, and motivation for success of the biofeedback practice. Ongoing use of the behavioral technique may be needed to control the condition after biofeedback sessions end. This should be made very clear before training is initiated.

USES

Biofeedback has been used in the treatment of many medical and psychological problems. For example, neurofeedback is used for attention and learning disabilities, seizures, depression, brain injury, substance abuse, and anxiety. HRV biofeedback, another relatively new approach, is possibly efficacious for depressive disorders, asthma, coronary heart disease, and myocardial infarction (Yucha & Montgomery, 2008). The AAPB website lists many conditions in which biofeedback has been empirically studied, and has resulted in an efficacy rating of 3 (probably efficacious) to 5 (efficacious and specific). Biofeedback has been shown to be efficacious in multiple observational, clinical, and wait-list controlled studies, including replications. A visitor to the AAPB website can click on the health condition of interest and obtain information on the level of evidence, the reason biofeedback would help, and the supporting evidence (www.aapb.org/i4a/pages/index .cfm?pageID=3404)

Researchers reviewed the efficacy ratings for many disorders that have been treated with biofeedback (Yucha & Montgomery, 2008). The health condition for which the best evidence is available is urinary incontinence in women (level 5— efficacious and specific). Biofeedback treatment of hypertension in adults, anxiety, and chronic pain are at level 4 (efficacious), whereas diabetes mellitus, fecal incontinence, and insomnia are at level 3 (probably efficacious).

Inspection of the PubMed database reveals that nurses have authored biofeedback studies on health problems that are of interest to nurses and are commonly seen in nursing care. These problems include labor stress, pelvic floor muscle strength after delivery, poststroke footdrop, chemotherapy, stress in mastectomy, climacteric symptoms, incontinence, blood glucose in diabetes, stress in nurses, pediatric migraine, hemodialysis, overactive bladder, hypertension, movement in hemiplegia, anxiety, and chronic lumbar pain.

Tension Headache

Controlled clinical and follow-up studies have shown that biofeedback reduces tension headaches in adults and children. Tension headaches are caused by prolonged tension in the face, jaws, neck, and shoulders. Muscle tension feedback is used to teach patients to recognize their level of tension and relax the muscles using relaxation therapy. Yucha and Montgomery (2008) found that several meta-analyses reporting biofeedback to have a stable medium effect for migraine and is as good as current medications for both migraine and tension headaches (Andrasik, 2007; Secic, Cvjeticanin, & Kes, 2016). The effects for most people last as long as they continue to practice the behavioral techniques they have learned.

Fecal Incontinence

A Cochrane review of 21 eligible randomized or quasirandomized trials evaluated biofeedback and/or anal sphincter exercises in 1,525 adults with fecal incontinence. They reported that the limited number of trials and their methodological weaknesses do not allow a definitive assessment of the possible role of anal sphincter exercises and biofeedback therapy in this population (Norton & Cody, 2012). These findings were supported by a subsequent Cochrane review (Woodward, Norton, & Chiarelli, 2014).

Motor Function After Stroke

An early Cochrane review found that 13 small trials of EMG biofeedback plus standard physiotherapy (269 people) provided weak evidence of effectiveness for motor function after stroke. Nevertheless, a small number of individual studies continued to suggest that EMG biofeedback plus standard physiotherapy improved motor power, functional recovery, and gait quality compared with physiotherapy alone (Woodford & Price, 2007; Yucha & Montgomery, 2008). A recent systematic review with meta-analysis of randomized trials found that biofeedback was superior to usual therapy/placebo in improving lower limb activities following stroke. Furthermore, these benefits were largely maintained in the longer term (Stanton, Ada, Dean, & Preston, 2011). Recent studies continue to be conducted for various poststroke issues such as hand motion (Dogan-Aslan, Nakipoglu-Yuzer, Dogan, Karabay, & Ozgirgin, 2012; Hsu, et al. 2012) and locomotion by using cycling (Ferrante et al., 2011), functional gait training (Jonsdottir et al. 2012), or a treadmill (Druzbicki, Kwolek, Depa, & Przysada, 2010).

Caregiver Stress

Stress accompanies many life experiences. For example, the stress experienced by grandmothers who are raising grandchildren in the absence of the parents has been found to have adverse effects of the grandmother's health. HRV biofeedback has been examined in that population in four small studies in which the grandmothers were taught slow-paced breathing to increase their HRV using a portable biofeedback device in their homes for 4 weeks (Zauszniewski, Au, & Musil, 2013; Zauszniewski & Musil, 2014; Zauszniewski, Musil & Variath, 2015; Zauszniewski, Musil, Herbell, & Givens, 2017). In addition, HRV biofeedback is being studied as a health self-management intervention in a study of family caregivers of patients with bipolar disorder (Zauszniewski, Sajatovic, & Burant, 2016- 2020); the study was funded by the National Institutes of Health (NIH).

Children and Adolescents

Age-appropriate biofeedback can be used to treat many conditions, such as migraine, hypertension, and fecal incontinence, in children and adolescents. Biofeedback, combined with self-hypnotherapy, helps them change their thoughts and bring about changes in their bodies. Olness (2008) describes special biofeedback equipment, explanations, and inductions for children. She reports the use of many imaginative techniques that appeal to children. Recent studies have reported successful use of EEG neurofeedback in children to improve attention deficit disorder (Bakhtadze, Beridze, Geladze, Khachapuridze, & Bornstein, 2016) and overactive bladder syndrome (Ebiloglu et al., 2016). An electronic breath game improved breath awareness among children with cystic fibrosis (Bingham, Bates, Thompson-Figueroa, & Lahiri, 2010).

CULTURAL APPLICATIONS

Biofeedback therapy has been used and studied around the world. In Thailand, for example, it has been used for a variety of conditions, as shown in Sidebar 10.1.

SIDEBAR 10.1. USE OF BIOFEEDBACK IN THAILAND

Nutchanart Bunthumporn

Many kinds of biofeedback—including galvanic skin response, electromyography, electroencephalography, and HRV—are used in Thailand. However, electromyography feedback is used most widely. Biofeedback is most often used with relaxation techniques to decrease stress and anxiety in students, staff nurses, and patients with chronic diseases. Along with autogenic training, it has also helped decrease aggressive behaviors in drug abusers and improve behaviors in children with attention deficit hyperactivity disorder. In a randomized study, an HRV biofeedback training program with support for paced breathing decreased older patients' depressive symptoms, negative affect, and depressive cognitions and enhanced their resourceful behaviors ($N = 100$; Bunthumporn, 2012). The first of three biofeedback studies by nurse researchers in Thailand reported that progressive relaxation and group supportive psychotherapy reduced depressive symptoms and muscle tension in older adults with chronic illness (Muijeen, Ruchiwit, & somprasert, 2012). The second found that meditation training with biofeedback training reduced stress in patients with chronic disease (Thongkhum, Ruchiwit, & sompraserts, 2015). The third study showed that HRV biofeedback significantly decreased depressive symptom scores in adults with depressive disorders (Ngamlers et al., 2018).

The benefits of biofeedback are limited by practitioner issues such as complexity of use, availability of training, and overall cost of some devices. To improve the training issues, biofeedback concepts have been integrated into courses for nursing and psychology graduate students. Interestingly, challenges of biofeedback technology did not deter Thai older adults, as there was no attrition during the Bunthumporn study (2012).

There are national biofeedback associations in 15 countries in North and South America, Europe, Asia, the Middle East, and Russia (Biofeedback Resources International, 2008). Although the number of articles published outside the United States cannot be easily estimated, the PubMed database identifies scientific articles about biofeedback that have been written in Japanese, German, Dutch, French, Spanish, Chinese, Norwegian, Finnish, Czech, Hebrew, Korean, Russian, and other languages. In the Russian and Japanese languages, for example, there are studies on many different health problems, including epilepsy, asthma, itch, sleep, and mandibular dysfunction. Many of these studies are written in English.

Using their native languages, nurses have authored or coauthored research reports on biofeedback for a variety of health problems of interest to nurses. Nurses in England reviewed how biofeedback is used to treat bowel dysfunction in adults with constipation (Burch & Collins, 2010). In the Chinese language, nurses reported that biofeedback training in adults with functional constipation improved bowel symptoms, quality of life, and psychological

(continued)

status (Zhu et al. 2011). Nurse researchers in Taiwan used a quasiexperimental design and demonstrated that biofeedback relaxation reduced the pain associated with continuous passive motion after total knee arthroplasty (Wang et. al., 2015).

HRV, heart rate variability.

FUTURE RESEARCH

There continues to be great need for randomized controlled clinical trials to determine the effectiveness, acceptability, and durability of biofeedback in treating physiological and psychological conditions in adults, children, and minorities worldwide. Biofeedback studies of prevalent local health problems are needed in developing countries. However, large multicenter studies with similar inclusion criteria, biofeedback protocol, and research methods are needed to show overall efficacy (Yucha, 2002). In addition, the perspective of biofeedback recipients regarding factors that are needed for ongoing self-care practice need further study. Nurses can address the following questions:

- What is the availability of biofeedback training in various countries?
- What culturally acceptable behavioral treatments can be provided with biofeedback?
- What are the predictors of improvement in using biofeedback for managing health?
- Do potential biofeedback recipients believe that biofeedback is necessary, acceptable, feasible, effective, and safe and that it can be performed by following a specified protocol (i.e., fidelity)?

REFERENCES

Andrasik, F. (2007). What does the evidence show? Efficacy of behavioural treatments for recurrent headaches in adults. *Neurological Sciences, 28*(Suppl. 2), S70–S77.

Association for Applied Psychophysiology and Biofeedback. (2016). 2018 AAPB 49th Annual Scientific Meeting. Retrieved from http://www.aapb.org

Bakhtadze, S., Beridze, M., Geladze, N., Khachapuridze, N., & Bornstein, N. (2016). Effect of EEG biofeedback on cognitive flexibility in children with attention deficit hyperactivity disorder with and without epilepsy. *Applied Psychophysiology and Biofeedback, 41*(1), 71–79.

Bingham, P. M., Bates, J. H., Thompson-Figueroa, J., & Lahiri, T. (2010). A breath biofeedback computer game for children with cystic fibrosis. *Clinical Pediatrics (Philadelphia), 49*(4), 337–342.

Bunthumporn, N. (2012). *Effects of biofeedback training on negative affect, depressive cognitions, resourceful behaviors, and depressive symptoms in Thai elders.* Retrieved from OhioLINK ETD Center (https://etd.ohiolink.edu/!etd.send_file?accession=case1333479530&disposition=inline).

Burch, J., Collins, B. (2010). Using Biofeedback to treat constipation, faecal incontinence and other bowel disorders. Nursing Times, 106(37), 20-21,

Dogan-Aslan, M., Nakipoglu-Yuzer, G. F., Dogan, A., Karabay, I., & Ozgirgin, N. (2012). The effect of electromyograph biofeedback treatment in improving upper extremity functioning of patients with hemiplegic stroke. *Journal of Stroke and Cerebrovascular Diseases, 21*(3), 187–192.

Druzbicki, M., Kwolek, A., Depa, A., & Przysada, G. (2010). The use of a treadmill with biofeedback function in assessment of relearning walking skills in post-stroke hemiplegic patients: A preliminary report. *Neurologia i neurochirurgia polska, 44*(6), 567–573.

Ebiloglu, T., Kaya, E., Kopru, B., Topuz, B., Irkilata, H. C., & Kibar, Y. (2016). Biofeedback as a first-line treatment for overactive bladder syndrome refractory to standard urotherapy in children. *Journal of Pediatric Urology, 12*(5), 290.e1–290.e7.

Ferrante, S., Ambrosini, E., Ravelli, P., Guanziroli, E., Molteni, F., Ferrigno, G., & Pedrocchi, A. (2011). A biofeedback cycling training to improve locomotion: A case series study based on gait pattern classification of 153 chronic stroke patients. *Journal of Neuroengineering and Rehabilitation, 8,* 47.

Hsu, H.-Y., Lin, C.-F., Su, F.-C., Kuo, H.-T., Chiu, H.-Y., & Kuo, L.-C. (2012). Clinical application of computerized evaluation and re-education biofeedback prototype for sensorimotor control of the hand in stroke patients. *Journal of Neuroengineering and Rehabilitation, 9,* 26. doi:10.1186/1743-0003-9-26

Jonsdottir, J., Cattaneo, D., Recalcati, M., Regola, A., Rabuffetti, M., Ferrarin, M., & Casiraghi, A. (2012). Task-oriented biofeedback to improve gait in individuals with chronic stroke: Motor learning approach. *Neurorehabilitation and Neural Repair, 24*(5), 478–485.

McGrady, A., & Bailey, B. (2005). Diabetes mellitus. In M. S. Schwartz & F. Andrisik (Eds.), *Biofeedback: A practitioner's guide* (3rd ed., pp. 727–750). New York, NY: Guilford Press.

McKee, M. G. (2008). Biofeedback: An overview in the context of heart-brain medicine. *Cleveland Clinic Journal of Medicine, 75*(Suppl. 2), S31–S34.

Muijeen, K., Ruchiwit, M., & Sompraset, C. (2012 January–April). The effect of progressive muscular relaxation program and group supportive psychotherapy on depression levels of the elderly with chronic illness. *Journal of Psychiatric Nursing and Mental Health, 26*(1), 19–34.

Neurodevelopment Center Inc. (2016, December 14). What is neurofeedback? Retrieved from https://neurodevelopmentcenter.com/neurofeedback-2

Ngamlers, D., Bunthumporn, N., & Somprasert, C. (2018 January–April). The effects of a heart rate variability biofeedback training program on depression symptoms of adults with depression disorder. *Journal of Psychiatric Nursing and Mental Health, 61*(1).

Norton, C., & Cody, J. D. (2012). Biofeedback and/or sphincter exercises for the treatment of faecal incontinence in adults. *Cochrane Database Systematic Reviews, 7,* CD002111.

Olness, K. (2008, March). Helping children and adults with hypnosis and biofeedback. *Cleveland Clinic Journal of Medicine, 75*(Suppl. 2), S39–S43.

Peper, E., Tylova, H., Gibney, K. H., Harvey, R., & Combatalade, D. (2009). *Biofeedback mastery—An experiential teaching and self-training manual.* Wheat Ridge, CO: Association for Applied Psychophysiology and Biofeedback.

Schwartz, M. S., & Andrisik, F. (Eds.). (2003). *Biofeedback: A practitioner's guide* (3rd ed.). New York, NY: Guilford Press.

Secic, A., Cvjeticanin, T., & Kes, V. B. (2016). Biofeedback training and tension-type headache. *Acta Clinica Croatia, 55*(1), 156–160.

Stanton, R., Ada, L., Dean, C. M., & Preston, E. (2011). Biofeedback improves activities of the lower limb after stroke: A systematic review. *Journal of Physiotherapy, 57*(3), 145–155.

Thongkhum, K., Ruchiwit, M., & Somprasert, C. (2015 January–March). The effect of meditation training together with biofeedback training program on the stress levels of chronic disease patients. *Nursing Journal, 42*(1), 25–37.

Wang, T., Chang, C., Lou, M., Ao, M. et al. (2015). Biofeedback relaxation for pain associated with continuous passive motion in Taiwanese patients after total knee arthroplasty. Research in Nursing & Health,38 (1), 39-50.

Woodford, H., & Price, C. (2007, April 18). EMG biofeedback for the recovery of motor function after stroke. *Cochrane Database of Systematic Reviews, 2,* CD004585.

Woodward, S., Norton, C., & Chiarelli, P. (2014). Biofeedback for treatment of chronic idiopathic constipation in adults. *Cochrane Database of Systematic Reviews, 3,* CD008486. doi:10.1002/14651858.CD008486.pub2

Yucha, C., & Montgomery, D. (2008). *Evidence-based practice in biofeedback and neurofeedback.* Wheat Ridge, CO: Association for Applied Psychophysiology and Biofeedback.

Yucha, C. B. (2002). Problems inherent in assessing biofeedback efficacy studies. *Applied Psychophysiology and Biofeedback, 27*(1), 99–106.

Zauszniewski, J. A., Au, T.Y., & Musil, C. M. (2013). Heart rate variability biofeedback in grandmothers raising grandchildren: Effects on stress, emotions, and cognitions. *Biofeedback, 41*(2), 144–149.

Zauszniewski, J. A., & Musil, C. M. (2014). Interventions for grandmothers: Comparative effectiveness of resourcefulness training, HRV biofeedback, and journaling. *Biofeedback, 42*(3), 131–129.

Zauszniewski, J. A., Musil, C. M., Herbell, K., & Givens, S. (2017). Heart rate variability in grandmothers: Evaluation of intervention parameters. *Issues in Mental Health Nursing, 38(6)*, 493-499.

Zauszniewski, J. A., Musil C. M., & Variath, M. (2015). Biofeedback in grandmothers raising grandchildren: Correlations between subjective and objective measures. *Biofeedback, 44*(4), 193–199.

Zauszniewski, J. A., Sajatovic, M., & Burant, C. J. (2016–2020). *Tailored health self-management interventions for highly distressed family caregivers.* National Institute of Nursing Research, RO1-NR6817.

Zhu, F., Lin, Z., Wang, M. (2011). Changes in quality of life during biofeedback for people with puborectalis dyssynergia: gereric and disease-specific measures. Journal of Advanced Nursing, 67(6), 1285-1293.

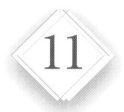

Meditation

CYNTHIA R. GROSS, MICHAEL S. CHRISTOPHER,
AND MARYANNE REILLY-SPONG

Meditation is the quintessential mind–body practice and the foundation for a number of widely used training programs, each with a rapidly growing evidence base to support health benefits (Creswell, 2017). Between 2002 and 2007, the number of U.S. adults turning to meditation for health reasons significantly increased, and in 2012 an estimated 8% of U.S. adults practiced meditation—nearly 18 million people (nccih.nih.gov/health/meditation). Primary reasons for meditating are to enhance well being, mitigate symptoms such as anxiety or pain, and self-manage chronic conditions (P. M. Barnes, Bloom, & Nahin, 2008). Among the most widely used and well-researched meditation programs are mindfulness-based stress reduction (MBSR) and transcendental meditation (TM; Kabat Zinn, 1990; Rosenthal, 2011). This chapter focuses on these and closely related programs and includes experimental findings of structural, physiological, cognitive, and emotional effects from meditation training. Although some definitions of *mindfulness meditation* consider practices such as yoga, tai chi, qigong, and meditation within the context of religious observance and prayer (e.g., chanting, use of prayer [Rosary] beads), these practices are covered elsewhere in this book and are therefore not included in this chapter.

In recent years, there has been a veritable explosion of research on meditation. Whereas in 2007 a major evidence report concluded that no firm conclusions could be drawn regarding the therapeutic impacts of any meditative practice or program based on available evidence (Ospina et al., 2007), recent meta-analyses, including research from the past decade, have confirmed benefits for selected health outcomes (Bai et al., 2015; Goyal et al., 2014; Hilton et al., 2016). There are many indications that this field is rapidly maturing. Currently funded grants have heeded calls for rigorously designed and adequately powered clinical trials, in-depth and replicable investigations of mechanisms of change, and tailored interventions. We recommend *Leaves Falling Gently: Living Fully with Serious and Life-Limiting Illness through Mindfulness, Compassion, and Connectedness* (Bauer-Wu, 2011), a brief and engaging introduction to mindfulness meditation for patients and health providers. Written by a nurse researcher, this book has detailed examples of how to integrate mindfulness into one's life and healthcare practice, and it is based on experience teaching meditation practices to hundreds of patients.

DEFINITION

For thousands of years and in many civilizations, meditation practices have played an important role in religious observances and as a means of cultivating well-being. *Meditation* can be defined as a set of attentional practices leading to an altered state or trait of consciousness characterized by expanded awareness, greater presence, and a more integrated sense of self (Davis, Lau, & Cairns, 2009). These practices are used to self-regulate the mind and body, thereby affecting mental events by engaging a specific attentional set. There are many distinct meditative techniques, but self-regulation of attention is a major component that is common among all of them, and it is possible to classify meditative style on a continuum, depending on how attentional processes are directed (Cahn & Polich, 2006).

Lutz, Slagter, Dunne, and Davidson (2008) proposed a theoretical framework in which meditation practices are categorized in two main groups—mindfulness and concentration. Mindfulness meditation strategies involve bringing one's attention in a nonjudgmental or in an accepting way to whatever experience arises in the present moment. In mindfulness, practitioners are instructed to allow any thought, feeling, or sensation to arise in consciousness while maintaining a nonreactive awareness to what is being experienced. Mindfulness practice was developed primarily in Buddhism, where it has been an integral component of a 2,500-year-old system of training that leads to insight and the overcoming of suffering (Bodhi, 2011). In the West, mindfulness has been integrated into medicine, nursing, psychology, and related fields, with the goal of teaching patients a more mindful approach to reducing distress, preventing relapse, and enhancing quality of life (e.g., MBSR).

Concentrative meditation processes involve focusing attention on a selected mental or sensory object. The object of focus may be breath or body sensations, a subvocal repeated sound or word (mantra), or an imagined mental image. In concentration meditation, awareness is narrowed so that the mind attends only to the object of focus. The mind is gently returned to the object of meditation when the meditator notices that it has wandered. Similar to mindfulness, concentration meditation was developed primarily in Buddhism, but it is also a core element in Sufism, Hinduism, and many other religious traditions. It has also become a widely practiced meditation in the West, beginning in the 1960s with the development of TM (Yogi, 1963).

In comparing the two types of meditation, Germer (2005) noted that mindfulness meditation is akin to a searchlight that illuminates a wider range of objects as they arise in awareness, one at a time, whereas concentration meditation is like a laser light beam that highlights whatever object on which it is directed. It has been hypothesized that meditators pass through stages, from effortful to effortless maintenance of a meditative state (Tang & Posner, 2013). Consistent with this conceptualization, the concentrative and guided-meditation techniques taught to novices have been termed "scaffolding" by Jon Kabat-Zinn, and others have commented on mantras with the phrase "you use it to lose it."

SCIENTIFIC BASIS

Understanding how meditation works is the basis for groundbreaking research by leading neuroscientists. Tang (2011) summarized the findings from a series of clinical trials they conducted to examine the effects of Integrative Body-Mind Training (IBMT), a brief meditation training program that he developed. In the first trial, 80 undergraduate students in China were randomly assigned to 5 days of 20 minutes of training per day with IBMT or to relaxation training. Findings showed that meditation, compared to relaxation, improves mood and abilities to self-regulate emotions and efficiently deploy cognitive resources. The IBMT group had significantly better attentional control (important for executive functioning); more energy/vigor; less anxiety, depression, anger, and fatigue on the Profile of Mood States (POMS); less stress reactivity to a mental arithmetic stressor based on cortisol levels; and greater immunoreactivity. Additional clinical trials have been conducted using the same treatment and a range of outcomes, including brain imaging (measures of regional cerebral blood flow), EEG, heart rate, and respiratory rate. Findings supported hypotheses that meditation improved regulation of the autonomic nervous system via systems in the ventral midfrontal brain system. In a series of controlled experiments with patients, clinician-scientists Park, Lyles, and Bauer-Wu (2014) have shown that a 14-minute mindfulness meditation acutely lowers blood pressure and muscle sympathetic nerve activity in Black men with chronic kidney disease. Other investigators have explored neuroplasticity: changes in brain morphology following meditation training. A meta-analytic review of 21 neuroimaging studies in about 300 meditation practitioners concluded that particular brain regions are consistently altered in meditators, although methodological limitations and possible publication bias likely impact estimates of morphological changes (Fox et al., 2014).

Hölzel et al. (2011) synthesized self-report, brain imaging, and experimental evidence on meditation's impacts and proposed four distinct but interrelated mechanisms of action for mindfulness meditation: attention regulation, body awareness, emotional regulation, and change in perspective on the self. These authors note that mindfulness techniques may differ in the extent they activate each mechanism, which suggests an opportunity to tailor practices to specific health needs. Evidence of physiological and structural impacts of meditation provide a powerful stimulus for new clinical trials to establish the therapeutic value of meditation, and elucidating the mechanisms responsible for the health benefits of meditation continues to be a dynamic area of inquiry.

The scientific literature on meditation has virtually exploded in recent years. A search of Ovid MEDLINE and PsycINFO from 2012 to January 2017 found 178 systematic reviews or meta-analyses addressing the health impacts of meditation for common disorders and symptoms (e.g., anxiety, depression, pain), specific diseases (e.g., heart disease, diabetes, multiple sclerosis), harmful health behaviors (e.g., binge eating, smoking cessation, substance abuse), populations (e.g., cancer survivors, adolescents, older adults), or settings (e.g., schools, prisons, workplaces). One of the largest and most rigorous of these reviews was conducted by Goyal et al. (2014) to evaluate the efficacy of meditation training programs for reducing psychological distress and improving outcomes for clinical populations. Goyal et al. examined evidence from 47 randomized controlled trials (RCTs) representing 3,515 participants with a variety of conditions (including stressed populations) published through 2012. Findings were summarized according to type of meditation (mindfulness, TM, and/or mantra), control group (time/attention/expectancy vs. specific alternative therapy), and outcome. Outcomes included emotional and physical symptoms (anxiety, depression, pain, insomnia), stress-related behaviors (weight loss, substance abuse), and overall quality of life. Meta-analyses found moderate evidence to support findings that mindfulness meditation, compared with a time and attention control, reduces anxiety, depression, and pain, with small to medium (0.23–0.38) treatment effect sizes. Low or insufficient evidence was found for TM and for other outcomes. Interestingly, Goyal et al. found no evidence that meditation training improves attention, a finding the authors attribute to the inadequacy of self-report measures. Strengths of this review include the range of outcomes evaluated, estimation of effect sizes, and assignments of levels of evidence to findings. An earlier meta-analysis by Bohlmeijer, Prenger, Taal, and Cuijpers (2010) focused exclusively on estimating the impact of mindfulness training on anxiety, depression, and psychological distress in adults with chronic medical diseases (chronic back pain, heart disease, chronic fatigue syndrome, fibromyalgia, rheumatoid arthritis, and cancer) and considered only studies with outcomes assessed by widely used, psychometrically strong, self-report measures such as the State-Trait Anxiety Inventory Scale and Hospital Anxiety and Depression Scale. Consistent with Goyal et al.'s findings, Bohlmeijer et al.'s meta-analyses found significant treatment impacts on anxiety and depression, with medium effect sizes. Notably, when only studies of high or medium quality were included, Bohlmeijer et al. found their effect sizes were still significant, but smaller.

There is growing evidence that mindfulness meditation can improve psychological functioning among cancer survivors. Shennan, Payne, & Fenlon (2011) reviewed the evidence for use of mindfulness-based interventions, based on 13 studies published from 2007 to 2009, in patients with varying types of cancer. They included quantitative, qualitative, and mixed-methods reports, concluding that mindfulness interventions have promising results for subjectively (e.g., anxiety, sexual dysfunction) and objectively (e.g., physiological arousal, immune function) measured outcomes. They suggested that mindfulness interventions may be useful across the cancer trajectory but noted that most studies they reviewed were small, had limited follow-up, and were not randomized trials. Between 2010 and 2014, six randomized trials of MBSR representing 1,004 breast cancer patients were published, and all found some positive effects on psychological or physiological outcomes related to stress (Rush & Sharma, 2017). Further work is needed to establish the durability of these impacts and refine protocols to optimize benefit.

The effects of meditation on psychological outcomes has also been studied in healthy adults (Sedlmeier et al., 2012). This review included 163 studies of mantra-concentrative, mindfulness, or guided-meditation interventions conducted between 1970 and 2011. Outcomes evaluated included measures of emotion, personality, cognition, affect, behavior, and well-being. To provide an overall summary of impact, effects were pooled across all outcomes in which meditation could be regarded as having either a positive or negative impact. This global analysis revealed medium beneficial effects for meditation compared with active controls (such as relaxation) and no-treatment comparison groups. Examination of individual outcomes showed the largest effect sizes were for emotional (e.g., anxiety reduction) and relationship outcomes. Findings varied by type of meditation.

There is very promising evidence that mindfulness meditation can benefit people with chronic pain. Hilton et al. (2016) conducted a systematic review and meta-analysis to investigate the efficacy and safety of mindfulness meditation for patients with chronic pain due to headache, migraine, back pain, arthritis, irritable bowel syndrome, cancer, or neuralgias. They examined evidence from 38 RCTs trials representing 3,536 randomized participants who had pain for at least 3 months. Interventions were MBSR (21 trials), mindfulness-based cognitive therapy (MBCT; six trials), or other programs that included some formal mindfulness meditation practices. Mindfulness interventions were used as an adjunct therapy (18 trials), used as monotherapy (13 trials), or did not specify other pain therapies. Outcomes included pain (primary outcome), depression, use of analgesics, and overall quality of life. Comparison groups included treatment as usual, education, support groups, or waiting lists. Trials were evaluated for quality and classified as good (11 trials), fair (14 trials), or poor (13 trials) based on issues such as dropouts, use of intention-to-treat analyses, and gaps in reporting. Meta-analyses were conducted based on poolable data from 30 studies representing 2,292 patients. Data from a variety of pain-appraisal measures were aggregated for this meta-analysis. A statistically significant, small effect on pain was found for meditation compared with all controls (standardized mean difference = 0.32, 95% confidence interval [CI]: 0.09, 0.54). Although substantial heterogeneity of effects was found across trials, there was no evidence of publication bias. Hilton et al. concluded that the quality of the evidence for pain reduction is low for both short- (less than 12 weeks) and longer-term outcomes. Additional meta-analyses confirmed impacts on secondary outcomes of depression (a small impact with a high level of evidence) and quality of life (small impact with moderate evidence for mental health–related quality of life, low evidence for physical health–related quality of life). No safety concerns were identified, but only seven trials reported monitoring for adverse events. No impact of meditation on use of analgesics was found. Based on these findings, one can be cautiously optimistic about the value of mindfulness training for chronic pain, associated symptoms of depression, and quality of life. Because large variations in effect sizes for pain were found across studies, more research is needed to identify the factors that predict better outcomes and to refine meditation training protocols to optimize outcomes.

A trial of MBSR for low back pain conducted by Morone et al. (2016) was one of the largest and most recent in the review by Hilton et al. (2016). This trial provides a useful exemplar of meditation for pain research, as the meta-analysts rated this trial as good quality with low risk of bias. The purpose of this RCT was to determine the effectiveness of MBSR on improving functioning and reducing pain among older adults with chronic low back pain. Participants were 282 adults aged 65 or older experiencing daily chronic pain and related functional limitations for at least the past 3 months. Some 66% of participants were women, 28% were Black, and the average age was 75. The intervention was an 8-week MBSR program followed by six monthly booster sessions, and the control was a health education program delivered in a similar format to MBSR. The primary outcome was the Roland–Morris Disability Questionnaire score for functional limitations caused by lower back pain. Secondary outcomes included pain (present, average, and most severe assessed by numeric rating scale), quality of life, and pain self-efficacy. At the end of the 8-week program, the MBSR group had significantly improved function (fewer pain limitations) compared with controls (effect size –0.23, p = .01), and more clinically meaningful reductions in limitations, defined as greater than 2.5 points on the Roland–Morris Disability Questionnaire (57% vs. 45%, p = .051). Ratings of current and most severe pain in the past week at 6-month follow-up were also better in the MBSR group than in the control group. No serious adverse events related to the interventions were reported. Morone et al. (2016) concluded that mindfulness training resulted in short-term improvements in physical functioning and encouraged more work to improve durability of meditation's benefit to function.

Experimental evidence of meditation's impact on blood pressure and other physiological parameters provide a strong rationale for clinical trials to evaluate its clinical potential among those with hypertension and other cardiovascular risk factors. Bai et al. (2015) conducted a systematic review and meta-analysis of the effects of TM as a primary intervention on blood pressure. They identified 12 RCTs published between 1989 and 2012 representing 996 patients. Ten of these trials compared TM with health education controls, and two compared TM with a waiting list. Duration of the TM interventions ranged from 3 to 60 months. Most participants were hypertensive or had blood pressures in the range of high normal, and some trials included patients on antihypertensive medications. Approximately 60% of participants were men; samples included adolescents, younger adults, and older adults; and more than half of the participants were Blacks. Nine of the trials were funded by the National Institutes of Health. Bai et al.'s primary meta-analyses estimated that TM groups had significantly greater blood pressure reductions than controls: systolic blood pressure (SBP) of –4.26 mmHg (95% CI –6.09, –2.42) and diastolic blood pressure (DBP) of –2.33 mmHg (95% CI –3.70, –0.97). A series of subgroup meta-analyses suggested that TM is most effective with adults aged 65 or older, those with SBP greater than 140 mmHg, and women. Overall, these authors judged trial quality as acceptable, noting some trials had limitations such as unclear attrition rates or gaps in reporting randomization sequence generation, but all were judged to have low risk of reporting bias. Bai et al. concluded that TM may reduce risks from cardiovascular disease by lowering blood pressure but called for additional rigorously designed TM trials with improved blood pressure measurement techniques to confirm these results.

One of the largest and most recent studies in the review by Bai et al. (2015) was conducted by Schneider et al. (2012). This was a randomized controlled prevention clinical trial to evaluate the impact of TM on cardiovascular mortality in Blacks with cardiovascular disease. Participants were 201 Blacks with angiographic evidence of 50% or more stenosis of at least one coronary artery. Secondary outcomes included nonfatal cardiovascular events and lifestyle variables (smoking, alcohol use, diet, body mass index, and psychological distress). Participants were randomized to either TM or cardiovascular health education. The TM technique was taught by a certified instructor in a series of six 90-minute to 2-hour individual or group meetings, with home practice expectations of 20 minutes per day throughout follow-up. The health education program included information about diet, exercise, and stress and was taught by professional health educators in a format designed to be similar in time and attention to the TM intervention. With an average of 5.4 years of follow-up, the TM group had a significant 42% risk reduction for cardiovascular mortality in a survival analysis stratified by age, gender, and lipid-lowering medications. Significant impacts for TM were also found for SBP, and no serious adverse events related to the interventions were reported. These authors concluded that TM may be clinically useful in the secondary prevention of cardiovascular disease among Blacks.

The effectiveness of mindfulness-based meditation interventions on patients with vascular diseases, including diabetes, hypertension, heart disease, and stroke, has also been examined in systematic reviews (Abbott et al., 2014). These mindfulness trials contributed to the evidence that established impacts on psychological outcomes in patients (Goyal et al., 2014), but evidence is not yet sufficient to establish benefits from mindfulness meditation to physical outcomes among patients with vascular diseases (Abbott et al., 2014). Two of the largest trials reviewed by Abbott et al. examined a wide array of outcomes for patients with diabetes: the Heidelberger Diabetes and Stress Study (HEDIS; Hartmann et al., 2012) clinical trial in Heidelberg, Germany, and the DiaMind (van Son et al., 2012) trial of MBCT in the Netherlands. HEDIS is a 5-year trial of MBSR to reduce emotional distress and progression of nephropathy in patients with type 2 diabetes and albuminuria. Patients were randomized to the MBSR group or the treatment-as-usual control group. All participants received standard diabetes care. The primary outcome was change in albuminuria, a measure of nephropathy and a risk factor for cardiovascular disease. Secondary outcomes included the Patient Health Questionnaire-9 (PHQ-9) depression scale and the Short-Form Health Survey (SF-12; German version). Groups of six to eight participants attended 8 weekly MBSR sessions, plus a booster session at 6 months, led by a psychologist and a resident in internal medicine. The MBSR curriculum was integrated with discussion about diabetes-specific thoughts and feelings. Findings at year 1 showed no differences in progression of albuminuria, based on intention-to-treat analyses adjusted for baseline values, age, and gender. However, the MBSR group reported less depression, better mental health, and lower DBP. Because HEDIS is a 5-year study, the authors remain optimistic. The year-1 treatment impact on albuminuria was in the correct direction and encouraging in magnitude (effect size of 0.40). Unlike some interventions, which wane with time, it has been posited that MBSR's benefits increase with time.

DiaMind (van Son et al., 2012) was designed to test the short-term effectiveness of MBCT on stress, mood, and health-related quality of life in patients with diabetes. The study sample comprised 139 outpatients with type 1 or 2 diabetes, who reported low levels of emotional well-being. Participants were randomized to either MBCT or treatment as usual; all received standard diabetes care throughout the study. MBCT consisted of eight weekly, 2-hour group sessions with four to eight participants led by certified mindfulness instructors who were also psychologists with a personal mindfulness practice. Program adaptations specific to diabetes were detailed in the design paper (van Son, Nyklíček, Pop, & Pouwer, 2011). Results indicated better outcomes for the MBCT group compared with controls for measures of stress, depression, anxiety, fatigue, and health-related quality of life, with medium to large effects from baseline to postintervention based on mixed models and an intention-to-treat sample. Most outcomes showed some improvement by 4 weeks (mid intervention), and greater improvement by 8 weeks, the end of the intervention period. Hemoglobin A1c (HbA1c) results were not significant. Inability to detect improvements in HbA1c levels may be partly explained by relatively good glycemic control at baseline (mean HbA1c = 7.6%). There is also some question about the acceptability of the intervention because approximately 80% of those eligible declined to participate. These authors conclude the MBCT adapted for diabetes may be effective in reducing emotional distress and enhancing health-related quality of life for patients with diabetes.

Findings of medium to large effects for psychosocial outcomes from the HEDIS and DiaMind trials are encouraging; however, enthusiasm must be tempered by the fact the each used an inactive control. Treatment effects tend to be biased upward when there are no controls for nonspecific effects such as the time and attention from an instructor, group support, or expectations of benefit (placebo effect; Chiesa & Serretti, 2009; Ospina et al., 2007). Establishing active control groups for meditation interventions is feasible, as evidenced by the work of Tang and colleagues (Tang, Lu, Fan, Yang, & Posner, 2012; Tang & Posner, 2013) and by our trial, which tested the impact of MBSR on the symptoms of anxiety, depression, and insomnia in solid organ transplant recipients (Gross et al., 2010). In the latter trial, 150 recipients were randomized into one of three groups: MBSR; Health Education—a peer-led, chronic disease self-management program conducted to match MBSR for time, attention, and group support; and a wait-list. Primary outcomes were the State-Trait Anxiety Inventory, Center for Epidemiologic Studies Depression Scale, and the Pittsburgh Sleep Quality Index. Results demonstrated that those receiving active interventions had better outcomes than those on the wait-list at 8 weeks (the end of the active intervention period). Over 1 year, MBSR ($n = 63$) was superior to Health Education ($n = 59$) in reducing anxiety and sleep dysfunction based on mixed-model regression analyses. A notable finding in this trial was that outcomes continued to improve in the MBSR group over the entire follow-up period, whereas the active control group had an initial benefit but then returned to baseline levels.

In summary, there is solid evidence based on rigorous clinical trials of meditations' benefits, particularly to psychological symptoms that include anxiety and depression; across many clinical and healthy populations; and with rapidly mounting evidence of specific benefits to a wide array of other outcomes, including pain, quality of life, and cardiovascular risk factors. However, without exception, authors of meta-analyses have called for improved designs, larger samples, longer follow-up, and more rigorous methods to strengthen the evidence base (Abbott et al., 2014; Bai et al., 2015; Goyal et al., 2014; Hilton et al., 2016; Huang, He, Wang, & Zhou, 2016). Systematic reviewers cite issues such as wait-list control groups, no measurement of meditation adherence, no blinding or no blinded assessment of outcomes, and limited follow-up to assess durability of benefit. Reviewers also call for greater attention to optimizing intervention impacts in terms of type and duration of meditation training. Interestingly, Goyal et al. (2014) concluded that there is insufficient evidence to assert that meditation programs are superior to any established treatments, such as sedatives approved by the Food and Drug Administration (FDA) or cognitive behavioral therapy for insomnia. Bohlmeijer et al. (2010) suggested that integrating mindfulness with other therapies specific for each condition may enhance overall efficacy because mechanisms of action are apt to differ. Along these lines, there is some evidence that adding mindfulness may improve the efficacy of cognitive behavioral therapy for insomnia (Ong et al., 2014). Moreover, given the side effects of sedative medications and the identified benefits of meditation for anxiety, depression, and pain without concomitant treatment-related adverse events, clinicians may consider recommending meditation training to those with insomnia unwilling or unable to take sedatives. Meditation training may also be an appropriate adjunct therapy for other therapeutically challenging patients, such as those with chronic renal failure, those requiring multiple medications to control blood pressure or seizures, and those with psychological comorbidities.

INTERVENTION

Techniques and Guidelines

Although there are numerous meditation programs, four of the most widely used and well-researched meditation programs in Western healthcare are MBSR and several related programs, IBMT, TM, and loving-kindness.

MBSR and Related Programs

MBSR was developed by Jon Kabat-Zinn at the Stress Reduction Clinic at the University of Massachusetts Medical Center (www.umassmed.edu/cfm) more than 30 years ago. It is a particular way of learning mindfulness meditation that emerged in a hospital system and was fashioned as a complement to traditional medical care for patients with chronic pain conditions (Kabat-Zinn, 1990). The program is theoretically grounded in secularized Buddhist meditation practices, mind-body medicine, and the transactional model of stress that suggests people can be taught to manage their stress by adjusting their cognitive perspective and increasing their coping skills to build self-confidence in handling external, stressful situations. MBSR is an 8-week, generic skills-based program led by an instructor in a classroom format. The course comprises eight weekly 2.5-hour classes, one 7.5-hour meditation retreat, and 30 to 45 minutes of daily homework practicing the techniques learned in the course. Sessions include information about stress, cognition, and health but primarily concentrate on learning to focus attention through a variety of meditative techniques, such as focusing on the breath, body scan, sitting and walking meditations, and gentle yoga. Participants are trained to perceive their immediate emotional and physical state, including pain or discomfort, and to let thoughts come and go into awareness with no attempt to change, suppress, or ruminate on them.

Through mindfulness training, participants come to view their thoughts as temporary mental events. In this way, they become exposed to the positive and negative content of their thoughts but do not get absorbed in thought—caught up in planning for the future, or worrying about the past. By incorporating mindfulness techniques into their daily lives, practitioners learn to find breathing space to respond skillfully to stressors with appropriate action, as opposed to reacting on automatic pilot with conditioned responses that can be emotionally arousing or unhelpful. The goal of MBSR is lifelong self-management. Although MBSR was originally developed for people with chronic pain, it was later applied to patients with a variety of conditions, such as cancer (Hoffman et al., 2012), diabetes (Hartmann et al.,

2012), fibromyalgia (Schmidt et al., 2011), irritable bowel syndrome (Gaylord et al., 2011), and social anxiety (Goldin & Gross, 2010). Moreover, MBSR has expanded beyond medical settings, and courses are now widely available in community settings, at universities, and in the workplace. Referral by a health provider and medical oversight are not required. Becoming a certified MBSR instructor (for details see www.umassmed.edu/cfm/training/MBSR-Teacher-Education/) requires intensive experiential and didactic training, including a practicum and supervised work.

Over the past two decades, a number of similar programs have been developed that integrate core elements of mindfulness practices with existing evidence-based therapies. Unlike MBSR, which is a generic stress-reduction program, most of these programs target a specific physical or mental illness. The first of these to emerge was MBCT (Segal, Teasdale, & Williams, 2012). MBCT is an 8-week group intervention that integrates elements of cognitive therapy (CT) with the MBSR program to prevent depressive relapse in patients with a history of major depressive disorder. Unlike CT, there is no attempt to challenge or change the content of thoughts; rather, the emphasis is on changing the awareness of and relationship to thoughts, feelings, and bodily sensations. Aspects of CT included in MBCT are primarily those designed to facilitate a detached or decentered view such as "thoughts are not facts" and "I am not my thoughts." Increased mindfulness allows early detection of relapse-related patterns of negative thinking, feelings, and bodily sensations, allowing them to be stopped at a stage when this may be much easier than if such warning signs were noticed later or ignored (Segal, Teasdale, & Williams, 2004, p. 56). The MBCT program has added several techniques to MBSR that have been widely disseminated, including the 3-minute breathing space (see Exhibit 11.1). In addition, the MBCT protocol is clear and concise and includes all necessary materials to begin an MBCT group.

Similar to MBCT, mindfulness-based relapse prevention (MBRP; Witkiewitz, Marlatt, & Walker, 2005) was developed to integrate mindfulness into cognitive behavioral treatment (CBT) of substance use and the prevention of relapse. In MBRP, mindfulness practices provide a unique opportunity to decrease habitual responding and avoidance by cultivating an attitude of curiosity and attention to ongoing cognitive, affective, and physical stimuli (Bowen, Chawla, & Marlatt, 2011). The goal of MBRP is to develop awareness of thoughts, feelings, and sensations (including urges or cravings) by developing mindfulness skills that can be applied in high-risk situations for relapse.

Mindfulness-based eating awareness training (MB-EAT; Kristeller & Hallet, 1999) was developed by integrating elements from MBSR and CBT with guided-eating meditations. The program draws on traditional mindfulness meditation techniques, as well as guided meditation, to address specific issues pertaining to shape, weight, and eating-related self-regulatory processes, such as appetite, and both gastric and taste-specific satiety (Kristeller, Baer, & Quillian-Wolever, 2006). The meditative process is integrated into daily activity related to food craving and eating. Similar to MBCT and MBRP, mindfulness meditation is conceptualized as a way of training attention to help individuals first to increase awareness of automatic patterns and then to disengage from undesirable reactivity.

Exhibit 11.1.   MBSR and MBCT Sample Intervention Techniques

Breath Awareness

Breath awareness is a practice in which passive breathing is carefully observed. Breath awareness may be used as needed or can be practiced as a technique to promote awareness and health. Continued practice of breath awareness is an anchor for mindfulness, which helps the practitioner to remain in the moment, bringing calm and creativity to situations requiring perspective (Kabat-Zinn, 1990). The practice of breath awareness requires a beginner's mind, open to observation without attempts to change the breath. Kabat-Zinn (1990) describes a simple process that can be used to teach breath awareness to patients:

1. Sit or lie in a comfortable position. If sitting, keep a straight spine and let the shoulders drop.
2. Close your eyes if that is comfortable, or gaze ahead without focusing.
3. Bring attention to your full in-breath and out-breath. Notice the sensation of the breath, especially in the rising and falling abdomen.
4. Don't try to change the breath, just notice the waves of your own breathing.
5. When your mind wanders away from the breath (e.g., you notice that you are thinking of something else) just return your focus to the breath.

Body Scan

Body scan is a technique that promotes the mind's ability to focus and adapt and is a powerful tool for reconnecting with the body. This practice involves lying down or sitting comfortably in a chair and focusing attention through the parts of the body, noticing the sensations there and directing the breath, as if breathing in and out of each body part. In this practice, unwelcome sensations such as discomfort, tension, or fatigue are noticed and let go, or they are imagined to flow out of the body with the breath. The typical sequence for the scan follows: toes of left foot, left foot, left ankle, leg, pelvis, then toes of the right foot progressing up to the right hip, pelvis, low back and belly, high back and chest, fingers of both hands (simultaneously), and then both arms, shoulders, neck, face, back of the head, and top of the head (Kabat-Zinn, 1990). At the end of the body scan, one visualizes that the breath goes through the whole body, through the toes, and in and out of an imaginary blow hole at the top of the head. As in other mindfulness practices, unrelated thoughts or interruptions are noted and let go, and the practitioner brings attention back to the scan. The body scan is deeply relaxing for some, and so taking some time to move slowly afterward is helpful. Meditation novices may find that they fall asleep while practicing body scan or have concerns they are not doing it right. These are normal responses, and practitioners may be encouraged to continue practicing and to bring themselves back to the scan with awareness and acceptance when they notice that their minds have wandered.

Breathing Space

Breathing space can be used routinely to cultivate awareness and self-compassion, or it can be used as needed when experiencing unwanted thoughts or feelings. A three-step, 3 minute Breathing Space practice designed by Segal and colleagues is part of MBCT (Segal, Teasdale, & Williams, 2002).

(continued)

> 1. Awareness: Bring awareness to the breath and thoughts, feelings, and sensations of this moment, observing carefully and describing the experience silently, in words (e.g., "Noticing tension in the body and feeling anxious.").
> 2. Redirecting attention: Bring your attention to the breath and experience it fully.
> 3. Expanding attention: Let awareness grow to include the whole body, breathing into areas of discomfort (thoughts, feelings, sensations), breathing out discomfort, and making accepting statements (e.g., "Whatever it is, it's okay.").
>
> MBCT, mindfulness-based cognitive therapy; MBSR, mindfulness-based stress reduction.

Mindfulness-Based Resilience Training

Mindfulness-based resilience training (MBRT; Christopher et al., 2016) is designed to enhance physiological and psychological resilience for acute and chronic stressors common to law enforcement and other first responders. Based on a MBSR framework, it is an 8-week course with experiential and didactic exercises, including body scan, sitting and walking meditations, mindful movement, and other MBSR practices (Kabat-Zinn, 1990). Weekly classes last 2 hours, and the seventh week is an extended 6-hour class, as opposed to MBSR's 7-hour silent retreat in the sixth week of the program.

Each class contains experiential and didactic exercises, as well as discussion and homework. Content and language of experiential exercises were altered to be more relevant to first responders, and much of the curriculum is focused on learning strategies to manage stressors inherent to this type of work. These include critical incidents, chronic stress, and public scrutiny, as well as interpersonal, affective, and behavioral challenges in first responders' personal lives. Didactic learning is much more prominent than in MBSR. This was found to be very helpful for first responders as they sought to enhance their intention to endure the challenges of the training. An additional adaptation, in the tradition of typical first responder meetings, is the inclusion of a debriefing at the conclusion of each class, in which participants ask questions and give frank feedback about the class. The mindful encounters exercise is a derivation of the martial arts exercises (e.g., conversational Jujitsu) used in the MBSR curriculum to practice mindful interpersonal conflict. The exercise is framed as an important skill to be used when interacting with coworkers, family, and friends. In another exercise, reactivity awareness, participants settle into a sustained, reclined breath-awareness practice, and then with verbal instruction to sustain awareness, a 911 call center recording with emergency audio tone is played for 60 seconds and then turned off. Participants are cued to continue sustained attention to body sensation and breath for a few more minutes, helping them gain an experiential sense of stress physiology. In addition, participants are invited to include a component of mindfulness during their regular exercise regimen, such as running, swimming, or biking, as part of their mindful movement homework.

Adaptations of MBSR or MBCT have also been developed or are in the developmental process for specific populations, such as adolescents, pregnant women, and couples, and for health conditions, such as cancer, diabetes, insomnia, and post-traumatic stress disorder (PTSD). It is now possible to find MBSR materials and homework assignments designed for specifically for children or teenagers, as well as curricula for delivery of MBSR in schools, prisons, rehabilitation centers, and other settings.

Integrative Body–Mind Training

Integrative body–mind training (IBMT; Tang, 2011) originates from traditional Chinese medicine, and also uses the idea of humans in harmony with nature from Taoism and Confucianism. IBMT was developed in the mid-1990s, and the goal of the practice is to enhance self-regulation for body–mind health, balance, and well-being (Tang et al., 2012). IBMT involves body relaxation, mental imagery, breath adjustment, and mindfulness training, which are accompanied by background music. It achieves the desired state by "initial mind setting" with a brief period of instructions, to induce a cognitive or emotional set that will influence the training. The method does not stress the control of thoughts but instead provides a state of restful alertness that allows a high degree of awareness of the body, breathing, and external instructions. IBMT stresses a balanced state of relaxation while focusing on attention. This is achieved gradually through posture and relaxation, body–mind harmony, and balance with the help of the coach rather than by making the trainee attempt an internal struggle to control thoughts. For adults, IBMT has three levels of training: body–mind health, body–mind balance, and body–mind purification. For children, there are two levels: health and wisdom. Across age groups, in each level there are several core techniques that are instructed and guided by a qualified coach. A person who achieves the three levels of full training after theoretical and practical tests can apply for instructor (for details see imcenter.net) status.

Transcendental Meditation

The TM technique is the principal mind–body modality of the Maharishi Vedic Approach to Health, a comprehensive traditional system of natural healthcare derived from the ancient Vedic tradition. A much-publicized program, TM was developed and introduced into the United States in the early 1960s by Maharishi Mahesh Yogi. It is estimated that there are now more than five million practitioners worldwide, and the TM organization has grown to include educational programs, health products, and related services (Rosenthal, 2011). According to the TM movement, it is a method for relaxation, stress reduction, and self-development. Certified instructors teach TM in a seven-step course that is outlined on the TM website (www.tm.org). A TM teacher presents general information about the technique and its effects during a 90-minute introductory lecture. This is followed by a second 60-minute lecture in which more specific information is given. People interested in learning the technique then attend a 10- to 15-minute interview and a 1- to 2-hour session. Following a brief ceremony, prospective practitioners receive mantras, which they are told to keep confidential. Over the next 3 days, learners attend three more 1- to 2 hour sessions. In these sessions, the teacher explains the practice in greater detail, offers corrective advice if needed, and provides information about the benefits of regular practice. Over the next several months, the teacher regularly meets with practitioners to ensure correct technique.

TM practice involves two components: a suitable sound (mantra) specifically chosen for its facilitation of the process of settling the mind and a precise technique for using it (Haaga et al., 2011). Thinking the sound leads the meditator to experience quieter and quieter aspects of awareness, eventually experiencing complete silence (Nidich et al., 2009). In this way, the mantra serves as scaffolding for the developing practice but eventually fades away as the practitioner's skills are enhanced. TM practice is intended to take the mind from active levels of thinking to the state of least mental activity. This is practiced for 20 minutes, twice per day (in the morning, and in the evening). The TM technique can be taught only by a certified instructor through the seven-step course of instruction.

Loving-Kindness Meditation

Loving-kindness meditation (LKM), a core Buddhist meditation practice, refers to a mental state of unselfish and unconditional kindness to all beings. It is used to develop an affective state of increased feelings of warmth and caring for the self and others (Salzberg, 1995). Like other meditation practices, LKM involves quiet contemplation in a seated posture, often with eyes closed and an initial focus on the breath. Whereas mindfulness and similar types of meditation encourage nonjudgmental awareness of experiences in the present moment by focusing on bodily or other sensorial experience, affective states, thoughts, or images, LKM focuses on loving and kind concern for well-being. During LKM, the person typically proceeds through a number of stages that differ in focus and generally become more challenging. These include (a) focus on self, (b) focus on a good friend (i.e., a person who is still alive and who does not invoke sexual desires), (c) focus on a neutral person (i.e., a person who typically does not elicit either particularly positive or negative feelings but who is commonly encountered during a normal day), (d) focus on a difficult person (i.e., a person who is typically associated with negative feelings), and eventually, (e) focus on the entire universe (Hofmann, Grossman, & Hinton, 2011). As can be seen from this sequence, typically warm feelings are initially directed toward oneself and then extended to an ever-widening circle of others, ultimately radiating them in all directions (e.g., north, south, east, west), although the order can be changed to accommodate individual preferences. In LKM, people cultivate the intention to experience positive emotions during the meditation itself, as well as in their life more generally. Within traditional Buddhist practice, LKM is considered particularly helpful for people who have a strong tendency toward hostility or anger (Anālayo, 2003). Although there are no training requirements or guidelines for LKM, a number of Buddhist and secular resources are available to help develop practice.

Measurement of Outcomes

Meditation training with programs such as MBSR or TM is a low-risk activity that complements regular medical treatments, diet, exercise, and other lifestyle changes prescribed for known health conditions. Because these meditation practices have no known serious adverse effects, recommendations for monitoring patients who engage in meditation are consistent with general practice guidelines. Regular assessments to screen for depression, pain control, and changes in disease-specific symptoms are warranted. In research studies, meditation has been found to have impacts on mood, perceived stress, physiological markers of stress (including blood pressure, respiration, heart rate, and cortisol levels), and global indicators of health-related quality of life. Due to meditation's physiological effects, meditators with hypertension should be regularly monitored for possible dose adjustments (reductions). Also, nurses should be alert to changes in other conditions because anecdotal evidence suggests that meditation practice enhances adherence, enabling practitioners to better tolerate intrusive treatments such as nocturnal oxygen (continuous positive airway pressure [CPAP]) for obstructive sleep apnea or "put pain in its place" affirmations without exacerbating suffering with worries. One would speculate that present-moment attention and awareness lead to better symptom awareness, attention to cues to treating symptoms that wax and wane, and recognition of health changes in conditions such as asthma and diabetes. Under Scientific Basis, several specific instruments and methods for measuring these effects in a research setting were mentioned. Some instruments, such as the PHQ-9 (available from Pfizer Inc. at www.phqscreeners.com), are appropriate for clinical practice as well as for research. Other brief, valid, and reliable self-report instruments appropriate for measuring patient outcomes in clinical practice or research are available at no cost through the Patient-Reported Outcomes Measurement Information System (PROMIS) project of the National Institutes of Health (www.healthmeasures.net/explore-measurement-systems/promis).

PRECAUTIONS

Meditation practices are considered generally safe as a complementary therapy. They are appealing in medical settings because they are inherently portable, do not require a prescription, and can be personalized to meet the needs of the individual. Clinical research supports the use of awareness meditation combined with other behavioral approaches for the treatment of serious disorders such as borderline personality disorder (dialectical behavior therapy; Linehan et al., 1999) and addictions or psychosis (acceptance and commitment therapy; Hayes, Wilson, & Strosahl, 1999). There are few conditions for which we do not recommend meditation at the bedside: delirium, psychosis, drug or alcohol intoxication, and mania. People experiencing symptoms of post-traumatic stress or grief may find it difficult to practice awareness exercises because meditation might intensify their negative experience. Research in this area is ongoing, so consultation with a mental health provider is encouraged. People who practice meditation may experience decreased blood pressure and need for insulin or cardiovascular medications. Patients with low blood pressure or who are dizzy or light-headed should not meditate, and medication dose and levels should be considered if their effects could be potentiated by the relaxation response. In studies of organ transplant recipients, kidney transplant candidates, and people with chronic insomnia, no adverse events related to meditation were encountered (Gross et al., 2010, 2011).

USES

Meditation's health benefits are attributed largely to two over-arching, interacting mechanisms—reduced physiological arousal and increased mental clarity. These factors are thought to combine to change how individuals respond to stress and thereby reduce its harmful effects on health and well-being. In *Full Catastrophe Living*, Jon Kabat-Zinn (1990) provides an overview of how stressors can trigger automatic "fight or flight" reactions, causing rises in blood pressure, pulse rate, and stress hormones and igniting feelings of fear, anxiety, and anger. He goes on to describe how hyperarousal can become "a way of life," eventually leading to maladaptive, self-destructive behaviors and poor health outcomes. Kabat-Zinn proposes that practice of mindful meditation can prevent this harmful cycle of stress reactivity. He posits that with present-centered attention and awareness, choices can be made and actions taken to skillfully respond to potential stressors. These choices allow the meditator to maintain balance and equanimity and thereby avoid or diminish the negative impacts of stress that, over time, erode health and well-being.

The physiological processes leading to stress-induced disease and ways that meditation may change these processes are detailed in Vernon Barnes and David Orme-Johnson's (2012) biobehavioral model of how TM works to treat and prevent hypertension and cardiovascular disease. They explain that environmental and psychosocial stress contribute to the development of hypertension and cardiovascular disease through pathways of excessive cardiovascular reactivity, chronic sympathetic nervous system activation, hypothalamic–pituitary–adrenal dysfunction, and increased circulation of neurohormones. These processes cause vasoconstriction, increase blood pressure, and if sustained or repeated, lead to the structural changes of hypertension and cardiovascular disease. V. A. Barnes and Orme-Johnson posit that TM practice provides periods of "deep metabolic rest" that result in numerous psychological and physiological changes working in an integrated fashion to enable the body's homeostatic mechanisms to resume normal functioning. Herbert Benson, a pioneer in mind–body research, termed this the *relaxation response,* a state of physiological quietude in which blood pressure, metabolic rate, and respiratory rate are matched to physiological needs—essentially the opposite of the stress response (Benson & Klipper, 2000). Benson has shown that any number of meditative practices, as well as yoga, qigong, or recitation of a prayer, can induce the relaxation response; however, Benson's initial work was conducted with TM (Wallace & Benson, 1972).

Proposed physiological mechanisms responsible for meditation's effects on health are reductions in stress reactivity and sympathetic tone. Meditation practice reduces acute and chronic stress reactivity and sympathetic nervous system activity, thereby lowering the load on the heart and lowering blood pressure levels. As a result, risks for hypertension and cardiovascular disease are reduced. In their review, V. A. Barnes and Orme-Johnson (2012) cite evidence of the immediate and long-term physiological effects of TM that is consistent with their model. This evidence includes studies of adolescents at risk for hypertension who were trained in TM and demonstrated reduced ambulatory and resting blood pressures and no enlargement of left ventricular mass or increase in cardiovascular reactivity, and studies of hypertensive adults demonstrated reductions in blood pressure and use of medications that control blood pressure.

The psychological processes that enable meditators to change how they respond to stress have not been established. Cognitive and behavioral mechanisms include:

- Attention control
- Attention switching
- Meta-cognition (how one views one's thoughts)
- Meta-cognitive awareness (insight about one's attitudes and beliefs)
- Cognitive restructuring (changing of one's perspective on events/thoughts)
- Emotional regulation
- Decreased rumination

- Exposure and desensitization (enabling of recognition and exposure to painful states or discomfort without heightened arousal from "catastrophizing," as opposed to avoidance behaviors; Kabat-Zinn, 1990)
- Nonattachment (ability to not rely on objects or events to attain happiness)
- Acceptance
- Present-moment orientation

All of these mechanisms have been proposed to account for the impact of mindfulness meditation on health outcomes (Gu, Strauss, Bond, & Cavanagh, 2015; Tang, Hölzel, & Posner, 2015). Varying levels of evidence support each of these mechanisms; it is derived mostly from longitudinal intervention trials using self-report scales to measure mechanisms such as rumination or avoidance. Causal modeling of self-report data using structural equation models is another source of support for some of these mechanisms. A growing number qualitative studies contribute to our understanding of the effects of meditation as perceived by patients and offer insights about how patients used meditative practices to benefit their health (Hubbling, Reilly-Spong, Kreitzer, & Gross, 2014; Long, Briggs, Long, & Astin, 2016).

Portable Resources—Is There an App for That?

Tools for meditation instruction and practice are widely available as portable applications. Although many argue that the use of technology has resulted in a culture that is constantly wired or plugged in, these electronic resources can be useful for introducing patients to meditation practices at the bedside. It is recommended that practitioners always familiarize themselves with and use these tools before providing them to patients (see Exhibit 11.2). Portable app developers may not be experts in the content. Apps are frequently mislabeled, and user reviews do not provide enough information to gauge their content or quality. Mani, Kavanagh, Hides and Stoyanov conducted a systematic review of 700 mindfulness meditation apps for smartphones and tablets in 2014 (Mani, Kavanagh, Hides, & Stoyanov, 2015). Narrowing to English language, relevance, mindfulness training, and education (not merely a timer, relaxation, music, or guided imagery) resulted in only 23 unique apps in English with mindfulness training that were accessible and inexpensive. The systematic review identified only one mindfulness meditation app, "Headspace," that is high in quality and has efficacy data; it is included in Exhibit 11.2 with selected resources. Additional resources are described by Dr. Ruth Buczynski on her blog at the National Institute for the Clinical Application of Behavioral Medicine (www.nicabm.com/nicabmblog).

CULTURAL APPLICATIONS

Several meditation practices have been examined across a variety of different populations. For example, several small-sample quantitative and qualitative studies have generated some promising preliminary findings regarding the effectiveness of the standard MBSR protocol with ethnic minorities. Roth and colleagues (Roth & Creaser, 1997; Roth & Robbins, 2004) found that a Spanish version of MBSR for inner-city patients resulted in significant decreases in reported anxiety and medical

Exhibit 11.2.   Portable Resources for Meditation

Resource	Tool, Technology, Source	Description
Diaphragmatic breathing exercise	Breathe2Relax (portable app); National Center for Telehealth & Technology (t2health. org/apps/breathe2relax; available in iTunes and GooglePlay)	Includes instructions with diagrams, practice with an adjustable breath timer, audio prompts with music, and nature scenery choices. Free.
Mindfulness meditation tracks	MARC Mindfulness Meditation (podcasts and iTunes downloads); UCLA Mindful Awareness Center (marc.ucla.edu)	Instructions, 5-minute breathing meditation, LKM, body scan for sleep. Free.
Mindfulness meditation	Headspace (portable app); Andy Puddicombe (www .headspace.com; available in iTunes, GooglePlay, and Amazon)	Instruction and guidance through mindfulness meditation practices. Ten 10-minute practices are free.
MBSR information, training, and classes	CFM at the University of Massachusetts Medical School (www .umassmed.edu/cfm)	Search engine identifies MBSR programs worldwide, by state, or country. CFM offers MBSR teacher training, annual scientific conference, and MBSR courses.
TM information, training, and classes	Transcendental Meditation Program (www.tm.org)	Search engine will identify TM teachers and programs.

CFM, Center for Mindfulness; LKM, loving-kindness meditation; MARC, Mindfulness Awareness Research Center; MBSR, mindfulness-based stress reduction; TM, transcendental meditation.

symptoms, and a significant increase in self-esteem. Similarly, in an RCT, Palta et al. (2012) found statistically significant improvements in SBP and DBP among Black female MBSR group members compared with a social support control group. Sbinga et al. (2011) found reductions in hostility, general discomfort, and emotional discomfort among HIV-infected or at-risk Black youth after participation in an MBSR group. Several qualitative studies among racial/ethnic minority participants have also identified important benefits to MBSR, including receipt of social support from other group members (Abercrombie, Zamora, & Korn, 2007; Szanton, Seplaki, Thorpe, Allen, & Fried, 2010) and positive impact on family relationships (Sbinga et al., 2011). In addition to these quantitative and qualitative findings, several authors have suggested possible modifications to the standard MBSR protocol to enhance its appeal and effectiveness among racial/ethnic minority participants. These modifications include delivering the program in the native language of participants (if relevant to a particular group), locating the group at a community agency or center that is trusted by patients, and facilitating increased interaction among group members (Abercrombie et al., 2007; Roth & Robbins, 2004).

Meditation is practiced in countries around the globe. The experience and use of meditation in Thailand, including Thai studies and a case report, are described in Sidebar 11.1.

SIDEBAR 11.1. MEDITATION AS A NURSING INTERVENTION IN THAILAND

Sukjai Charoensuk

Meditation has long been considered to be a religious practice in Thailand. The application of meditation as a nursing intervention was first documented in 1992, when, for her master's thesis (Jitsuwan, 1992), Pattaya Jitsuwan examined the effects of anapanasati (mindfulness of breathing) training on anxiety and depression in 35 chronic renal failure patients. The effect of anapanasati was found to decrease anxiety and depression, as well as to improve mental health. Since then, there has been a strong trajectory of studies by faculty and students at a number of Thai universities that have added to the evidence base for the use of meditation for a variety of conditions among a variety of populations. These universities include, Ramkhamheng University, Mahidol University, Mahasarakham University, Khon Kaen University, Ratchabhut Nakhon Ratchasima University, Phuket Rajabhat University, and Chiangmai University.

Anapanasati has been used to improve the mental state of students, and meditation combined with cognitive behavioral therapy has been used for depressive disorders. Meditation has been studied with Thai youth and adolescents to enhance happiness, improve emotional well-being, and promote self-esteem and self-control. Studies have also used meditative practices to target indicators of poor health, including hypertension, HbA1c, hypercholesterolemia, tachycardia, anxiety, and pain. Meditation has also been used for specific patient groups with conditions such as diabetes, rheumatoid arthritis, end-stage cancer, and depression.

Types of Practice in Thailand

The most common type of meditation examined in Thai research has been aanapanasati. In the studies described earlier, meditation practice times ranged from 30 to 90 minutes daily. In Thailand, meditation includes sitting practices, such as anapanasati, and movement meditation, such as qigong.

(continued)

Recently, meditation interventions have been incorporated into palliative care as a spiritual dimension; meditation has been applied with other medical treatments and complementary therapies in the care of patients with end-stage cancer to improve clinical status and quality of life.

Case Study: Arokaya Sala

Arokaya Sala is a natural recovery center located at Kam Pramong temple in Sakol Nakorn province, Thailand. It was established to provide help and integrated treatments for cancer patients—including those who are in the final stages of illness—to aid in relief from stress and pain, and to improve patients' quality of life. Religious ceremonies, including chanting, sitting meditation, and walking meditation, are organized to cultivate faith and encourage patients to treat the illness. Arokaya Sala has served more than 3,300 cancer patients from across Thailand and from other countries since it was established.

Reference

Jitsuwan, P. (1992). *Effect of anapanasati practice on anxiety and depression of chronic renal failure patients with dialysis* (Unpublished master's thesis). Salaya, Thailand: Mahidol University.

FUTURE RESEARCH

To survey the lines of research being actively pursued, we searched the database of U.S. federally funded grants, using keywords of meditation or mindfulness, and identified 223 active grants, a remarkable 64% increase over the number yielded by the same search just 4 years earlier (projectreporter.nih.gov/reporter_searchresults. cfm, searched February 2017). Particularly noteworthy were the substantial number of large, multiyear research grants—47 individual or program project grants, each with annual funding over $500,000. Grants included clinical trials of MBSR, MBCT, and other meditation programs in diverse populations (including children, older adults, veterans, the underserved, and urban minorities) and for numerous conditions. These grants had the hallmarks of methodological rigor: randomization, adequate statistical power, active comparison groups, an array of self-reported and physiological outcomes, and longer follow-up to establish the durability of impact. There were also experiments and imaging studies to elucidate mechanisms, intervention-development studies to create or adapt meditation programs to particular populations, and use of qualitative or mixed-methods approaches to improve understanding of the patient experience.

To maximize the potential for meditation to improve health, more research is needed about *how* it works and to identify *who* it is most likely to benefit. Meditation is unlikely to be "one size fits all." It is not known whether the quality of the meditation state achieved differs by technique (concentration, mindfulness, or other) and to what extent all meditation approaches engage common pathways versus distinct cognitive and physiological systems. This information could form the foundation for matching specific meditative techniques to particular health problems. Specific personality or genetic factors may predict ability to learn and use each type of meditation. The roles of personal characteristics such as age, gender, personality traits, and genetics could be evaluated to determine the best age to begin meditation training or to tailor programs. With this information, it may be possible to match people to the type of meditation training most likely to work best for them.

REFERENCES

Abbott, R. A., Whear, R., Rodgers, L. R., Bethel, A., Thompson Coon, J., Kuyken, W., ... Dickens, C. (2014). Effectiveness of mindfulness-based stress reduction and mindfulness based cognitive therapy in vascular disease: A systematic review and meta-analysis of randomised controlled trials. *Journal of Psychosomatic Research, 76*(5), 341–351. doi:10.1016/j.jpsychores.2014.02.012

Abercrombie, P. D., Zamora, A., & Korn, A. P. (2007). Lessons learned: Providing a mindfulness-based stress reduction program for low-income multiethnic women with abnormal Pap smears. *Holistic Nursing Practice, 21*(1), 26–34.

Anālayo. (2003). *Satipatthāna: The direct path to realization.* Cambridge, UK: Windhorse Publications.

Bai, Z., Chang, J., Chen, C., Li, P., Yang, K., & Chi, I. (2015). Investigating the effect of transcendental meditation on blood pressure: A systematic review and meta-analysis. *Journal of Human Hypertension, 29*(11), 653–662. doi:10.1038/jhh.2015.6

Barnes, P. M., Bloom, B., & Nahin, R. (2008). Complementary and alternative medicine use among adults and children: United States, 2007. CDC National Health Statistics Report #12. Retrieved from http://nccam.nih.gov/news/camstats/2007/72_dpi_CHARTS/chart6.htm

Barnes, V. A., & Orme-Johnson, D. W. (2012). Prevention and treatment of cardiovascular disease in adolescents and adults through the Transcendental Meditation® Program: A research review update. *Current Hypertension Reviews, 8*(3), 227–242.

Bauer-Wu, S. (2011). *Leaves falling gently: Living fully with serious and life-limiting illness through mindfulness, compassion, and connectedness.* Oakland, CA: New Harbinger.

Benson, H., & Klipper, M. Z. (2000). *The relaxation response- updated and expanded.* New York, NY: HarperCollins.

Bodhi, B. (2011). What does mindfulness really mean? A canonical perspective. *Contemporary Buddhism, 12*(1), 19–39.

Bohlmeijer, E., Prenger, R., Taal, E., & Cuijpers, P. (2010). The effects of mindfulness-based stress reduction therapy on mental health of adults with a chronic medical disease: A meta-analysis. *Journal of Psychosomatic Research, 68*(6), 539–544.

Bowen, S., Chawla, N., & Marlatt, G. A. (2011). *Mindfulness-based relapse prevention for addictive behaviors: A clinician's guide.* New York, NY: Guilford Press.

Cahn, B. R., & Polich, J. (2006). Meditation states and traits: EEG, ERP, and neuroimaging studies. *Psychological Bulletin, 132*(2), 180–211.

Chiesa, A., & Serretti, A. (2009). Mindfulness-based stress reduction for stress management in healthy people: A review and meta-analysis. *Journal of Alternative and Complementary Medicine, 15*(5), 593–600.

Christopher, M. S., Goerling, R. J., Rogers, B. S., Hunsinger, M., Baron, G., Bergman, A. L., & Zava, D. T. (2016). A pilot study evaluating the effectiveness of a mindfulness-based intervention on cortisol awakening response and health outcomes among law enforcement officers. *Journal of Police and Criminal Psychology, 31*(1), 15–28.

Creswell, J. D. (2017). Mindfulness interventions. *Annual Review of Psychology, 68*, 491–516. doi:10.1146/annurev-psych-042716-051139

Davis, K. M., Lau, M. A., & Cairns, D. R. (2009). Development and preliminary validation of a trait version of the Toronto Mindfulness Scale. *Journal of Cognitive Psychotherapy, 23*(3), 185–197.

Fox, K. C., Nijeboer, S., Dixon, M. L., Floman, J. L., Ellamil, M., Rumak, S. P., ... Christoff, K. (2014). Is meditation associated with altered brain structure? A systematic review and meta-analysis of morphometric neuroimaging in meditation practitioners. *Neuroscience & Biobehavioral Reviews, 43*, 48–73.

Gaylord, S. A., Palsson, O. S., Garland, E. L., Faurot, K. R., Coble, R. S., Mann, J. D., ... Whitehead, W. E. (2011). Mindfulness training reduces the severity of irritable bowel syndrome in women: Results of a randomized controlled trial. *American Journal of Gastroenterology*, *106*(9), 1678–1688.

Germer, C. K. (2005). Mindfulness: What is it? What does it matter? In C. K. Germer, R. D. Siegel, & P. R. Fulton (Eds.), *Mindfulness and psychotherapy* (pp. 3–27). New York, NY: Guilford Press.

Goldin, P. R., & Gross, J. J. (2010). Effects of mindfulness-based stress reduction (MBSR) on emotion regulation in social anxiety disorder. *Emotion*, *10*(1), 83–91.

Goyal, M., Singh, S., Sibinga, E. M., Gould, N. F., Rowland-Seymour, A., Sharma, R., ... Haythornthwaite, J. A. (2014). Meditation programs for psychological stress and well-being: A systematic review and meta-analysis. *JAMA Internal Medicine*, *174*(3), 357–368. doi:10.1001/jamainternmed.2013.13018

Gross, C. R., Kreitzer, M. J., Reilly-Spong, M., Wall, M., Winbush, N. Y., Patterson, R., ... Cramer-Bornemann, M. (2011). Mindfulness-based stress reduction versus pharmacotherapy for chronic primary insomnia: A randomized controlled clinical trial. *Explore (NY)*, *7*(2), 76–87.

Gross, C. R., Kreitzer, M. J., Thomas, W., Reilly-Spong, M., Cramer-Bornemann, M., Nyman, J. A., ... Ibrahim, H. N. (2010). Mindfulness-based stress reduction for solid organ transplant recipients: A randomized controlled trial. *Alternative Therapies in Health and Medicine*, *16*(5), 30–38.

Gu, J., Strauss, C., Bond, R., & Cavanagh, K. (2015). How do mindfulness-based cognitive therapy and mindfulness-based stress reduction improve mental health and wellbeing? A systematic review and meta-analysis of mediation studies. *Clinical Psychology Review*, *37*, 1–12. doi:10.1016/j.cpr.2015.01.006

Haaga, D. A. F., Grosswald, S., Gaylord-King, C., Rainforth, M., Tanner, M., Travis, F., ... Schneider, R. H. (2011). Effects of the transcendental meditation program on substance use among university students. *Cardiology Research and Practice*, *2011*, 537101. doi:10.4061/2011/537101

Hartmann, M., Kopf, S., Kircher, C., Faude-Lang, V., Djuric, Z., Augstein, F., ... Nawroth, P. P. (2012). Sustained effects of a mindfulness-based stress-reduction intervention in type 2 diabetic patients: Design and first results of a randomized controlled trial (the Heidelberger Diabetes and Stress-study). *Diabetes Care*, *35*(5), 945–947.

Hayes, S. C., Wilson, K. G., & Strosahl, K. (1999). *Acceptance and commitment therapy: An experiential approach to behavior change*. New York, NY: Guilford Press.

Hilton, L., Hempel, S., Ewing, B. A., Apaydin, E., Xenakis, L., Newberry, S., ... Maglione, M. A. (2016). Mindfulness meditation for chronic pain: Systematic review and meta-analysis. *Annals of Behavioral Medicine*, *51*(2), 199–213. doi:10.1007/s12160-016-9844-2

Hoffman, C. J., Ersser, S. J., Hopkinson, J. B., Nicholls, P. G., Harrington, J. E., & Thomas, P. W. (2012). Effectiveness of mindfulness-based stress reduction in mood, breast-and endocrine-related quality of life, and well-being in stage 0 to III breast cancer: A randomized, controlled trial. *Journal of Clinical Oncology*, *30*(12), 1335–1342.

Hofmann, S. G., Grossman, P., & Hinton, D. E. (2011). Loving-kindness and compassion meditation: Potential for psychological interventions. *Clinical Psychology Review*, *31*(7), 1126–1132.

Hölzel, B. K., Lazar, S. W., Gard, T., Schuman-Olivier, Z., Vago, D. R., & Ott, U. (2011). How does mindfulness meditation work? Proposing mechanisms of action from a conceptual and neural perspective. *Perspectives on Psychological Science*, *6*(6), 537–559.

Huang, H.-P., He, M., Wang, H.-Y., & Zhou, M. (2016). A meta-analysis of the benefits of mindfulness-based stress reduction (MBSR) on psychological function among breast cancer (BC) survivors. *Breast Cancer*, *23*(4), 568–576. doi:10.1007/s12282-015-0604-0

Hubbling, A., Reilly-Spong, M., Kreitzer, M. J., & Gross, C. R. (2014). How mindfulness changed my sleep: Focus groups with chronic insomnia patients. *BMC Complementary & Alternative Medicine*, *14*, 50. doi:10.1186/1472-6882-14-50

Kabat-Zinn, J. (1990). *Full catastrophe living: Using the wisdom of your body and mind to face stress, pain, and illness*. New York, NY: Bantam Dell.

Kristeller, J. L., Baer, R. A., & Quillian-Wolever, R. (2006). Mindfulness-based approaches to eating disorders. In R. A. Baer (Ed.), *Mindfulness-based treatment approaches: A clinician's guide to evidence base and applications* (pp. 75–91). San Diego, CA: Academic Press.

Kristeller, J. L., & Hallet, B. (1999). Effects of a meditation-based intervention in the treatment of binge eating. *Journal of Health Psychology, 4*(3), 357–363.

Linehan, M. M., Schmidt, H., Dimeff, L. A., Craft, J. C., Kanter, J., & Comtois, K. A. (1999). Dialectical behavior therapy for patients with borderline personality disorder and drug-dependence. *American Journal of Addictions, 8*(4), 274–292.

Long, J., Briggs, M., Long, A., & Astin, F. (2016). Starting where I am: A grounded theory exploration of mindfulness as a facilitator of transition in living with a long-term condition. *Journal of Advanced Nursing, 72*(10), 2445–2456. doi:10.1111/jan.12998

Lutz, A., Slagter, H. A., Dunne, J. D., & Davidson, R. J. (2008). Attention regulation and monitoring in meditation. *Trends in Cognitive Science, 12*(4), 163–169.

Mani, M., Kavanagh, D. J., Hides, L., & Stoyanov, S. R. (2015). Review and evaluation of mindfulness-based iPhone apps. *JMIR Mhealth and Uhealth, 3*(3), e82. doi:10.2196/mhealth.4328

Morone, N. E., Greco, C. M., Moore, C. G., Rollman, B. L., Lane, B., Morrow, L. A., … Weiner, D. K. (2016). A mind-body program for older adults with chronic low back pain: A randomized clinical trial. *JAMA Internal Medicine, 176*(3), 329–337. doi:10.1001/jamainternmed.2015.8033

Nidich, S. I., Rainforth, M. V., Haaga, D. A. F., Hagelin, J., Salerno, J. W., Travis, F., … Schneider, R. H. (2009). A randomized controlled trial on effects of the Transcendental Meditation Program on blood pressure, psychological distress, and coping in young adults. *American Journal of Hypertension, 22*(12), 1326–1331.

Ong, J. C., Manber, R., Segal, Z., Xia, Y., Shapiro, S., & Wyatt, J. K. (2014). A randomized controlled trial of mindfulness meditation for chronic insomnia. *Sleep, 37*(9), 1553–1563. doi:10.5665/sleep.4010

Ospina, M., Bond, K., Karkhaneh, M., Tjosvold, L., Vandermeer, B., Liang, Y., … Klassen, T. (2007). *Meditation practices for health: State of the research.* Evidence Report/Technology Assessment No. 155. Rockville, MD: Agency for Healthcare Research and Quality.

Palta, P., Page, G., Piferi, R. L., Gill, J. M., Hayat, M. J., Connolly, A. B., & Szanton, S. L. (2012). Evaluation of a mindfulness-based intervention program to decrease blood pressure in low-income African American older adults. *Journal of Urban Health, 89*(2), 308–316.

Park, J., Lyles, R. H., & Bauer-Wu, S. (2014). Mindfulness meditation lowers muscle sympathetic nerve activity and blood pressure in African-American males with chronic kidney disease. *American Journal of Physiology, Regulatory, Integrative and Comparative Physiology, 307*(1), R93–R101. doi:10.1152/ajpregu.00558.2013

Rosenthal, N. E. (2011). *Transcendence: Healing and transformation through transcendental meditation.* New York, NY: Tarcher.

Roth, B., & Creaser, T. (1997). Mindfulness meditation-based stress reduction: Experience with a bilingual inner-city program. *Nurse Practitioner, 22*(3), 150–152, 154, 157 passim.

Roth, B., & Robbins, D. (2004). Mindfulness-based stress reduction and health-related quality of life: Findings from a bilingual inner-city patient population. *Psychosomatic Medicine, 66*(1), 113–123.

Rush, S. E., & Sharma, M. (2017). Mindfulness-based stress reduction as a stress management intervention for cancer care: A systematic review. *Journal of Evidence-Based Complementary & Alternative Medicine, 22*(2), 347–359. doi:10.1177/2156587216661467

Salzberg, S. (1995). *Loving-kindness: The revolutionary art of happiness.* Boston, MA: Shambhala.

Sbinga, E. M. S., Kerrigan, D., Stewart, M., Johnson, K., Magyari, T., & Ellen, J. M. (2011). Mindfulness-based stress reduction for urban youth. *Journal of Alternative & Complementary Medicine, 13*, 213–218.

Schmidt, S., Grossman, P., Schwarzer, B., Jena, S., Naumann, J., & Walach, H (2011). Treating fibromyalgia with mindfulness-based stress reduction: Results from a 3-armed randomized controlled trial. *Pain, 152*(2), 361–369.

Schneider, R. H., Grim, C. E., Rainforth, M. V., Kotchen, T., Nidich, S. I., Gaylord-King, C., … Alexander, C. N. (2012). Stress reduction in the secondary prevention of cardiovascular disease: Randomized, controlled trial of transcendental meditation and health education in Blacks. *Circulation: Cardiovascular and Quality Outcomes, 5*(6), 750–758.

Sedlmeier, P., Eberth, J., Schwarz, M., Zimmermann, D., Haarig, F., Jaeger, S., & Kunze, S. (2012). The psychological effects of meditation: A meta-analysis. *Psychological Bulletin*, *138*(6), 1139–1171.

Segal, Z. V., Teasdale, J. D., & Williams, J. M. G. (2002). *Mindfulness-based cognitive theory therapy for depression: A new approach to preventing relapse.* New York, NY: Guilford Press.

Segal, Z. V., Teasdale, J. D., & Williams, J. M. G. (2004). Mindfulness-based cognitive therapy: Theoretical rationale and empirical status. In S. C. Hayes, V. M. Follette, & M. Linehan (Eds.), *Mindfulness and acceptance: Expanding the cognitive–behavioral tradition* (pp. 45–65). New York, NY: Guilford Press.

Segal, Z. V., Teasdale, J. D., & Williams, J. M. G. (2012). *Mindfulness-based cognitive theory therapy for depression: A new approach to preventing relapse* (2nd ed.). New York, NY: Guilford Press.

Shennan, C., Payne, S., & Fenlon, D. (2011). What is the evidence for the use of mindfulness-based interventions in cancer care? A review. *Psycho-Oncology*, *20*(7), 681–697.

Szanton, S. L., Seplaki, C. L., Thorpe, R. J., Allen, J. K., & Fried, L. P. (2010). Socioeconomic status is associated with frailty: The women's health and aging studies. *Journal of Epidemiology and Community Health*, *64*(1), 63–67.

Tang, Y.-Y. (2011). Mechanism of integrative body-mind training. *Neuroscience Bulletin*, *27*(6), 383–388.

Tang, Y.-Y., Hölzel, B. K., & Posner, M. I. (2015). The neuroscience of mindfulness meditation. *Nature Reviews Neuroscience*, *16*(4), 213–225. doi:10.1038/nrn3916

Tang, Y.-Y., Lu, Q., Fan, M., Yang, Y., & Posner, M. I. (2012). Mechanisms of white matter changes induced by meditation. *Proceedings of the National Academy of Sciences USA*, *109*(26), 10570–10574.

Tang, Y.-Y., & Posner, M. I. (2013). Tools of the trade: Theory and method in mindfulness neuroscience. *Social Cognitive and Affective Neuroscience*, *8*(1), 118–120.

van Son, J., Nyklíček, I., Pop, V. J., Blonk, M. C., Erdtsieck, R. J., Spooren, P. F., … Pouwer, F. (2012). The effects of a mindfulness-based intervention on emotional distress, quality-of-life, and HbA1c in outpatients with diabetes (DiaMind): A randomized controlled trial. *Diabetes Care*, *36*(4), 823–830.

van Son, J., Nyklíček, I., Pop, V. J., & Pouwer, F. (2011). Testing the effectiveness of a mindfulness-based intervention to reduce emotional distress in outpatients with diabetes (DiaMind): Design of a randomized controlled trial. *BMC Public Health*, *11*, 131. doi:10.1186/1471-2458-11-131

Wallace, R. K., & Benson, H. (1972). The physiology of meditation. *Scientific American*, *226*, 84–90.

Witkiewitz, K., Marlatt, G. A., & Walker, D. (2005). Mindfulness-based relapse prevention for alcohol and substance use disorders. *Journal of Cognitive Psychotherapy*, *19*(3), 211–228.

Yogi, M. M. (1963). *The science of being and art of living.* New York, NY: Meridian Press.

12

Journaling

Mariah Snyder

Journal writing is one of a group of therapies that provides an opportunity for individuals to reflect on and analyze their lives and the events and people surrounding them, as well as to get in touch with their feelings. A term that is often used as a synonym for journal writing is *expressive writing*. Memoirs, life review, and storytelling are other interventions having a similar scientific basis. All of these therapies require individuals to be engaged in reflecting on and gaining insights about their lives and experiences.

Reeve Lindbergh (2008), Charles and Ann Lindbergh's daughter, states:

> To write as honestly as I can in my journals about my everyday life and the thoughts and feelings I have as I go along is an old tenacious yearning, maybe due to an early discomfort with the oddly intangible enormities of my family history. Or perhaps this effort is just something else my mother left to me; her belief that writing is the way to make life as perceptible as life can be perceived. (p. 80)

From the beginning of history, people have recorded the events of their lives, first in pictures and then in words. One of the most well-known journals of the 20th century is the journal kept by Anne Frank that details the life of the teenager while she and her family hid from Nazis during World War II.

DEFINITION

The terms *journaling, diary, reflective writing*, and *expressive writing* are often used interchangeably. Diaries more often only focus on recording the event or encounter, whereas journaling serves as a tool for reflecting on the event in terms of one's life. However, in reviewing the literature on the use of diaries in healthcare, they often include a reflective component. A key aspect of journaling and expressive or reflective writing is the person's reflections about the personal meaning given to the event or experience. In journal writing, interplay between the conscious and unconscious often occurs. Forms of expressive writing in addition to writing include poetry, stories, and scrapbooking that an individual may use to explore inner feelings and thoughts. Journaling may be used as an intervention for recovery from or dealing with a specific health condition or it may be selected by an individual to promote self-health.

SCIENTIFIC BASIS

Journaling is a holistic therapy because it involves all aspects of a person—physical (muscular movements), mental (thought processes), emotional (getting in touch with or expressing feelings), and spiritual (finding meaning). Through journal recordings, people are able to view the continuity of their lives and thus enhance wholeness. Writing may also aid individuals in identifying unconscious ideas and emotions that may be influencing their behaviors and lives. Awareness of these is furthered as subjects reflect on specific events, thoughts, or feelings while recording them; link them with past feelings and meanings; and consider present and future implications.

Journaling provides an opportunity for catharsis related to traumatic events in one's life (Sealy, 2012). Unlike merely venting one's feelings, journaling provides an avenue for a person to explore causes and solutions and gain insights. Sealy noted that "reflective journaling and meditation can provide an opportunity to 'socially reconstruct' past psychological injury" (p. 38).

Inhibiting expression of emotions may result in increased autonomic activity that may have long-lasting harmful effects on the body, such as precipitating hypertension. Therapies that assist one in venting feelings in a healthy manner may help lower stress and improve a person's health. In a review of three studies that had explored the efficacy of diary use by families of ICU patients, Ullman et al. (2015) found that the experimental group using diaries had reduced post-traumatic stress symptomatology when compared with the control group, who did not use diaries, although the differences between the groups was small. Likewise, Sayer et al. (2015) reported beneficial effects of journaling on distress in a veterans' group. Emotional disclosure in an online journaling study found that mothers of children with autism manifesting behavior problems had reduced stress compared with the control group (Whitney & Smith, 2015). However, Nyssen et al. (2017), in a meta-analysis of 64 studies of the use of therapeutic writing, did not find any significant positive outcomes in its use with patients with long-term care conditions.

Although much anecdotal evidence exists about the beneficial effects of journaling, research on the use of journals is sparse. Some studies exploring the use of journaling have been conducted with a number of the studies showing positive effects (Pepe et al., 2014; Proctor, Hoffmann, & Allison, 2012; Sayer et al., 2015). In addition to research conducted within nursing, journaling has been explored in other disciplines, including education, psychology, and medicine.

Although the precise mechanisms for why journaling may help some people reduce stress or decrease symptoms such as pain have not been identified, it is thought that the intervention may assist them in discovering patterns in their lives, particularly those that have a negative impact. This awareness may then prompt them to seek assistance. Journaling may further the discernment process by helping clarify thoughts and the emotions generated through encounters with specific events or people. It may also assist in generating possible solutions to the problem.

INTERVENTION

Various techniques for journaling exist—free-flowing writing, topical or focused journaling, and creative writing. The length of time that journaling is carried out (weeks, months, or years) depends on the specific purpose of the journaling. Sometimes, people initially write during a stressful situation or transition in their lives but become hooked and continue writing after the initial event has ended. The time spent on daily journaling can vary, with some recommending 15 to 30 minutes (Pennebaker, 2012). However, journaling during small spurts of time such as during coffee breaks may be a feasible option.

Some general guidelines for journaling are found in Exhibit 12.1. What is most important is that the person be honest. Knowing that the content is private and to be shared only if the writer so desires allows the individual to write about difficult topics or feelings. If, on the other hand, participants know that what they are writing has to be shared either with a healthcare professional or a group, an internal censor may be activated that impedes them from writing their true feelings. It was not always clear in reviewing studies if individuals did or did not have to share their journals which may have had an impact on the indices being measured. Journals used in educational settings often are shared with the instructor.

Entries should be made in a special notebook. This may be a special book designed exclusively for journaling or an inexpensive spiral or loose leaf notebook. These latter notebooks can be personalized by decorating the cover, or using pictures and colored markers. Because pencil recordings fade over time, a pen should be used to allow the person to reread past entries. Reviewing past entries provides a person with a mirror of one's past life and possible changes that may have occurred.

Developments in technology have created many new avenues for journal writing. Some may prefer using a computer to make entries. Use of passwords helps ensure privacy. With the advent of tablets and smart phones, it is easy to make entries during short breaks. Some may wish to use blogs to share their reflections with others. Shepherd and Aagard (2011) described the possible use of Web 2.0 tools with older adults to promote health.

Journaling needs to be the servant and not the master. Establishing a specific time of day to make entries is helpful. Some find early morning a good time to write when information in the unconscious seems to be closest to the surface.

Exhibit 12.1. Guidelines for Journaling

- Use a notebook specific to journaling
- Use a pen or a computer
- Date entries
- Choose a time of day to write, such as morning or evening
- Select a specific place to write, if possible, where there will be few interruptions
- Do not correct what is written; in reviewing the entry, comments may be added
- Remember, journaling is for you and does not need to be shared unless you choose to do so

Others prefer to do journaling in the evening to resolve pent-up stress or trouble-some events of the day before retiring.

Techniques

There are several different types of journaling, and each lends itself to specific goals. Over the course of treatment, individuals may use more than one type to accomplish what they need. Free-flow journaling, topical journaling, and creative writing are effective journaling techniques, and each has a different focus.

Free-Flow Journaling

Free-flow journaling is the most common type of journaling. Cortright (2008) suggested writing quickly and allowing words to just fall onto the page, without attention to grammar, punctuation, or spelling. The main goal is to put thoughts and feelings on paper. Journaling provides a vehicle for uncovering the wisdom already possessed and the feelings that have been dormant. Sometimes a person writes multiple pages on one topic or event. At other times, the mind flits from topic to topic. The latter may happen when one is distressed, and concentrating on one topic is difficult. There is no right or wrong way to journal. The main goal is to put words into written form and then reflect on them. One suggestion is, on finishing the day's entry, to reread it and then jot down an "insight line" about what the entry is telling you (Cortright, 2008).

Topical Journaling

Topical journaling focuses on a specific event or situation. It is often used in groups in which a specific topic is given for the participants. For example, individuals may be asked to write about when they were confronted with a challenge and how they reacted. Patients or family members may be asked to write about the way that a new diagnosis is affecting them, concerns they may have, and their fears and feelings. Instructions may include specific questions to which the person is to respond. For example, in using journaling with people who desire to lose weight, the following are a sample of questions that could be posed:

- What are your eating habits? For example, do you eat large meals or snack throughout the day?
- What is the meaning of food in your life?
- What are your favorite foods?
- What do you see as the biggest challenge you will face in trying to lose weight?
- Who or what will assist you in this endeavor?
- What is your motive for losing weight?

Creative Writing

Some people may be more comfortable writing in story form or in poetry rather than focusing on specific events or emotions in their lives. This type of writing can assist individuals in uncovering deeper thoughts or emotions in a safe man-ner because a story may have characters saying things that individuals would feel uncomfortable attributing to themselves. Stories allow for feelings to be seen initially in the people in the story and then as they relate to oneself. Pictures may be used as an initiator of a story.

Some prefer to do free-flowing journaling in a poetic form. This type of writing allows one to be creative and still explore feelings. Using short lines and spreading the content over a page make it easier to examine thoughts and emotions.

Combining journaling and art is another form of creative writing. Several authors described using scrapbooking and journaling for therapeutic purposes (Davidson & Robison, 2008; Subhani & Ifrah, 2012). Pictures or items used in creating the scrapbook served as the trigger for the journaling for the participants. Digital online pictures could be used for the journaling stimulus. Infinite possibilities exist and can be adapted to the preferences of the patient.

A number of websites provide helpful information about journaling. Some of these are noted in Exhibit 12.2.

Measurement of Outcomes

Many outcomes from journal writing may not be immediately discernible. Some of the possible areas to measure are improvement in self-esteem or quality of life, reduction in anxiety and/or negative feelings, and adaptation to a chronic condition. Physiological measures such as the immune system, weight loss, and blood pressure have also been used to determine the efficacy of journaling. Unless patients share, nurses are not aware of the content or focus of the journaling. Content analysis could be used to determine the themes generated in group journaling sessions.

PRECAUTIONS

Fear that others will find and read journal entries is a common concern and may deter people from being open in expressing themselves in a journal. A concern expressed at a corrections facility was that the journals would be confiscated and used in court. Care needs to be taken if individuals appear to be extremely introspective or scrupulous because journaling may deepen this inward focus. Passwords help ensure privacy of entries when technology is used for journaling.

USES

Journaling has been used with various conditions and populations, both in illness and in health promotion. Exhibit 12.3 lists some of the populations for whom journaling has been used. In those newly diagnosed with a chronic illness, journaling

---

Exhibit 12.2.   Online Resources About Journaling

- Penzu (penzu.com)
- Five top journal apps (lifestreamblog.com/top-5-smart-journal-apps/)
- Websites about various types and purposes of journaling (https://www.lifejournal.com/journal-writing-websites/)
- Conversations within: journal writing and inner dialog (www.journal-writing.com)

Exhibit 12.3. Uses of Journaling

- Cope with cancer (Baggs, Mckhann, Gessert, & Johnson, 2013; Milbury, et al., 2014)
- Decrease anxiety (Meshberg-Cohen, Svikis, & McMahon, 2014)
- Decrease distress/depression (Blasio et al., 2015; Milbury et al., 2014; Sayer et al., 2015)
- Decrease jail recidivism (Proctor et al., 2012)
- Cope with intensive care unit (Ullman et al., 2015)
- Manage maternal stress in caring for children with disabilities (Whitney & Smith, 2015)
- Decrease musculoskeletal pain (Pepe et al., 2013)
- Cope with palliative care (Penz & Duggleby, 2012)
- Manage psychological and physical health (Niles, Haltom, Mulvenna, Lieberman, & Stanton, 2013)
- Manage substance abuse (Proctor et al., 2012; Snead, Pakstis, Evans, & Nelson, 2015; Young, Rodriguez, & Neighbors, 2013)

---

about their perspectives on how the illness may affect their lives may help them uncover fears that could then be discussed with a health professional. Journaling also provides an avenue for people to identify hidden resources or strengths they may possess that will assist them in living with a chronic illness. Writing positive affirmations and then reading the statements may help them gain confidence in their abilities to manage the chronic condition. Milbury et al. (2014) used journaling to assist patients with cancer adjust to changes in their body image.

Research and anecdotal evidence support the use of journaling in recovery from substance abuse and crime. Procter et al. (2012) found interactive journaling to be helpful in reducing recidivism in jail inmates. Other investigators found that journaling assisted women recovering from substance abuse (Meshberg-Cohen, Svikis, & McMahon, 2014). Snead et al. (2015) elaborated on various ways that expressive writing may be effective in the treatment of substance abuse. Emotional writing, poetry writing (either individually or in groups), and free-flowing writing were some of the methods proposed.

A safe online environment was used by Baggs et al. (2013) for survivors of breast cancer to write or share with other women. The women could share, via postings, their feelings and challenges, or women were given the option to just read what others had posted. Many patients and the families of those who are faced with cancer often have many feelings. Sometimes, just putting these on paper assists them in recognizing these feelings and perhaps getting insights for handling the feelings. This may also be why journaling is helpful in individuals with high anxiety (Whitney & Smith, 2015).

CULTURAL APPLICATIONS

Although journaling is a therapy that many find helpful, others—particularly those from oral-based cultures—may find it daunting to reflect on their thoughts and experiences in writing. Painting and other forms of art may be alternative mechanisms that can be used to express feelings. The Hmong culture, an Asian ethnic group, has been an oral culture. The embroidered pieces of art created by Hmong women depict the history of the Hmong. This representational embroidery, or "story cloths," is used by members, especially women, to convey their experiences and history to future generations (Arkenberg, 2007).

Sidebar 12.1 describes the consideration of the use of journaling in the Philippines.

SIDEBAR 12.1. REFLECTIVE JOURNALING WRITING IN THE PHILIPPINES

Marlene Dohm and Leticia S. Lantican

Journal writing in the Philippines takes many forms as used in day-to-day living, educational settings, and therapeutic environments. In any situation, journaling becomes a way used to express thoughts, feelings, and insights. It gives a person a chance to reflect on life events and experiences and give meaning to them.

Before presenting the use of free-flowing journaling by a Filipino man who was diagnosed with cancer, the following statements describe several values, beliefs, and traditions that I believe, as a Filipino myself, are common among Filipinos; these may impact the use of journaling by Filipinos:

- Most Filipinos are modest and nonverbal when it comes to personal matters. Putting things in writing, as in journaling, works best for those who can express their sentiments in writing better than verbalizing them. Many prefer silence, which should be respected in relating with them.
- Many Filipinos are raised as Roman Catholics and have a strong faith in God. They feel strongly supported by the spirituality of their family, friends, church, and the community.
- Acceptance of a diagnosis and prognosis again is centered around a person's strength derived from faith and support from the family, which includes not only the nuclear family but also the extended family, consisting of brothers, sisters, aunts, uncles, and grandparents.

The following details the use of journaling by Mark (not actual name to protect privacy), a man and animation artist, who was born and raised in the Philippines. Mark was diagnosed at age 45 with an autoimmune disease that was in an advanced stage. He underwent almost a year of treatment consisting of intensive chemotherapy and bone marrow transplant. During the many times he waited at his clinic visits and during infusion times when he was having chemotherapy treatments that sometimes lasted 8 hours, Mark found time to do free-flow journaling using his tablet. He wrote on a variety of topics such as his experiences with treatment and perspectives on life, often punctuated with

(continued)

spiritual and religious themes. He provided periodic/monthly updates through-out his entire treatment duration to his family and close relatives through email. Most emails provided written expressions of his emotions, attitudes, and ways of coping with his treatment and its side effects. Often, these expressive writings reflected his strong faith in God and gratitude for family support and prayers. Even when he seemed to be in remission, Mark continued to engage in reflective writing while riding on a train. An example of his free-flowing jour-naling follows:

> One thing about being confined in a cancer treatment center (with other patients) is that your range of emotions can run the entire spectrum. Seeing so many people fight the same battle made me feel I am not alone. However, more often than not, I was constantly reminded of one's mortality. I remem-ber weeks prior to my transplant, I was told, due to the high dose chemo, there's a chance I might not make it. I have to admit, that information shook me a bit. It was circling around my head for days. I was restless to say the least.

> After a while, I was able to psyche myself up, that ultimately, I am going in that direction anyway. After all, my life is simply borrowed and not mine to keep. And then that started a slew of other questions. Knowing that my life is simply a borrowed one, why would I want an extension? Do I want to earn more money? Do I still want to see the rest of the world?

> Do I hunger for more achievements?

> As I thought about the answers to these questions, I realized, I've been so blessed to have the career that I have, the same career that allowed me to see the world, a career that allowed me to live comfortably. But most importantly, it's this same career that led me to meeting that very significant person in my life—my dear wife. I had a good run. I couldn't ask for anything more. I have more blessing than I could possibly count.

Mark found journaling to be helpful not only for himself personally, but also for his family members.

FUTURE RESEARCH

Exploration in the efficacy of journaling in healthcare is in its infancy. Journaling has often been used with other therapies, and hence its specific impact has been difficult to extract. Some of the areas in which research is needed include:

- Technology offers numerous possibilities for new avenues for journaling. Few studies have explored the use of technology as a means for journal-ing. Investigations in this arena are particularly needed with younger populations.
- Ethical and legal implications for journaling require study and need to be resolved, especially for those who are incarcerated. Fears about their jour-nals being "used against them" may inhibit people from being honest.

- Personal variables that may impact the effectiveness of journaling need to be identified.
- Few studies examined or reported how many subjects were faithful in journaling and how many quit journaling and the reasons for quitting.

REFERENCES

Arkenberg, R. (2007). Hmong story cloths. *SchoolArts: The Art Magazine for Teachers, 107*(2), 32–33.

Baggs, C., Mckhann, L., Gessert, C., & Johnson, B. (2013). Healing through reflective writing: Breast cancer survivor's experience. *Minnesota Medicine, 96*(7), 45–47.

Blasio, P., Camisasca, E., Caravita, S., Ionio, C., Milani, C., & Sacro, C. (2015). The effects of expressive writing on postpartum stress symptoms. *Psychological Reports, 117*(3), 856–882.

Cortright, S. M. (2008). Journaling: A tool for your spirit. Retrieved from http://www.journalforyou.com/full_article.php?article_id=7

Davidson, J., & Robison, B. (2008). Scrapbooking and journaling interventions for chronic illness: A triangulated investigation of approaches in the treatment of PTSD. *Kansas Nurse, 83*(3), 6–11.

Lindbergh, R. (2008). *Forward from here*. New York, NY: Simon & Schuster.

Meshberg-Cohen S., Svikis, D., & McMahon, T. (2014). Expressive writing as a therapeutic process in drug dependent women. *Substance Abuse, 35*(1), 80–88.

Milbury, K., Spelman, A., Wood, C., Matin, S., Tannir, N., Jonasch, E., ... Cohen, L. (2014). Randomized controlled trial of expressive writing for patients with renal cell carcinoma. *Journal of Clinical Oncology, 32*(7), 663–670.

Niles, A., Haltom, K., Mulvenna, C., Lieberman, M., & Stanton, A. (2014). Randomized controlled trial of expressive writing for psychological and physical health: The moderating role of motional expressivity. *Anxiety, Stress, & Coping, 27*, 1–17.

Nyssen, O., Taylor, S. J., Wong, G., Steed, E., Bourke, L., Lord, J., ... Meads, C. (2017). Does therapeutic writing help people with long-term conditions? Systematic review, realist synthesis and economic considerations. *Health Technology Assessment (No. 27)*. Retrieved from https://www.ncbi.nlm.nih.gov/books/NBK355726/

Pennebaker, J. (2012) Writing and health: Some practical advice. Retrieved from http://www.Homepage.psy.utexas.edu/homepage/Faculty/Pennebaker/Homepage

Penz, K., & Duggleby, W. (2012). "It's different in the home..." The contextual challenges and rewards of providing palliative care in community settings. *Journal of Hospice and Palliative Care, 14*, 365–373.

Pepe, L, Milani, R., De Trani, M., Di Folco, G., Lanna, V., & Solano, L. (2013). A more global approach to musculoskeletal pain: Expressive writing as an effective adjunct to physiotherapy. *Psychology, Health & Medicine, 19*(6), 687–697.

Proctor, S., Hoffmann, N., & Allison, S. (2012). The effectiveness of interactive journaling in reducing recidivism among substance-dependent jail inmates. *International Journal of Offender Therapy and Comparative Criminology, 56*, 317–332.

Sayer, N., Noorbaloochi, S., Frazier, P. A., Pennebaker, J. W., Orazam, R. J., Schnurr, P. P., ... Litz, B. T. (2015). Randomized controlled trial of online expressive writing to address readjustment difficulties among U.S. Afghanistan and Iraq War veterans. *Journal of Traumatic Stress, 28*(5), 381–390.

Sealy, P. (2012). Autoethnography: Reflective journaling and meditation to cope with life-threatening breast cancer. *Clinical Journal of Oncology Nursing, 16*, 38–41.

Shepherd, C., & Aagard, S. (2011). Journal writing with Web 2.0 tools: A vision for older adults. *Educational Gerontology, 37*, 606–620.

Snead, B., Pakstis, D., Evans, B., & Nelson, R. (2015). The use of creative writing interventions in substance abuse treatment. *Therapeutic Recreation Journal, 49*(3), 179–182.

Subhani, M., & Ifrah, I. (2012). Digital scrapbooking as a standard of care in neonatal intensive care units: Initial experience. *Journal of Neonatal Nursing, 31*, 162–168.

Ullman A. J., Aitken, L. M., Rattray, J., Kenardy, J., Le Brocque, R., MacGillivray, S., & Hull, A. M. (2015). Intensive care diaries to promote recovery for patients and families after critical illnesses: A Cochrane Systematic Review. *International Journal of Nursing Studies*, *52*(7), 1243–1253.

Whitney, R., & Smith, G. (2015). Emotional disclosure through journal writing: Telehealth intervention for maternal stress and mother-child relationships. *Journal of Autism and Development Disorders*, *45*(11), 3735–3745.

Young, C., Rodriguez, L., & Neighbors, C. (2013). Expressive writing as a brief intervention for reducing drinking intentions. *Addictive Behaviors*, *38*(12), 2913–2917.

Storytelling

Margaret P. Moss

The art and science of storytelling is presented in this chapter as a mechanism that can be used in alternative or complementary therapy. Its historical roots in orality (also known as *oralism*) are defined and explicated through examples from primary oral cultures. These are cultures that do not have a written language system (Sampson, 1980). In direct contrast, taking the art form into the future, digital storytelling is explored. Storytelling is then connected to its use as an alternative method in which to affect the path of one's health in terms of education, prevention, and intervention. Finally, concrete recommendations for health professionals close out the chapter.

DEFINITION

Orality

"The narratives we live and share everyday are our identity as a storied people and make visible what matters most in our lives" (Heliker, 2007, p. 21). Although there are around 3,000 languages in existence today, only 106 have ever been written and less than half of those are said to have literature (Edmondson, 1971). *Orality* is defined as a mostly verbal communication system used by whole cultures and devoid of the conventions or use of the written word (Olson & Torrance, 1991). The connection of orality or oralism to storytelling is intuitive. Storytelling is as universal in human communication as "the basic orality of language is permanent" (Ong, 2002, p. 7).

Literate societies evolved from oral societies. Each literate individual evolved from an oral beginning (Olson & Torrance, 1991). That is not to say that the formal and informal rules of orality are not as intricate as those in written communication. However, the majority of languages have never been translated into a written language (Edmondson, 1971).

The speaker, the process, and the aesthetics of orality are keys to imparting information (Lord, 1960). The rules concerning who speaks and when are defined by the culture. For instance, in some American Indian tribes, certain stories can be told only in the winter, others in the summer. Some words are not to be spoken at certain times of the day or to certain listeners. The process may be as in a prayer, a dance, or a story and can be in front of a large audience or one on one. Aesthetics may involve the use of masks, rattles, costumes, or specific surroundings. Finally, orality uses postural and gestural tools, as well as silence, as paralinguistic features in the transmission of the communication (Tedlock, 1983). "Formulaicness is valued when wisdom is seen as knowledge passed down through generations. Novelty is valued when wisdom is viewed as new information" (Tannen, 1982, p. 6). Therefore, anyone wishing to impart information through purposive oral means, such as through storytelling, needs to understand the key components, rules, and assigned power of oralism.

Storytelling

Storytelling is defined as the art or act of telling stories. A story is "a narrative, either true or fictitious, in prose or verse, designed to interest, amuse, or instruct the hearer or reader; [a] tale" (Dictionary.com, n.d.). Sociolinguist William Labov (as cited in Sandelowski, 1994) states that a complete story typically is composed of the:

- Abstract—what the story is about
- Orientation—the "who, when, where, and what" of the story
- Complicating action—the "then-what-happened" part of the story
- Evaluation—the "so-what" of the story
- Resolution—the "what-finally-happened" portion of the story
- Coda—the signal a story is over
- Return to the present (Sandelowski, 1994, p. 25)

It is the instructive nature of storytelling that is of interest for healthcare as an alternative means to an outcome: improved health. However, it must also be understood that lives, including our health, are "shaped by the stories we live" (Heliker, 2007, p. 21). Stories have shaped patients' current selves, and it is through stories that nurses can "interest, amuse, or instruct" them as listeners. Storytelling has paralleled human endeavors and will continue to evolve through future mechanisms.

Digital Storytelling

Digital storytelling is "the modern expression of the ancient art of storytelling. Digital stories derive their power by weaving images, music, narrative, and voice together, thereby giving deep dimension and vivid color to characters, situations, experiences, and insights" (Rule & Digital Storytelling Association, 2011, para. 1).

Although technology in digital storytelling provides the processes and aesthetics, it can also present some difficulties. For cultures with restrictions on word use, the 24-hour, 365-day availability of words via computer technology brings uncertainty. Matching the listener and the teller and their implicit contract is of utmost importance when choosing the type of conveyance.

Storytelling, whether traditional or digital, whether oral or written, serves multiple purposes across the life span and can be used by nurses. Nurses listen to stories when patients tell them what is going on in their lives, and they tell and retell stories every time they pass on information about patients (Fairbairn & Carson, 2002). Whether it is the person being cared for or the nurse, each individual telling the story *is* the story being told (Sandelowski, 1994). It is in the unfolding, intertwining, and connecting that a story becomes my story, your story, or our story. Stories are woven into the threads of life's fabric in our daily lives (Barton, 2004). We are all connected on a deeper or—if you prefer—higher level, and storytelling can take us to these levels.

SCIENTIFIC BASIS

Storytelling "is one of the world's most powerful tools for achieving astonishing results" in almost any industry (Guber, 2007, p. 55). Through an implicit contract between the storyteller and the listener (Guber, 2007), time is always a necessary ingredient. The storyteller must take the time to fully tell a story through all of its parts, using the necessary gestures, processes, and aesthetics. A story, as a sequence of events with discernible relations between those events and culminating in some conclusion, is a cognitive package (Bergner, 2007) that can be given to the listener. The listener must make time available to be present within the story to *hear* the message and absorb it. Successful transmission allows the listener to repeat the story to others in some form. Repetition, of course, leads to stronger transmission on both sides.

Effective storytellers understand their listener(s) and what they already know, what they care about, and what they want to hear (Guber, 2007). A great storyteller guides the story through essential elements based on the listener's understanding that the story is larger than the teller (Guber, 2007).

Language and Healing Beyond Health Literacy

"One of the few universals is that humans in all known cultures use language and tell stories" (Ramirez-Esparza & Pennebaker, 2006, p. 216). Storytelling without language is not possible. "Language embodies cultural reality" (Kramsch, 1998, p. 3). Language *itself* and healing may have a connection not yet fully explored or understood, beyond health literacy bounds. Most of the literature involving language and health surround the idea of health literacy, which has been defined as "the degree to which individuals have the capacity to obtain, process, and understand basic health information and services needed to make appropriate health decisions" (Nielsen-Bohlman, Panzer, & Kindig, 2004, p. 4). Although evidence points to greater understanding of health services and all that entails when spoken in the receiver's primary language (Koh et al., 2012), language as a healing tool and force are offered for consideration in this section.

In many indigenous cultures, for example, medicine and religion lines blur (Moss, 2000). Healing prayers are taken as a means to optimal health, whether in the physical, mental, spiritual, or emotional domain (Moss, 2000). These prayers are likely conducted in the traditional language. A recent study from South Africa offers that, "language creates an image of the unknown to which people attach meaning" (Lourens, 2013, abstract). There is comfort in hearing one's own language. It takes away a struggle and the required energy needed to accept either information or prayer, presumably allowing more energy to be used for healing.

Whereas indigenous examples of language use in prayer and healing may be specifically seen as other examples, the dominant cultures also use language in healing and prayer beyond their use as delivery of information only. We see this in the change in tone, speed, earnestness, and length of delivery that exceeds any aesthetic needed to merely deliver information. This can be from a mother to a sick child, a prayer group to a member, or another cultural convention or relationship.

American Indian Exemplar

The Zuni tribe of New Mexico use storytelling through all parts of their lives. It is used casually and formally. It is used in secular and sacred telling. The teller can be a priest, a *kiva* group, a grandmother, or another person. A *kiva* is a "medicine (i.e., priestly) society" to which men are initiated as youths and remain to carry out the work of the *kiva* (Moss, 2000). The purpose of the dances they perform can be solely to heal listeners from sickness. Through word of mouth, the news may spread that a Rain Dance is called. Unlike what Hollywood portrays, this dance calls listeners to one of the small plazas (flat dirt squares) in the village where they can receive needed healing prayers.

Time is part of the contract. The listener arrives at a loosely determined time and waits. The dancers and lead teller arrive some time later. The teller knows why the listeners are there: The contract is intact. There is respectful listening and targeted telling. The telling is in the form of prayer, song, and dance. The team is in full regalia, with masks and dress from centuries of performances. A formula is used in the telling. It can take hours. The teller(s), the process, and the aesthetics all come together in dance, silence, and singing to heal the listener.

Language Revitalization

So far, this chapter has explored present-day oral languages, written languages, and the use of digital "telling." The use of each of these modalities has pros and cons in storytelling. Oral languages represent millennia of information passed down faithfully from one generation to another. Some members' main roles in the society is to "remember" and "store" this information. However, there may be discrepancies over the years when key pieces of important stories may be lost, much like happens in the "telephone game." It is the addition of processes and aesthetics that seeks to temper those losses.

Equally important are the issues with written languages (whether scribed or digital). In this mode, there is reliance on a place (book, computer drive) rather than a person or persons storing and transmitting language/stories. If there is destruction of the person or place where the information is stored and there is no person or organic backup, huge amounts of information will be forever lost.

The digital age is largely described as proliferating anywhere from the 1970s or 1980s and continuing through to present. Written language is acknowledged from around 3500 to 3000 BCE, originating in southern Mesopotamia (Mark, 2011). A best guess on the origin of oralism (i.e., language use as a modality of information transmission) is around 100,000 years ago (Bolhuis, Tattersall, Chomsky, & Berwick, 2014).

What hasn't been discussed is the loss of language and the need for their revitalization, especially languages that were forced out of existence rather than fading naturally. Examples of this can be seen especially throughout the *settler states* of the United States, Canada, Australia, and New Zealand. Similar histories "hurried" indigenous languages to extinction or near-extinction and with it the loss of stories so vital to the societies and the health of their members.

In the United States, passage of the Native American Languages Act of 1990 was an effort to begin attempts to retain and revitalize language among indigenous communities (Whalen, Moss, & Baldwin, 2016). Little progress has been made, and these languages are still rapidly losing speakers and their knowledge (Whalen et al., 2016). Some of this knowledge contains healing aspects, whether the words themselves, medicines, or therapies specific to the language and its use. "Language programs in indigenous communities hold the promise of improving the mental and physical health of those who participate in them" (Whalen et al., 2016, para. 19). One advantage to these programs are that young and old can participate, thereby bringing together another important intergenerational aspect to many indigenous cultures.

INTERVENTION

Bergner (2007) writes about the "staying power of stories," which has obvious benefits when delivering therapeutic messages. He tells of stories that patients have recounted as far back as 8 years earlier.

Technique

Stories in therapy draw from the general culture of the patient, integrate common knowledge sequences, and therefore do not require the acquisition of new knowledge to participate (Bergner, 2007). Code words can then be used to recall the entire story for the patient at later dates. Stories can be targeted to specific diagnoses in increasing meaning for the patient. This allows taking away aspects that do not apply and bringing in aspects that may be unique to the patient.

Guidelines

The following guideline sequence has been presented in the literature for storytelling in therapy: Present the story, elaborate as needed to increase understanding, and then discuss application to this particular patient situation (Bergner, 2007). In some cultures, there are situations in which reality can be "spoken into being." Again, often these types of stories are strongest in oral cultures. However, even in the dominant culture in the United States, people may shush a person who speaks about death, cancer, or some bad thing happening.

In primarily oral cultures, such as traditional indigenous societies, it would be difficult to explain advance directives or informed consent in the manner in which they are presented in Western medical facilities. This applies whether in caring for a patient or in conducting research. As an example, it might be the task of a healthcare provider to tell a traditional American Indian older adult from the Southwest that this individual could die, lose a leg, or get an infection if the suggested traditional treatments were completed. The patient would perceive harm in even hearing this message. The subject certainly would not want to review or sign a consent form that contained these facts. In this case, one would be wise to use a hypothetical story instead. The harm would be taken away from the patient, and instead, the teller would describe to the listener facts about "another" person in a similar situation, drawing from cultural norms and common knowledge and asking the listener whether the hypothetical person would be willing to go through the procedure.

Using these guidelines, there would be elaboration, as needed, in a context familiar to the patient. For instance, one might describe the following:

> Mr. Vigil was an older Pueblo man who had diabetes. He had it for 20 years and lived fairly comfortably with his family on the pueblo and saw his doctor regularly. There came a time when Mr. Vigil's leg began to bother him more and more. He tried several things with his doctor to increase blood flow and promote nerve health. Even though he did what he could for his health, it became apparent that he might have to lose the leg to continue living and being with his family. The doctor told him that he would still be able to participate in ceremonies and get around after the surgery with the use of a prosthetic leg and physical therapy. Mr. Vigil was worried. What do you think he was worried about? What do you think he might have decided? What questions would you ask if you were Mr. Vigil?

The use of vignettes such as this one has been introduced in research, as well as in practice.

When using stories as an intervention, one should use the ideas of orality, in which repetition, setting, esthetics, and process are important in the transmission of information. Implementing these assists the listener in retaining the information.

Suggestions for Implementing Storytelling

Suggestions for healthcare practitioners, educators, or researchers contemplating using storytelling include:

- Learn the difference between orality and literacy:
  - It is much more than one group reads and the other writes.
  - A whole system of rules for the use of each exists.
  - Each uses differing paths to arrive at the desired outcomes.
  - Orality and literacy may be used separately or together.
- Understand differences in response to storytelling by age and culture:
  - Younger *and* older patients may be more attuned to traditional, oral, face-to-face storytelling.
  - The teenage through middle-adult patient may be more open and attuned to digital storytelling techniques.
  - Use of vignettes and anecdotes in the third person takes the pressure off the listener.

- Use technology as appropriate:
  - Certain cultures may not access the computer for fear of encountering a word deemed inappropriate at certain times or to certain people.
  - Interactive media can be used with almost all people *if geared specifically to* their age, culture, and level of technological proficiency.

Measurement of Outcomes

A variety of tools can be used to measure outcomes of storytelling. Depending on the purpose for which storytelling is being used, instruments that measure anxiety, depression, social isolation, spirituality, caring, and sense of well-being may be appropriate. Qualitative research methods may also be used to measure the effectiveness or changes brought about through storytelling, including increased understanding of the information.

PRECAUTIONS

Those using storytelling need to be prepared to deal with the strong emotions stories may evoke. Health professionals should be ready to assist and support the participants because diverse reactions can occur. A list of available resources for making referrals for follow-up are helpful. Only practitioners trained in psychotherapy should use storytelling with people who have psychological problems. The health sciences represent disciplines that attempt to understand humans from their various perspectives and philosophies, but these disciplines have grown so specialized in their jargon that the message to the patient may easily be lost (Evans, 2007). The use of storytelling in the common vernacular can be an antidote to this loss of message.

USES

The use of storytelling in healthcare settings, healthcare research, and teaching is unlimited. Nurses can use storytelling in multiple situations across the life span for a variety of purposes. Stories can be used in family therapy and can assist members in tapping into the flow of meaning of the past, present, and future, and help patients open up possibilities for "making meaning" and healing (Roberts, 1994).

Another aspect of using storytelling is when the *teller* of the story is the one to benefit from it. In Ramirez-Esparza and Pennebaker's article "Do Good Stories Produce Good Health?" (2006), evidence for a link between expressive writing (storytelling) and markers for both mental and physical health are described. The stories do not even have to be coherent, but just the ability of the person to express the story is beneficial (Ramirez-Esparza & Pennebaker, 2006). Analysis of the story down to which type of pronoun is used (i.e., first person or not) can point to health indicators around depression, for example (Ramirez-Esparza & Pennebaker, 2006).

This use and resulting phenomena have been seen in digital storytelling as well. The *teller* of the story receives a feeling of greater well-being or other health-related benefit. Sharing experiences, lightening a burden, and helping others allowed participants to report feeling better (www.patientvoices.org.uk; Haigh & Hardy, 2011).

Older Adults: Practice

To increase the reciprocity of care between nursing home staff and residents, *story sharing* has been used as an intervention strategy. To lessen the almost totally task-oriented nature of caring, the use of story sharing has been shown to increase the quality of life of residents in six different nursing homes (Heliker, 2007). Through story sharing, the staff was encouraged to come to know the patients, their backgrounds, interests, and likes. Active listening and expressions of concern are key elements. This is a mutual process in which each learns about the other and trust and shared experiences become evident. The intervention suggested by Heliker used three 1-hour sessions between six nurse aides and a facilitator. In session 1, staff learn about confidentiality, respectful and attentive listening, and role playing. In session 2, staff bring an object that holds personal meaning for themselves, to better understand the residents and what few possessions residents may have with them, as well as the monumental meaning of these possessions. In session 3, staff learn about "sharing informs care" practices. Both residents and aides reported being in a better relationship with each other, which can be seen as a "best practice" in the care of older, frail adults (Heliker, 2007).

Older Adults: Education

"Many older adults were raised in an era when learning occurred primarily through reading, discussion, and retelling stories" (Cangelosi & Sorrell, 2008, p. 19). Often, it is through storytelling, whether formal or informal, that otherwise missed information is shared. Many older patients detail numerous topics and events until they hit on pertinent information in describing their current problem. Unless this wandering is not only allowed but encouraged, especially with older subjects, crucial data needed for their care will be missed. When questions requiring only *yes* and *no* answers are asked and are hurried in encounters with older clients, they will not be able to share vital information with the healthcare professional. Probing questions require time, patience, and empathy. In addition, older adults need time to *hear* and process what the healthcare provider is telling them. One strategy is to share health information in a group setting, allowing for support from others in the group (Cangelosi & Sorrell, 2008). When storytelling is used as an intervention for teaching older individuals, unique learning needs will be met (Cangelosi & Sorrell, 2008).

Digital Storytelling

Digital storytelling may be an effective way of educating younger people, whether in the classroom or in patient education, in this world of ever-changing technology. Visual and audio media may stimulate deeper learning in this population, which is largely familiar and comfortable with the use of technology (Sandars, Murray, & Pellow, 2008). Sandars et al. have used digital storytelling with medical students. As a guideline, they suggest the following 12-step sequence of events for digital storytelling:

1. Decide on the topic of the story
2. Write the story

3. Collect a variety of multimedia to create a story
4. Select which medium to use to create the story
5. Create the story
6. Present the digital story
7. Encourage reflection at each stage of the project
8. Avoid being too ambitious
9. Provide adequate technical support
10. Develop a relevant assessment framework
11. Embed it within existing teaching and learning approaches
12. Persuade others of its value

Building the story encourages active learning and constant reflection for the teller. This process could be used with other populations such as patient groups. Although the storyteller is in many ways the learner in this situation, the same orality notions are in play. The storyteller, the process, and the aesthetics are of great import. Rather than regalia, video and audio supply the aesthetics.

When looking ahead to digital delivery and/or storytelling in the future, it is probable that, "growth in technology is actually likely to increase health disparities for those with limited health, computer, and reading literacy, unless effort is devoted to the development of IT [information technology] specifically designed for these disadvantaged groups, and issues of technology access are addressed" (Bickmore & Paasche-Orlow, 2012, p. 23).

CULTURAL APPLICATIONS

In many indigenous societies, especially when they are described as primarily oral cultures, Western health practices are seen as the alternative and complementary modalities (Moss, 2000). This is important because the practitioner—or the storyteller—must understand that to patients coming from a basically oral culture, storytelling is already seen as primary to their well-being. A number of health-related studies use storytelling in various cultures (Crawford O'Brien, 2008; Finucane & McMullen, 2008; Inglebret, Jones, & Pavel, 2008; Larkey & Gonzalez, 2007; Leeman, Skelly, Burns, Carlson, & Soward, 2008).

In a narrative analysis of 115 stories of women of African descent, Banks-Wallace (2002) found storytelling useful for learning more about the historical and contextual factors affecting the well-being of these women. The major functions storytelling served were contextual grounding, bonding with others, validation and affirmation of experiences, venting and catharsis, resistance to oppression, and education of others. See Sidebar 13.1 for a vivid personal account of the use of storytelling in Kenya illustrating these major functions.

Rogers (2004) found storytelling at the heart of 11 Pacific Northwest African American widows, 55 years of age and older, who described their experiences of bereavement after their husbands' deaths. During the interviews, the widows took on various mannerisms and speech patterns of people who were part of the story. These included changed tones; mimicking the voices of those involved; and use of hands, body language, and facial expressions. Nurses should be aware of storytelling as a means to gain in-depth understanding and cultural insight into African American experience.

SIDEBAR 13.1. HEALING THROUGH THE ORAL TRADITION: CONTEXTUALIZING PATIENT NARRATIVES IN KENYA

Eunice M. Areba

Presenting health messages in a manner that patients can easily understand and incorporate into their lives is our obligation. Communicating effectively means *transforming* health messages into pieces of information that are not only easily understood, but that can also be put into *action* by recipients to attain mutually agreed-on health outcomes (Silver, 2001). Key to effective communication is use of mechanisms familiar to members of the target community, which ensures the ownership and sustainability of the intervention. A notable example is the use of oral narratives (e.g., folklore) or simply storytelling, an art that has been used for eons in communities across the world. Nurses and other healthcare providers in Kenya and beyond have been great proponents and facilitators of storytelling, especially in chronic disease management. These stories usually detail patients' lived experiences.

I grew up surrounded by stories depicting characters that I could easily relate to, and children were encouraged to participate in the storytelling process through song, dance, and rehearsed phrases such as these roughly translated ones:

Paukwa? Pakawa! (Who wants to be served? Me!)
Sahani? Ya mchele! (A plate? Of rice!)

Now as an adult, I vividly remember not just the stories, but also the lessons that were imparted. The storyteller is most often an elder who aims to instill a virtue, rectify a vice, and educate the young on the history or origin of a community or practice. Some examples in the Kisii, Luhya, Coastal, and Maasai tribes in Kenya include *the prophetess Moraa and Otenyo* (a historical event), *Simbi and Nashikufu* (beauty and humility), *hekaya za Abunuwasi* and *Mekatilili Wa Menza* (social justice and leadership), and *Naiterukop and Maasae* (the origin of cattle ownership in the Maasai community). Oral narratives—especially from tribes whose mother tongue might soon become extinct—are being recorded both on paper and digital platforms. Storytelling in any form is a powerful and versatile health-teaching tool that can easily be implemented by healthcare providers across many settings, as illustrated in these examples.

HIV is not killing anybody unless you close your mouth (Leon, 2012, p. 28). HIV-positive women are healing with the help of their peers whose stories have helped them conquer social stigma, fear, and denial. Participants in the programs organized by the nongovernmental organization (NGO) Women Fighting Aids in Kenya (WOFAK) and its affiliates draw strength from one another's stories and, in so doing, develop a shared identity that comforts and assures them that they are not alone (Leon, 2012). Storytelling in this setting takes on a communal nature and encourages them to adhere to treatment programs. Healthcare providers also organize storytelling workshops targeting high-risk groups such as transport workers in specific geographical locations.

(continued)

Trauma, restorative justice, and mental health. No matter where or how it happens, exposure to violence and trauma negatively impact psychosocial, emotional, and physical well-being. The destruction of social institutions and the tapestry of shared values during and after war denies victims of trauma essential tools needed to cope. Widescale violence disrupts everyday way of life and, most important, deconstructs the meaning of life. Narratives of the atrocities meted out and the physical and psychological wounds and scars of victims have been used in peace and reconciliation tribunals to rebuild relationships and reestablish trust. Narratives are most often shared in communal settings (e.g., in Rwanda's gacaca courts that addressed the acts of violence committed during the 1994 genocide; Ingelaere, 2012). In South Africa, the Truth and Reconciliation Commission established after the abolition of apartheid in 1994 was a court system infused with communal values, illustrating the use and importance of narratives in the quest for peace, restitution, and healing. However, these efforts are not used in isolation; effective interventions are multipronged, and adaptive coping and healing can be elusive if efforts do not acknowledge culturally acceptable interventions and because the atrocities have lifelong implications (Hamber, 2015).

Storytelling is seen as *familiar ground*, a tradition that many are exposed to during their upbringing and is, in turn, perceived as *safe ground*. Some participants in these traditional setups have expressed feelings of relief, empowerment, and personal and communal healing. In cases of community reintegration, storytelling has been critical in accepting people back into the community. Conversely, there is the danger of retraumatization, so adequate provisions for mental healthcare have to be instituted.

In multicultural societies we religiously include snippets of how to be culturally competent. In doing so we run into the danger of reducing patients' rich and diverse cultures into a catalog of what they identify with (Le, Miller, & McMullin, 2017). Focusing on just the cultural context is shortsighted, and we are prone to create stereotypical accounts of our patients' narratives. It is essential to consider the social, structural, and institutionalized factors that render treatment and care plans impractical (Singer, Dressler, George, & NIH Expert Panel, 2016). Care providers need to consider if relevant resources are available, accessible, and adequate to patients (immigrant, minority, poor) before labeling them as difficult or noncompliant and need to critically examine their ability to consider the effect of these complex factors on patient outcomes (Le, Miller, & McMullin, 2017).

Creating a space for storytelling empowers patients, creates rapport, and places decisions in the hands of the patients—thus building the capacity to identify and acknowledge practical solutions. Care providers need to listen intently, learn from patients on how to best give care, and create care plans that acknowledge difficult circumstances that impede positive patient outcomes.

References

Hamber, B. (2015). Dealing with painful memories and violent pasts: Towards a Framework for Contextual Understanding. In B. Austin & M. Fischer (Eds). *Transforming war-related identities*. Berghof Handbook Dialogue Series No. 11. Berlin: Berghof Foundation.

(continued)

Leon, K. (2012). *Storytelling and healing: The influence of narrative on identity construction among HIV positive individuals in Kisumu,* Kenya (Unpublished manuscript). Retrieved from http://digitalcollections.sit.edu/isp_collection/1385

Ingelaere, B. (2012). From model to practice: Researching and representing Rwanda's "modernized" gacaca courts. *Critique of Anthropology, 32*(4), 388–414.

Le, A., Miller, K., & McMullin, J. (2017). From particularities to context: Refining our thinking on illness narratives. *AMA Journal of Ethics, 19*(3), 304.

Silver, D. (2001). Songs and storytelling: Bringing health messages to life in Uganda. *Education for Health, 14,* 51–60.

Singer, M. K., Dressler, W., George, S., & NIH Expert Panel (2016). Culture: The missing link in health research. *Social Science & Medicine, 170,* 237–246.

Culturally appropriate communication methods, such as storytelling, have been found to be effective in health-promotion activities. The *talking circle* is one format in which the art of storytelling occurs. Indigenous Ojibwa and Cree women healers use talking circles as instruments of healing and storytelling in their everyday traditional practice (Struthers, 1999). Storytelling was preferred as a natural pattern of communication for the Yakima tribe to learn about health promotion related to cervical cancer prevention (Strickland, Squeoch, & Chrisman, 1999).

FUTURE RESEARCH

Technology will certainly play a larger role in storytelling. However, the orality of storytelling with which we are familiar will always be retained. Therefore, integrating future trends will keep the modality in line with evolving human endeavors. Wyatt and Hauenstein (2008) explore "how technology and storytelling can be joined to promote positive health outcomes" (p. 142). They recognize that although storytelling is widely used to teach children in the classroom, it has been minimally used in the health arena as a teaching–learning tool. With advances in technology—and its ubiquitous presence—interactive, digital storytelling may provide one mechanism to help enhance health promotion.

Explorations are needed to determine the efficacy of vignettes in both research and practice, particularly with individuals from other cultures and with older adults. Triangulation of qualitative and quantitative measures will provide a more complete examination of a patient's reflection, understanding, and outcomes. Specific questions that require investigation include:

- What are strategies to use to help nurses become more comfortable using storytelling as an intervention?
- What are some ways in which vignettes can be used with people from diverse cultures and age groups?

REFERENCES

Banks-Wallace, J. (2002). Talk that talk: Storytelling and analysis rooted in African American oral tradition. *Qualitative Health Research, 12*(3), 410–426.

Barton, S. S. (2004). Narrative inquiry: Locating Aboriginal epistemology in a relational methodology. *Journal of Advanced Nursing, 45*(5), 519–526.

Bergner, R. M. (2007). Therapeutic storytelling revisited. *American Journal of Psychotherapy*, *61*(2), 149–162.

Bickmore, T. W., & Paasche-Orlow, M. K. (2012). The role of information technology in health literacy research. *Journal of Health Communication: International Perspectives*, *17*(Suppl. 3), S23–S29.

Bolhuis, J. J., Tattersall, I., Chomsky, N., & Berwick, R. C. (2014). How could language have evolved? *PLOS Biology*, *12*(8), e1001934. doi:10.1371/journal.pbio.1001934

Cangelosi, P. R., & Sorrell, J. M. (2008). Storytelling as an educational strategy for older adults with chronic illness. *Journal of Psychosocial Nursing and Mental Health Services*, *46*(7), 19–22.

Crawford O'Brien, S. (Ed.). (2008). *Religion and healing in Native America: Pathways for renewal*. Westport, CT: Praeger.

Dictionary.com Unabridged. (n.d.). Story. Retrieved from www.dictionary.com/browse/story

Edmondson, M. E. (1971). *Lore: An introduction to the science of folklore and literature*. New York, NY: Holt, Rinehart, & Winston.

Evans, J. (2007). The science of storytelling. *Astrobiology*, *7*(4), 710–711.

Fairbairn, G. J., & Carson, A. M. (2002). Writing about nursing research: A storytelling approach. *Nurse Researcher*, *10*(1), 7–14.

Finucane, M. L., & McMullen, C. K. (2008). Making diabetes self-management education culturally relevant for Filipino Americans in Hawaii. *Diabetes Educator*, *34*(5), 841–853.

Guber, P. (2007). The four truths of the storyteller. *Harvard Business Review*, *85*(12), 52–59, 142.

Haigh, C., & Hardy, P. (2011). Tell me a story—A conceptual exploration of storytelling in healthcare education. *Nurse Education Today*, *31*(4), 408–411.

Heliker, D. (2007). Story sharing: Restoring the reciprocity of caring in long-term care. *Journal of Psychosocial Nursing and Mental Health Services*, *45*(7), 20–23.

Inglebret, E., Jones, C., & Pavel, D. M. (2008). Integrating American Indian/Alaska native culture into shared storybook intervention. *Language, Speech, and Hearing Services in Schools*, *39*(4), 521–527.

Koh, H. K., Berwick, D. M., Clancy, C. M., Baur, C., Brach, C., Harris, L. M., & Zerhusen, E. G. (2012). New federal policy initiatives to boost health literacy can help the nation move beyond the cycle of costly 'crisis care.' *Health Affairs*, *31*(2), 434–443.

Kramsch, C. (1998). *Language and culture*. Oxford, UK: Oxford University Press.

Larkey, L. K., & Gonzalez, J. (2007). Storytelling for promoting colorectal cancer prevention and early detection among Latinos. *Patient Education and Counseling*, *67*(3), 272–278. doi:10.1016/j.pec.2007.04.003

Leeman, J., Skelly, A. H., Burns, D., Carlson, J., & Soward, A. (2008). Tailoring a diabetes self-care intervention for use with older, rural African American women. *Diabetes Educator*, *34*(2), 310–317.

Lord, A. (1960). *The singer of tales* (2nd ed.). Cambridge, MA: Harvard University Press.

Lourens, M. (2013). An exploration of Xhosa speaking patients' understanding of cancer treatment and its influence on their treatment experience. *Journal of Psychosocial Oncology*, *31*, 103–121.

Mark, J. J. (2011). Writing. *Ancient History Encyclopedia*. Retrieved from http://www.ancient.eu/writing

Moss, M. P. (2000). *Zuni elders: Ethnography of American Indian aging* (Unpublished doctoral dissertation). University of Texas Health Science Center at Houston, Houston, TX. Retrieved from http://digitalcommons.library.tmc.edu/dissertations/AAI9974591

Native American Languages Act of 1990, Pub. L. No. 101-477, 104 Stat. 1152 (1990).

Nielsen-Bohlman, L., Panzer, A., & Kindig, D. (Eds.). (2004). *Health literacy: A prescription to end confusion*. National Research Council. Washington, DC: National Academies Press.

Olson, D. R., & Torrance, N. (Eds.). (1991). *Literacy and orality*. Cambridge, UK: Cambridge University Press.

Ong, W. J. (2002). *Orality and literacy*. New York, NY: Routledge.

Ramirez-Esparza, N., & Pennebaker, J. W. (2006). Do good stories produce good health? Exploring words, language, and culture. *Narrative Inquiry*, *16*(1), 211–219.

Roberts, J. (1994). Tales and transformations: Stories in families and family therapy. New York, NY: Norton.

Rogers, L. S. (2004). Meaning of bereavement among older African American widows. *Geriatric Nursing, 25*(1), 10–16.

Rule, L., & the Digital Storytelling Association. (2011). Digital storytelling. Retrieved from http://electronicportfolios.com/digistory

Sampson, G. (1980). *Schools of linguistics*. Stanford, CA: Stanford University Press.

Sandars, J., Murray, C., & Pellow, A. (2008). Twelve tips for using digital storytelling to promote reflective learning by medical students. *Medical Teacher, 30*(8), 774–777.

Sandelowski, M. (1994). We are the stories we tell: Narrative knowing in nursing practice. *Journal of Holistic Nursing, 12*(1), 23–33.

Strickland, C. J., Squeoch, M. D., & Chrisman, N. J. (1999). Health promotion in cervical cancer prevention among the Yakima Indian women of the Wa'Shat Longhouse. *Journal of Transcultural Nursing, 10*(3), 190–196.

Struthers, R. (1999). *The lived experience of Ojibwa and Cree women healers* (Unpublished doctoral dissertation). University of Minnesota, Minneapolis, MN.

Tannen, D. (Ed.). (1982). *Spoken and written language: Exploring orality and literacy*. New York, NY: Ablex.

Tedlock, D. (1983). *The spoken word and the work of interpretation*. Philadelphia: University of Pennsylvania Press.

Whalen, D. H., Moss, M., & Baldwin, D. (2016). *Healing through language: Positive physical health effects of indigenous language use*. F1000Research, 5, 852. doi:10.12688/f1000research.8656.1

Wyatt, T. H., & Hauenstein, E. (2008). Enhancing children's health through digital story. *Computers, Informatics, Nursing: CIN, 26*(3), 142–148; quiz, 149–150.

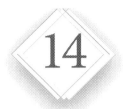

Animal-Assisted Therapy

Susan O'Conner-Von

The domestication of animals began more than 14,000 years ago and continues today because animals play a significant role in human life (Lear, 2012). Much of what was known about the animal–human bond was anecdotal in nature until recently. Research examining the use of animals as a complementary or alternative therapy is based on studies about pet ownership. It is evident—with approximately 70 million pet dogs and 74 million pet cats in the United States—that pets play an important role in people's lives (American Veterinary Medical Association, 2012). Pets can provide companionship, promote dialogue and social interaction, facilitate exercise, increase feelings of security, mitigate the effects of stress, be a source of consistency, and be a comfort to touch (Arkow, 2015). The healing power of pets is "their capacity to make the atmosphere safe for emotions, the spiritual side of healing; whatever you are feeling, you can express it around your pet and not be judged" (Becker, 2002, p. 80).

In a comparative study examining the impact of pet ownership in childhood on young adults' social characteristics and professional choices, those who owned a pet in childhood retrospectively rated their pet higher than television, relatives, and neighbors in terms of social support received during childhood (Vizek, Arambasic, Kerestes, Kuterovac, & Vlahovic-Stetic, 2001). The sample comprised 356 college students at a mean age of·21 years (68% women, 32% men). A total of 74% of the sample had pets (mostly dogs) during childhood and were found to be more empathetic and expressed more altruistic attitudes than those students who did not own a pet in childhood. Moreover, students who had a pet in childhood were more likely to choose a career in the helping professions.

The role that animals play in healing environments was first documented in records from 9th-century Belgium, where animals were used with individuals with physical disabilities, followed by 18th-century England where animals were used by people with mental illness (Serpell, 2015). Florence Nightingale wrote of the connection between animals and health in 1860 by suggesting that pets were perfect companions for the sick, especially individuals with chronic health conditions (Nightingale, 1859/1992).

The 1970s launched the beginning of widespread interest in the interaction between animals and humans in the healthcare setting. In 1976, Elaine Smith, an American registered nurse, observed the benefits of pets in the healthcare setting while working in England. She noticed how patients reacted positively to the visits of a chaplain and his golden retriever. On returning to the United States, Smith introduced the concept of pet therapy into healthcare settings and founded Therapy Dogs International (TDI; 2017). The goal of creating TDI was to formally test dogs so that they could be certified, insured, and registered as volunteer therapy dogs. In 1977, the Delta Foundation (now Pet Partners) was established to study the human–animal bond and the potential use of animal-assisted therapy (AAT). Scientific research in this area began in the 1980s, when the National Institutes of Health convened a conference in 1987 on the health benefits of pets (Fine & Beck, 2015). During the 1990s, the focus was the establishment of professional standards and guidelines with the development of the *Standards of Practice for Animal-Assisted Activities and Animal-Assisted Therapy* (Delta Society, 1996). In 2008, the National Institute of Child and Human Development convened a conference to discuss the need for clarity and well-designed research examining the animal–human bond (Fine & Beck, 2015). Carefully designed studies continue to provide the evidence needed to increase acceptance of AAT as a credible intervention (Stern & Chur-Hansen, 2013).

DEFINITION

The International Association of Human-Animal Interaction Organizations (IAHAIO; 2014) is a global association of 60 multidisciplinary organizations that engage in practice, research, and/or education in AAT, animal-assisted activity (AAA), and service animal training. In an effort to provide consistency of terminology and guidelines for research and practice, a white paper was developed and approved, and which includes the following definitions.

Animal-Assisted Intervention (AAI)

"An animal-assisted intervention is a goal-oriented and structured intervention that intentionally includes animals in health, education, and human service for the purpose of therapeutic gains in humans" (IAHAIO, 2014, p. 5). AAT, education, and activities are examples of types of animal-assisted interventions (IAHAIO, 2014).

Animal-Assisted Therapy

"Animal-assisted therapy is a goal-oriented, planned and structured therapeutic intervention directed and/or delivered by health, education and human service professionals" (IAHAIO, 2014, p. 5). Some key features of AAT are (a) specific goals and objectives are set for each patient, (b) progress is measured, and (c) interactions are documented. The goals are designed by a nurse, occupational therapist, physical therapist, counselor, physician, or other healthcare professional who uses AAT in the treatment process (American Veterinary Medical Association, 2017a). A physical goal would include, for example, improved mobility by walking with a dog. Examples of cognitive goals include improved verbal expression (via normal interaction with the animal) and improved short- and long-term memory (via recalling the animal's name and activity at last visit). Social goals could include improved social skills and building rapport with others through the animal. Animals may also help increase socialization by facilitating discussion of pets one may have had in the past. An illustration of an emotional goal would be improved motivation shown by getting dressed or walking to see the animal. Although a variety of animal species and breeds, such as cats, birds, rabbits, horses, and dolphins, are involved in AAT, dogs account for the highest percentage of animals (Grandin, Fine, O'Haire, Carlisle, & Bowers, 2015).

Animal-Assisted Activity

"Animal-assisted activity (AAA) is a planned and goal-oriented informal interaction and visitation conducted by the human–animal team for motivational, educational, and recreational purposes" (IAHAIO, 2014, p. 5). Some key features of AAA are (a) specific goals and objectives are not planned for each patient, (b) visit activities are spontaneous and last as long as needed, and (c) interactions are not necessarily documented. AAAs are less structured and provide human and animal contact for recreation, education, or pleasure. Examples include an informal visit by a friendly pet to a residential care center, hospice, hospital, school, or prison with the intent to bring joy, comfort, and companionship to the residents (Rivera, 2010).

Service Animals

A service animal was originally defined in the Americans with Disabilities Act of 1990 as any animal trained to do work for the benefit of an individual with a disability, including physical, psychiatric, sensory, intellectual, or mental conditions (American Disabilities Act National Network, 2014). As of March 15, 2011, only dogs are recognized as service animals under Title II (state and local government services) or Title III (public accommodations and commercial facilities) of the Americans with Disabilities Act. Service dogs or guide dogs are trained specifically for the service they are providing: sight, sound, movement, or support. Once service animals are certified, they have federally approved access to accompany their owners anywhere. Service dogs are considered working animals, not pets. Although there is increased awareness and acceptance of therapy dogs in healthcare and public settings, such dogs do not receive federal protection or the same rights as service dogs who assist people with physical or emotional disabilities (American Disabilities Act National Network, 2014).

SCIENTIFIC BASIS

Many studies indicate that there are physical and/or psychological benefits derived from human–animal bonds. Most of the research that has examined the physical benefits of AAT has focused on an animal's ability to attenuate a person's response to stress. When an individual becomes stressed, the sympathetic nervous system releases a cascade of hormones such as cortisol, aldosterone, and adrenaline. Stress-reduction strategies, such as petting an animal, can assist in reducing the build-up of these stress hormones (Wolff & Frishman, 2005). Likewise, the hormone oxytocin can lower blood pressure, lower cortisol levels, increase the pain threshold and have an antianxiety effect. One of the best ways to increase oxytocin levels is through positive physical touch, such as petting an animal (Chandler, 2017). In turn, research has revealed a similar increased level of oxytocin in dogs after interaction with humans (Odendaal & Meintjes, 2003). Research that has examined the psychological benefits of AAT has explored the stress-reducing outcomes and improved quality of life that the animal provides through social support (Arkow, 2015; Hart & Yamamoto, 2015).

INTERVENTION

AAT has been shown to be a successful intervention for patients of all ages with a variety of physical and psychological conditions. This intervention can be provided in many settings, including private homes, acute care and rehabilitation facilities, long-term and group care homes, schools, and correctional facilities.

Guidelines

Selecting an animal for AAT requires careful screening and extensive training (American Veterinary Medical Association, 2017b; IAHAIO, 2014). Although some animals are considered good pets, not all animals are appropriate candidates for AAT. There is no ideal animal for AAT, but the animal must be calm, tolerant, and reliable (Arkow, 2015). Furthermore, all animals must complete yearly veterinary screening to ensure that they are healthy, current on vaccinations, and parasite free (IAHAIO, 2014). AAT requires that the animal and handler work together as a team. To provide safe and effective AAT, the AAT team should abide by established standards of practice for AAA and AAT. Examples from the Standards of Practice (Delta Society, 1996) for the handler include (a) demonstrating appropriate treatment of people and animals, (b) using appropriate social skills, (c) acting as the animal's advocate, (d) having the ability to read the animal's cues, and (e) maintaining confidentiality.

AAT Training

Most national therapy dog organizations require the Canine Good Citizen test (American Kennel Club [AKC], 2017) as a basic skills requirement for acceptance into a therapy dog training program. This test, developed by the AKC in 1989, is a certification program that tests dogs in everyday situations and requires a dog to have mastered a basic set of skills. Dogs are tested in ten areas that include response to a friendly stranger and another dog, ability to walk with a loose leash, and reaction to distraction and separation. (For the complete list, see www.akc.org/dog-owners/training/canine-good-citizen/training-testing.)

Additional requirements may include didactic content for the human partner to understand the theory and research supporting AAT, standards of practice, and ethical considerations. The animal partner receives training in simulated healthcare settings that include activities such as (a) learning how to leave alone an object such as food or medication; (b) being bumped while walking in a crowded space; (c) being comfortable around hospital equipment such as wheelchairs, walkers, or crutches; (d) receiving petting from several people at once; and (e) sitting quietly as paws, ears, and tail are examined.

Measurement of Outcomes

The effects of AAT have been measured through qualitative and quantitative means. A variety of outcomes, such as cardiovascular benefits, decreased pain, lowered blood pressure, increased socialization and exercise, improved coordination and balance, and decreased stress, have been examined. Positive patient outcomes depend on the qualifications and experience of the AAT team. Specifically, the therapy team should complete adequate training, obtain national registration, and undergo yearly evaluation by a veterinarian and a professional therapy animal organization. The effectiveness of outcomes can be further complicated by the multidisciplinary nature of this intervention, along with the lack of standardized protocols and methods of evaluation. Therefore, frequent communication and collaboration are essential between the AAT team and the healthcare professionals or therapists involved in the patient's treatment plan (American Veterinary Medical Association, 2017b).

PRECAUTIONS

Although research supports the positive benefits and the safety of AAT for patients with various health conditions, the potential risks, such as disease transmission, allergies, and bites must be carefully taken into consideration (Tyberg & Frishman, 2008). As noted in the white paper titled *Animals in Healthcare Facilities: Recommendations to Minimize Potential Risks* (Murthy et al., 2015), a major concern for healthcare facilities is the transmission of infectious diseases. These potential risks can be decreased by using trained and registered AAT teams, along with enforcing standard hand hygiene before and after every visit for the handler and anyone who pets the animal (Murthy et al., 2015). Additional guidelines from the Centers for Disease Control and Prevention (2003) require that animals used for AAT be clean, groomed, healthy, fully vaccinated, and free of parasites.

To prevent possible risks, a mechanism must be in place for regularly scheduled examinations and preventive care by a veterinarian to assess the physical and behavioral health and well-being of the animal. Results of these examinations must be shared with the appropriate animal regulatory agency and AAT organizations on an annual basis (American Veterinary Medical Association, 2017c; IAHAIO, 2014).

A comprehensive review specifically examining the potential health risks of animals in the healthcare setting found that the potential benefits far outweighed the insignificant risks (Brodie, Biley, & Shewring, 2002). As research findings continue to be reported in this area, it is important to be aware of potential concerns related to disease transmission if they arise.

USES

Physical Conditions

The research investigating the impact of AAT on physical conditions has concentrated on cardiovascular disease, seizure disorders, dementia, and pain management.

Cardiovascular Disease

The study of the relationship between pets and their positive health effects on a human's cardiovascular system dates back to 1929 (Wolff & Frishman, 2005). Several studies demonstrated the effect of pet ownership on survival after myocardial infarction. Friedmann, Katcher, Lynch, and Thomas (1980) conducted the seminal longitudinal research examining the effect of pet ownership on survival for 92 adult patients after myocardial infarction. Only 5% of the subjects who owned pets died within 1 year after hospitalization, whereas 28% of those who were not pet owners died during the same interval.

Another study by Friedmann and Thomas (1995), examining pet ownership and 1-year survival after myocardial infarction, included the severity of cardiac disease. For the 368 patients in this investigation, disease severity and pet ownership were found to positively affect survival, whereas marital status and living situations did not.

In the Cardiac Arrhythmia Suppressions Trial (CAST) by Friedmann and Thomas (2003), the investigators examined the effect of owning a pet on heart rate variability (HRV) for patients after recovery from a myocardial infarction. As a noninvasive method of showing risk assessment after myocardial infarction, a depressed HRV predicts cardiac complications and increased mortality. Pet owners in this study had a higher HRV, thus supporting the hypothesis that survival differences between pet owners and non–pet owners were due to differences in the autonomic modulation of the heart, therefore providing long-term cardiac benefits and increased survival rates.

In work specifically examining the effects of AAT on hemodynamic measures and state anxiety, 76 adult patients (44 men and 32 women) with advanced heart failure were randomized to (a) a 12-minute AAT session with a therapy dog; (b) a 12-minute visit with a volunteer; or (c) the control group, which included usual care (Cole, Gawlinski, Steers, & Kotlerman, 2007). A repeated-measures experimental design was used to collect data at baseline, 8 minutes, and 16 minutes. The results revealed that, compared with the control group, the AAT group had significantly greater decreases in systolic pulmonary artery and pulmonary capillary wedge pressures during and after the AAT intervention. Moreover, after the intervention, patients in the AAT group had the greatest decrease in state anxiety, compared with the other two groups.

Seizure Disorders

The use of animals as an important component of the treatment plan for individuals with epilepsy was first documented in 1867 in Germany (Fontaine, 2015). Over the past several decades, a number of investigators have examined the value of dogs in caring for patients with seizure disorders. Of 122 families who had a dog and a child with epilepsy, 15% of the dogs could predict seizure onset at least 80% of the time (Kirton, Wirrell, Zhang, & Hamiwka, 2004). In addition, 50% of the dogs exhibited behaviors that were protective of the child, such as lying on the child during a seizure or pushing the child away from stairs.

Dogs that are specifically trained as seizure-response dogs can activate an alarm or alert a caregiver and then stay with the person to provide support during and after the seizure (Hart & Yamamoto, 2015).

Dementia

For more than two decades, studies have supported the use of AAT with patients with degenerative cognitive disorders. For patients with dementia, interacting with an animal can improve short-term memory and communication (Tyberg & Frishman, 2008) and trigger long-term memory (Laun, 2003). The presence of a therapy dog can decrease agitation and aggression while increasing social behaviors among patients with dementia (Filan & Llewellyn-Jones, 2006). Indeed, the presence of fish aquariums in a long-term care facility was associated with increased weights and improved nutritional status among 62 patients with Alzheimer's disease. These residents were more attentive in the presence of the aquarium, stayed at the dining room table longer, and required fewer nutritional supplements (Edwards & Beck, 2002). Research specifically examining problem behaviors in patients with dementia found significantly fewer problem behaviors after placement of a dog in the healthcare facility (McCabe, Baun, Speich, & Agrawal, 2002).

Dabelko-Schoeny et al. (2014) examined the impact of equine-assisted interventions on older adults with Alzheimer's disease and related dementias. A convenience sample of 16 residents from an adult day-care center participated in the study. A randomized pretest, posttest crossover design was used to compare equine-assisted interventions with standard care. The interventions consisted of opportunities for grooming and leading horses. Results revealed a significant reduction in behavior problems after the intervention in the experimental group.

Pain Management

Nurses are aware of the importance of including complementary therapies in providing pain management for patients. Most studies examining AAT in healthcare have been conducted in acute care settings. Researchers have studied the effects of the use of animals on pain management for both adults and children.

Adult Pain Management. Marcus et al. (2012) evaluated the effects of brief therapy dog visits in an outpatient adult chronic pain clinic compared with time spent in a waiting room without a therapy dog. The sample consisted of 235 patients, 34 family/friends, and 26 staff for a total of 295 therapy dog visits. Participants were able to spend clinic waiting time with a certified therapy dog or in the clinic waiting room. Significant improvements were reported on pain, mood, and other measures of distress among those patients who spent time with the therapy dog, compared with those who chose to remain in the clinic waiting room. Significant improvements were also reported by family/friends and staff after therapy dog visits. Study results revealed that therapy dog visits can significantly improve the feelings of well-being in this patient population.

Havey, Vlasses, Vlasses, Ludwig-Beymer, and Hackbarth (2014) conducted a retrospective study examining the impact of AAT on the use of oral pain medication (morphine equivalents) by adults (mean age of 66 years) after total joint replacement surgery. The study subjects in the intervention group ($n = 46$) were matched with the control group ($n = 46$) on age, gender, ethnicity, length of stay, and diagnosis code for type of joint replacement. Patients in the intervention group received daily AAT for 5 to 15 minutes postsurgery; patients in the control group did not. Results revealed that the patients who received AAT after surgery had statistically significant less pain medication use than the control group.

Pediatric Pain Management. Sobo, Eng, and Kassity-Krich (2006) examined the effectiveness of canine visitation therapy (CVT) on children's postoperative pain in a pediatric hospital. The convenience sample consisted of 25 English-speaking children, age 5 to 18 years. Each patient received a one-time visit after surgery by a West Highland terrier named Lizzy and could choose the level of interaction with the dog. At high-interaction levels, the child actively played and walked with the dog; at low-interaction levels, the dog would do an occasional trick for the child; and at passive-interaction levels, the dog would sit quietly with the child. Despite the small sample size, there was a significant decrease in pain perception after the dog visitation. Moreover, post-CVT interviews with each child revealed eight themes: The dog (a) brought pleasure or happiness, (b) provided distraction from the pain, (c) was fun, (d) provided company, (e) was calming, (f) reminded them of home, (g) was nice to cuddle with, and (h) eased the pain.

Psychological Conditions

The use of animals for the treatment of people with mental conditions dates back to 1792 at the York Retreat in England. It was observed that the farm animals helped enhance the humanity of those with emotional disorders (Altschiller, 2011). The goal was to lessen the use of medications and physical restraints by helping residents learn self-control through the care of animals (Fontaine, 2015). More recently, in 1964, American child psychotherapist Boris Levinson (who is considered to be the father of AAT) coined the term *pet therapy*. Levinson first described the therapeutic effects of companionship with his dog, Jingles, for withdrawn children living in a residential mental health program. The dog served as an icebreaker and opened communication to establish a positive relationship for effective therapy (Altschiller, 2011). Since the 1960s, a number of studies have been conducted to examine the effects of AAT for patients hospitalized on psychiatric units. It has been found that AAT can promote feelings of safety and comfort, along with a nonevaluative external focus for patients who are not fearful of animals or do not have a negative attitude toward them (Odendaal, 2000). Specifically, older patients with schizophrenia who were exposed to AAT showed growth in communication, interpersonal contact with others, and activities of daily living (Barak, Savorai, Mavashev, & Beni, 2001).

Military Personnel

Veterans can experience negative physical, emotional, and psychological effects from their experiences in war. As early as the 1940s, the beneficial effect of working with animals was evident in returning World War II veterans who recovered at the Army Air Corps Convalescent Hospital in New York (Fontaine, 2015). Today, there are several million veterans in our country, many of whom suffer from post-traumatic stress disorder (PTSD; Matuszek, 2010). Over the past decade, AAT has become more commonplace in veterans' hospitals, with the Department of Defense allocating funding to examine the effectiveness of its use. In addition, in March 2011, the Americans with Disabilities Act approved PTSD as a qualification of need for a service dog (Arkow, 2015). Veterans suffering with PTSD can apply for a service dog through organizations such as Veterans Moving Forward (2012; www .vetsfwd.org). Although research to support the use of a service or therapy dog for individuals with PTSD is at an early stage, veterans report that these dogs help manage their PTSD symptoms such as anxiety, panic attacks, and fear (Arkow, 2015).

A recent pretest, posttest nonrandomized control group study evaluated the effects of AAT on wounded warriors in transition (N = 24) attending an occupational therapy life skills program (Beck et al., 2012). Although significant differences were not found between the groups on most measures (mood, stress, resilience, fatigue, and function), anecdotal information indicated the participants expressed pleasure being with the dogs and did not want the experience to end.

Additional Uses

In addition to the types of interventions already mentioned, the variety of ways and settings in which AAT can be used are virtually limitless. One only has to be creative in the design of the intervention. The following is a partial list of ways that AAT can be used and populations in which AAT has been studied (see Exhibit 14.1).

Exhibit 14.1. Populations in Which Animals and AAT Have Been Used

- Adults after joint replacement surgery (Havey et al., 2014)
- Adult female abuse survivors (Porter-Wenzlaff, 2007)
- Adults in a residential substance-abuse therapy program (Wesley, Minatrea, & Watson, 2009)
- Adults in the community to promote adherence to walking (Johnson & Meadows, 2010)
- Adults undergoing electroconvulsive therapy (Barker, Pandurangi, & Best, 2003)
- Adults with fibromyalgia (Marcus et al., 2013)
- Adults with heart failure (Cole et al., 2007)
- Children undergoing dental procedures (Havener et al., 2001)
- Children with pain (Barker, Knisely, Schubert, Green, & Ameringer, 2015; Braun, Stangler, Narveson, & Pettingell, 2009)
- Children with attention deficit hyperactivity disorder (Cuypers, De Ridder, & Strandheim, 2011)
- Children with autism (Bass, Duchowny, & Llabre, 2009; O'Haire, 2013)
- Children with cancer (Gagnon et al., 2004)
- Children with cerebral palsy (Zadnikar & Kastrin, 2011)
- Children with pervasive developmental disorders (Martin & Farnum, 2002)
- Children with special healthcare needs (Gasalberti, 2006)

(continued)

- Older adults in a rehabilitation facility using psychoactive medications (Lust, Ryan-Haddad, Coover, & Snell, 2007)
- Older adults in long-term care facilities (Banks & Banks, 2002)
- Older adults with Alzheimer's disease and nutritional deficits (Edwards & Beck, 2002)
- Older adults with dementia (Dabelko-Schoeny et al., 2014; Richeson, 2003)
- Older adults with mental illness (Moretti et al., 2011)
- Older adults with schizophrenia (Barak et al., 2001)
- Older men with aphasia (Macauley, 2006)
- U.S. Army soldiers dealing with the stressors of living in a deployed environment (Fike, Najera, & Dougherty, 2012)

AAT, animal-assisted therapy.

CULTURAL APPLICATIONS

There is great diversity in culturally held attitudes about animals, especially pets, both among cultures and within them (Chandler, 2017). To understand the various attitudes about animals, it is important to consider the evolution of the domestication of animals and their role in society. Historically, only royalty and the wealthy were able to keep companion animals. Also significant is the influence of religious beliefs; for example, in some religions, cows are considered to be sacred and dogs are considered to be unclean.

Before implementing AAT, it is vital to be aware of and consider the influence of cultural and personal attitudes about animals. Although one cannot stereotype people's views of animals based on their ethnic or cultural backgrounds, it is important to be aware of the possibility of cultural differences. For example, Koreans in their native country rarely have cats or dogs as pets because they have been viewed for a long time as a source of food (Chandler, 2017). In contrast, European Americans have integrated cats and dogs into their family system as pets for hundreds of years. Native Americans, on the other hand, may allow their cats and dogs to roam freely, and members of their community share in caring for the animals. Moreover, these animals may never be spayed or neutered, out of respect for the animals' purpose and spirit (Chandler, 2017).

The interest in AAT has grown around the world, following the United States. The Animals Asia Foundation introduced the Dr. Dog program in Hong Kong, China, the Philippines, Japan, India, and Taiwan, with more than 300 dogs visiting hospitals and schools. In Japan, the Companion Animal Partnership Program was developed by the Japan Animal Hospital Association in 1986. It is the most well-known and largest AAT program in Japan with AAT teams visiting schools, nursing homes, and hospitals. In fact, multiple studies examining the impact of AAT and AAA on older patients have been conducted in Japan (Kanamori et al., 2001; Kawamura, Niiyama, & Niiyama, 2009; Mano, Uchizono, & Nishimura, 2003).

In India, Saraswathi Kendra—in collaboration with the Blue Cross of India—pioneered the use of AAT for children with autism beginning in 1996; in 2001, Dr. Dog AAT programs were introduced in schools and nursing homes (Krishna, 2009). Also in India, Minal Kavishwar and therapy dog Kutty were the first registered therapy dog team. Kavishwar founded the Animal Angels Foundation of India, the first in the country to consist of mental health professionals who provide AAT for special-needs children in schools, hospitals, and psychiatric settings. This organization is also active in disaster response (Chandler, 2017). Perspectives on the use of AAT in Taiwan are included in Sidebar 14.1, and its use in Brazil is included in Sidebar 14.2 and in Norway in Sidebar 14.3.

SIDEBAR 14.1. ANIMAL-ASSISTED CARE IN LONG-TERM CARE FACILITIES IN TAIWAN

Jing-Jy Sellin Wang and Miaofen Yen

Within the Oriental culture, especially from the older generation's point of view, there are some taboos on the interaction between humans and animals; thus, compared to the West, using animals in the treatment of human health can be restricted. For example, although relationships with cats can be very intimate in the West, many Taiwanese believe that cats have nine lives with negative meanings. Some superstitions say that cats can reduce a person's *yang spirit*. After one's death, the corpse would have negative resonance with the cat. Moreover, there are legends, such as if a black cat jumps over a dead body, within 7 days, the body will be resurrected. Sometimes these legends make workers or older patients in long-term care facilities fearful. In addition, although a dog is very loyal, Taiwan is an island country, which may cause public environmental health problems due to the humidity, such as when an animal touches human skin. Having dogs is only suitable for the home. As a result, the most widely accepted animals in long-term care facilities are fish and birds. System planning and targeted use of animal intervention can help the older subject, and professionals assist residents in long-term care facilities through breeding fish and birds. This can modestly enhance residents' physiological, psychological, and spiritual well-being.

During her graduate studies, Jing-Yi Lee completed a thesis focused on the use of fish-assisted care in long-term care facilities. In her study, 60 people with normal cognitive function were included. Older residents were selected from the same facility and randomly assigned to an experimental group and a control group of 30 individuals each.

Those in the experimental group were each given a small plastic fish tank containing water, plants, 12 guppies, and a fish feedbox to keep in

(continued)

their rooms. Institutional caregivers assisted residents with changing the water weekly, and residents had to feed the fish, observe them, and record their observations daily. Residents also participated in a weekly half-hour group-sharing session. If caregivers found dead fish, they secretly replaced them with new fish when the resident was not in the room. However, if residents found dead fish by themselves, caregivers helped them to replace these with new fish immediately and record the incident. Those in the control group were each given a small plastic fish tank with water and plants to keep in their rooms. They were required to take care of and observe the plants, and also to record and share their observations. The residents of both groups lived on the same floor but in different rooms. After 3 months of intervention, the measures of quality of life, self-esteem, vitality, and sense of self-control within the experimental group were better than in the control group. In addition, the level of depression was significantly lower in the experimental group than in the control group. Clearly, the experimental group had a meaningful experience of life and expectations in the weekly sharing. According to residents: "Now breeding [these] this fish is like raising children, so you have to take care [of] them very carefully, and some time you will worry that they eat not enough or the water is too dirty...." "Breeding a fish as treating a woman, need attentive care...." "I become very busy since I have [been] breeding fish daily...." "Every day I look at my fish and worry about whether there is a dead fish or not, because it will infect [the] to other fish. Also, I compare with other people to see if I keep them well..." "I am very happy when the fish give birth." A resident of the control group said, "I also want to have fish, because friends who breed fish become more active."

Another example is of an 80-year-old man with dementia was agitated and aggressive. The resident and caregivers received health services in the Dementia Care Clinic at the university hospital, and the caregiver indicated that the subject had serious problem behaviors. Due to severe delusion, the resident did not sleep at night. After an interview, it was discovered that the resident had loved birds in the past. Therefore, the suggestion was given to the caregiver to purchase a birdcage and help the resident breed a parrot. Because this resident was in a middle stage of dementia, his caregiver had to help in feeding the bird, changing the water, and cleaning up. The birdcage was hung at the resident's eye level, and he was encouraged to speak to the bird and to teach the bird to say "hello" and "thank you." Daily, after breakfast, the music of bird voices was played so that the subject could listen to this music with the bird. Caregivers were encouraged to write down their observations of interaction between the resident and bird and to note any changes in problem behaviors. After 3 months of the bird-assisted care intervention, it was reported that the subject's problem behaviors had improved and he had become less irritable. Due to the focus on the interactions with the bird during the day, the resident could fall asleep at night. Clearly, the resident's quality of life was enhanced when he developed a close link with the bird. Thus, it was demonstrated that animal-assisted measures could be useful for older people or those with dementia and problem behaviors.

SIDEBAR 14.2. A PET THERAPY PROJECT IN A BRAZILIAN HOSPITAL

Pediatric Oncology Unit

Isabel Rossato[a]
Paula Eustáquio[a]
Amália de Fátima Lucena[b]
Lisiane Pruinelli[b]

In Brazil, as well as in other places in the world, pet therapy has been increasingly used as a way to provide patients with pleasure and happiness and thus enable better conditions for the improvement and recovery of their health challenges. The presence of animals surrounded by adequate health and hygiene care is permitted in several hospitals, such as the Hospital de Clínicas de Porto Alegre, located in southern Brazil. In this hospital, one of several playful therapeutic projects is the Pet Project, which was recently implemented and is offered to pediatric oncology patients. The activities are provided in a therapeutic recreation room for patients and family members once a month. For the Pet Project, a dog that is accompanied by a trainer and up to date with immunizations and a recent bath, is transported in a suitable box to the therapeutic recreation room. During the dog visit day, the medical and nursing teams are advised of the visit, and children who have conditions that can receive the dog visit are allowed to interact with the dog.

Once in the therapeutic recreation room, the trainer removes the dog from the box so that children can cuddle and watch and participate in games played by the dog and its trainer. Children are instructed to sanitize their hands with alcohol gel every time they have contact with the dog. Preliminary results of this interaction among the dog, trainer, and patient demonstrate that the hospital environment becomes lighter, happier, and relaxed, reducing solitude and inhibition of patients, with improvement in their interpersonal relationships and social behavior. These benefits also extend to caregivers/family members and health professionals involved in the treatment of these children, who are subjected to suffering caused by witnessing childhood illness.

[a]Pet Therapy Project Developers
[b]Sidebar Writing Collaborators

FUTURE RESEARCH

Although there has been great enthusiasm for AAT and a proliferation of therapy teams worldwide, these interventions often lack evidence to support their efficacy (Arkow, 2015). Most research to date supports AAT as making a significant contribution to quality of life for patients of all ages and a variety of physical and

SIDEBAR 14.3. ANIMAL-ASSISTED ACTIVITIES IN NORWEGIAN NURSING HOMES

Ingeborg Pedersen

In Norway, many nursing homes have animal visit programs or have animals living within the facility, such as aquarium fish, caged birds, cats, or dogs. The purpose is to enhance the residents' engagement and social contact via animal-assisted activities, thereby preserving their well-being and quality of life. In a survey among 282 nursing homes in Norway, 10% of the wards had an animal visitation program, whereas almost 20% had animals living permanently in the facility (Myren, Kvaal, & Braastad, 2011). In the survey, nursing home staff rated the importance of the animals regarding a variety of factors, and the most important factor was the animals' contribution to a positive social environment. Other factors were improved communication abilities among the residents and better mood among residents and staff. Negative consequences, such as allergic reactions and enhanced workload for the healthcare staff, were rated of low importance.

Important research examining animal-assisted activities in nursing homes is being conducted by investigators at the Norwegian University of Life Sciences. Olsen, Pedersen, Bergland, Enders-Slegers, Patil, & Ihlebaek (2016) conducted a prospective, cluster randomized multicenter trial with follow-up 3 months after the animal-assisted intervention. A total of 58 participants, age 65 years and older, with dementia or a cognitive deficit, received an animal-assisted activity group session for 30 minutes twice weekly over 12 weeks. Data collection was completed at baseline, at 12 weeks when finishing the intervention, and 3 months after the last intervention was provided. Validated Norwegian versions of the following measure were used: Cornell Scale for Depression in Dementia, Brief Agitation Rating Scale, Quality of Life in Late-Stage Dementia Scale, and Clinical Dementia Rating Scale. Results revealed a statistical and clinical improvement in depression symptoms and quality of life for participants with severe dementia, from baseline to follow-up at 3 months after the intervention. No effect on agitation was noted. Of great value for these patients, the research team noted that the intervention may have contributed to an increased social interaction between the healthcare staff and participants.

Another important study that was part of the randomized controlled trial by Olsen, Pedersen, Bergland, Enders-Slegers, and Ihlebaek (2016), focused on 21 older adults with dementia living in nursing homes and 28 home-dwelling seniors with dementia attending a day-care center. The individuals with dementia (mean age 84 years) received therapy dog visits by a qualified dog handler, for 30 minutes twice weekly, over 12 weeks. Video recordings of the dog visits were completed at week 2 and week 10, with behaviors being categorized with an ethogram. Based on the high duration of behaviors connected to contact and activity with the dog and high level of laughter and smiles, it was determined that animal-assisted activities created engagement in individuals with dementia. The research team

(continued)

suggested the degree of dementia be carefully considered when planning animal-assisted activities for this population.

References

Myren, I., Kvaal & Braastad, B. (2011). Hund og katt i sykehjem—et bidrag til miljøøbehandling? [In Norwegian]. *Demens & Alderspsykiatri, 15*(2), 24–26.
Olsen, C., Pedersen, I., Bergland, A., Enders-Slegers, M., & Ihlebaek, C. (2016). Engagement in elderly persons with dementia attending animal-assisted group activity. *Dementia*, 1–17, doi:10.1177/1471301216667320
Olsen, C., Pedersen, I., Bergland, A., Enders-Slegers, M., Patil, G., & Ihlebaek, C. (2016). Effect of animal-assisted interventions on depression, agitation, and quality of life in nursing home residents suffering from cognitive impairment or dementia: A cluster randomized controlled trial. *International Journal of Geriatric Psychiatry*, 1–10. doi:10.1002/gps.4436

psychological health conditions; however, most studies tend to have small sample sizes and lack adequate control groups (Fine, 2015). Investigations are needed that use random assignment to an AAT intervention group and a standard care group to determine which intervention led to the better outcome. Explorations are also needed to examine the physiological mechanisms contributing to the positive effects of AAT on specific conditions, as well as the duration and frequency of AAT needed to provide maximum improvements. For example, because cardiovascular disease is the leading cause of death in the United States, the role of AAT within cardiovascular disease–prevention programs needs to be examined. Additional research is needed to help identify which patients would most benefit from AAT.

Studies are needed to examine the relationships among the AAT team, patients, and staff in creating healing environments. Further research is needed in settings such as schools, homeless shelters, outpatient clinics, and community health agencies. Additional work is necessary to examine the ethical use, potential fatigue, and healthcare needs of animals used for AAT. Given that animals have no voice in this intervention, it is imperative that their human companions ensure their physical and emotional well-being (Altschiller, 2011).

Nurses can take the lead in advocating for the appropriate use of AAT in their healthcare and school settings. Additional resources to assist in the implementation of AAT are listed in Exhibit 14.2.

Exhibit 14.2. Additional Resources

Breitenbach, E., Stumpf, E., & Lorenzov, E. (2009). Dolphin-assisted therapy: Changes in interaction and communication between children with severe disabilities and their caregivers. *Anthrozoos, 22*(3), 277–289.
Burch, M. (2010). *Citizen canine: Ten essential skills every well-mannered dog should know.* Freehold, NJ: Kennel Club Books.
Chur-Hansen, A., McArthur, M., Winefield, H., Hanieh, E., & Hazel, S. (2014). Animal-assisted interventions in children's hospitals: A critical review of the literature. *Anthrozoos, 27*(1), 5–18.

(continued)

DeCourcey, M., Russell, A., & Keister, K. (2010). Animal-assisted therapy: Evaluation and implementation of a complementary therapy to improve the psychological and physiological health of critically ill patients. *Dimensions of Critical Care Nursing*, *29*(5), 211–214.

Ernst, L. (2012, October). Animal-assisted therapy: Using animals to promote healing. *Nursing 2012*, *42*(10), 54–58.

Halm, M. (2008). The healing power of the human-animal connection. *American Journal of Critical Care*, *17*(4), 373–376.

Horowitz, S. (2008). The human-animal bond: Health implications across the lifespan. *Alternative and Complementary Therapies*, *14*(5), 251–256.

Howie, A. (2015). *Teaming with your therapy dog.* West Lafayette, IN: Purdue University Press.

Johnson, R., Odendaal, J., & Meadows, R. (2002). Animal-assisted interventions research. *Western Journal of Nursing Research*, *24*(4), 422–440.

Lind, N. (2009). *Animal-assisted therapy activities to motivate and inspire.* Lombard, IL: PYOW.

Perry, D., Rubinstein, D., & Austin, J. (2012). Animal-assisted group therapy in mental health settings. *Alternative and Complementary Therapies*, *18*(4), 181–185.

Pichot, T. (2012). *Animal-assisted brief therapy.* New York, NY: Routledge.

Rossetti, J., & King, C. (2010). Use of animal-assisted therapy with psychiatric patients: A literature review. *Journal of Psychosocial Nursing*, *48*(11), 44–48.

Winkle, M. (2013). *Professional applications of animal assisted interventions.* Albuquerque, NM: Dogwood Therapy Services.

WEBSITES

Alliance of Therapy Dogs

(www.therapydogs.com/alliance-therapy-dogs)

The Alliance of Therapy Dogs (ATD) is a volunteer organization of dedicated therapy dog handlers and their dogs on a mission of sharing smiles and joy. ATD's goal is to provide registration, support, and insurance for members who are involved in volunteer animal-assisted activities. These activities include visits to hospitals, special needs centers, schools, nursing homes, and airports. ATD teams may choose to be members of local therapy dog groups. They may also participate in nationwide therapy dog initiatives with organizations such as the Red Cross and Reading Education Assistance Dogs (R.E.A.D.).

American Hippotherapy Association

(www.americanhippotherapyassociation.org)

The mission of the American Hippotherapy Association is to educate and promote excellence in the field of equine-assisted therapy. This organization promotes the use of the movement of a horse as a treatment strategy in physical, occupational, and speech therapy sessions for individuals living with disabilities.

American Veterinary Medical Association

(www.avma.org/KB/Policies/Pages/default.aspx)

Established in 1863, the American Veterinary Medical Association (AVMA) recognizes and promotes the importance of the human–animal bond through clinical practice, service, and research. The policy section of this website includes guidelines for animal-assisted activity, AAT, and resident animal programs, including key definitions, guiding principles, preventive medical and behavioral strategies, and wellness guidelines.

Animal Behavior Institute

(www.animaledu.com)

The Animal Behavior Institute (ABI) was founded in 2004 by Dr. Gary Fortier and Dr. Janis Hammer to prepare adult students for careers in animal behavior. The ABI provides AAT certificate programs that require completion of 15 academic credits (online) and 40 hours of hands-on field experience. On graduation, students may use the designation of certified animal-assisted therapy professional (CAATP). The ABI is accredited by the International Association for Continuing Education and Training.

CENSHARE: Center to Study Human–Animal Relationships and Environments

(www.censhare.umn.edu)

Established in 1981, CENSHARE has become a national leader in promoting health and quality of life for individuals and animals through behavior research, educational opportunities, and a forum for public policy making. CENSHARE is a multidisciplinary group of individuals from the University of Minnesota and surrounding community dedicated to studying and improving human–animal relationships and environments.

Equine-Assisted Growth and Learning Association (EAGALA)

(www.eagala.org)

EAGALA is dedicated to improving the mental health of individuals, families, and groups around the world by setting the standard of excellence in equine-assisted psychotherapy and equine-assisted learning, also known as *horse therapy* or *equine therapy*. EAGALA is the largest professional association for equine therapy and has a comprehensive training and certification program to learn the EAGALA model of equine-assisted psychotherapy. EAGALA also provides a specialized program for service members, veterans, and their families, who are dealing with life challenges, including the treatment of PTSD, traumatic brain injury, depression, and anxiety.

Human–Animal Bond Research Institute

(www.habri.org)

The Human–Animal Bond Research Institute (HABRI) is a national research and education nonprofit foundation dedicated to promoting the positive role animals play in the health and well-being of people, families, and communities. This institute works to educate, inform, advocate, and support research and funding for human-animal–related initiatives. HABRI is an online hub that archives evidence on the benefits of the human–animal bond and is maintained by Purdue University under the direction of Dr. Alan Beck. The information focuses on human and animal health, AAT, and public policy.

Paws 4 Therapy

(www.paws4therapy.com)

Paws 4 Therapy specializes in the development of hospital-based AAT programs. Patty Kaplan, BSN, RN, founded Paws 4 Therapy in 2001 and is the director of AAT at Edward Hospital in Naperville, Illinois. In 2005 her AAT program was featured by The Joint Commission as a "best practice."

Pet Partners (Formerly Delta Society)

(www.petpartners.org)

In 1977, the Delta Foundation was created in Portland, Oregon, under the direction of Michael McCulloch, MD. In 1981, the name was changed to Delta Society; and in 2012 the name Delta Society was changed to Pet Partners to clearly reflect its mission, which is to improve human health through positive interactions with therapy, service, and companion animals. Pet Partners volunteers visit hospitals, hospices, schools, and veterans' centers with their animals to provide comfort to people in need. The Pet Partners Program provides comprehensive standardized training in animal-assisted activities and therapy for volunteers and healthcare professionals. It is the largest nonprofit organization that registers handlers of multiple species as volunteer teams to provide AAT. Dogs, cats, rabbits, horses, birds, and llamas are eligible for evaluation through Pet Partners.

Reading Education Assistance Dogs (R.E.A.D.)

(www.therapyanimals.org/Read_Team_Steps.html)

The mission of the R.E.A.D. program is to improve the literacy skills of children through the assistance of a registered therapy team as literacy mentors. The R.E.A.D. program improves a child's reading and communication skills by employing a powerful method—reading to an animal. This program was begun by Intermountain Therapy Animals in 1999 in Salt Lake City, Utah. Today, more than 3,500 therapy teams have been trained and registered with the R.E.A.D. program and work throughout the United States, Canada, Italy, Finland, France, Norway, Slovenia, South Africa, Spain, and Sweden.

Therapet: AAT

(www.therapet.org)

Therapet was founded in 1998 by an occupational therapist in Texas to provide AAT in a rehabilitation center. Therapet is a nonprofit foundation whose mission is to use specially trained and certified animals to promote health, hope, and healing. Therapet assists with the establishment of AAT programs throughout the United States and provides education for healthcare professionals, along with AAT training and evaluation of animal and human volunteers.

Therapy Dogs International

(www.tdi-dog.org)

TDI is the oldest registry for therapy dogs in the United States. In 2012, there were 24,750 dog/handler teams registered with TDI. Founded in 1976 by Elaine Smith—an American RN who observed the benefits of pets in the healthcare setting during a visit to England—TDI is dedicated to the regulation, testing, selection, and registration of qualified dogs and handlers for the purpose of visitations to hospitals, nursing homes, facilities, or any place where therapy dogs are needed. Since the 1995 bombing of the Murrah Federal Building in Oklahoma City, Oklahoma, TDI has provided disaster stress relief dog teams in such places as New York City during the September 11, 2001 attack on the World Trade Center and New Orleans, Louisiana, during hurricane Katrina in 2005.

ACKNOWLEDGMENT

The author gratefully thanks her therapy dog, Libby, for showing her the true value of AAT.

REFERENCES

Altschiller, D. (2011). *Animal-assisted therapy.* Santa Barbara, CA: Greenwood.

American Disabilities Act National Network. (2014). Retrieved from https://adata.org/factsheet/service-animals

American Kennel Club. (2017). AKC canine good citizen program. Retrieved from http://www.akc.org/dog owners/training/canine-good-citizen/training-testing

American Veterinary Medical Association. (2012). U.S. pet ownership & demographics sourcebook. Retrieved from https://www.avma.org/KB/Resources/Statistics/Pages/Market-research-statistics-US-Pet-Ownership-Demographics-Sourcebook.aspx

American Veterinary Medical Association. (2017a). Animal-assisted interventions: Definitions. Retrieved from https://www.avma.org/KB/Policies/Pages/Animal-Assisted-Interventions-Definitions.aspx

American Veterinary Medical Association. (2017b). Guidelines for animal-assisted activity, animal-assisted therapy and resident animal programs. Retrieved from https://www.avma.org/KB/Policies/Pages/Animal-Assisted-Interventions-Guidelines.aspx

American Veterinary Medical Association. (2017c). *Wellness guidelines for animals in animal-assisted activity, animal-assisted therapy, and resident animal programs.* Retrieved from https://ebusiness.avma.org/files/productdownloads/wellness_AAA.pdf

Arkow, P. (2015). *Animal-assisted therapy and activities: A study and research resource guide for the use of companion animals in animal-assisted interventions* (11th ed.). Stratford, NJ: Therapy Animals.

Banks, M., & Banks, W. (2002). The effects of animal-assisted therapy on loneliness in an elderly population in long-term care facilities. *Journal of Gerontology, 57*(7), 428–432.

Barak, Y., Savorai, O., Mavashev, S., & Beni, A. (2001). Animal-assisted therapy for elderly schizophrenic patients: A one-year controlled trial. *American Journal of Geriatric Psychiatry, 9*(4), 439–442.

Barker, S., Knisely, J., Schubert, C., Green, J., & Ameringer, S. (2015). The effect of an animal-assisted intervention on anxiety and pain in hospitalized children. *Anthrozoos, 28*(1), 101–112.

Barker, S., Pandurangi, A., & Best, A. (2003). Effects of animal-assisted therapy on patients' anxiety, fear, and depression before ECT. *Journal of Electroconvulsive Therapy, 19*(1), 38–44.

Bass, M., Duchowny, C., & Llabre, M. (2009). The effect of therapeutic horseback riding on social functioning in children with autism. *Journal of Autism & Developmental Disorders, 39*, 1261–1267.

Beck, C., Gonzales, F., Sells, C., Jones, C., Reer, T., Wasilewski, S., & Zhu, Y. (2012, April–June). The effects of animal-assisted therapy on wounded warriors in an occupational therapy life skills program. *Army Medical Department Journal*, 38–45.

Becker, M. (2002). *The healing power of pets: Harnessing the amazing ability of pets to make and keep people happy and healthy*. New York, NY: Hyperion.

Braun, C., Stangler, T., Narveson, J., & Pettingell, S. (2009). Animal-assisted therapy as a pain relief intervention for children. *Complementary Therapies in Clinical Practice, 15*, 105–109.

Brodie, S., Biley, F., & Shewring, M. (2002). An exploration of the potential risks associated with using pet therapy in healthcare settings. *Journal of Clinical Nursing, 11*(4), 444–456.

Centers for Disease Control and Prevention. (2003). Guidelines for environmental infection control in healthcare facilities. *MMWR Recommendations & Reports, 52*(RR-10), 1–42.

Chandler, C. (2017). *Animal-assisted therapy in counseling*. New York, NY: Routledge.

Cole, K., Gawlinski, A., Steers, N., & Kotlerman, J. (2007). Animal-assisted therapy in patients hospitalized with heart failure. *American Journal of Critical Care, 16*(6), 575–585.

Cuypers, K., De Ridder, K., & Strandheim, A. (2011). The effect of therapeutic horseback riding on 5 children with attention deficit hyperactivity disorder: A pilot study. *Journal of Alternative and Complementary Medicine, 17*, 901–908.

Dabelko-Schoeny, H., Phillips, G., Darrough, E., DeAnna, S., Jarden, M., Johnson, D., & Lorch, G. (2014). Equine-assisted interventions for people with dementia. *Anthrozoos, 27*(1), 141–155.

Delta Society. (1996). *Standards of practice for animal-assisted activities and animal-assisted therapy*. Renton, WA: Author.

Edwards, N., & Beck, A. (2002). Animal assisted therapy and nutrition in Alzheimer's disease. *Western Journal of Nursing Research, 24*(6), 697–612.

Fike, L., Najera, C., & Dougherty, D. (2012, April–June). Occupational therapists as dog handlers: The collective experience with animal-assisted therapy in Iraq. *Army Medical Department Journal*, 51–54.

Filan, S., & Llewellyn-Jones, R. (2006). Animal-assisted therapy for dementia: A review of the literature. *Intelligence Psychogeriatric, 18*(4), 597–611.

Fine, A. (2015). *Handbook on animal-assisted therapy: Foundations and guidelines for animal-assisted interventions* (4th ed.). New York, NY: Academic Press.

Fine, A., & Beck, A. (2015). Understanding our kinship with animals: Input for health care professionals interested in the human-animal bond. In A. Fine (Ed.), *Handbook on animal-assisted therapy: Foundations and guidelines for animal-assisted interventions* (pp. 3–10). New York, NY: Academic Press.

Fontaine, K. (2015). *Complementary & alternative therapies for nursing practice*. Upper Saddle River, NJ: Pearson.

Friedmann, E., Katcher, A., Lynch, J., & Thomas, S. (1980). Animal companions and one-year survival of patients after discharge from a coronary care unit. *Public Health Reports, 95*(4), 307–312.

Friedmann, E., & Thomas, S. (1995). Pet ownership, social support, and one-year survival after acute myocardial infarction in the Cardiac Arrhythmia Suppression Trial (CAST). *American Journal of Cardiology, 76*, 1213–1217.

Friedmann, E., & Thomas, S. (2003). Relationship between pet ownership and heart rate variability in patients with healed myocardial infarcts. *American Journal of Cardiology, 91*, 718–721.

Gagnon, J., Bouchard, F., Landry, M., Belles-Isles, M., Fortier, M., & Fillion, L. (2004). Implementing a hospital-based therapy program for children with cancer: A descriptive study. *Canadian Oncology Nursing Journal, 14,* 217–222.

Gasalberti, D. (2006). Alternative therapies for children and youth with special health care needs. *Journal of Pediatric Health Care, 20*(2), 133–136.

Grandin, T., Fine, A., O'Haire, M., Carlisle, G., & Bowers, C. (2015). The roles of animals for individuals with Autism Spectrum Disorder. In A. Fine (Ed.), *Handbook on animal-assisted therapy: Foundations and guidelines for animal-assisted interventions* (pp. 225–236). New York, NY: Academic Press.

Hart, L., & Yamamoto, M. (2015). Recruiting psychosocial health effects of animals for families and communities: Transition to practice. In A. Fine (Ed.), *Handbook on animal-assisted therapy: Foundations and guidelines for animal-assisted interventions* (pp. 53–72). New York, NY: Academic Press.

Havener, L., Gentes, L., Thaler, B., Megel, M., Baun, M., Driscoll, F., . . . Agrawal, S. (2001). The effects of a companion animal on distress in children undergoing dental procedures. *Issues in Comprehensive Pediatric Nursing, 24*(2), 137–152.

Havey, J., Vlasses, F., Vlasses, P., Ludwig-Beymer, P., & Hackbarth, D. (2014). The effect of animal-assisted therapy on pain management use after joint replacement. *Anthrozoos, 27*(3), 361–369.

International Association of Human-Animal Interaction Organizations. (2014). *IAHAIO White paper: The IAHAIO definitions for animal-assisted intervention and guidelines for wellness of animals involved.* Retrieved from http://www.iahaio.org

Johnson, R., & Meadows, R. (2010). Dog walking: Motivation for adherence to a walking program. *Clinical Nursing Research, 19*(4), 387–402.

Kanamori, M., Suzuki, M., Yamamoto, K., Kanda, M., Matsui, Y., Kojima, E., . . . Oshiro, H. (2001). A day care program and evaluation of animal-assisted therapy for the elderly with senile dementia. *American Journal of Alzheimer's Disease & Other Dementias, 16*(4), 234–239.

Kawamura, N., Niiyama, M., & Niiyama, H. (2009). Animal-assisted activity experiences of institutionalized Japanese older adults. *Journal of Psychosocial Nursing, 47*(1), 41–47.

Kirton, A., Wirrell, E., Zhang, J., & Hamiwka, L. (2004). Seizure alerting and response behaviors in dogs living with epileptic children. *Neurology, 62*(12), 2303–2305.

Krishna, N. (2009). Dr. Dog A programme for children with autism. Retrieved from http://www.autismindia.com

Laun, L. (2003). Benefits of pet therapy in dementia. *Home Healthcare Nurse, 21*(1), 49–52.

Lear, J. (2012). Our furry friends: The history of animal domestication. *Journal of Young Investigators, 23*(2), 1–3. Retrieved from http://www.jyi.org/issue/our-furry-friends

Lust, E., Ryan-Haddad, A., Coover, K., & Snell, J. (2007). Measuring clinical outcomes of animal-assisted therapy: Impact on resident medication usage. *Consultant Pharmacist, 22*(7), 580–585.

Macauley, B. (2006). Animal-assisted therapy for persons with aphasia: A pilot study. *Journal of Rehabilitation Research & Development, 43*(3), 357–366.

Mano, M., Uchizono, M., & Nishimura, T. (2003). A trial of dog-assisted therapy for elderly people with Alzheimer's disease. *Journal of Japanese Society for Dementia Care, 2,* 150–157.

Marcus, D., Bernstein, C., Constantin, J., Kunkel, F., Breuer, P., & Hanlon, R. (2012). Animal-assisted therapy at an outpatient pain management clinic. *Pain Medicine, 13*(1), 45–57.

Marcus, D., Bernstein, C., Constantin, J., Kunkel, F., Breuer, P., & Hanlon, R. (2013). Impact of animal-assisted therapy for outpatients with fibromyalgia. *Pain Medicine, 14*(1), 43–51.

Martin, F., & Farnum, J. (2002). Animal-assisted therapy for children with pervasive developmental disorders. *Western Journal of Nursing Research, 24*(6), 657–670.

Matuszek, S. (2010). Animal-facilitated therapy in various patient populations: Systematic literature review. *Holistic Nursing Practice, 24*(4), 187–203.

McCabe, B., Baun, M., Speich, D., & Agrawal, S. (2002). Resident dog in the Alzheimer's special care unit. *Western Journal of Nursing Research, 24*(6), 684–696.

Moretti, F., DeRonchi, D., Bernabel, V., Marchetti, L., Ferrari, B., Forlani, C., . . . Atti, A. (2011). Pet therapy in elderly patients with mental illness. *Psychogeriatrics, 11,* 125–129.

Murthy, R., Bearman, G., Brown, S., Bryant, K., Chinn, R., Hewlett, A., . . . Weber, D. (2015). Animals in healthcare facilities: Recommendations to minimize potential risks. *Infection Control & Hospital Epidemiology, 36*(5), 495–516.

Nightingale, F. (1992). *Notes on nursing.* Philadelphia, PA: J. B. Lippincott. (Original work published 1859)

Odendaal, J. (2000). Animal-assisted therapy: Magic or medicine? *Journal of Psychosomatic Research, 49,* 275–280.

Odendaal, J., & Meintjes, R. (2003). Neurophysiological correlates of affiliative behavior between humans and dogs. *Veterinary Journal, 165*(3), 296–301.

O'Haire, M. (2013). Animal-assisted intervention for autism spectrum disorder: A systematic literature review. *Journal of Autism and Developmental Disorders, 43*(7), 1606–1622.

Porter-Wenzlaff, L. (2007). Finding their voice: Developing emotional, cognitive, and behavioral congruence in female abuse survivors through equine facilitated therapy. *Explore, 3*(5), 529–534.

Richeson, N. (2003). Effects of animal-assisted therapy on agitated behaviors and social interactions of older adults with dementia. *American Journal of Alzheimer's Disorders and Other Dementias, 18*(6), 353–358.

Rivera, M. (2010). *On dogs and dying: Inspirational stories from hospice hounds.* West Lafayette, IN: Purdue University Press.

Serpell, J. (2015). Animal-assisted interventions in historical perspective. In A. Fine (Ed.), *Handbook on animal-assisted therapy: Foundations and guidelines for animal-assisted interventions* (pp. 11–19). New York, NY: Academic Press.

Sobo, E., Eng, B., & Kassity-Krich, N. (2006). Canine visitation (pet) therapy: Pilot data on decreases in child pain perception. *Journal of Holistic Nursing, 24*(1), 51–57.

Stern, C., & Chur-Hansen, A. (2013). Methodological considerations in designing and evaluating animal-assisted interventions. *Animals, 3*(1), 127–141.

Therapy Dogs International. (2017). Mission statement and history. Retrieved from http://www.tdi-dog.org

Tyberg, A., & Frishman, W. (2008). Animal-assisted therapy. In M. Weintraub, R. Mamtani, & M. Micozzi (Eds.), *Complementary and integrative medicine in pain management* (pp. 115–123). New York, NY: Springer Publishing.

Veterans Moving Forward. (2012). About us. Retrieved from www.vetsfwd.org/about-us

Vizek, V., Arambasic, L., Kerestes, G., Kuterovac, G., & Vlahovic-Stetic, V. (2001). Pet ownership in childhood and socio-emotional characteristics, work values and professional choices in early adulthood. *Anthrozoos, 14*(4), 224–231.

Wesley, M., Minatrea, N., & Watson, J. (2009). Animal-assisted therapy in the treatment of substance dependence. *Anthrozoos, 22*(2), 137–148.

Wolff, A., & Frishman, W. (2005). Animal-assisted therapy and cardiovascular disease. In W. Frishman, M. Weintraub, & M. Micozzi (Eds.), *Complementary and integrative therapies for cardiovascular disease* (pp. 362–368). St. Louis, MO: Elsevier Mosby.

Zadnikar, M., & Kastrin, A. (2011). Effects of hippotherapy and therapeutic horseback riding on postural control or balance in children with cerebral palsy: A meta-analysis. *Developmental Medicine & Child Neurology, 53,* 684–691.

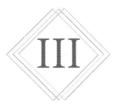

Manipulative and Body-Based Therapies

The National Center for Complementary and Integrative Health (NCCIH) includes therapies in this section in the larger category of mind and body practices. Three of the therapies are among the most commonly used complementary therapies: massage (Chapter 15), tai chi (Chapter 16), and relaxation therapies (Chapter 17). Exercise (Chapter 18), although not specifically included as a complementary therapy in the list of therapies on the NCCIH website, it is a body-based practice (also shown to impact mood and cognition) that is often recommended by nurses to patients to include in their daily health regimens; hence, exercise is included in this section of the text. It is also a therapy that many nurses include in promotion of their personal health.

Manipulative and body-based therapies not included in this text include chiropractic and osteopathic manipulation and movement therapies such as Feldenkrais method, Alexander technique, Pilates, rolfing structural integration, and Trager psychophysical integration (NCCIH, 2016). Both spinal manipulation and massage have been used for centuries in the treatment of illness and the promotion of health. Massage has had a long history in nursing and was included as a nursing intervention in many of the early nursing texts. A variety of massage techniques have been part of health care systems in many countries: Japan, China, Greece, Egypt, and Italy.

Although a number of the therapies in this category are administered by specially trained therapists such as chiropractors and massage therapists, a number of the procedures can be and are administered by nurses, particularly certain types of massage and relaxation therapies. Massage can range from simple hand or foot massage to back rubs or full-body massages, the latter provided by nurses who have been trained as massage therapists. A large number of relaxation therapies exist, and nurses choose from among these to fit the needs and preferences of patients.

Although tai chi could be classified as an energy therapy, it has been placed in this section because it involves movement. Tai chi classes are common in community settings and long-term care. One outcome from tai chi, decreased falls in older patients, has a growing body of scientific research to support its use with elders.

Nurses will find more uses for manipulative and body-based therapies as exploration grows and as these treatments are investigated with more conditions and populations, particularly with children. Nurses also need to be aware of therapies or nuances of these therapies that exist in other healthcare systems and cultures so that they can either include and accommodate preferences or use of such practices in the plan of care or so that they can caution patients about their use because some may be contraindicated with specific illnesses or conditions.

REFERENCE

National Center for Complementary and Integrative Health. (2016). *NCCIH facts-at-a-glance and mission*. Retrieved from https://www.nih.gov/about/ataglance

Massage

Melodee Harris

Massage is a widely used complementary therapy that has been employed by nurses since the time of Florence Nightingale. Early nurse specialists in massage traced the history of massage in textbooks such as *The Theory and Practice of Massage* (Goodall-Copestake, 1919); *Massage: An Elementary Text-book for Nurses* (Macafee, 1917); *Fundamentals of Massage for Students of Nursing* (Jensen, 1932); and *A Textbook of Massage for Nurses and Beginners* (Rawlins, 1933). The authors devoted extensive histories of massage "to teach the student appreciation for the subject" (Jensen, 1932, p. v). Macafee (1917) wrote, "The history of massage is as old as that of man …" (p. 5). Both Eastern and Western cultures are a part of the history of the traditional nursing practice of massage.

In 3000 BCE, the Chinese documented the use of massage in *Cong Fau of Tao-Tse*. There is evidence in *Sa-Tsai-Tou-Hoei*, written in 1000 BCE and published in the 16th century, that the Japanese also used massage (Calvert, 2002; Jensen, 1932). Goodall-Copestake (1919) records how massage is associated with ancient Hindu writings. The Japanese translated massage or shampooing as *amma*. Natives from the Sandwich Islands used *lomi-lomi*, the Maoris of New Zealand used the term *romi-romi*, and the natives of Tong Island used *toogi-toogi* to mean massage (Kellog, 1895, p. 12). The French word *masser,* or "to shampoo," was applied to massage (Goodall-Copestake, 1919, p. 1; Jensen, 1932, p. 20).

The Greeks and Romans influenced the use of massage in Western civilizations. Hippocrates, the Father of Medicine, incorporated massage into the practice of medicine. In 380 BCE, Hippocrates wrote, "A physician must be experienced in … rubbing" (Goodall-Copestake, 1919, p. 2). Galen used massage principles with gladiator students in Pergamos (Jensen, 1932; Rawlins, 1933). In 1813, Per Henrik Ling of Sweden developed Swedish massage movements at the Royal Central Institute of Stockholm. In 1860, Dr. Johan Mezger of Amsterdam used massage on King Frederick VII (then crown prince) of Denmark, and his success promoted the popularity of massage across Scandinavia, the Netherlands, and Germany (Jensen, 1932). Although throughout history it has been known as an art and a complementary/alternative therapy, the practice of massage continues to build on a robust foundation, and evidence-based practices related to massage are evolving. In the

Western world, massage may be used to treat a disease or syndrome diagnosed by a healthcare provider. Eastern or Asian massage is recommended by Eastern medical providers to treat disharmony and imbalance in the human body (Massage Therapy Body of Knowledge [MTBOK Task Force], 2010; Wieting & Cugalj, 2011). Western massage may use effleurage, petrissage, tapotement, or deep friction (Wieting & Cugalj, 2011). Eastern massage practices include shiatsu and may combine several techniques (Wieting & Cugalj, 2011). Today, across all cultures, massage is a holistic intervention that uses the natural healing process to connect the body, mind, and spirit.

DEFINITION

Massage is a part of almost every civilization. The definition and meaning of massage is influenced and interpreted by culture and the healing philosophy of the predominant healthcare discipline.

The term *massage* is derived from the Greek word *massein*, which means "to knead" (Calvert, 2002). The Arabic word *mass* or *mas'h*, "to press softly," also means "massage" (Goodall-Copestake, 1919, p. 1). The definition of massage varies by discipline. Nursing was among the first disciplines to use massage. Physicians, physical therapists, massage therapists, and even cosmetologists use massage.

Physicians term massage as medical massage. The Greeks and Romans influenced physicians to use massage. Hippocrates used the word *friction* for massage in the treatment of sprains (Jensen, 1932). Norstroëm (1868/1896) claimed that the use of massage came from bonesetters. Today, massage is used widely by doctors of osteopathic medicine.

Massage is within the scope of practice of physical therapy, and therapists use it across many settings (American Physical Therapy Association [APTA], 2013). Physical therapists use massage in sports medicine to reduce pain, rehabilitate, and boost physical performance for athletes (Brummitt, 2008).

According to the MTBOK Task Force (2010), massage therapists have a broad interpretation of massage. *Massage, body massage, body rub, somatic therapy,* and other similar terms are equivalent to massage therapy. The terms *massage therapy* and *bodywork* are often used interchangeably. The use of bodywork by massage therapists also includes a more holistic approach to enhance awareness of the mind–body–spirit connection. Clinical massage entails more extensive assessment and techniques focused on symptoms to mean treatment, orthopedic, and medical massage (MTBOK Task Force, 2010, p. 40).

Licensed nurse massage therapists use nursing theory and the nursing process with massage techniques (National Association of Nurse Massage Therapists, 2011). Bedside nurses are taught to use effleurage or slow-stroke back massage that does not require a separate license or training beyond nursing school. More than any other healthcare discipline, nurses have adopted massage into their curricula. In 1932, the National League for Nursing Education recommended 15 hours of lecture and training in massage for nursing curriculum (Ruffin, 2011). Today, the National Council of State Boards of Nursing (NCSBN) includes complementary and alternative therapies in the NCLEX-RN® examinations. The NCSBN specifically mentions massage therapy in the 2013 NCLEX-RN test plan (NCSBN, 2012). Swedish massage movements such as effleurage or slow-stroke back massage continue to be taught in schools of nursing.

Overall, massage is a broad term. Attempts to operationalize a definition that includes art and science, and also covers interpretations from culture and discipline are challenging. The American Massage Therapy Association (AMTA) defined *massage* as "manual soft tissue manipulation, and includes holding, causing movement, and/or applying pressure to the body" (Fletcher, 2009, p. 59). Simply put, "massage is a therapeutic manipulation of the soft tissues of the body with the goal of achieving normalization of those tissues" (Wieting & Cugalj, 2011, para. 5).

SCIENTIFIC BASIS

Although massage is both an art and a science, the early nurse massage specialists recognized massage as a science. Rawlins (1933) stated, "Massage is a science, not a fad of the times" (p. 19). Jensen (1932) defined massage as "the scientific manipulation of body tissue as a therapeutic measure" (p. 2).

Florence Nightingale based the use of nonpharmacological interventions such as massage on the Environmental Adaptation Theory. Nightingale believed that nurses should promote the best possible environment that would allow natural laws to improve the healing process (Dossey, Selanders, Beck, & Attewell, 2005).

Today, perhaps because of the relative lack of its study by rigorous research methods, massage is often thought of as more of an art than a science. Nurse researcher Dr. Tiffany Field established the first center in the world devoted to the science of touch and massage. The Touch Research Institute was established in 1992 at the University of Miami School of Medicine (Touch Research Institute, n.d.). Field was one of the first to study the effects of massage on weight gain in preterm infants (Field, 2002) and build the capacity for nursing science on massage.

Massage is used by nurses to promote health and wellness. It is used to increase circulation, relieve pain, induce sleep, reduce anxiety or depression, and improve quality of life (Rose, 2010). Massage produces therapeutic effects on multiple body systems: integumentary, musculoskeletal, cardiovascular, lymph, and nervous. Manipulating the skin and underlying muscle makes the skin supple. Massage increases or enhances movement in the musculoskeletal system by reducing swelling, loosening and stretching contracted tendons, and aiding in the reduction of soft tissue adhesions. Friction to the cutaneous and subcutaneous tissues releases histamines that, in turn, produce vasodilation of vessels and enhance venous return (Snyder & Taniguki, 2010).

Massage is a proposed mechanism for relaxation to reduce psychological and physiological stress (Harris & Richards, 2010). Stress is also an individual subjective experience. When the body interprets a physiological or psychological response as stressful, the sympathetic nervous system stimulates the hypothalamic–pituitary–adrenal (HPA) axis in the brain. There is a release of stress hormones such as cortisol and epinephrine. Tactile stimulation in the body tissues causes neurohormonal responses throughout the nervous system. Mechanoreceptors cause impulses to travel from the peripheral nervous system, up the ascending spinal cord to the brain. The stimulus is then interpreted in the higher brain, resulting in a neurological or biochemical response (Lawton, 2003). Massage activates the parasympathetic nervous system to decrease the heart rate, blood pressure, and respirations, resulting in relaxation (Moraska, Pollini, Boulanger, Brooks, & Teitlebaum, 2010).

Studies show that massage produces physiological and psychological indicators for the relaxation response (Harris & Richards, 2010). Using foot massage with cardiac patients, Hattan, King, and Griffiths (2002) found that subjects receiving this therapy reported feeling much calmer. In a quasiexperimental study ($n = 24$), Holland and Pokorny (2001) showed a statistically significant difference ($p = .05$) in vital signs before and after slow-stroke massage. The decrease in vital signs indicates that massage may mediate the stress response (Harris & Richards, 2010).

Reduction of pain, a frequent desired outcome of massage, is closely related to the relaxation response. Through the relaxation response, massage relieves pain by stimulating the large-diameter nerve fibers that have an inhibitory input on T-cells (Furlan, Imamura, Dryden & Irvin, 2008). According to Wang and Keck (2004), "massaging the hands and feet stimulates the mechanoreceptors that activate the nonpainful nerve fibers, preventing pain transmission from reaching consciousness" (p. 59). Studies have validated that patients were more comfortable after the administration of massage (Frey Law et al., 2008; Wang & Keck, 2004).

In addition, research is emerging on how massage impacts the psychoneuro-immunological functions of the body and mind. There was higher natural killer (NK) cytotoxicity and higher daily weight in preterm infants who received massage in a randomized placebo-controlled trial (Ang et al., 2012). Billhult, Lindholm, Gunnarsson, and Stener-Victorin (2008) explored the effect of massage on CD4[+] and CD8[+] T-cells in women with cancer. Findings revealed that massage had no effect on these indices.

Massage is a holistic therapy that promotes overall health, including emotional well-being (Currin & Meister, 2008); decreases pain and anxiety during labor (Chang, Wang, & Chen, 2002); and increases quality of life (Williams et al., 2005).

INTERVENTION

Various strokes are used to produce friction and pressure on cutaneous and subcutaneous tissues. The type of stroke and the amount of pressure chosen depend on the desired outcomes and the body part being massaged.

There are a number of types of massage: *Swedish* (a massage using long, flowing strokes), *Esalen* (a meditative massage using light touch), *deep tissue or neuromuscular* (an intense kneading of the body), *sports massage* (a vigorous massage to loosen and ease sore muscles), *shiatsu* (a Japanese pressure-point technique to relieve stress), and *reflexology* (a deep foot massage that relates to parts of the body). The different types of massage incorporate a variety of strokes, varying levels of pressure, and a multitude of procedures. Massage strokes can be administered to the entire body or to specific areas of the body, such as the back, feet, or hands.

The environment in which massage is administered is important. The room must be warm enough for the person to be comfortable because shivering could negate the effects of the massage. In addition, privacy needs to be ensured. Adding music and aromatherapy to sessions has been thought to increase the effectiveness of massage. Before administering massage, the nurse should explain the intervention, obtain a history, and secure the permission of the patient.

Massage Strokes in Nursing

In 1895, Dr. J. H. Kellog from Battle Creek, Michigan, wrote *The Art of Massage* to teach nurses and other practitioners how to use massage techniques (Calvert, 2002; Kellog, 1895). Although massage was prescribed by physicians early in nursing history, nurses responded by showing leadership to specialize in massage.

Commonly used strokes in administering massage include effleurage, friction, pressure, petrissage, vibration, and percussion.

Effleurage

Effleurage is a slow, rhythmic stroking, with light skin contact. Effleurage may be applied with varying degrees of pressure, depending on the part of the body being massaged and the outcome desired. The palmar surface of the hands is used for larger surfaces and the thumbs and fingers for smaller areas. On large surfaces, long, gliding strokes approximately 10 to 20 inches in length are applied.

Friction Movements

In *friction movements*, moderate, constant pressure to one area is made with the thumbs or fingers. The fingers may be held in one place or moved in a small circumscribed area.

Pressure Stroke

The *pressure stroke* is similar to the friction stroke. However, pressure strokes are made with the whole hand.

Petrissage

Petrissage, or kneading, involves lifting a large fold of skin and the underlying muscle and holding the tissue between the thumb and fingers. The tissues are pushed against the bone, then raised and squeezed in circular movements. The grasp on the tissues is alternately loosened and tightened. Tissues are supported by one hand while being kneaded with the other. Variations include pinching, rolling, wringing, and kneading with fists or fingers. Petrissage is limited to tissues having a significant muscle mass.

Vibration Strokes

Vibration strokes can be administered with either the entire hand or with the fingers. Rapid, continuous strokes are used. Because administering vibration strokes requires a significant amount of energy, mechanical vibrators are sometimes used.

Percussion Strokes

For *percussion strokes*, the wrist acts as a fulcrum for the hand, with the hand hitting the tissue. Strokes are made with a rapid tempo over a large body area. Tapping and clapping are variants of percussion strokes.

Slow-Stroke Back Massage

Slow-stroke back massage, or *effleurage*, is a technique taught in nursing schools. See Exhibit 15.1 for a description of how to perform slow-stroke back massage.

Hand Massage

Techniques for performing hand massage are outlined in Exhibit 15.2. The techniques are easy to use with many populations, including older adults (Kolcaba,

---

Exhibit 15.1. Technique for Slow-Stroke Back Massage

1. **Environment**
   - The room should be at a comfortable temperature
   - The lights should be dimmed
   - Noise should be eliminated
   - The nurse should keep talking at a minimum
2. **The Patient**
   - Ask the patient whether there is a need to use the bathroom or whether there is any way the nurse can assist to promote relaxation before beginning the massage
   - The patient should be assisted to a comfortable position
   - Clothing should be removed so the back is exposed
   - Modesty should be respected.
3. **The Slow-Stroke Back Massage**
   - Palms of the hands and fingers are used (effleurage)
   - The nurse warms her hands
   - The nurse applies nonallergenic lotion to her hands
   - Palms of the hands are placed in the sacral area on each side of the spine
   - Gentle pressure is applied
   - Long, slow, rhythmic, circular strokes are used to move upward on each side of the spine toward the base of the neck
   - Then long, slow, rhythmic, circular strokes are used to move downward on each side of the spine toward the sacral area
   - The masseur applies 12 to 15 strokes per minute to perform a rhythmic movement
   - The massage should continue until completion without removing the hands from the back
4. **Completion**
   - Remove hands from the spine
   - Replace clothing to the back
   - Replace bedcovers
   - Instruct the patient to rise slowly
   - Instruct the patient to stay hydrated
   - Quietly leave the room

Source: Protocol adapted from Harris, M., Richards, K. C., and Grando, V. T. (2012). The effects of slow-stroke back massage on minutes of nighttime sleep on persons with dementia in the nursing home. *Journal of Holistic Nursing, 30*(4), 255–263. doi:10.1177/08980101112455948

Exhibit 15.2. Techniques for Hand Massage

Each hand is massaged for 2½ minutes. Do not massage if the hand is injured, reddened, or swollen. Protocols from 5 to 10 minutes for each hand have also been recommended (Kolcaba et al, 2006; Remington, 2002).

1. **Back of hand**
   - Short, medium-length, straight strokes are done from the wrist to the fingertips; moderate pressure is used (effleurage).
   - Large, half-circle, stretching strokes are made from the center to the side of the hand, using moderate pressure.
   - Small, circular strokes are made over the entire hand, using light pressure (make small *o*s with the thumb).
   - Featherlike, straight strokes are made from the wrist to the fingertips, using very light pressure.

2. **Palm of hand**
   - Short, medium-length, straight strokes are made from the wrist to the fingertips, using moderate pressure (effleurage).
   - Gentle milking and lifting of the tissue of the entire palm of the hand is done using moderate pressure.
   - Small circular strokes are made over the entire palm, using moderate pressure (making little *o*s with index finger).
   - Large, half-circle, stretching strokes are used from the center of the palm to the sides, using moderate pressure.

3. **Fingers**
   - Each finger is gently squeezed from the base to the tip on both sides and the front and back, using light pressure.
   - Gentle range of motion is performed on each finger.
   - Gentle pressure is applied to each nail bed.

4. **Completion**
   - The patient's hand is placed on yours and covered your other hand. The top hand is gently toward you several times. The patient's hand is turned over, and your other hand is gently drawn toward you several times.

Schirm, & Steiner, 2006; Snyder, Eagan, & Burns, 1995) as well as infants and children (Field, 2002). A suggested period for administering massage is 2½ minutes per hand. The length of time is individualized for each patient, based on response.

Measurement of Outcomes

Both physiological and psychological outcomes have been used to measure the effectiveness of massage. Indices of relaxation—heart rate, blood pressure, respiratory rate, skin temperature, cortisol level, and muscle tension— have been measured in many studies. Anxiety inventories and scales to determine pain level and quality of sleep, as well as quality-of-life indices, have been used to determine the efficacy of massage. Protocols for the duration of massage are needed. Typically, massage is dosed at 30- or 60-minute intervals because this is the duration of time used by massage therapists. The results of a randomized controlled trial ($n = 125$)

used a 60-minute, once-weekly dose of massage in an 8-week protocol for osteoarthritis of the knee (Perlman et al., 2012). This was an optimal standard for future dose-finding studies. More research is needed to guide implementation and standardize massage protocols for other conditions. It is important that both short- and long-term effects of massage be measured.

PRECAUTIONS

Ernst (2003) reviewed the literature to determine adverse reactions to massage. Although a number of negative reactions were noted, the majority of these were associated with exotic types of massage and not with the Swedish massage technique. Another review of the literature (Batavia, 2004) indicated the following contraindications to performing massage: arteritis, esophageal varices, unstable hypotension, advanced respiratory failure, postmyocardial infarction, aneurysm, emboli, arrhythmia, anticoagulant therapy/disease, heart failure, phlebitis, varicose veins, deep vein thrombosis, atherosclerosis, tumor, and cancer.

The patient's history of massage gathered by the nurse prior to the intervention provides information about past use of massage and any adverse responses. It is also important to determine the person's overall response to touch. Some people may be averse to being touched because of past negative experiences. Others may be hypersensitive to touch. One method for overcoming this sensitivity is beginning with light touch and slowly increasing the pressure. The area to be massaged is assessed for redness, bruises, edema, or rashes prior to performing massage.

Age-related changes are important considerations for massage. Older adults have more fragile skin and may take anticoagulants, which could cause bruising with massage. Osteoporosis and corticosteroids also place the older adult at risk for fracture. Arthritis, Parkinson's disease, and stroke may limit mobility. The nurse may need to modify massage techniques, positioning, and protocols when considering age-related changes and comorbidities (Rose, 2010).

Massage therapists and nurses have been reluctant to use massage with cancer patients (Gecsedi, 2002) because of the belief that the therapy may initiate or accelerate metastases. A physician's order is needed for body region and technique to be used. Factors considered are the location of the tumor, the stage of the cancer, and the location of any metastatic lesions. Pressure in the immediate area of the cancer is to be avoided. A pilot study ($n = 12$) comparing reflexology and Swedish massage to reduce physiological stress and pain and improve mood was conducted on nursing home residents with cancer (Hodgson & Lafferty, 2012). The results revealed that both techniques were feasible and produced measurable improvements on cortisol levels, pain, and mood. The study supports the need to develop guidelines for older adults with cancer in the nursing home.

Because blood pressure may be lowered during massage, monitoring for light-headedness is suggested after the initial massage sessions, particularly in older adults. If light-headedness does occur, allowing the person to remain recumbent for several minutes at the conclusion of the massage may help decrease the likelihood of hypotension and falls. Monitoring of blood pressure and pulse rate are required in patients with cardiac conditions to determine whether adverse effects are being experienced.

In patients with burns, relief from itching precedes evidence of a therapeutic effect on scar formation. However, skin breakdown can occur if massage is initiated too early. If there is fragile skin breakdown, massage should be temporarily discontinued. Simultaneous use of massage and creams should be monitored closely for skin irritation (Agency for Clinical Innovation [ACI], 2014).

USES

Exhibit 15.3 is a list of selected conditions for which massage is used. Evidence related to relaxation, pain, sleep, and other conditions is discussed in this section.

Relaxation

Nurses use massage as an intervention to relieve physiological and psychological stress and promote relaxation (Harris & Richards, 2010). In a review of 22 studies in which massage had been used, Richards, Gibson, and Overton-McCoy (2000) found that the most commonly reported outcome was a reduction in anxiety.

Depression and Anxiety

A 20-minute effleurage with essential oils implemented 3 times a week for 2 weeks showed statistically significant reductions ($p < .001$) in State-Trait Anxiety Inventory scores and in heart and respiratory rates in patients ($n = 50$) in a psychiatric hospital (da Silva Domingos & Braga, 2015). In a quasiexperimental study ($n = 30$), there were statistically significant differences in anxiety ($p = .002$) and positive trending with a large effect size ($d = 1.3$) on the Hospital Anxiety and Depression Scale on patients in the intervention group after they received 5-minute hand massages

---

Exhibit 15.3. Uses of Massage

- Agitation (Remington, 2002)
- Comfort (Kolcaba et al., 2006)
- Decrease aggressive behaviors (Garner et al., 2008)
- Facilitate communication (Kolcaba et al., 2006)
- Increase psychological well-being (Hattan et al., 2002)
- Increase weight in preterm infants (Field, 2002)
- Lessen anxiety (Currin & Meister, 2008)
- Lessen fatigue (Currin & Meister, 2008)
- Lessen pain (Chang et al., 2002; Wang & Keck, 2004)
- Promote relaxation/reduce stress (Harris & Richards, 2010)
- Promote sleep (Harris et al., 2012; Richards, 1998)

(Prichard & Newcomb, 2015). Another study (Chen et al., 2013) revealed statistically significant decreases—after back massage—in systolic blood pressure ($p <.01$), diastolic blood pressure ($p <.01$), pulse ($p <.01$), and respiratory rate ($p <.01$), as well as a statistically significant difference in anxiety ($p = .02$) in participants ($n = 64$) with congestive heart failure.

Agitation

Several studies using hand massage reported a decrease in psychological indicators for stress (Hicks-Moore & Robinson, 2008; Kolcaba et al., 2006; Remington, 2002). Two randomized controlled trials on hand massage (Hicks-Moore & Robinson, 2008; Remington, 2002) used the Cohen Mansfield Agitation Index (CMAI) to test the effects of hand massage on reducing agitation. Hicks-Moore and Robinson (2008) and Remington (2002) reported statistically significant decreases in agitation 1 hour after hand massage in older participants. Kolcaba et al. (2006) showed statistically significant results for comfort using hand massage in the nursing home environment.

Burns

Massage is used in burn patients to control pain, anxiety, and scarring. There are physiotherapy and occupational therapy guidelines to break up collagen bundles, soften tissues, decrease itching, and prevent adhesions caused by burns (ACI, 2014). One randomized controlled trial ($n = 90$) with burn patients who received aromatherapy massage and inhalation massage showed statistically significant decreases in anxiety ($p = .007$) and pain ($p <.001$) compared with the control group (Seyyed-Rasodi, Salehi, Mohammadpoorosi, Goljaryan, & Seyyedi, 2016).

HIV

Cochrane reviewers (Hillier, Louw, Morris, Uwimana, & Stathum, 2010) found four randomized controlled trials. One study was associated with improvements in $CD4^+$ and killer cells. Other studies showed improvement in quality of life, especially when massage was used with other modalities.

Preterm Infants

In a research review, Dr. Tiffany Field (2014) outlined the benefits of massage on weight gain in preterm infants. Preterm infants experience significant stress. In one study in which preterm infants (n = 30) were randomly assigned to a massage therapy or exercise group, results suggested increased weight gain for the combination of tactile or kinesthetic stimulation (Diego, Field, & Hernandez-Reif, 2014).

Pain

Reduction of pain is another condition for which massage is often used. Numerous studies have found that massage does result in reduced pain. A Cochrane review ($n = 13$) revealed benefits for individuals with low back pain when massage was combined with exercise and education (Furlan et al., 2008). In a review of research on the use of massage and aromatherapy in patients with cancer, Wang and Keck (2004) reported a lessening of pain in postoperative patients, and Mok and Woo (2004) found that massage lessened pain in patients with strokes.

Sleep

A randomized controlled trial of massage on participants (n = 57) after coronary artery bypass graft surgery showed decreased fatigue and more effective sleep (Nerbass, Feltrim, de Souza, Ykeda, & Lorenzi-Filho, 2010). Two studies used objective measures for sleep to determine the effects of massage in older adults. Richards (1998) used polysomnography as an objective measure for sleep in hospitalized older men (n = 69) to compare a slow-stroke back massage intervention group between participants using relaxing music and a control group. Another randomized controlled pilot study (Harris et al., 2012) with patients with dementia in the nursing home (n = 40) used actigraphy to objectively measure sleep in participants receiving a 3-minute, slow-stroke back massage compared with a usual-care control condition. Although there were no statistically significant differences between participants in the intervention and control groups in either study, results provided evidence for clinical significance for the use of slow-stroke back massage for relaxation and sleep in the geriatric population.

CULTURAL APPLICATIONS

Shiatsu, a pressure-point type of massage, is popular in Japan and other Asian countries. Its underlying purpose is to rebalance the energy system in the body through pressure on specific points. Although shiatsu may not be comforting during administration, relaxation is often felt at the conclusion. Shiatsu may be used to help alleviate other conditions. Taniguki (2008) found shiatsu therapy to be highly efficacious in managing constipation in six elderly patients (from 81 to 93 years old) who were on bed rest and receiving home care.

In countries such as Japan, acupuncture and moxibustion are often used, in addition to massage, by massage therapists, who also often have a license to practice acupuncture and moxibustion. Therefore, in some research studies, because of the cultural implications, massage cannot be separated from acupuncture and moxibustion (Hirakawa et al., 2005).

In a multicultural qualitative study (Kilstoff & Chenoweth, 1998), hand massage was conducted on Chinese-, Italian-, Vietnamese-, Arab-, French-, and English-speaking participants (n = 39; 16 dyads of patients with dementia and caregivers; 7 day-care staff) in a dementia-care patient setting. The results showed reduction in stress, decreased agitation, increased alertness, improved self-hygiene, and improved sleep. Family caregivers also reported less distress, improved sleep, and feelings of calm.

Massage is widely used around the world as illustrated in the accounts of nursing students (see Sidebar 15.1).

SIDEBAR 15.1. ACCOUNTS OF MASSAGE OF INTERNATIONAL NURSING STUDENTS AT CARR COLLEGE OF NURSING, HARDING UNIVERSITY, SEARCY, ARKANSAS

Larissa Hubbard, Canada

As a missionary who lived in the Ukraine, I have traveled a lot and learned about many cultural practices and traditions. Among numerous home remedies and treatments that I have seen, the use of massage therapy seemed quite common, especially in care for the elderly. Some older people who cannot afford, or are afraid to seek, healthcare often turn to less-costly options, such as using massage for pain relief. In everyday living, it is also used in the home to relieve anxiety and correct bad posture. Some people even attend extracurricular massage courses to gain the professional skills that could better help their sick loved ones at home.

Esi Fosua Yeboah, Ghana

The use of massage therapy in Ghana and the United States is similar. In Ghana, it is used for relaxation, increasing circulation, decreasing pain, and inducing sleep. It is also used for the treatment of fibromyalgia and depression. The following comment was written in 2011 in a blog (www.massageprofessionals. com/profiles/blogs/initiating-our-association-in-africa) by Yaw Boateng, who has established a massage therapy school in Ghana: "the profession of massage has not been given attention in Africa, most especially in Ghana."

Azel Peralta, Philippines

In the Southeast Asian islands of the Philippines, one massage technique is called *hilot*. This means "healer" or "to rub." *Manghihilots*, those who practice the hilot technique, usually learn their art through teachings and practices that have been passed down through the generations. Hilot is not something learned through schooling. People in the Philippine villages visit Manghihilots to look for a cure instead of traveling many miles to the cities to see a doctor. Hilot is a holistic art of healing and is used to correct imbalances in the body such as fluid, energy, fractures, sprains, and dislocations. Hilot is also used for inducing labor of pregnant women. Natural banana leaves and coconut oil, which are staples of these islands, are used in the process of locating the problem areas and diagnosing health problems. Techniques can range from a combination of a deep-tissue massage to manipulate muscle tissue, bones, and joints to the use of only a stroking or rubbing motion of the fingers.

Sivchhun Hun, Cambodia

Massage therapy is a big part of the lives of Cambodian people. It is used for various reasons, including the benefits of relaxation. My parents have a massage therapist visit them at home daily around evening time. They believe that by receiving massage therapy before their bedtime, it helps them to relax, to sleep better at night, and to feel better when they wake up in the morning.

FUTURE RESEARCH

There is a lack of rigorous research on complementary therapies such as massage. Specific techniques, questions related to the person who should administer the massage, specific protocols, dose-finding studies, qualitative research, and studies to support the clinical significance of massage are all areas for further investigation to build nursing science in massage. One challenge in conducting research on massage is having a comparable control group. McNamara, Burnham, Smith, and Carroll (2003) compared massage and standard care in patients undergoing a diagnostic test.

Reflexology and Swedish massage (Hodgson & Lafferty, 2012) were compared on nursing home residents with cancer. A randomized controlled trial ($n = 125$) that compared structural and relaxation massage for low back pain used blinding to test the effectiveness of treatment for low back pain (Cherkin et al., 2012). More studies are needed that compare massage techniques for developing evidence-based practices. The results of a randomized controlled trial ($n = 125$; Perlman et al., 2012) showed that a 60-minute, once-weekly dose of massage was an optimal standard for future dose-finding studies in patients with osteoarthritis of the knee.

The following are suggestions for research that is needed so that practitioners may have more direction in using massage in clinical settings:

- Well-designed studies using blinding, randomization, and attention control groups with large sample sizes are needed.
- Few investigators have explored the impact that massage has on psychoneuroimmunological indices. Studies on the use of massage with patients with HIV infection and cancer would guide nurses in its use with these groups.
- Dose-finding studies for administering massage and the number of sessions that produce the best results need to be established. There is great variation in these two parameters in published studies. Because of time constraints in practice settings, this information would be very helpful to busy practitioners.
- Research studies on the benefits of massage using multimodal protocols, including exercise, aromatherapy, music, and other nonpharmacological interventions, are needed in the development of evidence-based practices.
- What, if any, is the effect of the gender of the therapist administering massage on the outcomes obtained? Few studies have reported on this factor.

REFERENCES

Agency for Clinical Innovation. (2014). *ACI statewide burn injury service: Physiotherapy and occupational therapy clinical practice.* Chatswood, Australia: Author.

American Physical Therapy Association (APTA). (2013). Minimum required skills of physical therapists graduates at entry-level. Retrieved from http://www.apta.org/uploadedFiles/APTAorg/About_Us/Policies/Education/MinimumRequiredSkillsPTGrads.pdf

Ang, J. Y., Lua, J. L., Mathur, A., Thomas, R., Asmar, B. I., Savasan, S., ... Shankaran, S. (2012). A randomized placebo-controlled trial of massage therapy on the immune system of preterm infants. *Pediatrics, 130*(6), e1548–e1549. doi:10.1542/peds.2012-1096

Batavia, M. (2004). Contraindications for therapeutic massage: Do sources agree? *Journal of Bodywork and Movement Therapies, 8,* 48–57. doi:10.1016/S1360-8592(03)0008-6

Billhult, A., Lindholm, C., Gunnarsson, R., & Stener-Victorin, E. (2008). The effect of massage on cellular immunity, endocrine and psychological factors in women with breast cancer—A randomized controlled clinical trial. *Autonomic Neuroscience Basic and Clinical, 140,* 88–95. doi:10.1016/j.autneu.2008.03.006

Brummitt, J. (2008). The role of massage in sports performance and rehabilitation: Current evidence and future direction. *North American Journal of Sports Physical Therapy, 3,* 7–21.

Calvert, R. N. (2002). *The history of massage.* Rochester, VT: Healing Arts Press.

Chang, M.-Y., Wang, S.-Y., & Chen, C.-H. (2002). Effects of massage on pain and anxiety during labour: A randomized controlled trial in Taiwan. *Journal of Advanced Nursing, 38,* 68–73.

Chen, W.-L., Liu, G.-J., Yeh, S.-H., Chiang, M.-C., Fu, M.-Y., & Hsieh, Y.-K. (2013). Effect of back massage intervention on anxiety, comfort, and physiologic responses in patients with congestive heart failure. *Journal of Alternative and Complementary Medicine, 19,* 464–470. doi:10.1089/acm.2011.0873

Cherkin, D. C., Sherman, K. J., Kahn, J., Wellman, R., Cook, A. J., Erro, J., … Deyo, R. A. (2012). A comparison of the effects of 2 types of massage and usual care on chronic low back pain. *Annals of Internal Medicine, 155*(1), 1–9.

Currin, J., & Meister, E. A. (2008). A hospital-based intervention using massage to reduce distress among oncology patients. *Cancer Nursing, 3,* 214–221. doi:10.1097/01.NCC.0000305725.65345.f3

da Silva Domingos, T., & Braga, E. M. (2015). Massage with aromatherapy: Effectiveness on anxiety of users with personality disorders in psychiatric hospitalization. *Journal of School of Nursing USP, 49*(3), 450–456. doi:10.1590/30080-6234201500003000013

Diego, M. A., Field, T., & Hernandez-Reif, M. (2014). Preterm infant weight gain is increased by massage therapy and exercise via different underlying mechanisms. *Early Human Development, 90*(3), 137–140. doi:10.1016/j.earlhumdev.2014.01.009

Dossey, B. M., Selanders, L. C., Beck, D., & Attewell, A. (2005). *Florence Nightingale today: Healing, leadership, global action.* Silver Spring, MD: American Nurses Association.

Ernst, E. (2003). The safety of massage therapy. *Rheumatology, 42,* 1101–1106. doi:10.1093/rheumatology/keg306

Field, T. (2002). Preterm infant massage therapy studies: An American approach. *Seminars in Neonatology, 7,* 487–494.

Field, T. (2014). Massage therapy research review. *Complementary Therapies in Clinical Practice, 20,* 224–229.

Fletcher, B. (2009). A bridge between the mind and body: The effects of massage on body image state. *Undergraduate Review, 5,* 58–63. Retrieved from http://vc.bridgew.edu/undergrad_rev/vol5/iss1/13

Frey Law, L. A., Evans, S., Kundston, J., Nus, S., Scholl, K., & Sluka, K. A. (2008). Massage reduces pain perception and hyperalgesia in experimental muscle pain: A randomized, controlled trial. *Journal of Pain, 9,* 714–721. doi:10.1016/j.jpain.2008.03.009

Furlan, A. D., Imamura, M., Dryden, T., & Irvin, E. (2008). Massage for low-back pain. *Cochrane Database of Systematic Reviews, 4,* CD001929. doi:10.1002/14651858.CD001929.pub2

Garner, B., Phillips, L. J., Schmidt, H. M., Markulev, C., O'Connor, J., Wood, S. J., … McGorry, P. D. (2008). Pilot study evaluating the effect of massage therapy on stress, anxiety, and aggression in a young adult psychiatric inpatient unit. *Australian & New Zealand Journal of Psychiatry, 42*(5), 414–422. doi:10.1080/00048670801961131

Gecsedi, R. A. (2002). Massage therapy for patients with cancer. *Clinical Journal of Oncology Nursing, 6,* 52–54. doi:10.1188/02.CJON.52-54

Goodall-Copestake, B. M. (1919). *The theory and practice of massage* (2nd ed.). New York, NY: Paul B. Hoeber.

Harris, M., & Richards, K. C. (2010). The physiological and psychological effects of slow-stroke back massage and hand massage on relaxation in the elderly. *Journal of Clinical Nursing, 19,* 917–926.

Harris, M., Richards, K. C., & Grando, V. T. (2012). The effects of slow-stroke back massage on minutes of nighttime sleep on persons with dementia in the nursing home. *Journal of Holistic Nursing, 30*(4), 255–263. doi:10.1177/08980101112455948

Hattan, J., King, L., & Griffiths, P. (2002). The impact of foot massage and guided relaxation following cardiac surgery: A randomized controlled trial. *Journal of Advanced Nursing, 37*, 199–207.

Hicks-Moore, S., & Robinson, B. (2008). Favorite music and hand massage. *Dementia, 7*(1), 95–108. doi:10.1177/1471301207085369

Hillier, S. L., Louw, Q., Morris, L., Uwimana, J., & Statham, S. (2010). Massage therapy for people with HIV/AIDS. *Cochrane Database of Systematic Reviews,* (1), CD007502. doi:10.1002/14651858.CD007502.pub2

Hirakawa, Y., Masuda, Y., Kimata, T., Uemura, K., Kuzuya, M., & Iguchi, A. (2005). Effects of home massage rehabilitation for the bed-ridden elderly: A pilot trial with a three-month follow up. *Clinical Rehabilitation, 19*, 20–27. doi:10.1191/0269215505cr795oa

Hodgson, N. A., & Lafferty, D. (2012). Reflexology versus Swedish massage to reduce physiological stress and pain and improve mood in nursing home residents with cancer: A pilot study. *Evidence-Based Complementary & Alternative Medicine, 2012*, 1–5. doi:10.1155/2012/456897

Holland, B., & Pokorny, M. E. (2001). Slow stroke back massage on patients in a rehabilitation setting. *Rehabilitation Nursing, 26*, 182–186.

Jensen, K. L. (1932). *Fundamentals of massage for students of nursing.* New York, NY: Macmillan.

Kellog, J. H. (1895). *The art of massage.* Battle Creek, MI: Good Health Publishing.

Kilstoff, K., & Chenoweth, L. (1998). New approaches to health and well-being for dementia daycare clients, family carers and day-care staff. *International Journal of Nursing Practice, 4*(2), 70–83. doi:10.1046/j.1440-172X.1998.00059.x

Kolcaba, K., Schirm, V., & Steiner, R. (2006). Effects of hand massage on comfort of nursing home residents. *Geriatric Nursing, 27*, 85–91.

Lawton, G. (2003). *Toward a neurophysiological understanding of manual therapy neuro-manual therapy.* Retrieved from http://www.americanmanualmedicine.com

Macafee, N. F. (1917). *Massage, an elementary text-book for nurses.* Pittsburgh, PA: Reed & Witting.

Massage Therapy Body of Knowledge (MTBOK Task Force). (2010). *Massage therapy body of knowledge* (MTBOK) version 1.0.

McNamara, M. E., Burnham, D. C., Smith, C., & Carroll, D. L. (2003). The effects of back massage before diagnostic cardiac catheterization. *Alternative Therapies in Health and Medicine, 9*(1), 50–57.

Mok, E., & Woo, C. P. (2004). The effects of slow-stroke massage on anxiety and shoulder pain in elderly stroke patients. *Complementary Therapies in Nursing & Midwifery, 10*, 209–216.

Moraska, A., Pollini, R. A., Boulanger, K., Brooks, M. Z., & Teitlebaum, L. (2010). Physiological adjustments to stress measures following massage therapy: A review of the literature. *Evidence-Based Complementary and Alternative Medicine, 7*, 409–418. doi:10.1093/ecam/nen029

National Association of Nurse Massage Therapists. (2011). About us: philosophy. Retrieved from http://www.nanmt.org/index-1philosophy.html

National Council of State Boards of Nursing. (2012). *National Council of State Boards of Nursing: 2013 NCLEX-RN® detailed test plan: item writer/item reviewer/nurse educator version.* Chicago, IL: Author.

Nerbass, F. B., Feltrim, M. I. Z., de Souza, S. A., Ykeda, D. S., & Lorenzi-Filho, G. (2010). Effects of massage therapy on sleep quality after coronary artery bypass graft surgery. *Clinicals, 65*, 1105–1110. doi:10.1590/S1807-59322010001000008

Norstroëm, G. M. (1868/1896). *The handbook of massage.* New York, NY: Leland Stanford Junior University, reprinted in 1896 by the Lane Medical Library.

Perlman, A. I., Ali, A., Njike, V. Y., Hom, D., Davidi, A., Gould-Fogeite, S., … Katz, D. L. (2012). Massage therapy for osteoarthritis of the knee: A randomized dose-finding trial. *PLOS ONE, 7*(2), e30248. doi:10.1371/journal.pone.0030248

Prichard, C., & Newcomb, P. (2015). Benefit to family members of delivering hand massage with essential oils to critically ill patients. *American Journal of Critical Care Nurses, 24*(5), 446–449. doi:10.4037/ajcc2015767

Rawlins, M. (1933). *A textbook of massage for nurses and beginners* (2nd ed.). St. Louis, MO: Mosby.

Remington, R. (2002). Calming music and hand massage with agitated elderly. *Nursing Research, 51*(5), 317–323.

Richards, K. C. (1998). Effect of a back massage and relaxation intervention on sleep in critically ill patients. *American Journal of Critical Care, 7*, 288–299.

Richards, K. C., Gibson, R., & Overton-McCoy, A. L. (2000). Effects of massage in acute and critical care. *AACN Clinical Issues, 11*, 77–96.

Rose, M. K. (2010). *Comfort touch.* Philadelphia, PA: Wolters Kluwer/Lippincott Williams & Wilkins.

Ruffin, P. T. (2011). A history of massage in nurse training school curricula (1860–1945). *Journal of Holistic Nursing, 29*, 61–67. doi:10.1177/0898010110377355

Seyyed-Rasodi, A., Salehi, F., Mohammadpoorosi, A., Goljaryan, S., & Seyyedi, A. (2016). Comparing the effects of aromatherapy massage and inhalation aromatherapy on anxiety and pain in burn patients. *Burns, 42*(8), 1774–1780. doi:10.1016/j.burns.2016.06.014

Snyder, M., Egan, E. C., & Burns, K. R. (1995). Efficacy of hand massage in decreasing agitation behaviors associated with care activities in persons with dementia. *Geriatric Nursing, 16*(2), 60–63.

Snyder, M., & Taniguki, S. (2010). Massage. In M. Snyder & R. Lindquist (Eds.), *Complementary & alternative therapies in nursing* (6th ed., pp. 337–448). New York, NY: Springer Publishing.

Taniguki, S. (2008). Use of Shiatsu with home care patients (Unpublished manuscript).

Touch Research Institute. (n.d.). *Touch Research Institute.* Retrieved from http://www6.miami.edu/touch-research

Wang, H. L., & Keck, J. F. (2004). Foot and hand massage as an intervention for postoperative pain. *Pain Management Nursing, 5*, 59–65.

Wieting, J. M., & Cugalj, A. P. (2011). Massage, traction, and manipulation. Retrieved from http://emedicine.medscape.com

Williams, A. L., Selwyn, P. A., Liberti, L., Molde, S., Njike, V. Y., McCorkle, R., … Katz, D. L. (2005). A randomized controlled trial of meditation and massage effects on quality of life in people with late-stage disease: A pilot study. *Journal of Palliative Medicine, 8*, 939–952.

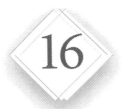

Tai Chi

Kuei-Min Chen

Time pressure is emerging as a contemporary malaise. Lack of time is the major barrier to exercising regularly. Failure to exercise may lead to mental strain, nervous breakdown, or inefficiency in daily work (Booth, Roberts, & Laye, 2012). Good health is essential; how to acquire and maintain a healthy mind and body are vital concerns. It is commonly recognized that exercise and other forms of physical activity have a wide range of health benefits, both physiological and psychological, for all age groups (Dogra, Shah, Patel, & Tamim, 2015). However, it is not easy to find an exercise that suits people of all ages.

Tai chi is one intervention that is receiving increasing attention among many professionals: nurses, physicians, occupational therapists, physical therapists, and recreational therapists. It is a manipulative and body-based therapy that can heighten individuals' awareness of their bodies and take advantage of their body structure for expressing feelings and ideas. Gradually, people become more aware of their total being, and harmony is enhanced.

DEFINITION

Tai chi, which means "supreme ultimate," is a traditional Chinese martial art (Koh, 1981) and a mind–body exercise. It involves a series of fluid, continuous, graceful, dance-like postures, and the performances of movements are known as *forms* (J. M. Yang, 2010). The graceful body movements engage continuous body and trunk rotation, flexion/extension of the hips and knees, postural alignment, and the coordination of the arms—integrated by mental concentration, the balanced shifting of body weight, muscle relaxation, and breath control. Movements are performed in a slow, rhythmic, and well-controlled manner (Clark, 2011).

Several styles of tai chi are practiced: chen (quick and slow large movements), *yang* (slow large movements), *wu* (midpaced, compact movements), *sun* (quick, compact movements), and *wu hao* (small, subtle movements; Douglas & Douglas, 2012). Each style has a characteristic protocol that differs from the other styles in the postures or forms included, the order in which they appear, the pace at which movements are executed, and the level of difficulty; however, the basic principles are the same (J. M. Yang & Liang, 2016). For example, one significant difference between the chen and yang styles is that Yang movements are relaxed, evenly paced, and graceful. Yang is the most popular tai chi practiced by older adults (Liang & Wu, 2014). In comparison, the chen style is characterized by alternating slow, gentle movements with quick and vigorous ones, as well as restrained and controlled actions, that reflect a more martial origin (Gu, 2011). Most tai chi movements were named after animals, such as "white crane spreads its wings" and "grasp the bird's tail" (Koh, 1981).

There are a few simplified forms of the ancient tai chi. For example, the simplified tai chi exercise program (STEP), developed by Chen, Chen, and Huang (2006), encompasses three phases: warm-up, tai chi exercises, and cool-down. In the warm-up phase, nine exercises are designed to loosen the body from head to toe; the second phase includes 12 easy-to-learn and easy-to-perform tai chi movements; three activities during the cool-down phase help the body to return to a preintervention state of rest. STEP differs from traditional tai chi styles in that it incorporates fewer leg movements, fewer knee bends, and less-complicated hand gestures. It was specifically designed for older adults suffering from chronic illness (Chen et al., 2006).

SCIENTIFIC BASIS

Tai chi practice is closely linked to Chinese medicine theory, in which the vital life energy, chi (or *qi*), is thought to circulate throughout the body in discrete channels called meridians. Using correct postures and adequate relaxation, tai chi promotes the free flow of chi throughout the body, which improves the health of an individual. The movements of tai chi are regulated by the timing of deep breathing and the movement of the diaphragm. It offers a balanced exercise to the muscles and joints of various parts of the body (Clark, 2011). In addition, a peaceful state of mind and spiritual dedication to each movement during the exercise ensure that the central nervous system (CNS) is given sufficient training and is consequently toned up with time as the exercise continues. A strong CNS is essential for a healthy body, and the various organs depend largely on its soundness (Clark, 2011).

INTERVENTION

In Asian countries such as Taiwan, it is common and popular for older adults to practice tai chi as a group, in the early morning, in parks or on the athletic grounds of elementary schools. Tai chi practice groups are usually led by masters who are pleased to share its essence with others. People who are interested in tai chi are welcome to join the groups and learn the movements from these masters. In Western countries such as the United States, there is a growing interest in the practice of tai chi. Various tai chi clubs are available to the public through community centers, health clinics, or private organizations. General information is widespread through websites, books, and videos. Tai chi is a convenient exercise that can be practiced in any place, at any time, and without any equipment.

Technique

Although various styles of tai chi are practiced, the underlying practice principles are the same. Five essential principles of movement are (Schaller, 1996):

- Hand and leg movements should be synchronous
- The emphasis should be on a soft, relaxed, rather than on a hard, tense position
- Moves should be practiced with a quiet and open mind
- The soles of the feet should be rooted to the ground, with the knees bent in a low stance and the primary focus of awareness within the lower abdomen
- The physical force should be rooted in the feet, passed up through the legs as weight is shifted, and distributed by the pivoting of the waist

In the physical performance, an individual must relax and think of nothing else before starting. The movements should be slow and rhythmic with natural breathing. Every action becomes easy and smooth, the waist turns freely, and the feelings of comfort and relaxation are gradually developed (Clark, 2011). In the spiritual aspect, tai chi is an exercise that produces harmony of body and mind. Each movement should be guided by thought instead of physical strength. For instance, to lift up the hands, an individual must first have the necessary mental concentration, and then the hands can be raised slowly in a proper manner. Hence, the breathing will become deeper and the body will be strengthened (Clark, 2011).

Guidelines

The steps for performing the movement called "white crane spreads its wings" are presented in Exhibit 16.1.

Exhibit 16.1. Procedure for Performing "White Crane Spreads Its Wings"

- Bring your right foot next to your left while your left palm circles clockwise up, palm down. At the same time, turn your body slightly to your left and rotate your right palm up.
- Bring your left foot a half step forward. Shift all your weight onto your right foot. At the same time, bring your right palm up past your left elbow and lift your left foot up slightly.
- Complete the movement by lowing your left palm down to waist level, palm down. Raise your right palm up to head level, palm facing inward, and touch down with your left foot into empty stance.

Source: Adapted from Liang, S. Y., & Wu, W. C. (2014). *Simplified tai chi chuan: 24 postures with applications & standard 48 postures* (2nd ed.). Wolfeboro, NH: Ymaa Publication Center.

Various videos on tai chi are also available. The following DVDs and/or books are useful for learning tai chi:

- *Tai Chi Chuan Classical Yang Style: The Complete Form Qigong* (J. M. Yang, 2010) is an in-depth guide for beginners to learn tai chi chuan properly. It offers a general plan for practicing tai chi chuan, and then goes into great depth to present enough content for proper learning. Each movement is presented in a series of large photographs with clear same-page instructions for each tai chi posture.
- *The Complete Illustrated Guide to Tai Chi: A Step-by-Step Approach to the Ancient Chinese Movement* (Clark, 2011) contains a complete introduction to the principles and practices of tai chi and is accompanied by clear and instructive photography throughout. It includes sections on the basic principles of movement and the body, ways that tai chi can help heal, life energies, meridians, the seven major chakras, and step-by-step guides to the complete movement sequence.
- *Complete Tai-Chi: The Definitive Guide to Physical and Emotional Self-Improvement* (Huang, 2011) includes a detailed guide to the 36 postures (with more than 250 photographs) of the *wu*-style tai chi, which stresses the development of internal energy for self-healing and has gained enormous popularity as a healing exercise.
- *Seated Tai Chi and Qigong: Guided Therapeutic Exercises to Manage Stress and Balance Mind, Body, and Spirit* (Quarta & Vallie, 2012) emphasizes that tai chi and qigong are the perfect antidote to the stresses of modern life and a great way to stay healthy. This illustrated guidebook provides an explanatory introduction to these forms of exercise and shows how to build up a program from easy to more challenging steps.
- *The Complete Idiot's Guide to T'ai Chi & Qigong Illustrated* (Douglas & Douglas, 2012) includes nearly 150 online videos that support the book and 300 richly detailed illustrations, giving it a highly effective how-to focus.
- *Simplified Tai Chi Chuan: 24 Postures with Applications & Standard 48 Postures* (Liang & Wu, 2014) is designed for self-study and can help people learn both the simplified tai chi chuan 24 posture form and the simplified tai chi chuan 48 posture form quickly and accurately.
- *Tai Chi Chuan Martial Applications: Advanced Yang Style* (J. M. Yang & Liang, 2016) includes a new, easy-to-follow layout. Each technique is presented in four to six large photographs with detailed instructions on how to perform the movements. Motion arrows are used on the photographs to help you execute the movements correctly.

Measurement of Outcomes

According to Plummer (1983), mind concentration and breathing control are two of the major tenets of tai chi practice. When practicing tai chi with a peaceful, focused mind and incorporating smooth breathing into each movement, a person experiences physical and psychological relaxation, which leads to enhanced well-being in both states (Plummer, 1983). With this conceptual framework in mind, the measurement of the effects of tai chi should include both physical and psychological well-being. More studies have been done to measure the physical outcomes of tai chi practice (such as cardiovascular functioning), with little emphasis on psychological well-being outcomes (such as mood states).

Exhibit 16.2.   Selecting a Tai Chi Class

- If possible, find a studio or organization that specializes in tai chi.
- Find an experienced teacher (6–10 years of experience) who demonstrates and verbally explains the movements. Ask to observe a class before joining.
- Find a class with fewer than 20 students.
- Avoid purchasing any special clothing or equipment.

Source: Adapted from Downs, L. B. (1992). Tai chi. *Modern Maturity, 35,* 60–64.

PRECAUTIONS

Tai chi is unique for its slow graceful movements with low-impact, low-velocity, and minimal orthopedic complications and is a suitable conditioning exercise for older adults (Dogra et al., 2015; Wayne, Berkowitz, Litrownik, Buring, & Yeh, 2014). Although many research studies have shown the benefits of tai chi, there are some contraindications to its practice, such as an acute stage of angina, ventricular arrhythmia, or myocardial ischemia. The instructor and the student have to be aware of these contraindications, and an initial assessment is necessary to determine an individual's exercise tolerance and other limitations (Wang et al., 2016). While learning tai chi, a novice should be periodically evaluated in terms of progress, program adherence, cognitive response, muscular strength, balance, and level of flexibility at fairly regular (e.g., every 4 weeks) intervals for the first 60 days to 90 days of participation in such a program. Progression is individualized and is based on the preference of the instructor (L. Li & Manor, 2010). It is strongly suggested that one learn tai chi from an experienced master who is able to teach the movements based on individual needs and physical tolerance. Advice on choosing a class is provided in Exhibit 16.2.

USES

Tai chi is especially appropriate for older adults or for patients with chronic diseases because of its low intensity, steady rhythm, and low physical and mental tension (Lin et al., 2015; Y. Yang et al., 2015). It has been shown to enhance cardiovascular and respiratory functions, improve health-related fitness, and promote positive health status (Dogra et al., 2015; Tsai, Chang, Beck, Kuo, & Keefe, 2013; Wang et al., 2016). In addition, practicing tai chi has been effective in lowering blood pressure (Figueroa, Demeersman, & Manning, 2012; Pan, Yan, Guo, & Yan, 2013; Sun & Buys, 2015). Studies also indicated that tai chi increases postural stability, enhances balance (Nguyen & Kruse, 2012; Wang, 2011, 2012), and improves muscle strength and endurance (Hwang et al., 2016; Song, Roberts, Lee, Lam, & Bae, 2010; Wang, 2011, 2012), which leads to a reduction in the risk of falls (Hwang et al., 2016; Maciaszek & Osinski, 2012; Merom et al., 2012; Taylor-Piliae et al., 2014). Tai chi also plays an important role in symptom control of chronic illnesses such as osteoarthritis (Tsai et al, 2013; Wang, 2011, 2012; Wang et al., 2016).

In addition, studies have indicated that tai chi practice may also provide psychological benefits, such as enhanced positive mood states (Hwang et al., 2016;

Irwin & Olmstead, 2012; Wang et al., 2016) and quality of sleep (Caldwell, Emery, Harrison, & Greeson, 2011; Chan et al., 2016; Hosseini, Esfirizi, Marandi, & Rezaei, 2011; Nguyen & Kruse, 2012).

Researchers have suggested that tai chi could be incorporated into community programs or senior center activities to promote the well-being of community-dwelling older adults. It could also be included as one of the activities in nursing homes or in rehabilitation programs in hospital settings (Desrochers, Kairy, Pan, Corriveau, & Tousignant, 2016; Moy et al., 2015). Furthermore, tai chi has been applied in other populations. For example, tai chi improves the pulmonary function of children with asthma (Caldwell, Harrison, Adams, & Triplett, 2009; Chang, Yang, Chen, & Chiang, 2008), serves as a therapy for patients with attention deficit hyperactivity disorder (Converse, Ahlers, Travers, & Davidson, 2014), increases functional capacity of people with myocardial infarction (Nery et al., 2015), and enhances balance, gait, and mobility of people with Parkinson disease (F. Li et al., 2012; Y. Yang et al., 2015). Tai chi has also been practiced in many countries, including the United States, the United Kingdom, Australia, Hong Kong, Singapore, and Taiwan. How tai chi is used in the United Kingdom, as an example, is illustrated in Sidebar 16.1.

SIDEBAR 16.1. USE OF TAI CHI IN THE UNITED KINGDOM

Graeme D. Smith

Although part of traditional Chinese medicine (TCM), tai chi appears to be increasingly used in the United Kingdom for health-related benefits and stress relief. To date, there is little UK-based research to support the popularity of this activity. Anecdotally, tai chi seems to be used mostly by older people for physical and mental health benefits. The National Health Service (NHS) in the United Kingdom notes that appropriate use of tai chi may prevent falls and improve overall psychological well-being in older adults. The basis of these claims may come from the improved balance control and flexibility those who practice tai chi may achieve. However, as with other forms of complementary and alternative medicine, high-quality rigorous research is required to substantiate these claims. Unfortunately, to date, such research is lacking.

Private healthcare providers in the United Kingdom also promote tai chi as a very low-impact, feel-good form of exercise. There would appear to be no real safety issues associated with using tai chi, although people who are pregnant or have a hernia, back pain, or severe osteoporosis are encouraged to speak to their family doctor before they start. Also, from a safety perspective, individuals are encouraged to find out about a tai chi instructor's qualifications and experience before they enroll in a program. At present, there is no statutory regulation of tai chi in the United Kingdom. Several tai chi bodies do exist, including the Tai Chi Union for Great Britain. This is the largest collective of independent tai chi instructors in the United Kingdom. They aim to unite

(continued)

tai chi practitioners and promote tai chi in all its aspects—health, aesthetic meditation, self-defense, and general improvement of standards. Tai Chi UK is another existing organization that claims tai chi can be "the ultimate holistic experience." Development of such groups is a clear indication of tai chi's increasing popularity in the United Kingdom.

FUTURE RESEARCH

Overall, practicing tai chi appropriately has various benefits, as evidenced in the literature, and it is highly recommended for the appropriate populations. More studies about the effects of tai chi from a nursing perspective are needed to provide guidance to nurses in its use with various populations. Some questions for further research include:

- Which populations can most benefit from practicing tai chi, and are there conditions that would preclude its use?
- What is the nature of change in the well-being status of older adults who practice tai chi?
- What are the differences on well-being outcomes of beginners (people who are just starting to learn tai chi movements), practitioners (people who have practiced tai chi regularly for more than a year), and masters (people who have practiced tai chi regularly for more than a decade and are licensed by the National Tai Chi Association to be instructors)?

WEBSITES

Additional information can be found through the following useful websites:

- www.supply.com/lee/tcclinks.html provides links to more than 100 other websites on tai chi and related topics.
- sunflower.signet.com.sg/~limttk/index.htm is a valuable site with complete historical and background information on tai chi.

REFERENCES

Booth, F. W., Roberts, C. K., & Laye, M. J. (2012). Lack of exercise is a major cause of chronic diseases. *Comprehensive Physiology, 2*(2), 1143 1211.

Caldwell, K., Emery, L., Harrison, M., & Greeson, J. (2011). Changes in mindfulness, well-being, and sleep quality in college students through taijiquan courses: A cohort control study. *Alternative and Complementary Medicine, 17*, 931–938.

Caldwell, K., Harrison, M., Adams, M., & Triplett, N. T. (2009). Effects of Pilates and taiji quan training on self-efficacy, sleep quality, mood, and physical performance of college students. *Journal of Bodywork and Movement Therapies, 13*, 155–163.

Chan, A. W. K., Yu, D. S. F., Choi, K. C., Lee, D. T. F., Sit, J. W. H., & Chan, H. Y. L. (2016). Tai chi qigong as a means to improve night-time sleep quality among older adults with cognitive impairment: A pilot randomized controlled trial. *Clinical Interventions in Aging, 11*, 1277–1286.

Chang, Y. F., Yang, Y. H., Chen, C. C., & Chiang, B. L. (2008). Tai chi chuan training improves the pulmonary function of asthmatic children. *Journal of Microbiology, Immunology, and Infection, 41,* 88–95.

Chen, K. M., Chen, W. T., & Huang, M. F. (2006). Development of the simplified tai-chi exercise program (STEP) for the frail older adults. *Complementary Therapies in Medicine, 14,* 200–206.

Clark, A. (2011). *The complete illustrated guide to tai chi: A step-by-step approach to the ancient Chinese movement.* Toronto, ON, Canada: HarperCollins.

Converse, A. K., Ahlers, E. O., Travers, B. G., & Davidson, R. J. (2014). Tai chi training reduces self-report of inattention in healthy young adults. *Frontiers in Human Neuroscience, 8*(13), 1–7.

Desrochers, P., Kairy, D., Pan, S., Corriveau, H., & Tousignant, M. (2016). Tai chi for upper limb rehabilitation in stroke patients: The patient's perspective. *Disability and Rehabilitation, 39,* 1313–1319. doi:10.1080/09638288.2016.1194900

Dogra, S., Shah, S., Patel, M., & Tamim, H. (2015). Effectiveness of a tai chi intervention for improving functional fitness and general health among ethnically diverse older adults with self-reported arthritis living in low-income neighborhoods: A cohort study. *Journal of Geriatric Physical Therapy, 38*(2), 71–77.

Douglas, B., & Douglas, A. W. (2012). *The complete idiot's guide to t'ai chi & qigong illustrated.* New York, NY: Alpha.

Downs, L. B. (1992). Tai chi. *Modern Maturity, 35,* 60–64.

Figueroa, M. A., Demeersman, R. E., & Manning, J. (2012). The autonomic and rate pressure product responses of tai chi practitioners. *North American Journal of Medical Sciences, 4,* 270–275.

Gu, Q. (2011). *Chen style taijiquan 56 form for competition.* Hong Kong, China: Hong Kong Study Society.

Hosseini, H., Esfirizi, M. F., Marandi, S. M., & Rezaei, A. (2011). The effect of tai chi exercise on the sleep quality of the elderly residents in Isfahan, Sadeghieh, elderly home. *Iranian Journal of Nursing and Midwifery Research, 16,* 55–60.

Huang, A. (2011). *Complete tai-chi: The definitive guide to physical and emotional self-improvement.* North Clarendon, VT: Tuttle.

Hwang, H. F., Chen, S. J., Lee-Hsieh, J., Chien, D. K., Chen, C. Y., & Lin, M. R. (2016). Effects of home-based tai chi and lower extremity training and self-practice on falls and functional outcomes in older fallers from the emergency department: A randomized controlled trial. *Journal of the American Geriatrics Society, 64*(3), 518–525.

Irwin, M. R., & Olmstead, R. (2012). Mitigating cellular inflammation in older adults: A randomized controlled trial of tai chi chin. *American Journal of Geriatric Psychiatry, 20*(9), 764–772.

Koh, T. C. (1981). Tai chi chuan. *American Journal of Chinese Medicine, 9,* 15–22.

Li, F., Harmer, P., Fitzgerald, K., Eckstrom, E., Stock, R., Galver, J., . . . Batya, S. S. (2012). Tai chi and postural stability in patients with Parkinson's disease. *New England Journal of Medicine, 366,* 511–519.

Li, L., & Manor, B. (2010). Long term tai chi exercise improves physical performance among people with peripheral neuropathy. *American Journal of Chinese Medicine, 38*(3), 449–459.

Liang, S. Y., & Wu, W. C. (2014). *Simplified tai chi chuan: 24 postures with applications & standard 48 postures* (2nd ed.). Wolfeboro, NH: YMAA Publication Center.

Lin, S. F., Sung, H. C., Li, T. L., Hsieh, T. C., Lan, H. C., Perng, S. J., & Smith, G. D. (2015). The effects of tai-chi in conjunction with thera-band resistance exercise on functional fitness and muscle strength among community-based older people. *Journal of Clinical Nursing, 24,* 1357–1366.

Maciaszek, J., & Osinski, W. (2012). Effect of tai chi on body balance: Randomized controlled trial in elderly men with dizziness. *American Journal of Chinese Medicine, 40*(2), 245–253.

Merom, D., Pye, V., Macniven, R., van der Ploeg, H., Milat, A., Sherrington, C., . . . Bauman, A. (2012). Prevalence and correlates of participation in fall prevention exercise/physical activity by older adults. *Preventive Medicine, 55*(6), 613–617.

Moy, M. L., Wayne, P. M., Litrownik, D., Beach, D., Klings, E. S., Davis, R. B., & Yeh, G. Y. (2015). Long-term exercise after pulmonary rehabilitation (LEAP): Design and rationale of a randomized controlled trial of tai chi. *Contemporary Clinical Trials, 45,* 458–467.

Nery, R. M., Zanini, M., de Lima, J. B., Bühler, R. P., da Silveira, A. D., & Stein, R. (2015). Tai chi chuan improves functional capacity after myocardial infarction: A randomized clinical trial. *American Heart Journal, 169*(6), 854–860.

Nguyen, M. H., & Kruse, A. (2012). A randomized controlled trial of tai chi for balance, sleep quality and cognitive performance in elderly Vietnamese. *Clinical Interventions in Aging, 7,* 185–190.

Pan, L., Yan, J., Guo, Y., & Yan, J. (2013). Effects of tai chi training on exercise capacity and quality of life in patients with chronic heart failure: A meta-analysis. *European Journal of Heart Failure, 15*(3), 316–323. doi:10.1093/eurjhf/hfs170

Plummer, J. P. (1983). Acupuncture and tai chi chuan (Chinese shadow boxing): Body/mind therapies affecting homeostasis. In Y. Lau & J. P. Fowler (Eds.), *The scientific basis of traditional Chinese medicine: Selected papers* (pp. 22–36). Hong Kong, China: Medical Society.

Quarta, C. W., & Vallie, M. M. (2012). *Seated tai chi and qigong: Guided therapeutic exercises to manage stress and balance mind, body and spirit.* London, UK: Singing Dragon.

Schaller, K. J. (1996). Tai chi chih: An exercise option for older adults. *Journal of Gerontological Nursing, 22*(10), 12–17.

Song, R., Roberts, B. L., Lee, E. O., Lam, P., & Bae, S. C. (2010). A randomized study of the effects of tai chi on muscle strength, bone mineral density, and fear of falling in women with osteoarthritis. *Journal of Alternative and Complementary Medicine, 16,* 227–233.

Sun, J., & Buys, N. (2015). Community-based mind-body meditative tai chi program and its effects on improvement of blood pressure, weight, renal function, serum lipoprotein, and quality of life in Chinese adults with hypertension. *American Journal of Cardiology, 116*(7), 1076–1081.

Taylor-Piliae, R. E., Hoke, T. M., Hepworth, J. T., Latt, L. D., Najafi, B., & Coull, B. M. (2014). Effect of tai chi on physical function, fall rates and quality of life among older stroke survivors. *Archives of Physical Medicine and Rehabilitation, 95*(5), 816–824.

Tsai, P. F., Chang, J. Y., Beck, C., Kuo, Y. F., & Keefe, F. J. (2013). A pilot cluster-randomized trial of a 20-week tai chi program in elders with cognitive impairment and osteoarthritic knee: Effects on pain and other health outcomes. *Journal of Pain and Symptom Management, 45*(4), 660–669.

Wang, C. (2011). Tai chi and rheumatic diseases. *Rheumatic Diseases Clinics of North America, 37,* 19–32.

Wang, C. (2012). Role of tai chi in the treatment of rheumatologic diseases. *Current Rheumatology Reports, 14,* 598–603.

Wang, C., Schmid, C. H., Iversen, M. D., Harvey, W. F., Fielding, R. A., Driban, J. B., ... McAlindon, T. (2016). Comparative effectiveness of tai chi versus physical therapy for knee osteoarthritis. *Annals of Internal Medicine, 165*(2), 77–86.

Wayne, P. M., Berkowitz, D. L., Litrownik, D. E., Buring, J. E., & Yeh, G. Y. (2014). What do we really know about the safety of tai chi: A systematic review of adverse event reports in randomized trials. *Archives of Physical Medicine and Rehabilitation, 95*(12), 2470–2483.

Yang, J.-M. (2010). *Tai chi chuan classical yang style: The complete form qigong.* Wolfeboro, NH: Yang's Martial Arts Association.

Yang, J.-M., & Liang, T. T. (2016). *Tai chi chuan martial applications: Advanced yang style* (3rd ed.). Wolfeboro, NH: Ymaa Publication Center.

Yang, Y., Hao, Y.-L., Tian, W.-J., Gong, L., Zhang, K., Shi, Q.-G., ... Zhao, Z.-L. (2015). The effectiveness of tai chi for patients with Parkinson's disease: Study protocol for a randomized controlled trial. *Trials, 16,* 111. doi:10.1186/s13063-015-0639-8

Relaxation Therapies

Susan M. Bee, Elizabeth L. Pestka, and Michele M. Evans

Many people's lives are very stressful, so it is important to have techniques to help lower stress levels to maintain health. Relaxation therapies can be used to decrease stress by reducing muscle tension in the body. Relaxation therapies have been shown to manage stress, offer pain relief, and promote health. A great many relaxation therapies exist. The ones discussed in this chapter range from the simple and easily implemented diaphragmatic breathing (DB) to more complex methods such as progressive muscle relaxation (PMR) and autogenic training (AT). Using a combination of these therapies is common because they provide variety in terms of time to learn and to use. Evidence supporting the use of these strategies continues to grow, making them good options for health symptom management and promotion of wellness.

DEFINITION

Relaxation therapies help reduce the tension that exists in muscles, which often generalizes to other areas of the body, including the mind. Learning to relax can reduce the destructive effects and symptoms of stress-induced illnesses and improve a person's quality of life. Teaching patients relaxation techniques allows them to become more active partners in their healthcare.

Relaxed deep breathing or DB, uses the diaphragm when a breath is taken. The purpose of relaxed breathing is to slow breathing and to reduce the use of shoulder, neck, and upper chest muscles to breathe more efficiently, which improves oxygenation to the entire body. According to the National Center for Complementary and Integrative Health (NCCIH, 2016a), DB is the second most commonly used therapy.

PMR is the tensing and releasing of successive muscle groups. This treatment was introduced by Jacobson (1938) and is still used widely today. A person's attention is drawn to discriminating between the feelings experienced when a muscle group is relaxed and when it is tensed; eventually, the person is able to relax the muscles just by focusing on them. Progressive relaxation is one of the top-10 relaxation techniques people in the National Center for Health Statistics (NCHS) survey used (NCCIH, 2016a).

AT is a relaxation method that uses both imagery and body awareness to reduce stress and muscle tension. This technique was developed and published by the German neurologist Schultz (Schultz & Luthe, 1959) and addresses autonomic sensations that lead to muscle relaxation.

SCIENTIFIC BASIS

The aim of relaxation therapies is to reduce stress and the accompanying effects that stress has on the body. Real and perceived events and thoughts can create stress that activates the sympathetic nervous system. This begins a cascade of physical and chemical reactions. The heart pounds and blood pressure rises, respirations become shallow, pupils dilate, and the muscles tense as the body prepares to cope with the stressor. This is often called the *fight-or-flight* response. The parasympathetic nervous system is known as the rest-and-digest or rest-and-restore response. When one response is activated, the other is quiet. Prolonged activation of the sympathetic nervous system over time can have deleterious effects on the body. The desired outcome of relaxation strategies is the mitigation of persisting high levels of stress and activation of the parasympathetic nervous system.

When a person breathes, the body takes in oxygen and releases carbon dioxide. If the body detects an imbalance in these two gases, it signals for changes in breathing that may lead to fast, shallow breathing called *hyperventilation*, often in response to stressful events or pain. DB is a relaxation technique that uses the diaphragm to breathe deeply and improve oxygenation to the entire body. It is a learned skill, and practice is required for optimal benefit. Research from Schmidt, Joyner, Tonyan, Reid, and Hooten (2012) provides evidence that using DB for 10 minutes three times per day significantly reduces the self-rating of anxiety, depression, fatigue, sleep quality, and pain.

Jacobson (1938) reported that PMR decreased the body's oxygen consumption, metabolic rate, respiratory rate, muscle tension, premature ventricular contractions, and systolic and diastolic blood pressure and increased alpha brain waves. Subsequent studies, including that of Zhao et al. (2012), have validated Jacobson's findings, with results indicating a decrease in self-reported anxiety and depression and an increase in quality of life for women with endometriosis.

AT reduces excessive autonomic arousal, and it is effective in raising dysfunctionally low levels of autonomic functions such as a low heart rate. It is known as a self-regulatory model. AT may not only affect sympathetic tone, but may also activate the parasympathetic system. The increase in parasympathetic dominance results in peripheral vasodilation and increased feelings of warmth and heaviness in the body. An example of evidence supporting the use of AT to reduce stress is a study by Miu, Heilman, and Miclea (2009) that found heart rate volume and vagal control of the heart were positively impacted by the use of this therapy.

INTERVENTION

Relaxation means more than simply having peace of mind or resting. It means eliminating tension from the body and mind. Learning relaxation skills requires the person to focus on the mind–body connection, such as when muscles are tensed, and practice ways to relax the muscles to improve overall health and wellness.

Techniques

DB Technique

DB can be used before and during stressful situations, such as a painful procedure, or for overall health enhancement. It is a relatively simple relaxation technique that can be used in any healthcare setting and does not require extensive training of the instructor or the patient. The instructions for DB are found in Exhibit 17.1. Emphasis needs to be placed on the person practicing DB throughout the day until it becomes a natural way of breathing. For best effect, an individual should practice this technique frequently when neither anxious nor short of breath. Access naturalhealthperspective.com/resilience/deep-breathing.html for succinct information on DB.

PMR Technique

Numerous techniques for muscle relaxation have been developed since Jacobson published his technique in 1938. Often, the procedures include attention to breathing (Schaffer & Yucha, 2004). The instructor assists the individual in identifying a place that is quiet and restful in which to practice relaxation. A comfortable chair that provides support for the body is recommended. Clothing should be loose and not restrictive; shoes, glasses, and contact lenses should be removed. The person may wish to use the bathroom before practicing muscle relaxation.

The PMR therapy or variations of it, developed by Bernstein and Borkovec (1973) is widely used. They combined the 108 muscles and muscle groups of Jacobson's original technique into the initial tensing and relaxing of 16 muscle groups. Subsequently, the number of groups was reduced to seven and then four (Exhibit 17.2). Although Bernstein and Borkovec included instructions for tensing muscles of the feet, those are not included in Exhibit 17.2 because spasms in the foot may result when tensing these muscles. The ultimate goal is to achieve muscle relaxation throughout the body without initially having to tense the muscles. Through practice, the individual acquires a mental image of how the muscles feel when they are relaxed and is able to relax them using this image.

Exhibit 17.1. Instructions for Diaphragmatic (Deep) Breathing

1. Sit comfortably with feet flat on the floor
2. Loosen tight clothing around the abdomen and waist
3. Place hands in lap or at sides
4. Breathe in slowly (through nose if possible), allowing the abdomen to expand with inhalation
5. Exhale at the normal rate
6. Use pursed-lip breathing—which creates a very small opening between lips through which to breathe out—if desired

---

Exhibit 17.2.   Guidelines for Progressive Muscle Relaxation for 14 Muscle Groups

General Information

Instruct patients to tense a specific muscle group when they hear "tense" and to release the tension when they hear "relax." Tension is held for 7 seconds. Draw attention to the feeling of tension and relaxation. When muscles are relaxed, attention is drawn to the differences between the two states.

Tensing Specific Muscle Groups
- Dominant hand and forearm: Make a tight fist and hold it
- Dominant upper arm: Push elbow down against the arm of the chair
- Repeat instructions for the nondominant arm
- Forehead: Lift eyebrows as high as possible
- Central face (cheeks, nose, eyes): Squint eyes and wrinkle nose
- Lower face and jaw: Clench teeth and widen mouth
- Neck: Pull chin down toward chest but do not touch chest
- Chest, shoulders, and upper back: Take deep breath and hold it, pull shoulder blades back
- Abdomen: Pull stomach in and try to protect it
- Dominant thigh: Lift leg and hold it straight out
- Dominant calf: Point toes toward ceiling

Repeat instructions for the nondominant side.

Source: Adapted from Bernstein, D., & Borkovec, T. (1973). *Progressive relaxation training.* Champaign, IL: Research Press.

Education on the scientific basis for the use of PMR is provided during the first session. Stressors, the impact of stress on the body, and the signs and symptoms of high levels of stress are discussed. Descriptions and demonstrations for achieving tension of each muscle group are given, and participants then practice tensing each of the muscle groups.

After progressing through all the muscle groups, the instructor asks the patient to identify whether tension remains in any of them. The instructor observes the patient to assess for general relaxation, focusing on slowed, deeper breathing; arms relaxed and shoulders forward; and feet apart with toes pointing out. At the conclusion of the session, 2 or 3 minutes are provided for the patient to enjoy the feelings associated with relaxation. Terminating relaxation is done gradually. The instructor counts backward from four to one. The individual is given the opportunity to ask questions or discuss the feelings experienced.

Bernstein and Borkovec (1973) proposed using 10 sessions to teach PMR. However, in many studies, instruction has been limited to fewer sessions with positive results obtained. A critical factor in determining the number of teaching sessions needed is ensuring that people have mastered relaxing the muscle groups and have integrated PMR into their lifestyles.

An essential factor in the effectiveness of PMR and other relaxation techniques is daily practice. At least one 15-minute practice session a day is recommended.

Schaffer and Yucha (2004) suggest two 10-minute sessions. Helping patients find a time of day to practice relaxation is an important component of instruction. Often, an audiotape of the instructions is provided for home practice. Patients are also instructed to use the relaxation technique anytime they feel tense or before an event that may cause them to become anxious and tense. Refer to www.guidetopsychology.com/pmr.htm for comprehensive instructions on PMR.

Autogenic Training

AT is a relaxation method that is self-generated or self-guided using relaxation phases. A healthcare provider familiar with the therapy can provide assistance with learning the method. AT is gaining in worldwide use and is intended to create a feeling of warmth and heaviness throughout the body while a profound state of physical relaxation, bodily health, and mental health are experienced. AT is most effective when done in a quiet place while wearing loose clothing and not wearing shoes. Practice should be done at a time when the individual has not recently eaten a large meal. The person focuses intently on inner experiences and excludes external events. When the session finishes, people relax with their eyes closed for a few seconds and then get up slowly. Instructions for self-guided AT are given in Exhibit 17.3. Refer to www.guidetopsychology.com/autogen.htm for an example of in-depth instructions on phases to be used for relaxation. To maintain proficiency, practicing at least once a day is recommended.

Measurement of Outcomes

Although findings from many studies have shown positive outcomes from the use of relaxation techniques, positive results have not been reported in all the research in which these therapies were explored. Reasons for the differences in outcomes may relate to the wide variation in the types of relaxation techniques, the length and type of instruction, the degree of mastery of the therapy, and irregular or sporadic use of the procedures.

Exhibit 17.3. Instructions for Self-Guided AT

AT consists of a warm-up period of breathing and progressively learning six phases of relaxation that all together may take several months to fully master. On completion, a person will progress through and include:

- *Warm-up:* Focused breathing on slow exhalation
- *Phase 1:* Heaviness—arms and legs are heavy
- *Phase 2:* Warmth—arms and legs are warm
- *Phase 3:* A calm heart—heartbeat is calm
- *Phase 4:* Breathing—breathing is steady
- *Phase 5:* Stomach—stomach is soft and warm
- *Phase 6:* Cool forehead—forehead is cool
- *Completion:* Feel supremely calm

A variety of outcomes have been used to measure the efficacy of relaxation techniques. Physiological measurements that are often used include respiratory rate, heart rate, and blood pressure. Electromyogram readings are occasionally taken to determine the degree of tension in the specific muscle groups. Practitioners need to be alert to underlying pathology or medications that may interfere with reduction in physiological parameters.

Anxiety is the most frequently used subjective measure. The State-Trait Anxiety Inventory (STAI) Scale of Spielberger, Gorsuch, Luschene, Vagg, and Jacobs (1983) has been widely used. People's self-reports about feelings of relaxation have been included in many studies because satisfaction is a good indicator of whether an individual will continue to use an intervention. Reports of reduction of pain, symptoms of depression, increases in comfort, and improved sleep are other results that have been used to measure the effects of these techniques.

PRECAUTIONS

Although muscle-relaxation techniques have been used with multiple populations and have been proved to be an effective therapy for nurses to use, some cautions should be observed. It is important for practitioners to know whether patients practice the relaxation techniques on a regular basis because this may affect the pharmacokinetics of medications. Adjustment in doses of medication for hypertension, diabetes, and seizures may be indicated.

Relaxation of muscles may produce a hypotensive state. People are instructed to remain seated for a few minutes after practice. Movement in place and gradual resumption of activities helps raise the blood pressure. Taking a person's blood pressure at the conclusion of teaching sessions helps in identifying those who are prone to hypotensive states after muscle relaxation and AT because the relaxation therapy may have caused hypotension.

Some individuals with chronic pain have reported a heightened awareness of pain following the tensing and relaxing of muscles. Concentrating on tensing and relaxing muscles may draw attention to the pain rather than to the muscle sensation. A good assessment of patients is needed to determine whether negative outcomes are occurring.

Children younger than school age lack the discipline to do AT. Also, those with limited mental ability, acute central nervous system disorders, or uncontrolled psychosis may be unable to process the in-depth instructions (Linden, 2007). In some patients, AT may produce the side effects of anxiety, sadness, resurfaced memories and suppressed thoughts, or reawakened pain sensation from old illnesses or injuries. These effects may stem from disinhibition of various cortical processes due to the autogenic formulas and the focus on body sensations (Lehrer, 2009).

USES

Promoting an understanding of the anticipated positive benefits of the therapies is critical. Relaxation therapies have been used to achieve a variety of outcomes in diverse populations. Exhibit 17.4 lists conditions and populations, including the country in which the research was conducted, showing widespread use of these therapies. The use of DB, PMR, and AT in reduction of anxiety and stress, relief of

Exhibit 17.4.   Selected Studies Supporting Use of Therapies

Therapy	Health Condition	Study Authors	Country of Study
DB	Chronic pain and fibromyalgia	Busch et al. (2012)	Germany
		Schmidt, Hooten, Kerkvliet, Reid, and Joyner (2008)	United States
			United States
		Schmidt et al. (2012)	
DB	Anxiety	Chen, Huang, and Chen et al. (2012)	Taiwan
DB	Type 2 diabetes mellitus	Hedge et al. (2012)	India
DB	Pain and anxiety during burn care	E. Park, Oh, and Kim (2013)	South Korea
DB	Coronary heart disease	Chung et al. (2010)	Taiwan
DB	Chronic obstructive pulmonary disease	Yamaguti et al. (2012)	Brazil
DB	Gastroesophageal reflux disease	Eherer et al. (2012)	Austria
DB	Dysfunctional voiding (with children)	Zivkovic et al. (2012)	Serbia
DB and PMR	Multiple sclerosis	Artemiadis et al. (2012)	Greece
	Irritable bowel syndrome	S. Park, Han, and Kang (2014)	South Korea
			Iran
	Hypertension during pregnancy	Aalami, Jafarnejad, Modarres, and Gharavi (2016)	
PMR with music	Low back pain with pregnancy	Akmese and Oran (2014)	Turkey
PMR with guided imagery	Cancer (decreasing nausea and vomiting, pain, and depression)	Charalambous et al. (2016)	India
PMR	Chronic obstructive pulmonary disease	Sahin and Dayapoglu (2015)	Turkey

(continued)

Therapy	Health Condition	Study Authors	Country of Study
PMR	Night eating syndrome	Vander Wal, Maraldo, Vercellone, and Gagne (2015)	United States
PMR	Depression in females with multiple sclerosis	Safi (2015)	Iran
PMR	Migraine headaches	Meyer et al. (2016)	Germany
PMR	Pain and anxiety in older patients undergoing abdominal surgery	Rejeh, Heravi-Karimooi, Vaismoradi, and Jasper (2013)	Iran
PMR	Ectopic pregnancy	Pan, Zhang, and Li (2012)	China
PMR	Endometriosis	Zhao et al. (2012)	China
PMR	Schizophrenia	Melo-Dias, Apostolo, and Cardoso (2014)	Portugal
AT	Chest pain	Asbury, Kanji, Ernst, Barbir, and Collins (2009)	United Kingdom
AT	Psychiatric diagnoses (mood disorders, anxiety, and psychosis)	Malhotra et al. (2013)	India
AT	Poststroke anxiety	Golding, Kneebone, and Fife-Schaw (2016)	United Kingdom
AT	Anxiety disorder	Miu et al. (2009)	Netherlands
AT	Insomnia	Bowden, Lorenc, and Robinson (2012)	United Kingdom
AT	Chronic subjective dizziness	Goto, Tsutsumi, Kabeya, and Ogawa (2012)	Japan
AT	Breastfeeding	Vidas, Folnegovic-Smalc, Catipovic, and Kisic (2011)	Croatia
AT	Irritable bowel syndrome	Shinozaki et al. (2010)	Japan

AT, autogenic training; DB, diaphragmatic breathing; PMR, progressive muscle relaxation.

pain, and health promotion are discussed. As noted in the list of uses, studies have been carried out worldwide. Sidebar 17.1 describes how these relaxation therapies are used in the Republic of Singapore.

Reduction of Anxiety and Stress

As noted in Exhibit 17.4, these therapies have been effective in reducing the stress associated with a number of conditions. DB training significantly lowered anxiety measures in an experimental group of 51 participants in China (Chen et al., 2012). Golding et al. (2016) reported a reduction in anxiety scores using AT with post stroke patients. Miu et al. (2009) found that AT increased heart rate variability and facilitated vagal control of the heart, reducing symptoms of anxiety. Relaxation techniques can be used both to decrease and to prevent stress, which is a risk factor for many health conditions.

Cultural Applications

Almost every culture has therapies for reducing stress. These include the use of various herbal preparations or potions, use of muscle exercises such as yoga, or spiritual practices. The three relaxation therapies described in this chapter or variations of them are commonly used in a number of cultures. Sidebar 17.1 describes therapies used in Singapore.

SIDEBAR 17.1. USE OF RELAXATION THERAPIES IN THE REPUBLIC OF SINGAPORE

Siok-Bee Tan

In Singapore, relaxation techniques may be taught by nurses, psychologists, therapists, or other health professionals. Not a substantial number of practitioners use these strategies. At present, most nurses working in Singapore hospitals who use relaxation techniques employ deep diaphragmatic breathing. Fewer nurses use progressive muscle relaxation and autogenic training because a minority has been trained in these techniques and because these therapies are not suited to a fast-paced hospital environment. Nevertheless, in the mental health institutions, relaxation techniques are more widely used. In outpatient areas the relaxation techniques can also be better utilized. For example, nurses who attend the Chronic Disease Management Workshop teach both deep diaphragmatic breathing and progressive muscle relaxation.

Siok-Bee is an advanced practice nurse in Singapore, who uses a combination of medical, nursing, and therapy models in clinical care. She specializes in helping patients who have intractable pain and chronic neurological conditions by utilizing various relaxation techniques. Techniques are important, but

(continued)

it is also crucial to ensure that rapport is established first, for success of the relaxation therapies. For example, in the practice of autogenic training, the key is to access the subconscious mind with relaxation. This requires considerable time and discipline to learn. In a culture where patients mostly prescribe to medication and surgery, it is a challenge to get patients to adopt the technique for relaxation. With rapport, patients have the trust to commit their time to practice and, in turn, be able to bypass the critical factor of the conscious mind to access the subconscious mind to install the positive suggestions. Dr. Siok-Bee has successfully empowered many patients in using the healing powers of the mind as they get into a trance state during autogenic training.

It would be prudent to enable a greater number of nurses in Singapore to complete training in relaxation therapies, not only for the financial savings it may provide by shortening hospital stays, but also for the benefits it provides to patients by equipping them with tools to manage anxiety and concerns at home. However, there is a need to have a shift in the hospital culture for relaxation techniques to be fully used. Relaxation techniques must be viewed as advancement in pain and anxiety care and must be given an opportunity to be implemented by health professionals. The hospital culture in Singapore is focused on medication or surgery. However, there is some hope because mind–body interventions are slowly gaining entry into mainly medically dominated treatment. Patient care will be optimal if more healthcare professionals are willing to use complementary techniques as part of the recovery regimen.

Work-related demands result in poor health and well-being for a substantial number of nurses, which leads to increased absenteeism, high attrition, and reduced performance. Their stress also affects their working relationship with fellow nursing staff, their interactions with patients, and therefore, their delivery of care. Thus, nursing management in Singapore has explored ways to enable nurses to embrace tools of self-care that will promote resiliency in their work environment, such as mindfulness and deep breathing practices and strategies. Mindfulness is increasingly gaining recognition as a tool for improving care, competence, and compassion among healthcare practitioners and, as a result, their patients. The practice of mindfulness cultivates the ability to purposefully focus one's attention on internal experiences, as well as interaction with the external environment, and to view these experiences more objectively, accepting them without judgment.

Nursing management in one Singapore hospital engaged a psychologist to conduct an introductory mindfulness and deep-breathing program for nurse leaders. This psychologist also supports new nurses and leaders during orientation programs. The psychologist has also facilitated a 5-week mindfulness and deep-breathing course, 2 hours each session, with a group of 16 nurses. This course aimed to prepare nurse trainers, who will then facilitate courses for other nurses within their clinical areas.

Nurses who attended the program reported positive impact of mindfulness and its benefits applied to the context of their daily lives at home and at work. They were motivated to continue their practice after the end of the program. The hospital in Singapore hopes to form a culture that will promote the ongoing practice of mindfulness and deep breathing. There is a vision of creating a culture shift to an environment full of empathy, compassion, and kindness.

Although relaxation strategies are helpful in reducing stress and anxiety in many conditions, it is important to note that these interventions alone may not be the most effective treatment for generalized anxiety disorder. According to the NCCIH (2016b) website, a cognitive behavioral approach is found to be the most helpful for this condition.

Pain

Relaxation therapies have been used extensively in the management of many types of pain. Muscle tension increases the perception of pain, so lessening anxiety and tension may help in reducing it. Schmidt et al. (2008) reported that three 10-minute DB sessions each day in patients with chronic pain were associated with significant changes in a number of areas of physiological and psychological functioning. Results indicated significant improvements in fatigue, pain management, and self-efficacy and changes in pain severity. Mean pain severity scores changed from 4.56 to 3.78 (p <.05) on a 0-to-10 rating scale. Further supporting research by Schmidt et al. (2012) with patients with fibromyalgia found that the use of three 10-minute daily DB sessions showed significant improvements in pain severity, fatigue, pain self-efficacy, cold pressor tolerance, and heart rate variability in measurements 2 weeks apart. Significant reduction in pain levels were found in patients with burns using DB (E. Park et al., 2013) AT was used with 21 patients with irritable bowel syndrome, with results indicating a significant decrease in the rating of bodily pain (Shinozaki et al., 2010). In a 6-week PMR program, migraine headache frequency was significantly decreased. PMR was suggested to operate by enhancing self-efficacy in managing headaches and reducing associated pain episodes (Meyer et al., 2016).

Health Promotion

Nursing has been at the forefront in teaching patients about health-promotion practices. Reducing and managing stress is an important preventive health strategy, and these therapies can be used for reducing risks for numerous conditions. Although relaxation therapies may not reduce heart rate and blood pressure in those who have readings within the normal range, use of these techniques on a regular basis by healthy people may help to prevent the development of hypertension. PMR and DB were found to decrease both systolic and diastolic blood pressure in pregnant women (Aalami et al., 2016). Sleep is essential for overall health; Bowden et al. (2012) found that the use of AT resulted in significant improvement in sleep-onset latency and stated that study participants (N = 153) with insomnia reported feeling more refreshed and energized. Those with type II diabetes mellitus responded positively to DB, with significant reductions in fasting and postprandial plasma glucose and glycated hemoglobin levels (Hedge et al., 2012). This therapy may have the potential to be a preventive measure for a condition that is increasing in the United States.

There is considerable interest in promoting more independence for individuals to maintain their health and wellness. The relaxation strategies of DB, PMR, and AT are ways to relax the body and move from the sympathetic response of fight or flight into a calmer parasympathetic response. As interest in these methods has grown, the number of electronic applications and resources to instruct and support their use has also expanded. Healthcare providers may recommend various independent resources on the internet and mobile devices but must ensure the scientific integrity of the sources before making a recommendation.

FUTURE RESEARCH

Relaxation therapies discussed in this chapter have been used singly and in combination with other therapies to reduce and prevent stress. A scientific body of knowledge is emerging to guide the use of these techniques in practice, but more research is necessary. The following are several areas in which studies are needed:

- Many of the studies have been completed with relatively small samples. Replication with larger sample sizes will provide greater support for these interventions.
- Clinical evidence for the feasibility and effectiveness of mobile devices for learning and using relaxation therapies presents an important research opportunity (Blodt, Pach, Roll, & Wilt, 2014).
- As the focus of healthcare becomes more individualized, it is important to identify relaxation therapies most likely to be effective for people based on their genetic information, cultural background, and lifestyle preferences. Studies connecting phenotype with genotype will be informative.
- More research concentrating on using these therapies for health promotion and disease prevention in primary care settings may help improve the delivery of healthcare. Studies focusing on healthcare cost savings related to the use of relaxation strategies will be beneficial.

REFERENCES

Aalami, M., Jafarnejad, F., & ModarresGharavi, M. (2016). The effects of progressive muscular relaxation and breathing control technique on blood pressure during pregnancy. *Iranian Journal of Nursing and Midwifery Research, 21*(3), 331–336.

Akmese, Z., & Oran, N. (2014). Effects of progressive muscle relaxation exercises accompanied by music on low back pain and quality of life during pregnancy. *Journal of Midwifery & Women's Health, 59*(5), 503–509.

Artemiadis, A., Vervainioti, A., Alexopoulos, E., Rombos, A., Anagnostouli, M., & Darviri, C. (2012). Stress management and multiple sclerosis: A randomized controlled trial. *Archives of Clinical Neuropsychology, 27*, 406–416.

Asbury, E., Kanji, N., Ernst, E., Barbir, M., & Collins, P. (2009). Autogenic training to manage symptomatology in women with chest pain and normal coronary arteries. *Menopause, 16*(1), 1–6.

Bernstein, D., & Borkovec, T. (1973). *Progressive relaxation training.* Champaign, IL: Research Press.

Blodt, S., Pach, D., Roll, S., & Witt, C. (2014). Effectiveness of app-based relaxation for patients with chronic low back pain (Relaxback) and chronic neck pain (Relaxneck): Study protocol for two randomized pragmatic trials. *Trials, 15*, 490 doi:10.1186/1745-6215-15-490

Bowden, A., Lorenc, A., & Robinson, N. (2012). Autogenic training as a behavioural approach to insomnia: A prospective cohort study. *Primary Health Care Research & Development, 13*(2), 175–185.

Busch, V., Magert, W., Kern, U., Haas, J., Hajak, G., & Eichhammer, P. (2012). The effect of deep slow breathing on pain perception, autonomic activity, and mood processing–An experimental study. *Pain Medicine, 13*, 215–228.

Charalambous, A., Giannakopoulou, M., Bozas, E., Marcou, Y., Kitsios, P., & Paikousis, L. (2016). Guided imagery and progressive muscle relaxation as a cluster of symptoms management intervention in patients receiving chemotherapy: A randomized control trial. *PLOS ONE, 11*, e0156911. doi:10.1371/journal.pone0156911

Chen, Y., Huang, X., & Chen, C. (2012, July–August). *Performance of 10-minutes of diaphragmatic breathing relaxation training in relieving in outpatients and accompanied relatives.* Paper presented at Sigma Theta Tau 23rd International Nursing Research Congress, Brisbane, Australia.

Chung, L., Tsai, P., Liu, B., Chou, K., Lin, W., Shyu, Y., & Wang, M. (2010). Home based deep breathing for depression in patients with coronary heart disease: A randomized controlled trial. *International Journal of Nursing Studies, 47*, 1346–1353.

Eherer, A., Netolitzky, F., Hogenauer, C., Puschnig, G., Hinterleitner, T., Schneidl, S., … Hoffmann, K. (2012). Positive effect of abdominal breathing exercise on gastroesophageal reflux disease: A randomized, controlled study. *American Journal of Gastroenterology, 107*(3), 372–378.

Golding, K., Kneebone, I., & Fife-Schaw, C. (2016). Self-help relaxation for post-stroke anxiety: A randomized, controlled pilot study. *Clinical Rehabilitation, 30*(2), 174–180.

Goto, F., Tsutsumi, T., Kabeya, M., & Ogawa, K. (2012). Outcomes of autogenic training for patients with chronic subjective dizziness. *Journal of Psychosomatic Research, 72*(5), 410–411.

Hedge, S., Adhikari, P., Subbalakshmi, N., Nandini, M., Rao, G., & D'Souza, V. (2012). Diaphragmatic breathing exercise as a therapeutic intervention for control of oxidative stress in type 2 diabetes mellitus. *Complementary Therapies in Clinical Practice, 18*, 151–153.

Jacobson, E. (1938). *Progressive relaxation.* Chicago, IL: University of Chicago Press.

Lehrer, P. (2009). In L. Freeman (Ed.), Relaxation therapies (p. 148–150) In *Mosby's complementary and alternative medicine: A research-based approach* (3rd ed.). St. Louis, MO: Mosby Elsevier.

Linden, W. (2007). *Autogenic training.* New York, NY: Guilford Press.

Malhotra, S., Chakrabarti, S., Gupta, A., Mehta, A., Shah, R., Kumar, V., & Sharma, M. (2013). A self-guided relaxation module for telepsychiatric services: Development, usefulness, and feasibility. *International Journal Psychiatry in Medicine, 46*(4), 325–337.

Melo-Dias, C., Apostolo, J., & Cardoso, D. (2014). Effectiveness of progressive muscle relaxation training for adults diagnosed with schizophrenia: A systematic review protocol. *JBI Database of Systematic Reviews & Implementation Reports, 12*(10), 85–97.

Meyer, B., Keller, A., Wohlbier, H., Overath, C., Muller, B., & Krupp, P. (2016). Progressive muscle relaxation reduces migraine frequency and normalizes amplitudes of contingent negative variation (CNV). *J Headache Pain, 17*, 37. doi:10.1186/s10194-016-0630-0

Miu, A. C., Heilman, R. M., & Miclea, M. (2009). Reduced heart rate variability and vagal tone in anxiety; trait versus state, and the effects of autogenic training. *Autonomic Neuroscience-Basic & Clinical, 145*(1/2), 99–103.

National Center for Complementary and Integrative Health. (2016a). *NCCIH facts-at-a-glance and mission.* Retrieved from https://nccih.nih.gov/about/ataglance

National Center for Complementary and Integrative Health. (2016b). Relaxation techniques for health. Retrieved from https://nccih.nih.gov/health/stress/relaxation.htm

Pan, L., Zhang, J., & Li, L. (2012). Effects of progressive muscle relaxation training on anxiety and quality of life of inpatients with ectopic pregnancy receiving methotrexate treatment. *Research in Nursing & Health, 35*, 376–382.

Park, E., Oh, H., & Kim, T. (2013). The effects of relaxation breathing on procedural pain and anxiety during burn care. *Burns, 39*, 1101–1106. Retrieved from http://www.elsevier.com/locate/burns

Park, S., Han, K., & Kang, C. (2014). Relaxation therapy for irritable bowel syndrome: A systematic review. *Asian Nursing Research, 8*, 182–192.

Rejeh, N., Heravi-Karimooi, M., Vaismoradi, M., & Jasper, M. (2013). Effect of systematic relaxation techniques on pain and anxiety in older patients undergoing abdominal surgery. *International Journal of Nursing Practice, 19*(5), 462–470.

Safi, S. Z. (2015). A fresh look at the potential mechanisms of progressive muscle relaxation therapy on depression in female patients with multiple sclerosis. *Iranian Journal of Psychiatry and Behavioral Sciences, 9*, e340. doi:10.17795/ijpbs340

Sahin, Z., & Dayapoglu, N. (2015). Effect of progressive relaxation exercises on fatigue and sleep quality in patients with chronic obstructive lung disease (COPD). *Complimentary Therapies in Clinical Practice, 21*, 277–281.

Schaffer, S. D., & Yucha, C. B. (2004). Relaxation & pain management: The relaxation response can play a role in managing chronic and acute pain. *American Journal of Nursing, 104*(8), 75–82.

Schmidt, J., Hooten, W., Kerkvliet, J., Reid, K., & Joyner, M. (2008). Psychological and physiological correlates of a brief intervention to enhance self-regulation in chronic pain [Abstract]. *Journal of Pain, 9*(4), 55.

Schmidt, J., Joyner, M., Tonyan, H., Reid, K., & Hooten, W. (2012). Psychological and physiological correlates of a brief intervention to enhance self-regulation in patients with fibromyalgia. *Journal of Musculoskeletal Pain, 20*(3), 211–221.

Schultz, J. H., & Luthe, W. (1959). *Autogenic training: A psycho-physiological approach in psychotherapy*. New York, NY: Grune & Stratton.

Shinozaki, M., Kanazawa, M., Kano, M., Endo, Y., Nakaya, N., Hongo, M., & Fukudo, S. (2010). Effect of autogenic training on general improvement in patients with irritable bowel syndrome: A randomized controlled trial. *Applied Psychophysiology & Biofeedback, 35*(3), 189–198.

Spielberger, C., Gorsuch, R., Luschene, R., Vagg, P., & Jacobs, G. (1983). *Manual for STAI*. Palo Alto, CA: Consulting Psychological Press.

Vander Wal, J., Maraldo T., Vercellone, A., & Gagne, D. (2015). Education, progressive muscle relaxation therapy, and exercise for the treatment of night eating syndrome: A pilot study. *Appetite, 89*, 136–144.

Vidas, M., Folnegovic-Smalc, V., Catipovic, M., & Kisic, M. (2011). The application of autogenic training in counseling center for mother and child in order to promote breastfeeding. *Collegium Antropologicum, 35*(3), 723–731.

Yamaguti, W., Claudino, R., Neto, A., Chammas, M., Gomes, A., Salge, J., ... Carvalho, C. (2012). Diaphragmatic breathing training program improves abdominal motion during natural breathing in patients with chronic obstructive pulmonary disease: A randomized controlled trial. *Archives of Physical Medicine and Rehabilitation, 93*, 571–577.

Zhao, L., Wu, H., Zhou, X., Wang, Q., Zhu, W., & Chen, J. (2012). Effects of progressive muscular relaxation training on anxiety, depression and quality of life of endometriosis patients under gonadotrophin-releasing hormone agonist therapy. *European Journal of Obstetrics & Gynecology and Reproductive Biology, 162*, 211–215.

Zivkovic, V., Lazovic, M., Vlajkovic, M., Slavkovic, A., Dimitrijevic, L., Stonkovic, I., & Vacic, N. (2012). Diaphragmatic breathing exercises and pelvic floor retraining in children with dysfunctional voiding. *European Journal of Physical Rehabilitation Medicine, 48*(3), 413–421.

Exercise

DERECK L. SALISBURY, DIANE TREAT-JACOBSON, ULF G. BRONÄS,
AND RYAN J. MAYS

Exercise is well-recognized as a lifelong endeavor essential for energetic, active, and healthy living. In large, longitudinal studies, it has been established that morbidity and mortality are reduced in physically fit individuals compared with sedentary individuals (Samitz, Egger, & Zwahlen, 2011). Although the research supporting the benefits of exercise is substantial, it is often overlooked in the practice of conventional Western medicine.

Exercise, either alone or as an alternative or complementary therapy, has been linked to many positive physiological and psychological responses, from reduction in the stress response to an increased sense of well-being (Ehrman, Gordon, Visich, & Keteyian, 2013). Surprisingly, despite the tremendous benefits of exercise, it is an activity that is largely ignored by the general population. In 1996, the U.S. Surgeon General (USSG, 1996) issued a report identifying millions of inactive Americans as being at risk for a wide range of chronic diseases and ailments, including coronary heart disease (CHD), adult-onset diabetes, colon cancer, hip fractures, hypertension, and obesity. In 2007, the American Heart Association (AHA) and the American College of Sports Medicine (ACSM) issued several updates (Haskell et al., 2007; Nelson et al., 2007; Williams et al., 2007) to the USSG's 1996 guidelines. This was followed in 2008 by a report and revised guidelines from the U.S. Department of Health and Human Services (USDHHS) Physical Activity Advisory Committee (USDHHS-PAAC, 2008), and again in 2011 by the ACSM (Garber et al., 2011).

The USDHHS publication *Healthy People 2020* (USDHHS-PAAC, 2008) continues to specify several objectives for improving health, including physical activity and exercise. These include reducing the percentage of adults who do not participate in any physical activity; increasing the percentage of adults who engage in moderate physical activity on most days of the week; and increasing the percentage of adults participating in vigorous exercise, as well as exercise to improve strength and flexibility. The physical activity objectives in *Healthy People 2020* reflect the strong state of science supporting the health benefit of exercise as indicated by the USDHHS-PAAC (2008). There are additional objectives related to physical activity and exercise habits of children and adolescents, including goals to increase participation in daily school physical education classes, increase physical activity in childcare settings, and reduce television and computer use. The alarmingly low percentage of children participating in physical activity in school and outside of school (less than 27%) is reportedly contributing to the nation's growing childhood obesity problem (National Research Council, 2011).

It is important to recognize the role of exercise as a component of good health. Exercise *must* be an integral part of one's personal lifestyle if it is to have optimal effects. Maintaining physical fitness should be enjoyable and rewarding for people of all ages and can contribute significantly to extending longevity and improving quality of life (Kodoma et al., 2009; Slawinska, Posluszny, & Rozek, 2013). Nurses' knowledge of exercise and its application in multiple populations assists in the delivery of expert nursing care. This chapter discusses the definition, physiological basis, and application of exercise as a nursing intervention in a variety of populations, along with specific cultural applications.

DEFINITION

Physical activity is defined as "any bodily movement produced by skeletal muscles that results in caloric expenditure" (ACSM, 2017). Definitions of exercise are complex and vary according to the scientific discipline; however, they all incorporate physical activity into their descriptions. Exercise is commonly considered to be a planned, recurring subset of physical activity that results in improved physical fitness, a term used to describe cardiorespiratory fitness, muscle strength, body composition, and flexibility related to the ability of a person to perform physical activity (Thompson et al., 2003).

Exercise is commonly classified according to the rate of energy expenditure, which is expressed in either absolute terms as metabolic equivalents of task (METs) or in relative terms according to what percentage of maximal heart rate or maximal oxygen consumption (VO_2) is achieved (Astrand, Rodahl, Dahl, & Stromme, 2004; Thompson et al., 2003). Exercise is aerobic when the energy demand by the working muscles is supplied by aerobic adenosine triphosphate (ATP) production as allowed by inspired oxygen and mitochondrial enzymatic capacity (Astrand et al., 2004). In general, aerobic exercise increases demand on the respiratory, cardiovascular, and musculoskeletal systems. Sustained periods of work require aerobic metabolism of energy at a level compatible with the body's oxygen supply capabilities (i.e., oxygen uptake equals oxygen requirements of the tissues). *Anaerobic exercise* is the term used when energy demand exceeds what the body is able to produce through the aerobic process or when the body is performing short bursts of high-intensity exercise, such as in resistance and sprint training (Astrand et al., 2004).

SCIENTIFIC BASIS

Better understanding of exercise physiology and the body's response to various stages of physical activity assists in the development of exercise programs appropriate for the individual and the goal of the exercise training session. The response of the body to exercise occurs in stages. The initial response to acute exercise is a withdrawal of parasympathetic stimulation of the heart through the vagus nerve. This results in a rapid increase in heart rate (HR) and cardiac output (Tipton, Sawka, Tate, & Terjung, 2006). The sympathetic stimulation occurs more slowly and becomes a dominant factor once HR is above approximately 100 beats per minute. Sympathetic stimulation is fully completed after approximately 10 to 20 seconds, during which time a large sympathetic outburst occurs and the heart overshoots the rate needed but then returns to the rate required for increased activity.

The brain stimulates the initial cardiovascular response together with impulses from muscles being exercised, and these impulses are sent to the brain; an increase in HR is initiated and the blood flow is shunted toward the exercising muscles (Astrand et al., 2004). During this phase, there is a slow adjustment of respiration and circulation, resulting in an oxygen deficit; the initial energy needed by the exercising tissue is fueled mainly by the anaerobic metabolism of creatine phosphate and anaerobic glycolysis (Jones & Poole, 2005).

As exercise continues, VO_2 increases in a linear fashion in relation to the intensity of exercise. The increase in VO_2 is caused by an increase in oxygen extraction by the working muscles and an increase in cardiac output. Oxygen extraction by the working muscle tissues is approximately 80% to 85%, or a threefold increase from rest, in sedentary and moderately active individuals. This is caused by an increase in the number of open capillaries, thereby reducing diffusion distances and increasing capillary blood volume (Fletcher et al., 2001). Cardiac output is increased to meet the increased oxygen demands of the working muscle. The increase in cardiac output is caused by increased stroke volume, which is due to an increase in ventricular filling pressure brought on by increased venous return and decreased peripheral resistance offered by the exercising muscles. Together with the withdrawal of parasympathetic stimulation and increases in sympathetic stimulation, the increase in HR further accentuates the increase in cardiac output, as well as increased myocardial contractility (from positive inotropic sympathetic impulses to the heart) (Astrand et al., 2004). In normal individuals, cardiac output can increase four to five times, allowing for increased delivery of oxygen to exercising muscle beds and facilitating removal of lactate, CO_2, and heat. Respiration increases to deliver oxygen and to allow for elimination of CO_2. Blood pressure (BP) increases as a result of increased cardiac output and the sympathetic vasoconstriction of vessels in the nonexercising muscles, viscera, and skin. During this "steady state" exercise phase, oxygen uptake equals oxygen tissue requirement, aerobic metabolism of glucose and fatty acids occurs, and there is no accumulation of lactic acid (Tipton et al., 2006).

As exercise becomes more strenuous, there is a shift toward anaerobic metabolism, resulting in increased production of lactic acid (Tipton et al., 2006). The anaerobic threshold is a point during exercise at which ventilation abruptly increases despite linear increases in work rate (Beaver, Wasserman, & Whipp, 1986). As exercise goes beyond steady state, the oxygen supply does not meet the oxygen requirement, and energy is provided through anaerobic glycolysis and creatine phosphate breakdown. This increases proton release and phosphate accumulation, increasing acidosis (Robergs, Ghiasvand, & Parker, 2004; Westerblad, Allen, & Lannergren, 2002). Shortly beyond the anaerobic threshold, fatigue and dyspnea ensue and work ceases, coinciding with a significant drop in blood glucose levels. The breathlessness that coincides with maximal exertion is not the limiting factor of aerobic exercise performance in healthy adults. Exercise at a level that allows for a greater contribution of energy via aerobic metabolism and less involvement of the anaerobic system (and hence glucose as the primary fuel) may delay onset of these biochemical fatigue-inducing changes.

Following cessation of exercise, there is a period of rapid decline in oxygen uptake, followed by a slow decline toward resting levels. This slow phase of oxygen uptake return is called *excess postexercise* VO_2 (LaForgia, Withers, & Gore, 2006). During this period, the body attempts to resynthesize used creatine phosphate, remove lactate, restore muscle and blood oxygen stores, decrease body temperature, return to resting levels of HR and BP, and lower circulating catecholamines (Astrand et al., 2004). It is important to facilitate this phase of exercise by performing a 5- to 10-minute cool-down.

Tools for Monitoring the Intervention

Prior to a thorough description of the evidence-based recommendations in regard to the intervention, terminology commonly used in monitoring the intervention should be defined. Exercising individuals should monitor the response of their bodies to the activity to ensure that the intensity is appropriate (Table 18.1). This can be done in several ways, including monitoring target HR, rating of perceived exertion (RPE), and applying the talk test.

Table 18.1.   Monitoring Levels of Exercise

Intensity	% HR Method	% HRR	RPE
Light	57–<64	30–<40	9–11
Moderate	64–<76	40–60	12–13
Vigorous	>76	>60	14+

HR, heart rate; HRR, heart rate reserve; HR method: target HR, $HR_{max/peak}$ (intensity); RPE, rating of perceived exertion.

Note: HRR method: target heart rate ($HR_{max/peak} - HR_{rest}$) × (% intensity) + HR_{rest}; HR_{rest} is determined after 5 minutes of seated, quiet rest; $HR_{max/peak}$ is determined directly from a graded exercise or physical fitness test (i.e., 10-m shuttle walk or 6-minute walk test), or estimated from taking 220 and subtracting it from one's age. RPE is based off of Borg 15 Category RPE scale.

Source: Adapted with permission from Wolters Kluwer Health, Baltimore, MD. From American College of Sports Medicine. (2017). *Guidelines for exercise testing and prescription* (10th ed.). Baltimore, MD: Lippincott Williams & Wilkins.

Monitoring Target HR

The most common way to objectively monitor relative exercise intensity is through monitoring of HR. Two established methods are the HR method (Fox, Naughton, & Haskell, 1971) and heart rate reserve (HRR) method (Karvonen & Vuorimaa, 1988) based on the peak HR achieved on a graded exercise or physical fitness test or an age-predicted maximum HR estimated from a prediction equation (Table 18.1). The HR should be assessed a third of the way to halfway through the exercise session and immediately after stopping exercise. Exercise intensity can be increased or decreased based on this measurement.

Rating of Perceived Exertion

RPE is the subjective intensity of effort, strain, discomfort, and/or fatigue that is experienced during exercise (Noble & Robertson, 1996). The RPE can be quantified using a variety of scales, most notably the Borg 15 Category RPE scale (ranges from 6–20) (Borg, 1998) and the OMNI Picture System of Perceived Exertion scales (ranges from 0–10) (Robertson, 2004). In addition, differentiated (overall body) and undifferentiated (legs; chest/breathing) RPE can be assessed by the individual during the exercise session. This concept is important because the exercise modality used may influence the perceptual response, particularly the differentiated perceptual signal arising from the activated anatomical region (Mays et al., 2014).

The Talk Test

The Talk Test can replace target HR monitoring when an individual is exercising at a moderate intensity (Loose et al., 2012). If the exercise prevents the individual from talking comfortably, the intensity should be decreased. A variation of this technique is to whistle; if the individual is unable to whistle, the intensity is too great and should be decreased.

INTERVENTION

Healthy People 2020 is a continuing set of initiatives for the United States to achieve by the year 2020 through the use of the National Physical Activity Plan (NPAP). The NPAP aims to create a national culture that supports the incorporation of physical activity throughout everyday life, with the objective of improving health, fitness, and quality of life. Updated reviews and guidelines from the ACSM (Garber et al., 2011) and USDHHS-PAAC (2008), affirming the USSG's 1996 report (USSG, 1996), specifically state that exercise is considered to be beneficial to health, with a class IA (highest) evidence base, and that physical activity decreases the risk of the following:

1. Dying prematurely
2. Dying prematurely from heart disease
3. Acquiring type 2 diabetes
4. Incurring high BP
5. Developing colon cancer

The updated report further confirms that exercise also:

1. Aids in weight control
2. Helps strengthen and maintain the integrity of muscles, joints, and bones
3. Assists older adults with balance and mobility
4. Fosters feelings of psychological well-being
5. Reduces feelings of uneasiness and despair

Given that the benefits apply to all age groups across a broad spectrum of health and disease, it is important for nurses to recognize opportunities to promote exercise as a nursing intervention. There are countless activities included under the umbrella of exercise. When prescribing an exercise intervention, it is important to take into account the goals of the individual, health, medical, exercise and physical activity histories, as well as the patient's personal exercise preference, to ensure both safety and compliance during the exercise training program. Evidence suggests that exercise is more likely to be initiated if the individual (a) recognizes the need to exercise; (b) perceives the exercise to be beneficial and enjoyable; (c) understands that the exercise has minimal negative aspects, such as expense, time burden, or negative peer pressure; (d) feels capable and safe engaging in the exercise; and (e) has ready access to the activity and can easily fit it into the daily schedule (USDHHS-PAAC, 2008). A complete, multimodal exercise training program should involve each of the following modalities: resistance, flexibility, neuromuscular (i.e., functional fitness training), and aerobic; specific exercise selections within each given modality should be prescribed based on the needs of the individual.

Resistance Training

Resistance training is any exercise that causes the muscles to contract against an external resistance with the expectation of increases in strength, mass, and/or endurance (ACSM, 2009). This external resistance can be provided through the use of a variety of equipment, including machines and lower-cost alternatives such as free weights and rubber exercise tubing or bands. Furthermore, external resistance can be provided by one's own body weight or even household items such as bricks or jugs of water. Resistance training has physiological and healthy aging–promoting effects, which include increasing bone, muscle, and connective tissue strength and improving insulin sensitivity, BP, mental health, and body composition. Because of this, the ACSM has included it in its recommendations since 1998 (ACSM, 1998). The current guidelines state that resistance training should be performed 2 to 3 days per week, with specific recommendations based on the goals and experience of the individual. Briefly, for the novice to improve muscular strength, resistance training should involve eight to 10 of the major muscle groups with one set of eight to 12 repetitions performed at a resistance that induces moderate fatigue (RPE 12–13/20) (ACSM, 2009; Garber et al., 2011; USDHHS-PAAC, 2008).

Flexibility Training

Flexibility training (stretching) is an important, but often neglected part of an exercise training program. Stretching is particularly important for older adults to attenuate aging-related declines in joint range of motion and loss of skeletal muscle elasticity. Furthermore, stretching is important in the maintenance of postural stability and the prevention and management of nonspecific low back pain (Posadzki & Ernst, 2011). Flexibility exercises should be performed 2 to 3 days per week and target major muscles of the shoulder girdle, chest, neck, trunk, lower back, hips, and legs. Each stretch should be moved slowly into a position that induces mild discomfort (but not sharp pain) and held (static) for 10 to 30 seconds (Garber et al., 2011).

Neuromuscular Training

Neuromuscular exercise training focuses on the implementation of exercises designed to challenge balance and proprioception. During the past few decades, there has been an increase in the popularity of non-Western styles of exercise that fall under the category of neuromuscular exercise, including qigong and related movements in yoga and tai chi (Humberstone & Stuart, 2016). These forms of exercise build on meditative movement and, as such, may provide a more enjoyable form of exercise (Humberstone & Stuart, 2016). Furthermore, the dynamic movements and isometric muscle contractions performed in these exercises have been shown to increase muscular strength, physical fitness, and joint range of motion. particularly in novices, deconditioned people, and the elderly (Hagglund, Hagerman, Dencker, & Stromberg, 2017; Noradechanunt, Worsley, & Groeller, 2017; Zhao, Chung, & Tong, in press). Of note, neuromuscular exercise can be incorporated in select resistance training exercises such as step-ups, lunges, or select exercises (such as a dumbbell shoulder press) while standing on one leg. The optimal effectiveness and dose of neuromuscular exercise training has yet to be established; however, performing 60 minutes weekly (i.e., 20-minute sessions 3 days a week) has been shown to improve measures of neuromotor performance (Garber et al., 2011).

Aerobic Exercise Training

The focus of the exercise intervention hereafter is devoted to aerobic exercise training. Specific aerobic exercise prescription recommendations for healthy and clinical populations are discussed later and summarized in Table 18.2.

An exercise session, particularly one focused on aerobic exercise, should involve three phases: warm-up, aerobic exercise, and cool-down. These phases are designed to allow the body an opportunity to sustain internal equilibrium by gradually adjusting physiological processes to the stress of exercise and thus maintaining homeostasis.

Warm-Up Phase

The goal of swarm-up is to allow the body time to adapt to the rigors of aerobic exercise. Warming up results in an increase in muscle temperature, a higher need for oxygen to meet the increased metabolic demands of the exercising muscles, dilation of capillaries to increase circulation, adjustments within the neural respiratory center to the demands of exercise, and a shifting of blood flow from the splanchnic beds to the exercising muscles, resulting in increased venous return (Bishop, 2003). A good warm-up also increases flexibility and decreases the risk for developing arrhythmias and adverse myocardial ischemic events during the exercise session (ACSM, 2017). The warm-up, 5 to 10 minutes of low- to moderate-intensity aerobic exercise, should achieve a HR within 20 beats per minute of the target HR for the subsequent aerobic exercise portion of the training session. In addition, a warm-up may incorporate stretching exercises. If stretching is incorporated in the warm-up, it should be performed after the low-intensity aerobic activity. Specific recommendations for performing flexibility exercises were discussed previously.

Table 18.2. Evidence-Based, Population-Specific Aerobic Exercise Recommendations and Key References

Condition	Frequency	Intensity	Duration (minutes)	Special Considerations
Healthy Adults (Garber et al., 2011)	5 d/wk (moderate) 3 d/wk (vigorous)	Moderate or vigorous	30–60 (moderate) 20–60 (vigorous)	Select modes that maximize interest and tolerability.
Older Adults (Chodzko-Zajko et al., 2009)	Same as healthy	RPE 12–13 (moderate) RPE 14–15 (vigorous)	Same as healthy	Select modes that minimize fall risk in frail individuals or those with a fall history.
Children (USDHHS-PAAC, 2008)	Daily	Moderate and vigorous	≥60	Moderate corresponds to noticeable increases in RR and HR; vigorous corresponds to substantial increases in RR and HR. Youth should avoid exercise in hot, humid environments and be properly hydrated
Obese (Donnelly et al., 2009)	≥5 d/wk	40%–60% HRR (novice) ≥60% HRR (experienced)	Progress to 60	Maximize caloric expenditure, greater volume of exercise required. Target a minimal reduction in body weight of at least 5%–10% of initial body weight over 3–6 months. Incorporate concurrent dietary changes by reducing caloric intake by 500–1,000 kcal/day.

(continued)

Table 18.2.   Evidence-Based, Population-Specific Aerobic Exercise Recommendations and Key References *(continued)*

Condition	Frequency	Intensity	Duration (minutes)	Special Considerations
Attentive/cognitive decline (Hearing et al., 2016; Strohle et al., 2015)	3–5 d/wk	40%–80% HRR	30–60	Specific recommendations are not documented; the available evidence for aerobic exercise attenuating cognitive decline is limited to several randomized controlled trials. Improvements in measures of aerobic fitness are correlated to attenuated decline in cognition in adults with AD.
Dyslipidemia (USDHHS-PAAC, 2008; Donnelly et al., 2009)	≥5 d/wk	40%–75% HRR	30–60	Maximize caloric expenditure, greater volume of exercise required.
HTN (Pescatello et al., 2004)	≥5 d/wk	40%–60% HRR	30–60	Medical consultation in people with uncontrolled hypertension is recommended prior to start. Maintain BP ≤ 220/105 mmHg while exercising. BP-lowering effects of aerobic exercise are immediate (postexercise hypotension). Medications such as beta-blockers can limit aerobic capacity.
DM (Colberg et al., 2016)	3–7 d/wk	40%–60% HRR (novice) ≥60% HRR (experienced)	20–60	Greater benefits observed with greater volume of exercise. Timing of exercise should be considered in individuals taking antiglycemic agents. Measure glucose prior to and after exercise and adjust CHO intake as necessary.

(continued)

Table 18.2. Evidence-Based, Population-Specific Aerobic Exercise Recommendations and Key References (*continued*)

Condition	Frequency	Intensity	Duration (minutes)	Special Considerations
CAD (Leon et al., 2005)	≥3 d/wk	40%–80% HRR	20–60	Exercise intensity should be prescribed 10 bpm under ischemic threshold if applicable. ECG monitoring is indicated based on risk stratification.
PAD (Gerhard-Herman et al., 2017)	3–5 d/wk	40%–60% HRR—see Special Consideration	Accumulate 30+ minutes of walking per session	Participant should walk to moderate claudication (3–4/5 rating), followed by seated rest until ischemic pain subsides. For individuals with severe PAD, contraindications to or low treadmill exercise capacity, use upper body ergometry.
COPD (Global Initiative for Chronic Obstructive Lung Disease, 2017)	3–5 d/wk	40%–60% HRR, progress to ≥60% HRR, further individualize based on dyspnea	Based on dyspnea, may be intermittent or continuous, accumulate 30+ minutes	Intensity should be further modified to promote 4–6 rating on Borg category (C) ratio (R) or CR 10 scale. Supplemental O_2 may be utilized during session when %SaO2 ≤ 88%. Individuals suffering from acute exacerbations should limit exercise until symptoms have subsided.

AD, Alzheimer's disease; BP, blood pressure; bpm, beats per minute; CAD, coronary artery disease; CHO, carbohydrate; COPD, chronic obstructive pulmonary disease; DM, diabetes mellitus; HR, heart rate; HRR, heart rate reserve; HTN, hypertension; kcal, kilocalorie; PAD, peripheral artery disease; RPE, rating of perceived exertion; RR, respiratory rate; %SaO2, percent oxygen saturation.

Note: Borg CR 10 scale; scale used to determine the magnitude of perceived exertion.

Source: Adapted with permission from Wolters Kluwer Health, Baltimore, MD. From the American College of Sports Medicine. (2017). *Guidelines for exercise testing and prescription* (10th ed.). Baltimore, MD: Lippincott Williams & Wilkins.

Aerobic Exercise Phase

The aerobic phase of exercise is also known as the *conditioning phase*. It consists of four essential components—frequency, intensity (which is usually measured a relative percentage of maximal aerobic capacity), time (session duration), and type (mode of exercise)—that are often collectively referred to in the literature as *FITT* (ACSM, 2017). The combination of these components determines the effectiveness of the exercise and is known as the *training volume* or *activity dose*. The mode of exercise should involve rhythmic, continuous movement of large muscle groups—walking, jogging, cycling, swimming, or cross-country skiing (Garber et al., 2011). The frequency should be 5 days per week, with a duration of at least 30 minutes for health benefits (Garber et al., 2011), 60 minutes for prevention of weight gain, and 60 to 90 minutes for aiding in weight loss and preventing weight regain following weight loss (Donnelly et al., 2009).

The current guidelines further reaffirm that the duration of exercise is cumulative and can be achieved by exercising three times for a minimum of 10 minutes each bout for a given day (Garber et al., 2011). The intensity of exercise can be either moderate or vigorous. If the exercise performed is vigorous, the duration can be shortened to 20 minutes. Moreover, the 2011 guidelines clarify that moderate and vigorous exercise can be combined to achieve the recommended activity dose per week (Garber et al., 2011). To simplify this concept, the current guidelines recommend using the activity dose of MET × minutes to meet the minimum physical activity recommendations of approximately 500 MET-minutes per week, with a recommended weekly target of 500 to 1,000 MET-minutes per week (Garber et al., 2011). To find the specific MET that each activity requires, the reader is encouraged to visit the University of South Carolina's Prevention Research Center website (prevention.sph.sc.edu/tools/compendium.htm). For individual determination of intensity, target HRs and RPE should be used (Table 18.1). For most people, physical fitness improvements may be gained with moderate-intensity exercise.

As physical fitness improves, it may be necessary to increase one of the FITT components (i.e., frequency, intensity, or duration) to gain additional benefits (Garber et al., 2011; Haskell et al., 2007; USDHHS-PAAC, 2008). The accumulated amount of daily moderate to vigorous physical activity and exercise is what is important. Although those who perform 30 minutes of accumulated moderate physical activity show significant health benefits compared with sedentary individuals, people who perform more exercise resulting in greater energy expenditures show additional health benefits (Lee & Skerrett, 2001). However, a balance still needs to be achieved to obtain maximal benefit with the least risk and discomfort. Adjustment of intensity is important not only for safety reasons, but also for comfort and enjoyment of the activity. If exercise can be kept at a comfortable level, the individual is more likely to continue to perform the activity. As tolerance develops, any or all of the exercise components can be increased to meet the person's aerobic capacity. For example, if an individual is comfortable with the intensity of the exercise, the duration and frequency can be increased to further improve training effect.

Cool-Down Phase

Immediately following endurance exercise, the person should engage in a cooling-down period. The cool-down allows the body to return to its normal resting state. This allows the HR and BP to return to resting levels and attenuates postexercise hypotension by improving venous return. The cool-down also improves heat dissipation and elimination of blood lactate and provides a means to combat any potential postexercise rise in catecholamines. Cooling-down exercises should last 5 to 10 minutes and may include walking slowly and deep breathing. It should be noted that the cool-down period is a great time to perform static flexibility exercises due to the increased compliance of the skeletal muscles induced by the aerobic exercise training session.

Maintenance

The maintenance phase begins after 6 months of regular training, with the goal of maintaining achieved improvements in physical fitness (USDHHS-PAAC, 2008). Maintaining the exercise program is the key to the effectiveness of the intervention. Setting both short- and long-term goals helps improve adherence. The individual can experience a sense of accomplishment on meeting short-term goals while still striving for overall goals (Ehrman et al., 2013). Keeping a record or graph supplies a visual demonstration of progress and may provide insight into adjustments to the exercise program that may assist in achievement of goals.

Reversibility and Detraining

Once participation in exercise has ceased, there is a rapid return to pre-exercise levels of physical fitness. Most of the rapid decline occurs during the first 5 weeks following cessation of exercise and is usually complete within 12 weeks (Mujika & Padilla, 2001). With disuse, the muscle tissues atrophy. In addition, the decreased caloric expenditure leads to a positive energy balance, which can result in increased accumulation of adipose tissue.

Specific Technique: Walking

One of the strategies identified by *Healthy People 2020* to improve health and quality of life through daily physical activity is promotion of an increase in "trips made by walking." Walking has declined rapidly in the United States and has reached the point at which 75% of all trips of 1 mile or less are made by car. Walking is an easy and enjoyable activity that has significant health benefits. Moreover, it is an exercise in which most people of all age groups and varying levels of ability can use to improve endurance. A major advantage is that walking requires no special equipment, facilities, or new skills. It is also safer and easier to maintain than many other forms of exercise. Intensity, duration, and frequency are easily regulated and adjusted to accommodate a wide range of physical capabilities and limitations. The initial intensity should be outlined at the start of the program and is dependent on baseline level of conditioning, physical, or disease-related limitations or precautions, and outcome goals.

A walking program can be approached in two ways. The exercise can be completed in one or more daily sessions. For example, a previously sedentary individual may wish to begin an exercise program consisting of 10-minute walks and progressively increase the time or intensity as physical fitness increases. The more traditional alternative is to engage in one longer session at least five times per week; the recommended frequency for optimal benefits is 60 to 90 minutes of enjoyable moderate physical activity 5 days of the week (USDHHS-PAAC, 2008; Haskell et al., 2007). These sessions would include a warm-up session of 5 to 10 minutes, an aerobic period that could start at 10 to 15 minutes and be gradually increased to 30 to 60 minutes and then to 90 minutes, and a cool-down period of 5 to 10 minutes (USDHHS-PAAC, 2008; Haskell et al., 2007). The AHA-sponsored website (startwalkingnow.org) contains many resources for individuals interested in starting a walking program. Tips for fitness walking are presented in Exhibit 18.1.

Exhibit 18.1.   Tips for Fitness Walking

- Warm-up by performing a few stretches.
- Think tall as you walk. Stand straight with your head level and your shoulders relaxed.
- Your heel will hit the surface first. Use smooth movements rolling from heel to toe.
- Keep your hands free and let your arms swing naturally in opposition to your legs.
- When you're ready to pick up the pace, quicken your step and lengthen your stride, but don't compromise your upright posture or smooth, comfortable movements.
- To increase your intensity, burn more calories, and tone your upper body, bend your arms at the elbows and pump your arms. Keep your elbows close to your body.
- Breathe in and out naturally, rhythmically, and deeply.
- Use the talk test to check your intensity, or take your pulse to see whether you are within your target heart rate.
- Cool-down during the last 3 to 5 minutes by gradually slowing your pace to a stroll.

Source: American Heart Association. (2013). Start walking now. Retrieved from http://www.startwalkingnow.org/home.jsp

---

Measurement of Outcomes

The appropriate measure of the effectiveness of an exercise intervention depends on the specific exercise prescribed and the goals of the intervention. Changes in atherosclerotic risk factors (i.e., cholesterol levels, triglycerides, insulin sensitivity, waist circumference, BP, body mass index [BMI]) may be measured if cardiovascular health is the primary outcome of the exercise program. If cardiovascular fitness is the targeted outcome, an aerobic exercise program would be prescribed, and improvements in the cardiovascular system such as increased cardiac output, VO_2, and improved local circulation would be used to determine the effectiveness of the intervention (Fletcher et al., 2001). Cardiovascular response to submaximal exercise may provide further information and may be even more beneficial in assessing the impact on quality of life, as most activities of daily living (ADL) are performed at submaximal intensity. Exercise prescribed to improve function may use parameters such as improved joint mobility, prevention or reduction of osteoporosis, and improved strength in determining exercise effectiveness.

Assessment may determine changes in physical functioning and disability (e.g., Short Physical Performance Battery, 6-Minute Walk Test, Timed Up and Go Test), ability to perform ADL, changes in symptoms and activity tolerance, and other variables that reflect the individual's ability to function in daily life. Lower-intensity programs, which may not demonstrate great changes in maximal exercise capacity, might produce sufficient changes in these outcome variables to make a difference in the individual's quality of life. Such programs would be especially appropriate in older and very sedentary individuals, for whom low-intensity exercise can produce a modest increase in fitness and more significant improvements in function. Development and implementation of programs designed to meet the specific needs of patients can help maximize functional and quality-of-life outcomes.

PRECAUTIONS

Before an exercise program is initiated, preparticipation screening procedures are recommended. These include questionnaires such as the Physical Activity Readiness Questionnaire (PAR-Q), designed to identify potential patients in need of medical advice prior to exercising (Adams, 1999). If a patient is identified as having potential or actual medical concerns, it is advisable that a graded exercise test be performed. The ACSM recommends that a graded exercise test be performed for any individual with more than two risk factors for CHD. This is done to rule out any potential contraindications to exercise and to provide a tool for determining initial exercise intensity (ACSM, 2017; Fletcher et al., 2001).

To avoid injury, it is important to begin an exercise program slowly, to follow safety guidelines, and to exercise consistently. Potential exercise-related injuries include muscle and joint pain, cramps, blisters, shin splints, low back pain, tendinitis, and other sprains or muscle strains. The most commonly reported adverse event of exercise is musculoskeletal injury; approximately 25% of adults between 20 and 85 years of age reported an injury occurring at least once during 1 year (Hootman et al., 2002). It is possible that some of these are misclassified as injuries instead of muscle soreness due to a rapid increase in volume or intensity of training without proper knowledge of the principles of training.

The AHA (2013) has listed general guidelines to help ensure exercise safety. These include (a) stretching the muscles and tendons prior to beginning exercise; (b) wearing appropriate footwear; (c) exercising on a surface with some give to it, especially during high-impact activities; and (d) learning the exercise properly and continuing good form even with increased speed or intensity. If exercise-related injuries occur, they can usually be treated with one or a combination of therapies, including rest, ice, compression, and elevation (AHA, 2013).

Previously sedentary older individuals and those with chronic disease, especially heart disease, should consult a physician prior to initiating an exercise program to ensure that an appropriate exercise prescription is given (ACSM, 2017). The warning signs of heart disease should be spelled out prior to initiation of an exercise program, especially to those in high-risk categories.

USES

Populations for whom exercise is particularly beneficial include, but are not limited to, children, older adults, and those with affective/cognitive, metabolic, cardiovascular, and pulmonary diseases. The application and demonstrated effects of exercise intervention (with a focus on aerobic exercise) in each of these populations are briefly discussed.

Overweight Children and Adolescents

The prevalence of overweight children and adolescents remains alarmingly high (Ogden, Carroll, Kit, & Flegal, 2014). Of particular concern are the increasing rates of type 2 diabetes mellitus (DM) and metabolic syndrome (MetS) diagnosed in overweight children and adolescents, problems that used to be limited primarily to adults. Lack of physical activity and excess caloric intake cause central obesity, which, in turn, is believed to promote development of these conditions (National Research Council, 2011). Treatment includes dietary modification and initiation of physical activity. Increased physical activity has been shown to improve insulin sensitivity, BP, cholesterol, and vascular function and prevent further weight gain (National Research Council, 2011). The current recommendations are essentially the same as for healthy adults: 60 to 90 minutes of enjoyable, moderate physical activity 5 days a week (Donnelly et al., 2009). The current guidelines also explicitly state that achieving weight loss by exercise alone is difficult and therefore recommend that a weight-loss regimen should be a combination of calorie restriction and increased physical activity (Donnelly et al., 2009). An additional goal is to achieve less than 2 hours per day of consecutive sedentary activity, and at least 90 minutes of physical activity to achieve weight loss and prevent weight regain (Donnelly et al., 2009; USDHHS-PAAC, 2008).

Older Adults

The fastest growing segment of the population in the United States is one with individuals older than the age of 65 (U.S. Census Bureau, 2010). The benefit of exercise as a therapy to prevent or delay functional decline and disease and improve quality of life is demonstrated by the numerous favorable changes occurring in response to exercise. Improvements in cardiovascular function have been shown to help lower risk factors for disease and reduce the need for assisted living (Cress et al., 2005). Older adults are especially prone to the "hazards of immobility" that affect many of the body's systems. Exercise, particularly resistance training, results in increased bone strength (Kohrt, Bloomfield, Little, Nelson, & Yingling, 2004) and increased total body calcium, as well as improved coordination, which may result in a reduction in falls (Chodzko-Zajko et al., 2009). Exercise has also been shown to improve body functioning, overall well-being, and quality of life in older adults (Chodzko-Zajko et al., 2009).

It is particularly important to tailor or customize exercise programs for older adults, who may have specific limitations. Exercise needs to be initiated at lower levels and increased gradually. The ACSM guidelines recommend using similar guidelines for people older than the age of 65, with one important modification—use of RPE instead of the MET level for determination of intensity (Chodzko-Zajko et al., 2009). Previously sedentary older individuals may be more comfortable initiating an exercise program with some supervision, which allows them to become accustomed to this new level of activity in a safe environment. Group exercise may be especially appealing to older adults. The current guidelines recommend—with the specific inclusion of resistance training 2 (or more) nonconsecutive days per week—using 8 to 10 major muscle groups and one set of 10 to 15 repetitions at a moderate intensity (12–13/20) based on the RPE scale (Chodzko-Zajko et al., 2009). Moreover, the updated guidelines recommend that older individuals should perform flexibility and balance (e.g., dancing) exercises a minimum of 10 minutes, two to three times per week, to prevent age-related reductions in range of motion and, hence, prevent falls (Chodzko-Zajko et al., 2009; USDHHS-PAAC, 2008).

Individuals With Affective and Cognitive Disorders

Exercise is an effective although underused intervention for individuals with affective disorders. There is considerable evidence supporting the positive effects of exercise in combating depression and anxiety (Carek, Laibstain, & Carek, 2011; Hearing, Chang, Szuhany, Nierenberg, & Sylvia, 2016; Herring, Puetz, O'Connor, & Dishman, 2012; Mason & Holt, 2012; Pope, 2017; Rimer et al., 2012). There are fewer, if any, side effects when compared with pharmacotherapy, and exercise is often more cost-effective than psychotherapy and pharmacotherapy. Although most studies have evaluated the effects of aerobic activity as an intervention, anaerobic activity has also been shown to be beneficial in alleviating depression (Levinger et al., 2011; Martins et al., 2011). This suggests that improvement in mood is associated with exercise in general, rather than increased aerobic capacity. Because of mixed effectiveness of medications, exercise has been considered as a treatment for preclinical and late-stage Alzheimer's disease, and as a prevention strategy (Cass, 2017; Northey, Cherbuin, Pumpa, Smee, & Rattray, 2017). Aerobic exercise appears to improve brain blood flow, increase hippocampal volume, and improve neurogenesis (Chen, Zhang, & Huang, 2016), all of which are believed to be contributing factors to the preservation of brain function with aging. Both aerobic and resistance training have shown promise as a treatment modality for Alzheimer's disease by attenuating declines in cognitive function, reducing neuropsychiatric symptoms, and increasing functional capacity (Strohle et al., 2015). As with affective disorders, exercise training has been shown to have fewer side effects and better adherence compared with pharmacotherapy. Although no specific exercise recommendations have been established to date, it appears that moderate- to vigorous-intensity aerobic exercise training holds the most promise in attenuating the cognitive decline seen in people with Alzheimer's disease (Strohle et al., 2015).

Individuals With Metabolic Syndrome

MetS is characterized by a grouping of risk factors associated with cardiovascular disease, stroke, and type 2 DM. Definitions of MetS vary, but the National

Cholesterol Adult Treatment Panel III *Guidelines* are most commonly used (Expert Panel on Detection, Evaluation, and Treatment of High Cholesterol in Adults, 2001). Typically, individuals with MetS have three of the following: overweight or obese (with central adiposity), dyslipidemia (elevated triglycerides and/or low high-density lipoprotein [HDL]), elevated BP (130/85 mmHg) or hypertension, and elevated blood glucose (fasting blood glucose over 100 mg/dL) or DM. The treatment guidelines for MetS focus on three interventions, including weight control, exercise, and pharmacotherapy, individually based on the cardiovascular risk factors present. Exercise training can favorably attenuate each component of the MetS, particularly when weight loss occurs; however, reductions in components of the MetS can been seen following aerobic exercise training even if not accompanied by weight loss. The exercise prescription may need to be tailored to the most severe MetS variable, the following discusses exercise prescription guidelines for each MetS component.

Dyslipidemia

Lifestyle change such as regular exercise and dietary changes should be implemented for the management of dyslipidemia (Stone et al., 2013). Focus should be on reductions in body weight and adiposity because these factors influence BMI scores, which correlate with total cholesterol concentrations, and an exercise program that focuses on weight loss can affect total cholesterol, low-density lipoprotein (LDL), HDL, and triglyceride levels (Ellsworth et al., 1998). The goal of the exercise program should be on maximizing caloric expenditure (USDHHS-PAAC, 2008), and therefore aerobic exercise should be the focus of the exercise prescription, as this mode enhances fat utilization. Specific recommendations are similar to those for weight-loss promotion and maintenance (Donnelly et al., 2009).

Hypertension

Aerobic exercise training is well known for its antihypertensive effects, influencing BP at rest and at submaximal exercise/activity workloads. As with dyslipidemia, emphasis should be placed on aerobic exercise training, as resting BP reductions of 5 to 7 and even up to 8 mmHg are seen following aerobic exercise training in individuals with hypertension (Corneilissen & Smart, 2013; Pescatello et al., 2004) and 2 mmHg in individuals considered prehypertensive (Corneilissen & Smart, 2013). Resistance training should be used as a supplement to aerobic exercise training because resistance training has also been shown to reduce resting BP by up to 4 mmHg in hypertensive participants (Corneilissen & Smart, 2013). Special factors to consider when prescribing exercise in individuals with hypertension are found in Table 18.2.

Diabetes Mellitus

Regular exercise in people with impaired glucose tolerance (prediabetes) and type 2 DM commonly results in several positive physiological adaptations, including improved glucose tolerance, increased insulin sensitivity, and reduced hemoglobin A1c (HbA1c; Colberg et al., 2016). In people with insulin-dependent type 2 DM, exercise training has been shown to lower requirements of exogenous insulin

(ACSM, 2017). Specific exercise prescriptions are based on healthy weight loss and maintenance because 90% of people with type 2 DM are obese. Moderate to high volumes of aerobic exercise are recommended, since they are associated with substantially lower cardiovascular and overall mortality risk in those with type 2 DM (Sluik et al., 2012). In addition, resistance training is more important in the treatment of hyperglycemia compared with the other MetS components and should be encouraged (Wood & O'Neill, 2012) because DM is an independent risk factor for low muscular strength (Nishitani et al., 2011) and an accelerated decline in functional status and muscle strength (Anton, Karabetian, Naugle, & Buford, 2013).

Individuals With Cardiovascular Disease

Cardiac rehabilitation is a common therapy that is prescribed for those with CHD, providing a safe environment for the initiation of an exercise program (Heran et al., 2011). Programs usually have several phases and are tailored to the specific needs, limitations, and characteristics of individuals, helping them resume active and productive lives (Kwan & Balady, 2012). Exercise has multiple protective mechanisms that contribute to the reduction of CHD risk, including antiatherosclerotic, antiarrhythmic, anti-ischemic, and antithrombotic effects (Leon & Bronäs, 2009; Leon et al., 2005).

Exercise training has been shown to improve symptom-limited exercise capacity in patients with CHD, primarily as a result of peripheral hemodynamic adaptations. Patients with CHD have a low skeletal muscle oxidative capacity, which is significantly improved with training, despite relatively low workloads and exercise intensities, consistent with other nonheart disease populations (Dorosz, 2009). Prior to training, patients with CHD are often unable to perform ADL without symptoms. Exercise-trained CHD patients function farther above the ischemic threshold in performing ADL and thus require a lower percentage of maximal effort to perform activities. This increases stamina and endurance and helps maintain independence (Dorosz, 2009). Even patients with heart failure, who typically have very poor cardiac function, have found that cardiac rehabilitation improves their exercise tolerance (Downing & Balady, 2011; Keteyian, Pina, Hibner, & Fleg, 2010).

Peripheral artery disease (PAD), a prevalent atherosclerotic occlusive disease, limits functional capacity and is related to decreased quality of life. Individuals with PAD typically experience exercise-induced ischemic pain in the lower extremities, known as claudication. Exercise training is one of the most effective interventions available for the treatment of claudication caused by PAD (Hamburg & Balady, 2011). Aerobic exercise training in the form of treadmill walking has been shown to improve walking distance up to 200% (Watson, Ellis, & Leng, 2008). Optimally, prior to program initiation, an exercise prescription should be generated based on a graded exercise test, and patients should start training at the intensity at which the onset of claudication occurs (Bronäs et al., 2009). During a typical session, patients exercise at a moderate pace until they experience moderate to moderately severe claudication. At that point they rest until the pain subsides. This exercise/rest pattern is repeated throughout the exercise session. The most effective exercise programs for the treatment of claudication include the following components: The patient should exercise to the point of moderate/moderately severe claudication (3–4 rating on a 5-point scale); the exercise session should be at least 30 minutes in length, with at least three sessions per week; and the exercise program should continue for at least 12 weeks with intermittent walking as the most effective mode of exercise (Gerhard-Herman et al., 2017). In addition, a number of studies have shown that modalities of exercise that avoid claudication (i.e., upper body ergometry) or walking performed at intensities that are pain-free or produce only mild levels of claudication can achieve health benefits comparable to walking at moderate or higher levels of claudication (Gerhard-Herman et al., 2017) and should be used by those for whom treadmill training is not suitable.

Individuals With Pulmonary Disease

Chronic obstructive pulmonary disease (COPD) is an umbrella term used to describe progressive lung diseases, including emphysema, chronic bronchitis, refractory (nonreversible) asthma, and some forms of bronchiectasis (Global Initiative for Chronic Obstructive Lung Disease, 2017). The hypoxic and inflammatory state induced by COPD results in skeletal muscle dysfunction, a condition characterized by reduced type I oxidative fibers and mitochondrial dysfunction (Mador & Bozkanat, 2001). Both the reduced capacity for alveolar gas diffusion and reduced oxidative capacity of the skeletal muscles attribute to the increasing breathlessness and muscular fatigue particularly seen on exertion. Upper body skeletal muscle fatigue is most commonly noted (McKeough, Velloso, Lima, & Allison, 2016) as activities such as changing a tire can become exceedingly difficult. The increased fatigue seen in the upper body skeletal muscles is most likely due to increase need to recruit this musculature to assist in ventilatory mechanics. As the disease progresses, inability to perform ADLs and disability are often seen. The benefits to COPD patients from pulmonary rehabilitation are considerable, and rehabilitation has been shown to be the most effective therapeutic strategy to improve shortness of breath, health status, and exercise tolerance (Global Initiative for Chronic Obstructive Lung DiseaseGOLD, 2017). The focus of pulmonary rehabilitation is aerobic exercise training, which most notably improves cardiovascular function and skeletal muscle oxidative capacity, thereby enhancing oxygen delivery, extraction, and utilization. In turn, these training effects can lower the demands and stress put on the pulmonary system during exertion. Light to moderate aerobic exercise is known to reduce fatigue, whereas vigorous aerobic exercise can improve select respiratory measurements such as minute ventilation during submaximal exercise (ACSM, 2017). Resistance training is also increasingly important for individuals with COPD to improve skeletal muscle strength and endurance in an attempt to attenuate the skeletal muscle dysfunction and disability and increase the performance of ventilatory accessory muscles (Liao et al., 2015).

CULTURAL APPLICATIONS

The benefits of exercise and physical activity appear to be equal across gender and race; however, this topic remains poorly studied and recommendations are based primarily on assumptions that findings in one population will carry over to another. It should be mentioned that there exist cultural preferences, including religious and ethnic preferences, in the use of exercise and physical activity. Although there has been little systematic investigation regarding these preferences, their potential influence should be considered when prescribing exercise and physical activity. For example, with certain ethnicities, it may be beneficial to modify an exercise program to allow exercise with a garment that covers the body.

The use of alternate exercise techniques has gained popularity during the past few decades, especially among older adults. These forms of physical activity include meditative forms of movement in the practice of qigong and its specific forms such as tai chi and yoga (discussed in separate chapters in this book). Within these alternative forms of physical activity, numerous styles and movements have been reported, but the overarching theme remains the same. Although the evidence base for this type of exercise is less strenuous than for structured Western-style exercise (e.g., walking), it appears that these forms of physical activity may provide health benefits, especially in improving balance and lowering fear of falling. However, most reported studies have been small and have used large variations of these techniques.

Other cultures have also been able to incorporate daily physical activity as part of their usual routine, either by necessity or by choice. For example, European countries have facilitated walking and cycling as modes of transportation by incorporating walkways and bicycle lanes in city planning. These forms of transportation are also culturally accepted as the primary modes of transportation in those countries, whereas in the United States, this is commonly not the case. Exercise in Sweden, as one example of activity incorporated into the European lifestyle, is presented in Sidebar 18.1. Sidebar 18.2 illustrates another country in which activity is incorporated into lifestyles; in Nigeria, the work life of farmers keeps them active and fit.

There is a clear need for future city planning to incorporate safe, accessible, and enjoyable walkways and bicycle lanes so that the American population can incorporate daily physical activity into their lives and gain the health benefits associated with increased physical activity levels. This will help change the cultural perspective of physical activity in this country and support walking and/or bicycling as a preferred mode of transportation.

SIDEBAR 18.1. EXERCISE IN SWEDEN

Ulf G. Bronäs

In Sweden (as in most of Europe), major cities are built to facilitate walking and cycling as the primary modes of transportation to and from work, school, day care, grocery shopping, and places of entertainment. Walkways and bicycle lanes are incorporated into city planning and allow for easy access for most people. It is common for parents to bring their children to day care by walking or using a specialized bicycle child seat assembled on the back of the bicycle. Once the child is older, the family bikes together to day care or school. Parents drop their children off at day care or school and continue biking either to work or to a mass-transit station. More than 60% of Swedes use public transportation to and from work, which facilitates both walking and bicycling. These modes of transportation are culturally accepted and used as primary methods of transportation in Sweden and throughout Europe. It is often said that to experience Europe, one must walk the cities. The cities are built to promote walking; it is the most convenient (and least expensive) form of transportation. Availability of multiple walkways and bicycle lanes is evident in the cities, allowing the population the option of incorporating daily physical activity into their lives.

SIDEBAR 18.2. EXERCISE IN NIGERIA

Gladys O. Igbo

As far as exercise is concerned, in my home country of Nigeria, people exercise at levels that are not all that different from the United States recommendations for exercise, and they use some elements of movement and exercise as part of their healing modalities. In considering exercise and activity, one must bear in mind that in Nigeria, most individuals exercise "naturally," as farmers; during cultivating seasons, there are a lot of vigorous movements involved in daily work activities. Likewise, exercise is commonly used as part of the recovery process when someone becomes ill. Growing up there, I witnessed a lot of early morning rising and walking out in nature, especially when someone was ill and was trying to recover fast and well. I continue to value exercise; I advocate exercise as part of health promotion as a nurse and in my role as a fitness trainer in a health club in the United States. In Nigeria, we may not have traditional "health clubs," so to speak, like most developed countries do, with required dues and memberships. However, most Nigerians do have the basic knowledge of how incorporating some activities of movement help in their quest for good health and health enhancement.

FUTURE RESEARCH

There are many gaps in our knowledge related to exercise, its measurement, the benefits, and methods for improving exercise adherence. Specific areas of needed research include:

- Investigations of cultural and ethnic differences in physical activity and response to exercise
- Investigations of the benefit of exercise in individuals with disabilities, including mental and physical disabilities
- Development of strategies to increase lifelong physical activity and exercise
- Determination of electronic or social media can improve short- and long-term adherence

WEBSITES

General Guidelines and Information

- Centers for Disease Control and Prevention (CDC) (www.cdc.gov/physicalactivity)
- President's Council on Physical Fitness and Sports (www.fitness.gov)
- U.S. Department of Health and Human Services, Physical Activity Guidelines (www.health.gov/paguidelines)

Guidelines and Information Pertaining to Individuals and Families

- CDC
  (www.cdc.gov/physicalactivity/index.html)
- Exercise and Physical Activity: Your Everyday Guide from the National Institute on Aging
  (nihseniorhealth.gov/exerciseforolderadults/healthbenefits/01.html)
- National Institutes of Health
  (nihseniorhealth.gov/exercise/toc.html)
- Office of the Surgeon General
  (www.surgeongeneral.gov/obesityprevention/index.html)
- President's Council on Physical Fitness and Sports
  (www.presidentschallenge.org)

School

- CDC, Division of Adolescent and School Health
  (www.cdc.gov/HealthyYouth/physicalactivity)

Communities

- Federal Highway Administration
  (www.fhwa.dot.gov/environment/bicycle_pedestrian)
- National Institutes of Health
  (www.nhlbi.nih.gov/health/public/heart/obesity/wecan)
- National Park Service
  (www.nps.gov/ncrc/programs/rtca/helpfultools/ht_publications.html)

Worksite

- CDC, Healthier Worksite Initiative
  (www.cdc.gov/nccdphp/dnpao/hwi/index.htm)

REFERENCES

Adams, R. (1999). Revised physical activity readiness questionnaire. *Canadian Family Physician, 45*, 992.

American College of Sports Medicine. (1998). American College of Sports Medicine position stand. The recommended quantity and quality of exercise for developing and maintaining cardiorespiratory and muscular fitness, and flexibility in healthy adults. *Medicine & Science in Sports & Exercise, 30*(6), 975–991.

American College of Sports Medicine. (2009). American College of Sports Medicine position stand. Progression models in resistance training for healthy adults. *Medicine & Science in Sports & Exercise, 41*(3), 687–708. doi:10.1249/MSS.0b013e3181915670

American College of Sports Medicine. (2017). *Guidelines for exercise testing and prescription* (10th ed.). Baltimore, MD: Lippincott Williams & Wilkins.

American Heart Association. (2013). *Start walking now.* Retrieved from http://www.startwalkingnow.org/home.jsp

Anton, S. D., Karabetian, C., Naugle, K., & Buford T. W. (2013). Obesity and diabetes as accelerators of functional decline: can lifestyle interventions maintain functional status in high risk older adults? *Experimental Gerontology, 48*, 888–897.

Astrand, P., Rodahl, K., Dahl, K., & Stromme, B. (2004). *Textbook of work physiology* (4th ed.). Champaign, IL: Human Kinetics.

Beaver, W. L., Wasserman, K. W., & Whipp, B. J. (1986). A new method for detecting anaerobic threshold by gas exchange. *Journal of Applied Physiology, 60*, 2020–2027.

Bishop, D. (2003). Warm up I: Potential mechanisms and the effects of passive warm up on exercise performance. *Sports Medicine (Auckland, N.Z.), 33*(6), 439–454.

Borg, G. (1998). *Borg's perceived exertion and pain scales.* Champaign, IL: Human Kinetics.

Bronäs, U. G., Hirsch, A. T., Murphy, T., Badenhop, D., Collins, T. C., Ehrman, J. K., ... Regensteiner, J. G. (2009). Design of the multicenter standardized supervised exercise training intervention for the claudication: Exercise vs endoluminal revascularization (CLEVER) study. *Vascular Medicine, 14*(4), 313–321.

Carek, P. J., Laibstain, S. E., & Carek, S. M. (2011). Exercise for the treatment of depression and anxiety. *International Journal of Psychiatry in Medicine, 41*(1), 15–28.

Cass, S. P. (2017). Alzheimer's disease and exercise: A literature review. *Current Sports Medicine Reports, 16*(1), 19–22.

Chen, W. W., Zhang, X., & Huang, W. (2016). Role of physical exercise in Alzheimer's disease. *Biomedical Reports, 4*(4), 403–407.

Chodzko-Zajko, W., Proctor, D., Fiatarone Singh, M., Minson, C., Nigg, C., Salem, G., ... Skinner, J. (2009). American College of Sports Medicine position stand. Exercise and physical activity for older adults. *Medicine & Science in Sports & Exercise, 41*(7), 1510–1530. doi:10.1249/MSS.0b013e3181a0c95c

Colberg, S. R., Sigal, R. J., Yardley, J. E., Riddell, M. C., Dunstan, D. W., Dempsey, P. C., ... Tate, D. F. (2016). Physical activity/exercise and diabetes: A position statement of the American Diabetes Association. *Diabetes Care, 39*(11), 2065–2079.

Corneilissen, V. A., & Smart, N. A. (2013). Exercise training for blood pressure: A systematic review and meta-analysis. *Journal of the American Heart Association, 2*(1), e004473. doi:10.1161/JAHA.112.004473

Cress, M. E., Buchner, D. M., Prohaska, T., Rimmer, J., Brown, M., Macera, C., ... Chodzko-Zajko, W. (2005). Best practices for physical activity programs and behavior counseling in older adult populations. *Journal of Aging & Physical Activity, 13*(1), 61–74.

Donnelly, J. E., Blair, S. N., Jakicic, J. M., Manore, J. W., Rankin, J. W., & Smith, B. K. (2009). American College of Sports Medicine position stand. Appropriate physical activity intervention strategies for weight loss and prevention of weight regain for adults. *Medicine & Science in Sports & Exercise, 41*(7), 459–471.

Dorosz, J. (2009). Updates in cardiac rehabilitation. *Physical Medicine & Rehabilitation Clinics of North America, 20*(4), 719–736.

Downing, J., & Balady, G. J. (2011). The role of exercise training in heart failure. *Journal of the American College of Cardiology, 58*(6), 561–569. doi:10.1016/j.jacc.2011.04.020

Ehrman, J. K., Gordon, P. M., Visich, P. S., & Keteyian, S. J. (2013). *Clinical exercise physiology* (3rd ed.). Champaign, IL: Human Kinetics.

Ellsworth, N., Haskell, W., Mackey, S., Sheehan, M., Stefanick, M., & Wood, P. (1998). Effects of diet and exercise in men and postmenopausal women with low levels of HDL cholesterol and high levels of LDL cholesterol. *New England Journal of Medicine, 339*, 12–18.

Expert Panel on Detection, Evaluation, and Treatment of High Cholesterol in Adults. (2001). Executive summary of the third report of the National Cholesterol Education Program (NCEP) Expert Panel on Detection, Evaluation, and Treatment of High Blood Cholesterol in Adults (Adult Treatment Panel III). *Journal of the American Medical Association, 285*(19), 2486–2497.

Fletcher, G. F., Balady, G. J., Amsterdam, E. A., Chaitman, B., Eckel, R., Fleg, J., ... Bazarre, T. (2001). Exercise standards for testing and training: A statement for healthcare professionals from the American Heart Association. *Circulation, 104*, 1694–1740.

Fox, S. M., Naughton, J. P., & Haskell, W. L. (1971). Physical activity and the prevention of coronary heart disease. *Annals of Clinical Research, 3*, 404–432.

Garber, C. E., Blissmer, B., Deschenes, M. R., Franklin, B. A., Lamonte, M. J., Lee, I. M., ... Swain, D. P.; American College of Sports Medicine. (2011). American College of Sports Medicine position stand. Quantity and quality of exercise for developing and maintaining cardiorespiratory, musculoskeletal, and neuromotor fitness in apparently healthy adults: Guidance for prescribing exercise. *Medicine & Science in Sports & Exercise, 43*(7), 1334–1359. doi:10.1249/MSS.0b013e318213fefb

Gerhard-Herman, M. D., Gornik, H. L., Barrett, C., Corrriere, M. A., Drachman, D. E., Fleisher, L. A., … Walsh, M. E. (2017). 2016 AHA/ACC guideline on the management of patients with lower extremity peripheral artery disease: A report of the American College of Cardiology/American Heart Association task force on clinical practice guidelines. *Circulation, 135*(12), e726–e779.

Global Initiative for Chronic Obstructive Lung Disease. (2017). *Pocket guide to COPD diagnosis, management, and prevention.* Retrieved from http://goldcopd.org/wp-content/uploads/2016/12/wms-GOLD-2017-Pocket-Guide.pdf

Hagglund, E., Hagerman, I., Dencker, K., & Stromberg, A. (2017). Effects of yoga versus hydrotherapy training on health-related quality of life and exercise capacity in patients with heart failure: A randomized controlled study. *European Journal of Cardiovascular Nursing, 16*, 381–389. doi:10.1177/1474515117690297

Hamburg, N. M., & Balady, G. J. (2011). Exercise rehabilitation in peripheral artery disease: Functional impact and mechanisms of benefits. *Circulation, 123*(1), 87–97. doi:10.1161/CIRCULATIONAHA.109.881888

Haskell, W. L., Lee, I. M., Pate, R. R., Powell, K. E., Blair, S. N., Franklin, B. A., … Bauman, A. (2007). Physical activity and public health: Updated recommendation for adults from the American College of Sports Medicine and the American Heart Association. *Circulation, 116*, 1081–1093.

Hearing, C. M., Chang, W. C., Szuhany, T., Nierenberg, A. A., & Sylvia L. G. (2016). Physical exercise for treatment of mood disorders: A critical review. *Current Behavioral Neuroscience Reports, 3*(4), 350–359.

Heran, B. S., Chen, J. M., Ebrahim, S., Moxham, T., Oldridge, N., Rees, K., & Taylor, R. S. (2011). Exercise-based cardiac rehabilitation for coronary heart disease. *Cochrane Database of Systematic Reviews,* (7), CD001800. doi:10.1002/14651858.CD001800.pub2

Herring, M. P., Puetz, T. W., O'Connor, P. J., & Dishman, R. K. (2012). Effect of exercise training on depressive symptoms among patients with a chronic illness: A systematic review and meta-analysis of randomized controlled trials. *Archives of Internal Medicine, 172*(2), 101–111. doi:10.1001/archinternmed.2011.696

Hootman, J. M., Macera, C. A., Ainsworth, B. E., Addy, C. L., Martin, M., & Blair, S. N. (2002). Epidemiology of musculoskeletal injuries among sedentary and physically active adults. *Medicine & Science in Sports & Exercise, 34*(5), 838–844.

Humberstone, B., & Stuart, S. (2016). Older women, exercise to music, and yoga: Senses of pleasure? *Journal of Aging and Physical Activity, 24*(3), 412–418.

Jones, A. M., & Poole, D. C. (2005). Oxygen uptake dynamics: From muscle to mouth—An introduction to the symposium. *Medicine & Science in Sports & Exercise, 37*(9), 1542–1550.

Karvonen, J., & Vuorimaa, T. (1988). Heart rate and exercise intensity during sports activities. Practical application. *Sports Medicine, 5*(5), 303–311.

Keteyian, S. J., Pina, I. L., Hibner, B. A., & Fleg, J. L. (2010). Clinical role of exercise training in the management of patients with chronic heart failure. *Journal of Cardiopulmonary Rehabilitation and Prevention, 30*(2), 67–76. doi:10.1097/HCR.0b013e3181d0c1c1

Kodoma, S., Saito, K., Tanaka, S., Maki, M., Yachi Y., Asumi, M., … Sone, H. (2009). Cardiorespiratory fitness as a quantitative predictor of all-cause mortality and cardiovascular events in healthy men and women: A meta-analysis. *Journal of the American Medical Association, 301*(19), 2024–2035.

Kohrt, W. M., Bloomfield, S. A., Little, K. D., Nelson, M. E., & Yingling, V. R. (2004). American College of Sports Medicine position stand: Physical activity and bone health. *Medicine & Science in Sports & Exercise, 36*(11), 1985–1996.

Kwan, G., & Balady, G. J. (2012). Cardiac rehabilitation 2012: Advancing the field through emerging science. *Circulation, 125*(7), e369–373. doi:10.1161/CIRCULATIONAHA.112.093310

LaForgia, J., Withers, R. T., & Gore, C. J. (2006). Effects of exercise intensity and duration on the excess post-exercise oxygen consumption. *Journal of Sports Sciences, 24*(12), 1247–1264. doi:10.1080/02640410600552064

Lee, I. M., & Skerrett, P. J. (2001). Physical activity and all-cause mortality: What is the dose-response relationship? *Medicine & Science in Sports & Exercise, 33*(Suppl. 6), S459–S467.

Leon, A. S., & Bronäs, U. G. (2009). Pathophysiology of coronary heart disease and biological mechanisms for the cardioprotective effects of regular aerobic exercise. *American Journal of Lifestyle Medicine, 3*(5), 379–385.

Leon, A. S., Franklin, B. A., Costa, F., Balady, G. J., Berra, K. A., Stewart, K. J., … Lauer, M. S. (2005). Cardiac rehabilitation and secondary prevention of coronary heart disease. *Circulation, 111,* 369–376.

Levinger, I., Selig, S., Goodman, C., Jerums, G., Stewart, A., & Hare, D. L. (2011). Resistance training improves depressive symptoms in individuals at high risk for type 2 diabetes. *Journal of Strength and Conditioning Research, 25*(8), 2328–2333.

Liao, W. H., Chen, J. W., Chen, X., Lin, L., Yan, H. Y., Zhou, Y. Q., & Chen R. (2015). Impact of resistance training in subjects with COPD: A systematic review and meta-analysis. *Respiratory Care, 60*(8), 1130–1145.

Loose, B. D., Christiansen, A. M., Smolczyk, J. E., Roberts, K. L., Budziszewska, A., Hollatz, C. G., & Norman, J. F. (2012). Consistency of the Counting Talk Test for exercise prescription. *Journal of Strength and Conditioning Research, 26*(6), 1701–1707. doi:10.1519/JSC.0b013e318234e84c

Mador, J. M. & Bozkanat, E. (2001). Skeletal muscle dysfunction in chronic obstructive pulmonary disease. *Respiratory Research, 2,* 216–224.

Martins, R., Coelho, E., Silva, M., Pindus, D., Cumming, S., Teixeira, A., & Verissimo, M. (2011). Effects of strength and aerobic-based training on functional fitness, mood and the relationship between fatness and mood in older adults. *Journal of Sports Medicine and Physical Fitness, 51*(3), 489–496.

Mason, O. J., & Holt, R. (2012). Mental health and physical activity interventions: A review of the qualitative literature. *Journal of Mental Health (Abingdon, England), 21*(3), 274–284. doi: 10.3109/09638237.2011.648344

Mays, R. J., Goss, F. L., Nagle, F. F., Gallagher, M., Schafer, M. A., Kim, K. H., & Robertson, R. J. (2014). Prediction of VO2 peak using OMNI ratings of perceived exertion from a submaximal cycle exercise test. *Perceptual Motor Skills, 118*(3), 863–881.

McKeough, Z. J., Velloso, M., Lima, V. P., & Allison J. A. (2016). Upper limb exercise training for COPD. *Cochrane Database Systematic Reviews, 11,* CD011434.

Mujika, I., & Padilla, S. (2001). Cardiorespiratory and metabolic characteristics of detraining in humans. *Medicine & Science in Sports & Exercise, 33*(3), 413–421.

National Research Council. (2011). *Early childhood obesity prevention policies.* Washington, DC: National Academies Press.

Nelson, M. E., Rejeski, J. E., Blair, S. N., Duncan, P. W., Judge, J. O., King, A. C., … Casteneda-Sceppa, C. (2007). Physical activity and public health in older adults: Recommendation from the American College of Sports Medicine and the American Heart Association. *Circulation, 116,* 1094–1105.

Nishitani, M., Shimada, K., Sunayama, S., Masaki, Y., Kure, A., Fukao, K., … Daida, H. (2011). Impact of diabetes on muscle mass, muscle strength, and exercise tolerance in patients after coronary artery bypass grafting. *Journal of Cardiology, 58*(20), 173–180.

Noble, B. J., & Robertson, R. J. (1996). *Perceived exertion.* Champaign, IL: Human Kinetics.

Noradechanunt, C., Worsley, A., & Groeller H. (2017). Thai yoga improves physical function and well-being in older adults: A randomised controlled trial. *Journal of Science and Medicine in Sport, 20*(5), 494–501.

Northey, J. M., Cherbuin, N., Pumpa, K. L., Smee, D. J., & Rattray, B. (2017). Exercise interventions for cognitive function in adults older than 50: A systematic review with meta-analysis. *British Journal of Sports Medicine.* pii: bjsports-2016-096587. doi: 10.1136/bjsports-2016-096587

Ogden, C. L., Carroll, M. D., Kit, B., & Flegal, K. M. (2014). Prevalence of childhood and adult obesity in the United States, 2011-2012. *Journal of the American Medical Association, 311*(8), 806–814.

Pescatello, L. S., Franklin, B. F., Fagard, R., Farquhar, W., Kelley, G. A., & Ray, C. A. (2004). American College of Sports Medicine position stand: Exercise and hypertension. *Medicine & Science in Sports & Exercise, 36*(3), 533–553.

Pope, K. S. (2017). *Exercise's effects on psychological health, disorders, cognition, & quality of life: 31 meta-analyses published in 2013-16.* Retrieved from https://kspope.com/ethics/exercise-meta-analyses.php

Posadzki, P., & Ernst, E. (2011). Yoga for low back pain: A systematic review of randomized controlled trials. *Clinical Rheumatology, 30*(9), 1257–1262.

Rimer, J., Dwan, K., Lawlor, D. A., Greig, C. A., McMurdo, M., Morley, W., & Mead, G. E. (2012). Exercise for depression. *Cochrane Database of Systematic Reviews, 7*, CD004366. doi:10.1002/14651858.CD004366.pub5

Robergs, R., Ghiasvand, F., & Parker, D. (2004). Biochemistry of exercise-induced metabolic acidosis. *American Journal of Physiology. Regulatory, Integrative, and Comparative Physiology, 287*, R502–R516.

Robertson, R. J. (2004). The OMNI Picture system of perceived exertion. In M. S. Bahrke (Ed.), *Perceived exertion for practitioners: Rating effort with the OMNI Picture system* (pp. 1–8). Champaign, IL: Human Kinetics.

Samitz, G., Egger, M., & Zwahlen, M. (2011). Domains of physical activity and all-cause mortality: Systematic review and dose-response meta-analysis of cohort studies. *International Journal of Epidemiology, 40*(5), 1382–1400. doi:10.1093/ije/dyr112

Slawinska, T., Posluszny, P., & Rozek, K. (2013). The relationship between physical fitness and quality of life in adults and the elderly. *Human Movement, 14*(3), 10–15.

Sluik, D., Buijsse, B., Muckelbauer, R., Kaas, R., Teucher, B., Johnsen, N. F., ... Nothlings, U. (2012). Physical activity and mortality in individuals with diabetes mellitus: A prospective study and meta-analysis. *Archives of Internal Medicine, 172*(12), 1285–1295.

Stone, N. J., Robinson, J. G., Lichtenstein, A. H., Bairey Mets, C. N., Blum, C. B., Echkel, R. H., ... Tomaselli, G. F. (2013). ACC/AHA guideline on the treatment of blood cholesterol to reduce atherosclerotic cardiovascular risk in adults: A report of the American College of Cardiology/American Heart Association task force on practice guidelines. *Circulation, 24*(129), (25 Suppl. 2), S1–S45.

Strohle, A., Schmidt, D. M., Schultz, F., Fricke, N., Straden, T. Hellweg, R., ... Rieckmann, N. (2015). Drug and exercise treatment of Alzheimer's disease and mild cognitive impairment: A systematic review and meta analysis of cognition in randomized controlled trials. *American Journal of Geriatric Psychiatry, 23*(12), 1234–1249.

Thompson, P. D., Buchner, D., Pina, I. L., Balady, G. J., Williams, M. A., Marcus, B. H., ... Wenger, N. K. (2003). Exercise and physical activity in the prevention and treatment of atherosclerotic cardiovascular disease: American Heart Association scientific statement. *Circulation, 107*, 3109–3116.

Tipton, C. M., Sawka, M. N., Tate, C. A., & Terjung, R. L. (2006). *ACSM's advanced exercise physiology.* Baltimore, MD: Lippincott Williams, & Wilkins.

U.S. Census Bureau. (2010). *2010 Census shows 65 and older population growing faster than total U.S. population.* Retrieved from https://www.census.gov/newsroom/releases/archives/2010_census/cb11-cn192.html

U.S. Department of Health and Human Services, Physical Activity Advisory Committee. (2008). *Physical activity guidelines advisory committee report, 2008.* Washington, DC: Author. Retrieved from http://www.health.gov/paguidelines/guidelines/default.aspx

U.S. Surgeon General. (1996). *Report on physical activity and health.* Retrieved from http://www.cde.800/nccdphd/sgr/mm.htm

Watson, L., Ellis, B., & Leng, G. C. (2008). Exercise for intermittent claudication. *Cochrane Database of Systematic Reviews, 2008*(4), CD000990. doi:10.1002/14651858.CD000990.pub2

Westerblad, H., Allen, D., & Lannergren, J. (2002). Muscle fatigue: Lactic acid or inorganic phosphate the major cause? *News in Physiological Science, 17*, 17–21.

Williams, M. A., Haskell, W. L., Ades, P. A., Amsterdam, E. A., Bittner, V., Franklin, B. A., ... Stewart, K. J. (2007). Resistance exercise in individuals with and without cardiovascular disease: 2007 update: A scientific statement from the American Heart Association Council on Clinical Cardiology and Council on Nutrition Physical Activity and Metabolism. *Circulation, 116*, 572–584.

Wood, R. J., & O'Neill, E. C. (2012). Resistance training in type II diabetes mellitus: Impact on areas of metabolic dysfunction in skeletal muscle and potential impact on bone. *Journal of Nutrition and Metabolism, 2012*, 268197, 1–13. doi:10.1155/2012/268197

Zhao, Y., Chung, P.-K., & Tong, T. K. (in press). Effectiveness of a balance-focused exercise program for enhancing functional fitness of older adults at risk of falling: A randomised controlled trial. *Geriatric Nursing, 38*, 491–497. doi:10.1016/j.gerinurse.2017.02.011

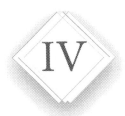

Biologically Based Therapies

The second major category of therapies listed on the website of the National Center for Complementary and Integrative Health (NCCIH) is *natural products*. This category includes herbal preparations (also called *botanicals*), vitamins, minerals, dietary supplements or nutraceuticals, essential oils, and live microorganisms (usually bacteria). One therapy that is becoming more commonly used by nurses is aromatherapy (Chapter 19). The essential oils used in aromatherapy are natural products. The most common use of essential oils by nurses is administration of aromatherapy externally—either by application to the skin or inhalation. The essential oils used in aromatherapy need to be differentiated from the artificial oils found in many popular bath-and-body shops.

Chapter 20 explores herbal preparations, whereas Chapter 21 focuses on functional foods and nutraceuticals. People from the earliest times have used herbal preparations to improve health or cure illnesses. Hildegard of Bingen, a Benedictine nun, wrote treatises in the 12th century detailing a large number of natural products such as herbs that could be used in healing (Encyclopedia of World Biography, 2004). Herbal product compounds for traditional Chinese medicine were documented in the Chinese *Materia Medica* as early as 400 BCE (Beijing Digital Museum of Traditional Chinese Medicine, 2012). Although the use of herbal preparations decreased in the 20th century as new medicines evolved, there has been resurgence in the public's use of natural products. The 2012 National Health Interview Survey (NHIS) included questions about the use of natural products (NCCIH, 2016). The report noted that 17.7% of those surveyed used one or more nonvitamin/nonmineral natural products.

The use of natural products in healing continues to be a part of the practices in many non-Western healthcare systems. For example, herbal preparations are a prominent part of Native American healing practices and traditional Chinese medicine; such preparations from natural products are also used in other parts of the world as illustrated in the international sidebars included within the chapters.

The majority of the products in the category of natural products (e.g., nonprescription supplements, food additives)—including nutraceuticals—are available over-the-counter. Since natural products do not require a prescription, healthcare professionals are often not actively involved in conversations and decisions regarding their use. As noted, natural products are an integral part of health practices in other cultures. Because a number of these products may interact with prescribed medications or other treatments, it is critical that the health care team be aware of a patient's use of natural products. Thus, careful, specific inquiry about their use needs to be a part of all patient assessments.

Research on natural products, especially herbal preparations, has only recently begun in the United States. However, a considerable body of research has been developed in other countries such as Germany. The German *Commission E Monographs* is akin to the *Physician's Desk Reference* (*PDR*) in the United States; specific monographs containing reliable information related to herbal preparations are included on the American Botanical Council website (cms.herbalgram.org/commissione/index.html).

REFERENCES

Beijing Digital Museum of Traditional Chinese Medicine. (2012). *Classic literature of traditional Chinese medicine.* Retrieved from http://en.tcm-china.info/culturehistory/literature/75830. shtml

Encyclopedia of World Biography. (2004). *Hildegard of Bingen.* Retrieved from http://www. encyclopedia.com/doc/1G2-3404708047.html

National Center for Complementary and Integrative Health. (2016). *NCCIH facts-at-a-glance and mission.* Retrieved from https://nccih.nih.gov/about/ataglance

Aromatherapy

LINDA L. HALCÓN

Aromatherapy is a relatively recent addition to nursing care in the United States, although it is growing in popularity within healthcare settings worldwide. Aromatherapy is offered by nurses in many countries, including Switzerland, Germany, Australia, Canada, Japan, Korea, and the United Kingdom, and it has been a medical specialty in France for many years. This modality is particularly well suited to nursing because it incorporates the therapeutic value of sensory experience (i.e., smell) and often includes the use of touch in the delivery of care. It also builds on a rich heritage of botanical therapies within nursing practice (Libster, 2002, 2012).

Aromatherapy has been part of herbal or botanical medicine for millennia. There is evidence of plant distillation and the use of essential oils and other aromatic plant products dating back 5,000 years. In ancient Egypt and the Middle East, plant oils were used in embalming, incense, perfumery, and healing. Therapeutic applications of essential oils were recorded as part of Greek and Roman medicine, and essential oils have been used in Ayurvedic medicine and in traditional Chinese medicine for more than 1,000 years. With the expansion of trade and improvements in distillation methods, essential oils became common elements of herbal medicine and perfumery in Europe during the Middle Ages (Keville & Green, 2009). In the late 1800s, scientists noted the association between environmental exposure to plant essential oils and the prevention of disease, and microbiologists conducted studies showing the in vitro activity of certain plant oils against microorganisms (Battaglia, 2003). More recent studies confirm the antimicrobial properties of essential oils (Solorzano-Santos & Miranda-Novales, 2012).

The development of clinical aromatherapy within the context of modern Western health science began in France just prior to World War I, when chemist René-Maurice Gattefossé was healed of a near-gangrenous wound with lavender essential oil. He subsequently championed its use for infections and battle wounds. Physician Jean Valnet and nurse Marguerite Maury followed Gattefossé in promoting the therapeutic value of essential oils in Europe, and, in the 1930s, interest in the anti-infective value of essential oils began to appear in the European and Australian medical literature (Price & Price, 2011). The use of essential oils continued sporadically as a nonconventional treatment modality in the West until the recent explosion of interest in botanical medicines, when its use became more visible and widespread. In their groundbreaking survey research on the use of complementary and alternative therapies in the United States, Eisenberg et al. (1998) reported that 5.6% of 2,055 adults surveyed used aromatherapy. Some large surveys estimating the overall prevalence of complementary therapies have not included aromatherapy as a separate modality (Barnes, Bloom, & Nahin, 2008; Tindle, Davis, Phillips, & Eisenberg, 2005); surveys of special populations, however, suggest its continuing and sometimes increasing use by the public (Akilen, Pimlott, Tsiami, & Robinson, 2014; Bowe, Adams, Lui & Sibbritt, 2015; Egan et al., 2012; Fisher, Adams, Hickman, & Sibbritt, 2016; Posadzki, Watson, Alotaibi, & Ernst, 2013).

DEFINITION

There are many operant definitions of aromatherapy, and some of them contribute to common misconceptions. The word *aromatherapy* can lead people to believe that it simply involves smelling scents, but this is incorrect. It is important to remember that the widespread use of synthetic scents in household and personal products is not considered aromatherapy. Styles (1997) defined aromatherapy as the use of essential oils for therapeutic purposes that encompass mind, body, and spirit—a broad definition that is consistent with holistic nursing practice. The National Cancer Institute (NCI, 2012) defines aromatherapy as the "therapeutic use of essential oils from flowers, herbs, and trees for the improvement of physical, emotional, and spiritual well-being." Buckle (2000) defined clinical aromatherapy in nursing as the use of essential oils for expected and measurable health outcomes. I define aromatherapy as "the scientific evidence informed use of plant essential oils for preventive or therapeutic purposes." Although aromatherapy clinical research has increased markedly in recent years, the evidence for using aromatherapy in nursing practice sometimes may be difficult to establish. There are findings for and against the use of a number of essential oils, however, and it is important to evaluate the available scientific data for individual essential oils and for specific conditions or symptoms.

Essential oils are obtained from a variety of plants worldwide, but not all plants produce essential oils. For those that do, the essential oils may be found in the plants' flowers, leaves, stems, bark, roots, seeds, resin, or peels. Most essential oils are obtained by steam distillation of a specific plant material. Steam-distilled essential oils are concentrated substances made up of the oil-soluble, lower-molecular-weight chemical constituents found in the source plant material. Essential oils from citrus fruit peels are usually obtained by expression (similar to grating or grinding), but they also may be distilled. Carbon dioxide extraction is increasingly accepted by scientists and practitioners as an acceptable method for obtaining certain essential oils; however, other types of solvent extraction generally are not preferred for clinical use. Expressed and CO_2-extracted essential oils contain a broader range of the chemicals present in the plant material; thus, they may have different therapeutic properties. Essential oils do not necessarily have the same medicinal properties as the plants from which they are derived because they do not contain the whole spectrum of chemicals present in the whole plant.

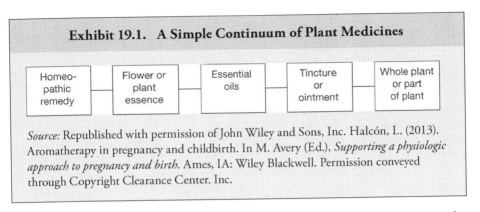

Exhibit 19.1.   A Simple Continuum of Plant Medicines

Homeo-pathic remedy	Flower or plant essence	Essential oils	Tincture or ointment	Whole plant or part of plant

Source: Republished with permission of John Wiley and Sons, Inc. Halcón, L. (2013). *Aromatherapy in pregnancy and childbirth.* In M. Avery (Ed.), *Supporting a physiologic approach to pregnancy and birth.* Ames, IA: Wiley Blackwell. Permission conveyed through Copyright Clearance Center. Inc.

Nurses have an important role in helping patients differentiate among the range of botanical products that are easily available. Misunderstanding the origin and makeup of these products can result in unnecessary risk. The most commonly used botanical products can be viewed as a continuum (Exhibit 19.1). On one end of the continuum are *whole herbs*, referring to unprocessed material from whole plants or parts of plants (Exhibit 19.1, far-right box). This is the oldest and most common form of botanical medicines worldwide. *Tinctures* and *ointments* are different from the whole plant and are also different from essential oils (Exhibit 19.1, second box from right). They are often confused with each other, and it is important that nurses understand the difference so that they can provide advice on their relative safety. Tinctures contain chemicals obtained from the plant material using alcohol as a solvent, and they include both water-soluble and oil-soluble chemicals. Tinctures are often taken orally or sublingually, with the dose and timing depending on the practitioner and the purpose. They are not as concentrated as essential oils. Ointments are made using vegetable oil (e.g., olive oil) rather than alcohol as the solvent. Plant-based tinctures and ointments are widely available. *Flower essences* (Exhibit 19.1, second box from left) are also often confused with essential oils. Essences contain some of the water-soluble chemicals present in the original plant material, and they also are thought to contain the vibrations or frequencies of the plants they are made from. *Homeopathy* (Exhibit 19.1, far-left box) was developed in Europe and was very popular in the United States in the late 1800s and early 1900s (Dooley, 2002). It declined in popularity as biomedicine became the dominant paradigm, although it is still an important healthcare paradigm in some European countries. Homeopathic remedies contain no molecules of the materials from which they are made. They are thought to work subtly on a vibrational level to promote balance and healing. Homeopathic remedies may be prescribed by a homeopathic physician or may be obtained over the counter. Homeopathy is becoming more popular in the United States once again; thus, nurses may benefit from understanding its basic concepts and differentiating it from other approaches.

SCIENTIFIC BASIS

Essential oils processed by any of these methods are highly volatile, complex mixtures of organic chemicals consisting of terpenes and terpenic compounds. The chemistry of an essential oil largely determines its therapeutic properties. There are 60 to 300 separate chemicals in each essential oil, and the proportions of the constituents for a particular plant species vary depending on a host of genetic and environmental factors. Knowing the plant species, the chemotype, the part of the plant used, the country of origin, and the method of extraction can provide information about an essential oil's chemical constituents using readily available aromatherapy textbooks.

The pharmacological activity of essential oils begins on entry into the body through the olfactory, respiratory, gastrointestinal, or integumentary systems. All body systems can be affected once the chemical molecules making up essential oils reach the circulatory and nervous systems. A proportion of the compounds within an essential oil finds its way into the body, however applied (Tisserand & Young, 2014), although the degree and rate of absorption vary depending on the route of administration. Inhaled aromas have the fastest effect, although compounds have been detected in the blood following massage (Cross, Russell, Southwell, & Roberts, 2008).

When inhaled, the many different molecules in each essential oil act as olfactory stimulants that travel via the nose to the olfactory bulb, and from there impulses travel to the brain. The amygdala and the hippocampus are of particular importance in the processing of aromas. The amygdala governs emotional responses. The hippocampus is involved in the formation and retrieval of explicit memories. The limbic system interacts with the cerebral cortex, contributing to the relationship between thoughts and feelings; it is directly connected to those parts of the brain that control heart rate, blood pressure, breathing, stress levels, and hormone levels (Kiecolt-Glaser et al., 2008). Although inhalation of essential oils affects the mind and body through the process of olfaction, most molecules from any inhaled vapor travel to the lungs, where they may be absorbed into the circulatory system (Tisserand, 2016). Tisserand and Young (2014, p. 139) cited several essential oils, including *Lavandula angustifolia* (true lavender), *Lavandula x intermedia* (lavandin), and *Citrus bergamia* (bergamot), that are thought to reduce the effect of external emotional stimuli by increasing gamma-aminobutyric acid (GABA). GABA inhibits neurons in the amygdala, producing a sedative effect. The literature increasingly supports physiological and psychological bases for the neurological actions of essential oils (Bagetta et al., 2010; Bikmoradi et al., 2015; Chien, Cheng, & Liu, 2012; Igarashi, Ikei, Song, & Miyazaki, 2014).

It is estimated that, at most, approximately 10% (5%–20%) of an essential oil may be absorbed through the skin on topical application (Cross et al., 2008; Tisserand, 2016), and there is controversy about skin penetration among essential oil researchers. Essential oils seem to be absorbed through the skin by working through the phospholipid bilayer via an intracellular route before the components of the essential oils reach the dermis and the bloodstream (Tisserand, 2016). In some instances, topically applied essential oil preparations have been used to enhance the dermal penetration of drugs (Nielsen, 2006; Valgimigli et al., 2012; Williams & Barry, 1989). There is some debate among essential oil experts about the rate and extent of penetration and absorption; however, there is evidence that penetration can vary depending on the condition of the skin, the age of the patient, the body part affected, and the carrier or vehicle for the essential oil. In addition, massage can enhance dermal penetration through heat and friction, and occlusion can enhance penetration. Essential oils are metabolized by the liver and excreted from the body mainly through the kidneys but also through respiration and insensate loss (Tisserand, 2016).

INTERVENTION

The choice of application method depends on patient characteristics and preferences, the symptom or condition being treated, the nurse's knowledge and practice parameters, the targeted outcome, and the properties and chemical components of the essential oil.

Although essential oils are not always pleasant smelling, inhalation is one of the simplest and most direct application procedures. With this method, one to five drops of an essential oil can be placed on a tissue or floated on hot water in a bowl and then inhaled for 5 to 20 minutes. Other inhalation techniques include the use of diffusers, burners, nebulizers, and vaporizers that can be operated by heat, battery, or electricity and may or may not include the use of water. Larger, portable aroma-inhalation systems are available commercially to provide a controlled release of essential oils into rooms of any size.

Inhalation, as well as skin, effects are experienced when essential oils are used in a bath. Baths have been found especially helpful for promoting relaxation and sleep in care settings and in the home. Lavender (*L. angustifolia*) is the essential oil most commonly used for these purposes, not only because it promotes relaxation, but also because it is generally well tolerated on the skin. For bath-use techniques, see Exhibit 19.2.

Compresses can be a useful method for applying essential oils to treat skin conditions or minor injuries. To prepare a compress, the nurse adds four to six drops of essential oil to warm water, soaks a soft cotton cloth in the mixture, wrings it out, and applies the cloth to the affected area, contusion, or abrasion. The nurse then covers the compress with plastic wrap to retain moisture, places a towel over the plastic wrap, and keeps it in place for as long as desired (up to 4 hours) (Buckle, 2003).

Massage also can facilitate the absorption of essential oils through the skin and can reduce the patient's perceived stress, thus enhancing the healing process and possibly communication. To create a mixture for massage, the nurse can dilute one to two drops of an essential oil in a teaspoon (5 mL) of cold-pressed vegetable oil and organic and scent-free lotion, cream, or gel. Mixtures for massage are generally 1% to 3% essential oil concentration (Tisserand & Young, 2014), using very low concentrations when massaging large areas of the body.

Exhibit 19.2. Therapeutic Bath With Essential Oils

Four to six drops of the essential oil may be dissolved first in a teaspoon of whole milk, rubbing alcohol, or carrier oil (cold-pressed) and then placed in the bath water. Because essential oils are not soluble in water, they float on top of the water if used without a dispersant, which could result in an uneven and too concentrated exposure. An essential-oil bath should last approximately 10 to 15 minutes. Essential oils also may be dissolved in salts (e.g., Epsom salts), which may be soothing to muscles and joints. One such recipe for bath salts consists of 1 tablespoon of baking soda, 2 tablespoons of Epsom salts, and 3 tablespoons of sea salt with four to six drops of essential oils mixed throughout. Salts should be added to the bath water just before immersion and after agitating the water to disperse them.

Essential oils should not be used undiluted on mucous membranes; even on intact skin they are generally used in concentrations seldom exceeding 5% to 10%. When used to treat conditions such as vaginal infections, essential-oil preparations can be created or purchased as pessaries or suppositories. Only essential oils high in alcohols, such as tea tree, are appropriate in pessaries; alcohols are less likely to cause skin irritation. If essential oils are applied via tampons, the tampons should be changed regularly (Buckle, 2003). Oral thrush (candidiasis) in adults also can be treated with diluted essential oils by the swish-and-spit method, taking care not to swallow (Jandourek, Vaishampayan, & Vazquez, 1998). Recent studies suggest that essential oils in a mouthwash solution can help prevent dental caries and treat periodontal disease (Carvalhinho, Costa, Coelho, Martins, & Sampaio, 2012; Charles, Cortelli, Aquino, Revankar, & Wu, 2015; Cortelli, Cortelli, Shang, McGuire & Charles, 2013).

General Guidelines for Use of Essential Oils

Nurses should be aware of general safety guidelines for patient education and in practice. These include:

- Store essential oils away from open flames; they are volatile and highly flammable.
- Store essential oils in a cool place away from sunlight; use amber- or dark blue-colored glass containers. Close the container immediately after use. Essential oils can oxidize in the presence of heat, light, and air, changing their chemistry and thus their actions in unpredictable ways.
- Be aware that essential oils can stain clothing and textiles and that undiluted essential oils can degrade some plastics. Take appropriate precautions.
- Keep essential oils away from children and pets unless you are well-versed in clinical aromatherapy. The literature contains cases of adverse reactions or deaths related to improper applications or accidental ingestion in young children and pets (Halicioglu, Astarcioglu, Yaprak, & Aydinlioglu, 2011).
- Use essential oils with care in pregnancy, especially in the first trimester (Halcón, 2013).
- Use essential oils from reputable suppliers. Seek the advice of a trained aromatherapist or the recommendation of a knowledgeable clinical provider. If using essential oils in clinical or research settings, test results verifying the chemical constituency should be obtained.
- Special care is needed when using essential oils with or around people who have a history of severe asthma or multiple allergies. Be sure to ask.
- Despite the relative safety of essential oils when used properly, sensitization and skin irritation can occur with topical application. In these cases, any residual essential oil solution should be removed with oil or whole milk and rinsed with water, and its use should be discontinued. Most such reactions resolve without treatment; however, a healthcare provider should be consulted if discomfort/itching is severe or persists.
- If an essential oil gets into the eyes, rinse it out with milk or carrier oil first and then with water. Remember that essential oils by themselves are not water soluble.

Measurement of Outcomes

The selection of suitable methods for assessing aromatherapy effects depends on the problem for which essential oils are used and the targeted outcomes of treatment. For example, if lavender is used to promote sleep, measures might include physiological markers, changes in sleep patterns, or comparison of signs and symptoms of insomnia between a treated group and another group that is similar in all ways other than the treatment. For psychological conditions such as depression or anxiety, many reliable survey instruments are available and can be further validated by adding physiological measures such as cortisol levels or skin temperature and conductance. For infectious disease outcomes, standard laboratory tests can be used to measure the effect of treatment on microbial load. Other useful measures could include digital photography, pain scales, quality-of-life scales, tests of cognitive performance, and electroencephalogram results. Using established measurement tools where possible is helpful in facilitating interpretation and comparing the effects of essential oils with those of other approaches.

Credentialing

There is neither a recognized national certification examination for aromatherapists nor a governing body. The Aromatherapy Registration Council, a nonprofit entity established in 2000, administers a national examination and can provide the public with a list of registered aromatherapy practitioners. Nurses and health professionals wishing to use aromatherapy in their practice should check with their licensing bodies; nurses should check with their state board of nursing. Many states allow nurses to use aromatherapy in their practice if they have received specialized education. Many courses are available, and health professionals should choose one that is relevant to their own clinical practice. Two large aromatherapy professional organizations in the United States are the National Association of Holistic Aromatherapy (www.naha.org) and the Alliance of International Aromatherapists (www.alliance-aromatherapists.org). There are no requirements in the United States at this time for a person administering aromatherapy to be certified or accredited; however, Canadian nurses have established criteria for practice. The length of training programs in aromatherapy may range from one weekend to several years. Generally, it is not necessary to be a health professional to enroll in these educational programs. Despite the lack of uniform credentialing, it is no longer unusual for hospitals and other clinical settings to include aromatherapy services, and nurses often have spearheaded the changes. Thus, nurses must insist that policies and procedures include good quality assurance and quality control.

PRECAUTIONS

Aromatherapy is a very safe complementary therapy if it is used with knowledge and within accepted guidelines. Many essential oils have been tested by the food and beverage industry for use as flavorings and preservatives, and much research has been carried out by the perfume and tobacco industries. Although most of the essential oils commonly used in clinical aromatherapy have been given generally-regarded-as-safe (GRAS) status, this only means that they are considered safe in minute amounts in foods and cosmetics. It does not give carte-blanche approval for all uses. Nurses should not administer essential oils orally, as this is outside a nurse's scope of practice, and poisonings have been documented (Jacobs & Hornfeldt, 1994; Janes, Price, & Thomas, 2005). According to Tisserand and Young (2014), most poisonings involve ingestion accidents with young children; however, adults also have been known to ingest toxic amounts and types of essential oils. Most essential oils should not be used during early pregnancy and should be used cautiously anytime during pregnancy. Nurses need to be aware of essential oils that can cause photosensitivity, such as bergamot (*C. bergamia*) and other citrus oils (Keljova, Jirova, Bendova, Gajdos, & Kolarova, 2010), and they should provide appropriate patient education and protection when these are used. Numerous cases of contact dermatitis following skin applications of essential oils have been reported (Brown & Browning, 2016; Fettig, Taylor, & Sood, 2014; Rudback, Islam, Borje, Nilsson, & Karlberg, 2015), underscoring the importance of diluting essential oils for topical use and knowing which essential oils are most likely to be irritating or sensitizing.

Essential oils are very concentrated and potent compounds, and in most cases, they must be diluted in carrier oils for topical use. Tea tree (*Melaleuca alternifolia*) and lavender (*L. angustifolia*) are among the few exceptions to this rule. These essential oils can be used full strength on minor cuts, abrasions, and small burns.

Some essential oils are known to be carcinogenic and others are contraindicated in people with specific conditions. Knowledge and common sense should guide nurses' thinking in this regard. For example, stimulant essential oils should not be used for patients with conditions for which stimulants are contraindicated. Essential oils can potentiate or decrease the effects of medications, often by increasing or decreasing metabolic enzymes (Tisserand, 2016). Extra care is needed when using essential oils with patients receiving chemotherapy because they may affect the absorption rate of cancer-treating and other drugs (Fox, Gerber, DuPlessis, & Hamman, 2011; Jain, Aqil, Ahad, Ali, & Khar, 2008; Lim, Liu, & Chan, 2009; Paduch, Kandefer-Szerszen, Trytek, & Fiedurek, 2007; Williams & Barry, 1989). In short, it cannot be assumed that all essential oils are safe in all situations simply because they are *natural*.

Product identity confusion is another potential threat to safety. As noted, essential oils should not be confused with herbal extracts, which are completely different chemical mixtures, and they cannot be used interchangeably. Besides their chemical dissimilarities, herbal extracts, and teas are usually taken internally, whereas essential oils generally are not. Nurses share responsibility for ensuring product integrity when essential oils are used in clinical practice. Chemical testing of essential oils used in patient care should be incorporated into ongoing quality assurance/quality control programs.

Nurses using essential oils regularly should protect themselves from unintended effects. Because essential oils are volatile, their molecules are inhaled by those applying them, as well as by patients. It has been demonstrated that hand dermatitis may be associated with long-term unprotected use of lotions and other products containing essential oils (Crawford, Katz, Ellis, & James, 2004; Uter et al., 2010).

Perhaps one of the greatest risks in aromatherapy is using an incorrect essential oil for a particular health outcome. This could stem from a nurse's lack of knowledge of plant taxonomy. Many essential oils have familiar common names such as lavender, rose, and rosemary, but it is important to know the full botanical name.

Exhibit 19.3.   Common and Botanical Names of Essential Oils Frequently Used in Aromatherapy

Common Name	Botanical Name
Chamomile Roman	*Chamaemelum nobile* or *Anthemus nobile*
Eucalyptus	*Eucalyptus globulus, Eucalyptus radiata*
Frankincense	*Boswellia carterii*
Ginger	*Zingiber officinale*
Lavender, true	*Lavandula officinalis* or *Lavandula angustifolia*
Lemon	*Citrus limon*
Mandarin	*Citrus reticulata*
Orange, sweet	*Citrus sinensis*
Peppermint	*Mentha x piperita*
Rosemary	*Rosmarinus officinalis*
Spearmint	*Mentha spicata*
Tea tree	*Melaleuca alternifolia*

For example, "lavender" is a common name that covers *three different kinds* of lavender *and* several hybrids. The genus of lavender is *Lavandula*, and all lavenders begin with this word. *L. angustifolia* is one of the most widely used and researched essential oils and is recognized as a relaxant and soporific. The other two species used in aromatherapy have very different properties. *Lavandula latifolia* (spike lavender) is a stimulant and expectorant; *Lavandula stoechas* is antimicrobial and not safe to use for long periods. The picture is further complicated by the hybrid *L. x intermedia* with its three chemotypes. Nurses who use aromatherapy clinically must know the full botanical name of an essential oil they intend to use. The botanical names of essential oils commonly used in clinical settings are found in Exhibit 19.3.

USES

Many health outcomes that fall within the domain of nursing practice can be addressed with essential oils, either alone or combined with other approaches. Essential oils can affect people psychologically and physically. They can increase or decrease sympathetic activity in individuals, affecting heart rate, blood pressure, plasma adrenaline, and plasma catecholamine levels (Chuang, Chen, Liu, Chuang, & Lin, 2014; Menezes, Barreto, Antoniolli, Santos, & de Sousa, 2010; Watanabe et al., 2015). The effect of essential oil odors can be relaxing or stimulating, depending on a person's previous experiences, likes and dislikes, and the chemistry of the essential oil used; therefore, it is important to explore patient preference and the purpose for which the oil is being used when selecting essential oils for therapeutic purposes.

Essential oils are used therapeutically to address a broad range of symptoms and body systems, and there are many aromatherapy texts describing their uses and recommending particular essential oils for specific conditions or symptoms. It is difficult to identify evidence other than case studies or historical anecdotes for some of these uses; however, with increased clinical use in recent years there is a more robust evidence base for a number of essential oils and clinical outcomes. The main applications of essential oils in conventional healthcare settings are to help address pain, symptoms of anxiety or depression, nausea, sleeplessness, or agitation and to prevent or treat infections. Nurse midwives have long incorporated essential oils into their practices, notably to reduce pain and aid relaxation during and after childbirth (Burns, Blamey, Ersser, Barnetson, & Lloyd, 2000; Conrad & Adams, 2012; Einion, 2016; Imura, Misao, & Ushijima, 2006; Musil, 2013; Sheikhan et al., 2012). In long-term care and hospital settings, essential oils are used to help reduce anxiety and agitation in patients with or without dementia (Bowles, Griffiths, Quirk, & Croot, 2002; Goes, Antunes, Alves, & Teixeira-Silva, 2012; Kritsidima, Newton, & Asimakopoulou, 2009; Lin, Chan, Ng, & Lam, 2007; Morris, 2008; O'Connor, Eppingstall, Taffe, & van der Ploeg, 2013; Woelk & Schlafke, 2010; Yoshiyama, Arita, & Suzuki, 2015), promote sleep and reduce nighttime sedation (Dyer, Cleary, McNeill, Ragsdale-Lowe & Osland, 2016; Lillehei, Halcón, Savik, & Reis, 2015), and promote wound healing (Culliton & Halcón, 2011; Lusby, Coombes, & Wilkinson, 2006). Aromatherapy can be a helpful intervention for palliative and end-of-life nursing care (Pounds, 2012).

Aromatherapy is used to address acute or chronic pain (de-Sousa, 2011; Gedney, Glover, & Fillingim, 2004; Ghelardini, Galeotti, Salvatore, & Mazzanti, 1999; Irmak et al., 2015; Kim et al., 2007), fatigue and nausea (Adib-Hajbaghery & Hosseini, 2015; Bagheri-Nesami, Shorofi, Nikkhah, Espahbodi, & Ghaderi, 2016; P. Lua, Salihah, & Mazlan, 2015; P. L. Lua & Zakaria, 2012; Pearson, 2015), infection (Bassol & Juliani, 2012; Gelmini, Belotti, Vecchi, Testa & Beretta, 2016; Paule, 2001; Thompson et al., 2011), and mood and cognition (Goes, Ursulino, Almeida-Souza, Alves, & Teixeira-Silva, 2015; Morris, 2008; Moss, Rouse, Wesnes, & Moss, 2010; Nagata et al., 2014). The literature also includes studies reporting the use of essential oils in the treatment of head lice and scabies (Barker & Altman, 2010; Choi, Yang, Lee, Clark, & Ahn, 2010; Gutierrez, Werdin-Gonzalez, Stefanazzi, Bras, & Ferrero, 2016; Thomas et al., 2016), and as an aid to smoking cessation (Rose & Behm, 1994) and drug withdrawal (Kunz, Schultz, Lewitzky, Driessen, & Rau, 2007; Lemme, 2009).

There is considerable and growing international literature on the use of plant essential oils against pathogenic microorganisms. The efficacy of essential oils in the treatment and prevention of infectious diseases has important implications for patient health as well as disinfection and hygiene (Edwards-Jones, Buck, Shawcross, Dawson, & Dunn, 2004; Enshaieh, Jooya, Siadat, & Iraji, 2007; Muthaiyan, Biswas, Crandall, Wilkinson & Ricke, 2012), especially with the increase in resistance bacteria (K. A. Hammer, Carson, & Riley, 2008). Methicillin-resistant *Staphylococcus aureus* and other microorganisms have been found to be sensitive to tea tree oil (*M. alternifolia*) (Carson, Hammer, Messager, & Riley, 2005; Halcón & Milkus, 2004; K. Hammer, Carson & Riley, 2012). Preliminary work suggests that essential oils may also be effective in other difficult-to-treat infections and wounds (Culliton & Halcón, 2011; Sherry, Sivananthan, Warnke, & Eslick, 2003).

Pediatric Applications

Aromatherapy has been one of the integrative therapies most used for and by children, as evidenced by prevalence studies (Adams et al., 2013; Grossoehme, Cotton, & McPhail, 2013; Simpson & Roman, 2001), the multitude of aromatherapy products advertised and sold for babies and children, and anecdotally by the increase in pediatric toxicity cases in emergency rooms and poison control centers. Knowledge and common sense are needed to guide nurses and parents in safe applications of essential oils in pediatrics. Hospital pediatric units generally limit aromatherapy to the safest essential oils and common symptoms such as pain (e.g., true lavender, Roman chamomile), nausea (e.g., ginger, spearmint, mandarin), and perceived anxiety (e.g., true lavender, sweet orange). Research suggests that essential oils may be quite helpful in addressing these symptoms (Kiberd, Clarke, Chorney, d'Eon, & Wright, 2016; Malachowska, Fendler, Pomkala, Suwala, & Mlynarski, 2016; O'Flaherty, van Dijk, Albertyn, Millar, & Rode, 2012). With vulnerable populations such as infants and small children, I recommend applying the precautionary principle (if a substance has not been proved safe, do not use it unless there is a compelling reason) and the integrative nursing principle that advises "moving from least intensive/invasive [therapies] to more, depending on need and context (Kreitzer & Koithan, 2014, p.12). As an example, if a child has postoperative nausea and vomiting, imagery or acupressure (neither of which involve chemical substance exposure) could be tried first and then followed by offering an inhalation of spearmint if they were not helpful. Extending this mode of thinking, if the aromatherapy is not helpful, the nurse could consider a pharmaceutical antiemetic.

Toxicity in children, as with others, is related to dose, meaning unsafe concentrations, inappropriate application methods, or unsafe essential oils. Essential oils are highly concentrated mixtures of many volatile chemicals, even though they are derived from plants. Chronic and acute reactions are usually caused by topical applications or ingestion. To avoid accidental ingestion of essential oils by small children, it is recommended that the oils be treated as medications and kept out of reach. They can be stored inside child-proof medication containers at home. In addition, essential oils should be sold and stored in bottles with integral drop dispensers and clearly labeled with all ingredients (Fitzgerald & Halcón, 2010). Allergic contact dermatitis is not uncommon (Brown & Browning, 2016; Storan, Nolan, & Kirby, 2016), and essential oil concentrations in skin or massage products should be lower for children than for adults. Tisserand and Young (2014) recommend concentrations of less than 0.2% for full-term infants up to 3 months, less than 0.5% up to 24 months, less than 2% up to 6 years, and no greater than 3% from 6 to 15 years. These guidelines assume that there is a good health rationale. Nurses who are knowledgeable about essential oils can introduce them in pediatric practice and remain within safety guidelines.

CULTURAL APPLICATIONS

There are regional, cultural, and religious traditions and preferences for the types of essential oils used therapeutically. For example, Ayurvedic practices include many essential oils that are produced in the Indian subcontinent, including those from sandalwood, jasmine, and other floral or spicy aromatic plants. Africa is the source of oils such as frankincense, myrrh, ylang ylang, ravensara, and others. In Europe and much of the United States, essential oil production focuses on herbs or flowers that grow and thrive in temperate climates, such as peppermint, lavender, and basil. Citrus oils are produced in warmer regions. However, the lines are not as distinct as in earlier times when the procurement of essential oils was more limited to native and local plants. Plants are routinely transported and grown in nonnative areas, and the essential oils most commonly used for therapeutic purposes are now readily available throughout the world, obtainable through global trade and Internet sales.

Cultural plant-healing traditions often have been altered and adopted by newcomers. The case of Australian tea tree oil provides an example of adaptation of cultural and regional health practices over time. *M. alternifolia* grows in one area of Australia as a native plant, and it was used as an herbal anti-infective medicine by Aboriginal peoples for centuries. More than 200 species of the genus *Melaleuca* are native to Australia and New Zealand, and only a few have been explored for modern medicinal uses as essential oils (Weiss, 1997). *M. alternifolia* is one of many plants referred to as "tea tree" in Australia and New Zealand; hence the importance of relying on Latin names for identification. The healing properties of this plant were noted by European explorers and settlers, and at some point, the foliage was distilled to produce a very concentrated antiseptic substance—tea tree oil. Since the early 1900s, there has been intermittent interest in tea tree oil on the part of the medical community. This interest has expanded in recent years, partly through partnerships between the Australian government and the private agricultural sector to expand tea tree oil's economic impact. Both public and private funding was provided for excellent scientific research on the antimicrobial properties of tea tree oil, subsequently added to by healthcare researchers and scientists around the world. Extensive information can be found at the website of the Tea Tree Oil Research Group, University of Western Australia (www.marshallcentre.uwa.edu.au). Tea tree is now an important plantation crop, and the antimicrobial properties of tea tree oil (*M. alternifolia*) are somewhat known in Western biomedical healthcare settings but more widely so by the public. Affordable, pure essential oil or health products with tea tree oil as a major ingredient are available worldwide, benefiting the Australian agricultural sector as well as healthcare. For a description of aromatherapy and issues relevant to its use in nursing practice in Australia, see Sidebar 19.1.

SIDEBAR 19.1. AROMATHERAPY IN NURSING PRACTICE IN AUSTRALIA

Trisha Dunning

Anecdotally, aromatherapy is one of the most popular complementary therapies Australian nurses use, often combined with massage. National population data about the use of complementary and alternative medicine (CAM) suggest approximately 70% of nurses use CAM, including aromatherapy; however, there are no national data about the number of nurses are qualified aromatherapists, work as aromatherapists in private practice, or incorporate aromatherapy in their nursing practice. One reason for the lack of such data is that aromatherapy is a self-regulated practice, unlike nursing. Currently, traditional Chinese medicine (TCM) is the only CAM regulated by the Australian Health Practitioner Regulation Agency.

Most Australians who use aromatherapy do so on a self-selected basis, and many may not understand the risks and benefits of essential oils or how to use them appropriately. In addition, aromatherapy products are often purchased from pharmacies, health food shops, local community markets, and supermarkets, where expert advice is not available and there is no guarantee of quality. Significantly, the public often confuses fragrances and essential oils, largely due to marketing of fragrance products in beauty and home care.

Many CAM professional groups—including the International Aromatherapy and Aromatic Medicine Association, the organization most aromatherapists in Australia (including nurses) belong to—have specific requirements for membership. Membership rules include completing accredited courses, ensuring knowledge is current, and holding professional indemnity. Aromatherapy training is delivered at certificate and diploma levels by various private education providers and can often be completed online. Many of these courses lead to qualifications in beauty therapy rather than clinical aromatherapy. Some university CAM courses include information about aromatherapy. The quality of these courses varies in course content, teaching quality, amount and quality of supervised clinical practice, and assessment criteria.

Aromatherapy is used in a variety of clinical settings in Australia; however, it may not always be truly integrated into care plans and the outcomes are not always monitored systematically. Key areas of practice in which aromatherapy is used include palliative and cardiovascular care to manage stress and pain, promote relaxation, and improve emotional well-being. Essential oils are mostly used externally in vaporizers and massage, applied to furnishings and clothing, or used in baths.

Until recently, aromatherapy was commonly used in older care facilities to address odor, reduce stress, promote sleep, and reduce the need for sedatives. One program, Creative Ways to Care, was developed to assist caregivers in home care for relatives with dementia. The program had been widely implemented in older care settings. However, CAM use (including aromatherapy) in such facilities has declined since the Aged Care Funding Instrument (ACFI) was introduced and residents now have to pay for CAM therapies. Introduction of the ACFI has also affected the enrollment in CAM courses.

A number of factors affect aromatherapy safety and quality:

- The individual (reason for using essential oils knowledge, health status, concomitant use of other CAM, conventional medicines)
- The practitioner (knowledge, competence)
- Essential oils and carrier substances (labels, quality, purity, storage conditions, manufacturing processes)
- Application method (internal or external use)
- Environment (where aromatherapy is delivered)
- Evidence base for use (articulated in policies and procedures or guidelines)
- Regulation of products and practitioners (Essential oils are regulated as medicines under the Therapeutic Goods Act [1989] and must meet a range of other regulations such as labeling and packaging.)

The growing interest in the discovery of new plant medicines that have health applications or profit possibilities has fueled expanded research on essential oils. In addition to laboratory and human studies aimed at improving health, research also is aimed at improved food preservation and the resultant prevention of food-borne illness and the eradication or control of insect-borne and parasitic diseases such as malaria (Samarasekera, Weerasinghe, & Hemalal, 2008; Singh et al., 2008). As new essential oils are produced and tested for their health and environmental applications (Baik et al., 2008; Dongmo et al., 2008), their production can provide international trade opportunities and improved agricultural sustainability, in addition to usually very affordable natural medicines. Sustainability of plant sources of essential oils is a growing concern, especially with essential oils derived from slow-maturing trees such as sandalwood, frankincense, myrrh, and rosewood. Integrative or holistic nurses have a role in this discussion.

FUTURE RESEARCH

The future of clinical aromatherapy is promising. Although aromatherapy researchers continue to face challenges related to the products themselves, such as smell blinding, synergistic and antagonistic effects when different oils are combined, possible confounding with aromatherapy massage, and natural variation in products, many more studies are being conducted and published, both in integrative therapies journals and in specialty journals. Nurses and other health professionals need to be aware of these challenges and critical about aromatherapy research reports, as they are about all research, as publication bias can occur in any direction. More work is needed to test the efficacy of essential oils already in common use and to extend the practice of aromatherapy in clinical settings where, for some conditions and individuals, it can be a cost-effective alternative or adjunct therapy with fewer side effects than pharmaceuticals and other biomedical treatments.

If current trends continue, aromatherapy (inhalation and topical) will be a standard care measure for addressing nursing diagnoses in acute, long-term, and community-based care. In some cities, most hospitals and nursing homes already have an aromatherapy program that is included in nursing protocols. Integrative nursing is a paradigm to guide and ground the growth of programs in healthcare settings and allow nurses to remain informed by evidence and view aromatherapy interventions in a larger context. Expanded applications, such as wound care and dermatological or oral preparations to address medical diagnoses, are very promising and will require multidisciplinary collaboration. Nursing perspectives will be important to ensure that essential oils are used to support health holistically.

WEBSITES

The following are websites that nurses may find helpful in identifying more information about essential oils:

- Alliance of International Aromatherapists
  (www.alliance-aromatherapists.org)
- Aromatherapy Registration Council
  (www.aromatherapycouncil.org)

* National Association of Holistic Aromatherapists (www.naha.org)

REFERENCES

Adams, D., Dagenais, S., Clifford, T., Baydala, L., King, W., Hervas-Malo, M., ... Vohra, S. (2013). Complementary and alternative medicine use by pediatric specialty outpatients. *Pediatrics, 131*(2), 225–232.

Adib-Hajbaghery, M., & Hosseini, F. (2015). Investigating the effects of inhaling ginger essence on post-nephrectomy nausea and vomiting. *Complementary Therapies in Medicine, 23*(6), 827–831.

Akilen, R., Pimlott, Z., Tsiami, A., & Robinson, N. (2014). The use of complementary and alternative medicine by individuals with features of metabolic syndrome. *Journal of Integrative Medicine, 12*(3), 171–174.

Bagetta, G., Morrone, L., Rombola, L., Amantea, D., Russo, R., Berliocchi, L., ... Corasaniti, M. (2010). Neuropharmacology of the essential oil bergamot. *Fitoterapia, 81*(6), 453–461.

Bagheri-Nesami, M., Shorofi, S., Nikkhah, A., Espahbodi, F., & Ghaderi Koolaee, F. (2016). The effects of aromatherapy with lavender essential oil on fatigue levels in haemodialysis patients: A randomized clinical trial. *Complementary Therapies in Clinical Practice, 22*, 33–37.

Baik, J., Kim, S., Lee, J., Oh, T., Kim J., Lee, N., & Hyun, C. (2008). Chemical composition and biological activities of essential oils extracted from Korean endemic citrus species. *Journal of Microbiology and Biotechnology, 18*(1), 74–79.

Barker, S. C., & Altman, P. M. (2010). A randomised, assessor blind, parallel group comparative efficacy trial of three products for the treatment of head lice in children—Melaleuca oil and lavender oil, pyrethrins and piperonyl butoxide, and a "suffocation" product. *BMC Dermatology, 10*(1), 6.

Barnes, P. M., Bloom, B., & Nahin, R. (2008). Complementary and alternative medicine use among adults and children: United States 2007. *National Health Statistics Report, 10*(12), 1–23.

Bassol, I. H. N., & Juliani, H. R. (2012). Essential oils in combination and their antimicrobial properties. *Molecules, 17*(4), 3989–4006. doi:10.3390/molecules17043989

Battaglia, S. (2003). *The complete guide to aromatherapy* (2nd ed.). Brisbane, Australia: International Centre of Holistic Aromatherapy.

Bikmoradi, A., Seifi, Z., Poorolajal, J., Araghchian, M., Safiaryan, R., & Oshvandi, K. (2015). Effect of inhalation aromatherapy with lavender essential oil on stress and vital signs in patients undergoing coronary artery bypass surgery: A single-blinded randomized clinical trial. *Complementary Therapies in Medicine, 23*(3), 331–338.

Bowe, S., Adams, J., Lui, C. W., & Sibbritt, D. (2015). A longitudinal analysis of self-prescribed complementary and alternative medicine use by a nationally representative sample of 19,783 Australian women, 2006-2010. *Complementary Therapies in Medicine, 23*(5), 699–704.

Bowles, E. J., Griffiths, M., Quirk, L., & Croot, K. (2002). Effects of essential oils and touch on resistance to nursing care procedures and other dementia-related behaviours in a residential care facility. *International Journal of Aromatherapy, 12*(1), 22–29.

Brown, M., & Browning, J. (2016). A case of psoriasis replaced by allergic contact dermatitis in a 12-year-old boy. *Pediatric Dermatology, 33*(2), e125–e126.

Buckle, J. (2000). The "M" technique. *Massage and Bodywork, 15*, 52–64.

Buckle, J. (2003). *Clinical aromatherapy: Essential oils in practice* (2nd ed.). New York, NY: Churchill Livingstone.

Burns, E. E., Blamey, C., Ersser, S. J., Barnetson, L., & Lloyd, A. J. (2000). An investigation into the use of aromatherapy in intrapartum midwifery practice. *Journal of Alternative and Complementary Therapies, 6*(2), 141–147.

Carson, C., Hammer, K., Messager, S., & Riley, T. (2005). Tea tree oil: A potential alternative for the management of methicillin-resistant *Staphylococcus aureus* (MRSA). *Australian Infection Control, 10*(1), 32–34.

Carvalhinho, S., Costa, A. M., Coelho, A. C., Martins, E., & Sampaio, A. (2012). Susceptibilities of *Candida albicans* mouth isolates to antifungal agents, essential oils and mouth rinses. *Mycopathologia*, *174*(1), 69–76.

Charles, C., Cortelli, J., Aquino, D., Revankar, R., & Wu, M. (2015). Gingival health benefits of essential oil, 0.075% cetylpyridinium chloride and control mouthrinses: A 4-week randomized clinical study. *American Journal of Dentistry*, *28*(4), 197–202.

Chien, L-W., Cheng, S., & Liu, C. (2012). The effect of lavender aromatherapy on autonomic nervous system in midlife women with insomnia. *Evidence-Based Complementary & Alternative Medicine*, *2012*, 1–8. doi:10.1155/2012/740813

Choi, H.-Y., Yang, Y.-C., Lee, S. H., Clark, J. M., & Ahn, Y.-J. (2010). Efficacy of spray formulations containing binary mixtures of clove and eucalyptus oils against susceptible and pyrethroid/malathion-resistant head lice (Anoplura: Pediculidae). *Journal of Medical Entomology*, *47*(3), 387–391.

Chuang, K. J., Chen, H. W., Liu, I. J., Chuang, H. C., & Lin, L. Y. (2014). The effect of essential oil on heart rate and blood pressure among solus por aqua workers. *European Journal of Preventive Cardiology*, *21*(7), 823–828.

Conrad, P., & Adams, C. (2012). The effects of clinical aromatherapy for anxiety and depression in the high risk postpartum woman—A pilot study. *Complementary Therapies in Clinical Practice*, *18*(3), 164–168.

Cortelli, S., Cortelli, J., Shang, H., McGuire, J., & Charles, C. (2013). Long-term management of plaque and gingivitis using an alcohol-free essential oil containing mouthrinse: A 6-month randomized clinical trial. *American Journal of Dentistry*, *26*(3), 149–155.

Crawford, G., Katz, K., Ellis, E., & James, W. (2004). Use of aromatherapy products and increased risk of hand dermatitis in massage therapists. *Archives of Dermatology*, *140*(8), 991–996.

Cross, S., Russell, M., Southwell, I., & Roberts, M. (2008). Human skin penetration of the major components of Australian tea tree oil applied in its pure form and as a 20% solution *in vitro*. *European Journal of Pharmaceutics & Biopharmaceutics*, *69*(1), 214–222.

Culliton, P., & Halcón, L. (2011). Chronic wound treatment with topical tea tree oil. *Alternative Therapies in Health and Medicine*, *17*(2), 46–47.

de-Sousa, D. (2011). Analgesic-like activity of essential oils constituents. *Molecules*, *16*(3), 2233–2252.

Dongmo, P., Tchoumbougnang, F., Sonwa, E., Kenfack, S., Zollo, P., & Menut, C. (2008). Antioxidant and anti-inflammatory potential of essential oils of some *Zanthoxylum* (Rutaceae) of Cameroon. *International Journal of Essential Oil Therapeutics*, *2*(2), 82–88.

Dooley, T. R. (2002). *Homeopathy: Beyond flat earth medicine* (2nd ed.). San Diego, CA: Timing Publications.

Dyer, J., Cleary, L., McNeill, S., Ragsdale-Lowe, M., & Osland, C. (2016). The use of aromasticks to help with sleep problems: A patient experience survey. *Complementary Therapies in Clinical Practice*, *22*, 51–58.

Edwards-Jones, V., Buck, R., Shawcross, S., Dawson, M., & Dunn, K. (2004). The effect of essential oils on methicillin-resistant *Staphylococcus aureus* using a dressing model. *Burns*, *30*(8), 772–777.

Egan, B., Gage, H., Hood, J., Poole, K., McDowell, C., Maguire, G., & Storey, L. (2012). Availability of complementary and alternative medicine for people with cancer in the British National Health Service: Results of a national survey. *Complementary Therapies in Clinical Practice*, *18*(2), 75–80.

Einion, A. (2016). Aromatherapy in midwifery practice. *Practising Midwife*, *19*(5), 12, 14–15.

Eisenberg, D. M., Davis, R. B., Ettner, S. L., Appel, S., Wilken, S., Van Rompay, M. I., & Kessler, R. C. (1998). Trends in alternative medicine in the USA, 1990–1997: Results of a follow-up national survey. *Journal of the American Medical Association*, *280*(18), 1569–1575.

Enshaieh, S., Jooya, A., Siadat, A., & Iraji, F. (2007). The efficacy of 5% topical tea tree oil gel in mild to moderate acne vulgaris: A randomized, double-blind placebo-controlled study. *Indian Journal of Dermatology, Venereology and Leprology*, *73*(1), 22–25.

Fettig, J., Taylor, J., & Sood, A. (2014). Post-surgical allergic contact dermatitis to compound tincture of benzoin and association with reactions to fragrances and essential oils. *Dermatitis*, *25*(4), 211–212.

Fisher, C., Adams, J., Hickman, L., & Sibbritt, D. (2016). The use of complementary and alternative medicine by 7427 Australian women with cyclic perimenstrual pain and discomfort: A cross-sectional study. *BMC Complementary & Alternative Medicine, 16*,129.

Fitzgerald, M., & Halcón, L. (2010). A pediatric perspective on aromatherapy. In T. Culbert & K. Olness (Eds.), *Integrative Pediatrics*. Oxford, UK: Oxford University Press.

Fox, L. T., Gerber, M., DuPlessis, J., & Hamman, J. H. (2011). Transdermal drug delivery enhancement by compounds of natural origin. *Molecules, 16*(12), 10507–10540.

Gedney, J., Glover, T., & Fillingim, R. (2004). Sensory and affective pain discrimination after inhalation of essential oils. *Psychosomatic Medicine, 66*(4), 599–606.

Gelmini, F., Belotti, L., Vecchi, S., Testa, C., & Beretta, G. (2016). Air dispersed essential oils combined with standard sanitization procedures for environmental microbiota control in nosocomial hospitalization rooms. *Complementary Therapies in Medicine, 25*, 113–119.

Ghelardini, C., Galeotti, N., Salvatore, G., & Mazzanti, G. (1999). Local anaesthetic activity of the essential oil of *Lavandula angustifolia*. *Planta Medica, 65*(8), 700–703.

Goes, T., Antunes, F., Alves, P., & Teixeira-Silva, F. (2012). Effect of sweet orange aroma on experimental anxiety in humans. *Journal of Alternative & Complementary Medicine, 18*(8), 798–804.

Goes, T., Ursulino, F., Almeida-Souza, T., Alves, P., & Teixeira-Silva, F. (2015). Effect of lemongrass aroma on experimental anxiety in humans. *Journal of Alternative & Complementary Medicine, 21*(12), 766–773.

Grossoehme, D., Cotton, S., & McPhail, G. (2013). Use and sanctification of complementary and alternative medicine by parents of children with cystic fibrosis. *Journal of Health Care Chaplaincy, 19*(1), 22–32.

Gutierrez, M., Werdin-Gonzalez, J., Stefanazzi, N., Bras, C., & Ferrero, A. (2016). The potential application of plant essential oils to control *Pediculus humanus capitis* (Anoplura: Pediculidae). *Parasitology Research, 115*(2), 633–641.

Halcón, L. (2013). Aromatherapy in pregnancy and childbirth. In M. Avery (Ed.), *Supporting a physiologic approach to pregnancy and birth*. Ames, IA: Wiley Blackwell.

Halcón, L., & Milkus, K. (2004). *Staphylococcus aureus* and wounds: A review of tea tree oil (*Melaleuca alternifolia*) as a promising antibiotic. *American Journal of Infection Control, 32*(7), 402–408.

Halicioglu, O., Astarcioglu, G., Yaprak, I., & Aydinlioglu, H. (2011). Toxicity of *Salvia officinalis* in a newborn and a child: An alarming report. *Pediatric Neurology, 45*(4), 259–260.

Hammer, K., Carson, C., & Riley, T. (2012). Effects of *Melaleuca alternifolia* (tea tree) essential oil and the major monoterpene component terpinen-4-ol on the development of single- and multistep antibiotic resistance and antimicrobial susceptibility. *Antimicrobial Agents & Chemotherapy, 56*(2), 909–915.

Hammer, K. A., Carson, C. F., & Riley, T. V. (2008). Frequencies of resistance to *Melaleuca alternifolia* (tea tree) oil and rifampicin in *Staphylococcus aureus, Staphylococcus epidermidis* and *Enterococcus faecalis*. *International Journal of Antimicrobial Agents, 32*(2), 170–173.

Igarashi, M., Ikei, H., Song, C., & Miyazaki, Y. (2014). Effects of olfactory stimulation with rose and orange oil on prefrontal cortex activity. *Complementary Therapies in Medicine, 22*(6), 1027–1031.

Imura, M., Misao, H., & Ushijima, H. (2006). The psychological effects of aromatherapy-massage in healthy postpartum mothers. *Journal of Midwifery & Women's Health, 51*(2), e21–e27.

Irmak, S., Uysal, M., Tas, U., Esen, M., Barut, M., Somuk, B., ... Ayan, S. (2015). The effect of lavender oil in patients with renal colic: A prospective controlled study using objective and subjective outcome measurements. *Journal of Alternative & Complementary Medicine, 21*(10), 617–622.

Jacobs, M., & Hornfeldt, C. (1994). Melaleuca oil poisoning. *Clinical Toxicology, 32*(4), 461–464.

Jain, R., Aqil, M., Ahad, A., Ali, A., & Khar, R. K. (2008). Basil oil is a promising skin penetration enhancer for transdermal delivery of labetolol hydrochloride. *Drug Development and Industrial Pharmacy, 34*(4), 384–389.

Jandourek, A., Vaishampayan, J., & Vazquez, J. (1998). Efficacy of melaleuca oral solution for the treatment of fluconazole refractory oral candidiasis in AIDS patients. *AIDS, 12*(9), 1033–1037.

Janes, S. E. J., Price, C. S. G., & Thomas, D. (2005). Essential oil poisoning: N-acetylcysteine for eugenol-induced hepatic failure and analysis of a national database. *European Journal of Pediatrics, 164*(8), 520–522.

Keljova, K., Jirova, D., Bendova, H., Gajdos, P., & Kolarova, H. (2010). Phototoxicity of essential oils intended for cosmetic use. *Toxicology In Vitro, 24*(8), 2084–2089.

Keville, K., & Green, M. (2009). *Aromatherapy: A complete guide to the healing art* (2nd ed.). Berkeley, CA: Crossing Press.

Kiberd, M., Clarke, S., Chorney, J., d'Eon, B., & Wright, S. (2016). Aromatherapy for the treatment of PONV in children: A pilot RCT. *BMC Complementary & Alternative Medicine, 16* (1), 450.

Kiecolt-Glaser, J., Graham, J., Malarkey, W., Porter, K., Lemeshow, S., & Glaser, R. (2008). Olfactory influences on mood and autonomic, endocrine, and immune function. *Psychoneuroendocrinology, 33*(3), 328–339.

Kim, J. T., Ren, C. J., Fielding, G. A., Pitti, A., Kasumi, T., Wajda, M., ... Bekker, A. (2007). Treatment with lavender aromatherapy in the post-anesthesia care unit reduces opioid requirements of morbidly obese patients undergoing laparoscopic adjustable gastric banding. *Obesity Surgery, 17*(7), 920–925.

Kreitzer, M., & Koithan, M. (2014). *Integrative nursing.* Oxford, UK: Oxford University Press.

Kritsidima, M., Newton, T., & Asimakopoulou, K. (2009). The effects of lavender scent on dental patient anxiety levels: A cluster randomised-controlled trial. *Community Dentistry and Oral Epidemiology, 38*(1), 83–87.

Kunz, S., Schultz, M., Lewitzky, M., Driessen, M., & Rau, H. (2007). Ear acupuncture for alcohol withdrawal in comparison with aromatherapy: A randomized-controlled trial. *Alcoholism: Clinical and Experimental Research, 31*(3), 436–442.

Lemme, P. (2009). The use of essential oils in psychiatric medication withdrawal. *International Journal of Clinical Aromatherapy, 6*(2), 15–23.

Libster, M. (2002). *Delmar's integrative herb guide for nurses.* Victoria, Australia: Delmar Thompson Learning.

Libster, M. (2012). *The nurse herbalist: Integrative insights for holistic practice.* Naperville, IL: Golden Apple Publications.

Lillehei, A., Halcón, L., Savik, K., & Reis, R. (2015). Effect of inhaled lavender and sleep hygiene on self-reported sleep issues: A randomized controlled trial. *Journal of Alternative & Complementary Medicine, 21*(7), 430–438.

Lim, P. F. C., Liu, X. Y., & Chan, S. Y. (2009). A review on terpenes as skin penetration enhancers in transdermal drug delivery. *Journal of Essential Oil Research, 21*(5), 423–428.

Lin, P., Chan, W., Ng, B., & Lam, L. (2007). Efficacy of aromatherapy (*Lavender angustifolia*) as an intervention for agitated behaviours in Chinese older persons with dementia: A cross-over randomized trial. *International Journal of Geriatric Psychiatry, 22*(5), 205–210.

Lua, P., Salihah, N., & Mazlan, N. (2015). Effects of inhaled ginger aromatherapy on chemotherapy-induced nausea and vomiting and health-related quality of life in women with breast cancer. *Complementary Therapies in Medicine. 23*(3), 396–404.

Lua, P. L., & Zakaria, N. S. (2012). A brief review of current scientific evidence involving aromatherapy use for nausea and vomiting. *Journal of Alternative & Complementary Medicine, 18*(6), 534–540.

Lusby, P. E., Coombes, A. L., & Wilkinson, J. M. (2006). A comparison of wound healing following treatment with *Lavandula x allardii* honey or essential oil. *Phytotherapy Research, 20*(9), 755–757.

Malachowska, B., Fendler, W., Pomykala, A., Suwala, S., & Mlynarski, W. (2016). Essential oils reduce autonomous response to pain sensation during self-monitoring of blood glucose among children with diabetes. *Journal of Pediatric Endocrinology & Metabolism, 29*(1), 47–53.

Menezes, I. A., Barreto, C. M., Antoniolli, A. R., Santos, M. R., & de Sousa, D. P. (2010). Hypotensive activity of terpenes found in essential oils. *Zeitschrift für Naturforschung C: A Journal of Biosciences, 65*(9), 562–566.

Morris, N. (2008). The effects of lavender (*Lavandula angustifolia*) essential oil baths on stress and anxiety. *International Journal of Clinical Aromatherapy, 5*(1), 3–7.

Moss, L., Rouse, M., Wesnes, K. A., & Moss, M. (2010). Differential effects of the aromas of *Salvia* species on memory and mood. *Human Psychopharmacology: Clinical & Experimental, 25*(5), 388–396.

Musil, A. (2013). Labor encouragement with essential oils. *Midwifery Today with International Midwife, 113* (Autumn), 57–58.

Muthaiyan, A., Biswas, D., Crandall, P., Wilkinson, B., & Ricke, S. (2012). Application of orange essential oil as an antistaphylococcal agent in a dressing model. *BMC Complementary & Alternative Medicine, 12*, 125.

Nagata, K., Iida, N., Kanzawa, H., Fujiwara, M., Mogi, T., Mitsushima, T., … Suqimoto, H. (2014). Effect of listening to music and essential oil inhalation on patients undergoing screening CT colonography: A randomized controlled trial. *European Journal of Radiology, 83*(12), 2172–2176.

National Cancer Institute (NCI), National Institutes of Health. (2012). *Aromatherapy and essential oils.* Retrieved from http://www.cancer.gov/cancertopics/pdq/cam/aromatherapy/patient/page1

Nielsen, J. (2006). Natural oils affect the human skin integrity and the percutaneous penetration of benzoic acid-dose dependency. *Basic & Clinical Pharmacology & Toxicology, 98*(6), 575–581.

O'Connor, D., Eppingstall, B., Taffe, J., & van der Ploeg, E. (2013). A randomized, controlled cross-over trial of dermally-applied lavender (*Lavandula angustifolia*) oil as a treatment of agitated behaviour in dementia. *BMC Complementary & Alternative Medicine, 13*, 315.

O'Flaherty, L., van Dijk, M., Albertyn, R., Millar, A. & Rode, H. (2012). Aromatherapy massage seems to enhance relaxation in children with burns: An observational pilot study. *Burns, 38* (6), 840–845.

Paduch, R., Kandefer-Szerszen, M., Trytek, M., & Fiedurek, J. (2007). Terpenes: Substances useful in human healthcare. *Archivum Immunologiae et Therapaie Experimentalis, 55*(5), 315–327.

Paule, A. (2001). Antimicrobial properties of essential oil constituents. *International Journal of Aromatherapy, 11*(3), 126–133.

Pearson. S. (2015). Essential oils for prenatal nausea and digestion. *Midwifery Today with International Midwife,* (116), 44–46.

Posadzki, P., Watson, L., Alotaibi, A., & Ernst, E. (2013). Prevalence of use of complementary and alternative medicine (CAM) by patients/consumers in the UK: Systematic review of surveys [Review]. *Clinical Medicine, 13*(2), 126–131.

Pounds, L. (2012). Art of aromatherapy for end-of-life care. *Beginnings, 32*(4), 20–23.

Price, S., & Price, L. (2011). *Aromatherapy for health professionals* (4th ed.). Edinburgh, Scotland: Churchill Livingstone.

Rose, J., & Behm, F. (1994). Inhalation of vapor from black pepper extract reduces smoking withdrawal symptoms. *Drug and Alcohol Dependence, 34*(3), 225–229.

Rudback, J., Islam, M., Borje, A., Nilsson, U., & Karlberg, A. (2015). Essential oils can contain allergenic hydroperoxides at eliciting levels, regardless of handling and storage. *Contact Dermatitis, 73*(4), 253–254.

Samarasekera, R., Weerasinghe, I., & Hemalal, K. (2008). Insecticidal activity of menthol derivatives against mosquitoes. *Pest Management Science, 64*(3), 290–295.

Sheikhan, F., Jahdi, F., Khoei, E. M., Shamsalizadeh, N., Sheikhan, M., & Haghani, H. (2012). Episiotomy pain relief: Use of lavender oil essence in primiparous Iranian women. *Complementary Therapies in Clinical Practice, 18*(1), 66–70.

Sherry, E., Sivananthan, S., Warnke, P., & Eslick, G. (2003). Topical phytochemicals used to salvage the gangrenous lower limbs of type 1 diabetic patients. *Diabetes Research and Clinical Practice, 62*(1), 65–66.

Simpson, N., & Roman, K. (2001). Complementary medicine use in children: Extent and reasons. A population based study. *British Journal of General Practice, 51*(472), 914–916.

Singh, G., Kiran, S., Marimuthu, P., de Lampasona, M., de Heluani, C., & Catalan, C. (2008). Chemistry, biocidal and antioxidant activities of essential oil and oleoresins from *Piper cubeba* (seed). *International Journal of Essential Oil Therapeutics, 2*(2), 50–59.

Solorzano-Santos, F., & Miranda-Novales, M. (2012). Essential oils from aromatic herbs as antimicrobial agents. *Current Opinion in Biotechnology, 23*(2), 136–141.

Storan, E., Nolan, U., & Kirby, B. (2016). Allergic contact dermatitis caused by the tea tree oil-containing hydrogel Burnshield. *Contact Dermatitis, 74*(5), 309–310.

Styles, J. (1997). The use of aromatherapy in hospitalized children with HIV. *Complementary Therapies in Nursing and Midwifery, 3*(1), 16–20.

Thomas, J., Carson, C., Peterson, G., Walton, S., Hammer, K., Naunton, M., … Baby, K. E. (2016). Therapeutic potential of tea tree oil for scabies [Review]. *American Journal of Tropical Medicine & Hygiene, 94*(2), 258–66. Retrieved from http://enhancementsaromatherapyllc.vpweb.com/upload/Tisserand%20flyer_2pg.pdf

Thompson, P., Jensen, T., Hammer, K., Carson, C., Molgaard, P., & Riley, T. (2011). Survey of the antimicrobial activity of commercially available Australian tea tree (*Melaleuca alternifolia*) essential oil products in vitro. *Journal of Alternative & Complementary Medicine, 17*(9), 835–841.

Tindle, H., Davis, R., Phillips, R., & Eisenberg, D. (2005). Trends in the use of complementary and alternative medicine by U.S. adults: 1997–2002. *Alternative Therapies in Health and Medicine, 11*(1), 42–49.

Tisserand, R. (2016). *Essential oil chemistry and pharmacology: The actions of aromatic compounds in the body.* Seminar, Boulder, CO. Retrieved from http://enhancementsaromatherapyllc.vpweb.com/upload/Tisserand%20flyer_2pg.pdf

Tisserand, R., & Young, R. (2014). *Essential oil safety* (2nd ed.). Edinburgh, UK: Churchill Livingstone.

Uter, W., Schmidt, E., Geier, J., Lessmann, H., Schnuch, A., & Frosch, P. (2010). Contact allergy to essential oils: Current patch test results (2000–2008) from the Information Network of Departments of Dermatology (IVDK). *Contact Dermatitis, 63*(5), 277–283.

Valgimigli, L., Gabbanini, S., Berlini, E., Lucchi, E., Beltramini, C., & Bertarelli, Y. L. (2012). Lemon (*Citrus limon*, Burm.f.) essential oil enhances the trans-epidermal release of lipid-(A, E) and water-(B6, C) soluble vitamins from topical emulsions in reconstructed human epidermis. *International Journal of Cosmetic Science, 34*(4), 347–356.

Watanabe, E., Kuchta, K., Kimura, M., Rauwald, H., Kamei, T., & Imanishi, J. (2015). Effects of bergamot (*Citrus bergamia* (Risso) Wright & Arn.) essential oil aromatherapy on mood states, parasympathetic nervous system activity, and salivary cortisol levels in 41 healthy females. *Forschende Komplementarmedizin, 22*(1), 43–49.

Weiss, E. (1997). *Essential oil crops.* Cambridge, UK: CAB International.

Williams, A., & Barry, B. (1989). Essential oils as novel skin penetration enhancers. *International Journal of Pharmaceutics, 57*(2), R7–R9.

Woelk, H., & Schlafke, S. (2010). A multi-center, double-blind, randomised study of the lavender oil preparation silexan in comparison to lorazepam for generalized anxiety disorder. *Phytomedicine, 17*(2), 94–99.

Yoshiyama, K., Arita, H., & Suzuki, J. (2015). The effect of aroma hand massage therapy for people with dementia. *Journal of Alternative & Complementary Medicine, 21*(12), 759–765.

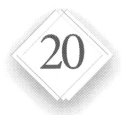

Herbal Medicines

GREGORY A. PLOTNIKOFF AND ANGELA S. LILLEHEI

Herbs and related natural products such as spices are the oldest and most widely used form of medicine in the world. The use of herbs for the treatment of disease and the promotion of well-being can be traced back in many cultures at least 2,500 years. In the 5th century BCE, Hippocrates recommended leaves and bark of the willow tree (genus *Salix*) for pain and inflammation. In the more recent past, in the 1850s, Florence Nightingale's medicine box that she brought to the Crimean War contained quinine and powdered rhubarb as well as other medicines to administer to the wounded and sick soldiers (Florence Nightingale Museum of London, 2016). However, herbal medicines are not restricted to historical use. Today, in addition to the well-known examples of aspirin from the willow tree, digoxin from the foxglove plant *Digitalis purpurea*, and paclitaxel from the pacific yew tree *Taxus brevifolia*, both over-the-counter and prescription plant-derived medications are frequently used; these include anticholinergic agents, anticoagulants, antihypertensives, and antineoplastic agents. Just a small percentage of the world's plant species provide medicines. There are likely many more waiting to be discovered. The most recently celebrated example is that of a potent antimalarial medication. Chinese scientists led by Dr. Tu Youyou, discovered and isolated artemisinin from sweet wormwood (*Artemesia annua* L), a plant used for medicinal purposes in China for more than 2,000 years. For her work, Dr. Tu was honored with the very prestigious Lasker-DeBakey Clinical Research Award in 2011 (Miller & Su, 2011).

The most comprehensive and reliable data on the use of herbal medicine in the United States come from the National Health Interview Survey (NHIS). Looking at combined data from 88,962 adults, nonvitamin, nonmineral dietary supplements were the most commonly used complementary health therapy used in 2002 (17.7%), 2007 (17.7%), and 2012 (18.9%). For the purpose of this survey, complementary health included a variety of therapies and products with a history of use or origins outside of conventional Western medicine (Clarke, Black, Stussman, Barnes, & Nahin, 2015)

The high prevalence of use in all regions of the United States and across all ages, genders, ethnicities, and medical diagnoses means that health professionals must address herbal medicine use in all patient encounters (Arcury et al., 2006;

Cherniack et al., 2008). In the 2012 NHIS study, 33.2% of adults reported the use of complementary and alternative medicines (CAM) in the previous year (Clarke et al., 2015). Most would support complementary approaches when used in combination with conventional medical treatments (P. M. Barnes, Powell-Griner, McFann, & Nahin, 2004). This is significant. The use of herbal medicines may not be disclosed unless specifically requested by the nurse, pharmacist, or physician. Even in 2008, as many as 62.5% of regular herbal medicine users also used prescription medicines; however, only 33% routinely reported their use to their care provider (Archer & Boyle, 2008). The 2004 Council for Responsible Nutrition's survey of 1,000 randomly selected U.S. adults documented that 90% looked to health-care professionals, including nurses, for guidance in herbal medicine use (Ward & Blumenthal, 2005). Thus, herbal medicine warrants significant attention by all nurses as a complementary, holistic therapy and as a potential risk for interaction with other conventional approaches.

DEFINITION

Herbal medicines, or plant-based therapies, continue to occupy a place of central importance in the world's many healing traditions. These include the use of single herbs in many Western traditions and multiple-herb combinations in traditional Asian medical systems. Frequently, herbs are part of an overarching belief system that may involve spiritual or metaphysical components. Herbal medicines are often included in the work of shamans and other traditional healers who serve as intermediaries with the spirit world. Herbal medicines are also a tool in traditional Asian medicine and are used, like acupuncture, to open blocked channels (meridians) for the free flow of qi (life spirit or force).

Herbal medicines, also known as *botanicals* or *phytotherapies*, are one component of the range of natural products sold in the United States as dietary supplements. Plant therapies for medicinal or health purposes include herbs from the whole plant or a part of the plant, plant extracts or tinctures, essential oils, flower essences, and homeopathic remedies. A variety of plant therapy types may be included in dietary supplements. In addition to herbal products, other dietary supplements include fungi-based products (mycotherapies) and vitamin, mineral, and nutritional therapies (nutraceuticals). Since the passage of the Dietary Supplement Health and Education Act of 1994 (DSHEA; U.S. Congress, 1994), these biological modifiers have been available over the counter as dietary supplements. Though neither food nor drug, these substances are still regulated by the Food and Drug Administration (FDA) but with less stringent requirements. Unlike foods and drugs, dietary supplements can be sold based on evidence of safety in the possession of the manufacturer and can only be removed from the market if the FDA can prove them unsafe under ordinary conditions of use.

Under DSHEA, herbal medicines can be sold for "stimulating, maintaining, supporting, regulating, and promoting health" rather than for treating disease. As dietary supplements rather than drugs, herbal medicines cannot claim to restore normal (or correct abnormal) function. In addition, herbs cannot claim to "diagnose, treat, prevent, cure, or mitigate" (U.S. Congress, 1994). Herbal medicine companies can assert that their product supports cardiovascular health but not that it lowers cholesterol. To do so would suggest that the product is intended for treating a disease (hypercholesterolemia) and is therefore subject to FDA pharmaceutical regulations.

This has raised questions about what constitutes a disease. The FDA originally defined a *disease* as any deviation, impairment, or interruption of the normal structure or function of any part, organ, or system of the body that is manifested by a characteristic set of one or more signs and symptoms. This definition generated many concerns. "Normal structure" appeared to be normed to a 30-year-old man and therefore did not account for gender or aging. For example, are menopause and menstrual cramps diseases? With no signs or symptoms, is hypercholesterolemia a disease or a risk factor? After significant public outcry, the FDA adopted the definition of *disease* found in the Nutrition Labeling and Health Act of 1990. Disease is considered damage to an organ, part, structure, or system of the body such that it does not function properly (e.g., cardiovascular disease) or a state of health leading to such (e.g., hypertension).

SCIENTIFIC BASIS

Significant research has been done on numerous single herbal agents using Western biomedical/scientific models. Beginning in 1978, the German government's *Bundesgesunheitsamt* (Federal Health Agency) began evaluating the safety and efficacy of phytomedicines. The health professionals charged with doing so, known as the Commission E, met until 1994 and evaluated 300 herbal medicines, of which they recognized 190 as suitable for medicinal use. The complete reports have been translated and are available from the American Botanical Council (2000).

Beginning in 1996, significant meta-analyses and review articles of single-herb products began appearing on a regular basis in leading Western medical journals. These are readily accessible via the National Library of Medicine's PubMed website (www.ncbi.nlm.nih.gov/PubMed). Compiling data from similar studies for analysis (meta-analysis) is complicated by the fact that many studies published to date have left out important information, including naming the specific plant species studied (e.g., echinacea versus *Echinacea purpurea*, *E. pallida*, or *E. angustifolia*), the parts used (stems, leaves, or roots), the form (pressed juice, powdered whole extract, aqueous extract, ethanol extract, or aqueous-ethanol extract), and the formulation (stated proportions of water to alcohol or specifically extracted fractions and concentrations).

Standardization of herbal medicines is crucial both for scientific study and consumer protection. Standardization is equated with reproducibility, guaranteed potency, quality of active ingredients, and documentable effectiveness. However, with herbal medicines, standardization presents several problems. First, the active ingredient may not be known. Second, there may be more than one active ingredient. Third, both the content and the activity of an herbal medicine may be related to the means of the herb's growth conditions, extraction, and processing. In addition, there is a lack of quality assurance along the distribution chain from growing and harvesting conditions to the end consumer product (Heinrich, 2015). This significantly complicates both research and counseling for health professionals and consumers.

A growing number of healthcare professionals are studying the effects of these substances. With an increase in the FDA's involvement, we can look forward to a more reliable herb market. Expanded knowledge of herbal indications may augment the safety and efficacy of herbal therapies for patients.

INTERVENTION

Herbal medicines and dietary supplements need to be addressed in clinical settings in the same manner one addresses pharmaceutical agents. Every health professional needs to be aware of the wide use of herbal medicines and other dietary supplements.

Technique

Efficient and effective patient advocacy means including questions on alternative therapies as a standard part of each patient interview. Reasonable questions include: "Are you using any herbs? Vitamins? Dietary supplements?" Follow-up questions could cover: "What dose? What source? What directions are you following? Why are you taking it?" Asking about the source of information can be quite helpful, as in, "Are you working with any other health professionals?" As with all good interviewing, listening for understanding rather than agreement or disagreement enhances the therapeutic alliance. In addition to knowing the type of herb used, the dose of each herb, and the intended purpose of each herb, gathering information regarding the duration of herb use is also helpful in assessing patients and providing the best possible care.

Unfortunately, professionals often do not ask such questions, and up to 69% of CAM-using patients do not volunteer such information (Graham et al., 2005). This "don't ask, don't tell" policy makes no sense in patient care. All health professionals need to create a safe environment that is conducive to patients' open sharing of important information, such as herbal use or use of other complementary/alternative therapies without fear of ridicule or other negative responses. "Ask, then ask again" is a practice policy foundational to safe and effective patient care.

PRECAUTIONS

A common misconception regarding herbal medicines is that herbs have no side effects because they are natural. However, herbs do indeed have side effects and may be toxic or poisonous if not used appropriately. Consider the toxicity of widely used natural products such as coffee, cocaine, and tobacco. Another dilemma is patient use of herbs in lieu of their prescribed medications. Although herbs may be a good option in particular cases and conditions, the decision to decline medications should be based on fully informed judgments in partnership with a health professional.

Interviewing for herbal medicine use is crucial for identifying patients at risk for interactions with prescription medications or for excessive bleeding in surgery. Patients with special risks of drug interactions and drug–herb interactions include those taking the following pharmaceutical agents: anticoagulants, hypoglycemics, antidepressants, sedative-hypnotics, antihypertensives, and medications with narrow therapeutic windows such as digoxin and theophylline. The significance of having knowledge of the ingestion of herbal medicines is illustrated in the list of known interactions of St. John's wort with commonly prescribed agents (see Exhibit 20.1).

Exhibit 20.1. Effect of St. John's Wort on Bioavailability of Selected Medications

St. John's wort decreases the bioavailability of:
- Calcium channel blockers
- Coumadin
- Cyclosporine
- Digoxin
- Irinotecan
- Oral contraceptives
- Protease inhibitors
- Simvastatin
- Tacrolimus
- Theophylline

Note: The effect can remain strong for weeks after stopping ingestion.

Pregnancy, lactation, breastfeeding, and childcare are special topics in herbal medicine use. For these situations, the most authoritative references are cited in Exhibit 20.2. In the absence of clinical trial data, use is guided by historical experience or breast milk analysis. Herbs that increase breast milk production, such as fenugreek, are frequently recommended by the International Board of Certified Lactation Consultants (IBLCE).

Nursing can play a critical role in patient assessment in regards to use of herbal medicines and in the education of patients on the safety and use of medicinal herbs. Exhibit 20.3 lists key teaching points regarding herbal medicines. Herbal therapies are safe only if herbs are prepared in the right way and used for the precise indication, in the correct amounts, for the exact duration, and with appropriate monitoring. Potential herb–herb and herb–drug interactions should be considered when patients are using herbal products. The lack of national standards in the collection and preparation of herbal products complicates this field in the United States. Because many herbs have potential or actual risks that need to be recognized, it is important for health providers to have reliable and accessible sources of information to prevent adverse herb-related reactions and to identify and manage complications of herbal therapies; selected reputable herbal references are provided at the end of this chapter (see Exhibit 20.2 and other resources at the end of this chapter).

All serious adverse reactions should be reported to the FDA through the MedWatch program at 1-800-332-1088 or at www.fda.gov/Safety/MedWatch/HowToReport/ucm167733.htm. An example of a complication associated with herbal therapy is illustrated in the case of the use of *Ma huang* (Ephedra), which was marketed in the United States as a major ingredient in formulations for weight reduction. Use of this herb had been linked to numerous adverse cardiovascular events, including stroke, myocardial infarction, and sudden death (Haller & Benowitz, 2000), and the FDA banned sales of this herb in April 2004.

Exhibit 20.2. Suggested Additional Reading for Pregnancy, Breastfeeding, Lactation, and Childcare

Hale, T. W. (2004). *Medications and mother's milk: A manual of lactational pharmacology* (11th ed.). Amarillo, TX: Pharmasoft Medical Publishers.
Humphrey, S. (2004). *The nursing mother's herbal*. Minneapolis, MN: Fairview Press.
Kemper, K. J. (2002). *The holistic pediatrician* (2nd ed.). New York, NY: Perennial Currents.
Romm, A. J. (2003). *The natural pregnancy book*. Berkeley, CA: Ten Speed Press.

Exhibit 20.3. Five Key Patient Teaching Points

1. Just because it is natural does not mean it is safe.
2. Just because it is safe does not mean it is effective.
3. Labels may not equal contents.
4. Self-diagnosis and self-treatment can result in self-malpractice.
5. Herbs are never a replacement for an emergency department.

USES

Given the volume and variety of products, herbal medicine knowledge relevant for nursing practice cannot be summarized quickly. This chapter addresses three of the most important herbs from an evidence-based perspective. There is a significant range in scientific data available on each, and the theoretical risks should be acknowledged and carefully considered both by patients and health professionals. Furthermore, the clinical knowledge related to combining herbal products with prescription and nonprescription drugs is only in the developmental stages; much remains to be known about interactions and side effects.

Chronic illness (such as cancer or autoimmune disease or chronic pain), surgery, and use of prescription medications are three situations in which herbal medicine reviews by nurses are important. Echinacea does stimulate the immune system, but this is not necessarily a positive effect. Ginkgo biloba's pharmacological activity places people at risk in surgery. St. John's wort is effective for depression but can render many prescription medications ineffective or even toxic. Many herbs have a sufficient evidence base and potential as alternatives to Western medicine. However, herbal medicine in the United States is a very broad and multicultural phenomenon; it is difficult to know all products used by or all products of potential benefit to patients. Readers should be aware that there are reputable clinical resources readily accessible for assistance in informed decision making (e.g., see Exhibits 20.2 and other resources at the end of this chapter).

The recent legalization of marijuana (*Cannabis sativa*) for distribution through approved dispensaries in 16 states and the District of Columbia deserves special attention. Medicinal marijuana is the first herbal medicine to require a prescription in the United States. Even before such changes in state laws, several prescription forms of cannabinoids existed in the United States and Canada.

Dronabinol and Nabilone were used for treatment of nausea and vomiting associated with chemotherapy or anorexia with weight loss in patients with AIDS. However, since 1970, marijuana as an herbal medicine has been considered a Schedule 1 substance and therefore illegal and without medical value. This understanding has been challenged by the discovery of what has been termed the endocannabinoid system. The presence of cannabinoid receptors CB1 and CB2 in the central nervous system (CNS) and elsewhere suggests the possibility of many promising pharmaceutical applications (Bostwick, 2012; Bostwick, Reisfield, & DuPont, 2013).

The most frequent medical use of the leaves and flowering tops of the marijuana plant is for pain and muscle spasticity (Borgelt, Franson, Nussbaum, & Wang, 2013). Safety concerns for all patients include dizziness, impaired memory and cognition, increased risk of schizophrenia in adolescents, and accidental ingestions by children and pets. A cannabis withdrawal syndrome has also been described (Crippa et al., 2013). Cannabis use disorders (CUDs) exist, especially among patients with a diagnosis of substance abuse and bipolar illness personality disorders. Nurses and all health professionals increasingly need to screen patients for appropriate medical use (Lev-Ran, Le Foll, McKenzie, George, & Rehm, 2013).

Echinacea (E. angustifolia, E. pallida, E. purpurea)

Echinacea is the most commonly used herbal medicine in the United States; it is used by people of all ages, genders, and ethnicities, including 19.8% of herbal medicine–using adults and 37.2% of herbal medicine–using children (P. M. Barnes, Bloom, & Nahin, 2008). North American gardens commonly contain *Echinacea*, also known as the *purple coneflower*. It was traditionally used by Native Americans and early settlers as a remedy for infections and for healing wounds. Several components, particularly the alkamides and caffeic acid derivatives, have clear pharmacological activity (J. Barnes, Anderson, Gibbons, & Phillipson, 2005). In vitro research suggests an immunostimulatory effect principally by macrophage, polymorphonuclear leukocyte, and natural killer cell activation (Barrett, 2003). Monocyte secretion of tumor necrosis factor-alpha (TNF-alpha) is particularly stimulated (Senchina et al., 2005).

Echinacea is promoted in the United States for the prevention and treatment of the common cold. In Europe, it is used topically for wound healing and intravenously for immunostimulation. Several methodologically valid clinical studies have been published in recent years with unimpressive results, suggesting that echinacea is not effective for the treatment or prevention of upper respiratory illness for adults. A 2014 meta-analysis by the prestigious Cochrane Collaborative stated that the echinacea products used in clinical trials differed greatly, finding that there is a weak benefit for some echinacea products for treating colds and a positive trend, although nonsignificant, for its use in prevention (Karsch-Völk et al., 2014). A previous meta-analysis of 14 randomized controlled trials documented that echinacea decreased the odds of developing a common cold by 58% and reduced the duration of symptoms by 1.4 days (Shah, Sander, White, Rinaldi, & Coleman, 2007). A recent randomized, controlled placebo study of echinacea followed 755 healthy participants for 4 months. The intervention used alcohol extract from freshly harvested *E. purpurea* leaves/roots. The active echinacea intervention significantly reduced the total number of cold episodes (149 vs. 188), cumulated episode days

(672 versus 850), and episodes with any pain medication use (58 vs. 88), all p <.05. Recurrent infections also appeared to be reduced, 65 episodes in 28 participants taking echinacea and 100 episodes in 43 participants taking placebo, p <.05 (Jawad, Schoop, Suter, Klein, & Eccles, 2012).

Echinacea has a good safety profile but has been associated (very infrequently) with gastric upset, rashes, and severe allergic reactions. It is not recommended for those with allergies to members of the Asteraceae family (formerly termed Compositae), which includes ragweed, daisies, thistles, and chamomile. More important, nonspecific immunostimulation may exacerbate pre-existing autoimmune disease or precipitate autoimmune disease in genetically predisposed individuals (Lee & Werth, 2004). TNF-alpha and interleukin-1 are proinflammatory cytokines, and recent evidence demonstrates that anti-TNF and anti–interleukin-1 therapies are effective for autoimmune diseases, including Crohn's disease and rheumatoid arthritis. Echinacea cannot be recommended for people with other chronic immunological diseases, including multiple sclerosis, lupus, and HIV. In a recent review and assessment of the safety of oral echinacea products, no significant inhibition of CYP2D6 or CYP3A4 isoforms were found, and adverse effects reported during clinical trials were generally mild. In addition, long-term published studies of up to 6 months did not report any toxicological issues (Ardjomand-Woelkart & Bauer, 2016).

There are no verifiable reports of drug–herb interactions with any echinacea product. *E. purpurea* products have a low potential for generating any cytochrome P450 drug–herb interactions (C. Freeman & Spelman, 2008; Hermann & von Richter, 2012). The median lethal dose (LD_{50}) of intravenously administered echinacea juice is 50 mL/kg in mice and rats. Regular oral administration to mice at levels greater than proposed human therapeutic doses has failed to demonstrate toxic effects (Mengs, Clare, & Poiley, 1991).

Ginkgo (Ginkgo biloba)

Ginkgo is the number-one-selling herb in Europe for improvement of blood flow and enhancement of cognition. Clinically, ginkgo is used for circulatory problems such as peripheral artery disease (Pittler & Ernst, 2005), impotence (Sikora, 1989), and cerebral insufficiency (Kleijnen & Knipschild, 1992). The German government's Commission E also approved its use for dementia syndromes with memory deficits, disturbances in concentration, depressive emotional conditions, dizziness, tinnitus, and headaches.

A Cochrane review in 2007 stated that ginkgo appears safe with no excess side effects compared with placebo. Benefits for mild cognitive impairment and dementia were seen at doses of 200 mg a day beginning at 12 weeks. However, they noted that, because of variability in trial design and quality, the evidence for predictable and clinically significant benefit is unconvincing (Birks & Grimley Evans, 2007). A follow-up systematic review noted that in all studies with active controls, ginkgo was at least as effective as the pharmaceutical intervention (May et al., 2009). In an overview of systematic reviews of *ginkgo biloba* extracts for mild cognitive impairment and dementia, findings in the 10 reviews identified included that *ginkgo biloba* extracts showed improved cognition, neuropsychiatric symptoms, and daily activities and that the effects were dose dependent. A high dose (240 mg) was needed to demonstrate efficacy.

In regards to safety, compared with placebo, overall adverse events were at the same level (Zhang et al., 2016).

European studies published in 1994 and 1996 demonstrated ginkgo's effectiveness in slowing or reversing dementia (Hofferberth, 1994; Kanowski, Herrmann, Stephan, Wierich, & Horr, 1996). A study published in 1997 affirmed these findings for patients with Alzheimer's disease and multi-infarct dementia in an American trial with 309 subjects (LeBars et al., 1997). Most recently, a double-blind, randomized, placebo-controlled trial of *ginkgo biloba* (as EGB761) at 240 mg daily for 24 weeks in 410 participants with mild to moderate dementia and neuropsychiatric symptoms suggests efficacy. The study demonstrated safety and clinically significant findings ($p < .001$) in favor of EBG761 for cognition by a short cognitive performance test (Syndrom-Kurztest [SKT] test battery; Erzigkeit, 1992) and neuropsychiatric symptoms (by the Neuropsychiatric Inventory). In addition, EGB761 administration improved functional measures and quality of life of patients (Herrschaft et al., 2012).

Recently, intriguing data have suggested possible use of ginkgo in Parkinson's disease (Ahmad et al., 2005; Kim, Lee, Lee, & Kim, 2004) and diabetic retinopathy (Huang, Jeng, Kao, Yu, & Liu, 2004). Additionally, there is interest in its use for cell phone users (Ilhan et al., 2004) and stressed adults (Walesiuk, Trofimiuk, & Braszko, 2005). However, larger trials are still needed to confirm such therapeutic benefit. In addition, there is no convincing evidence that ginkgo enhances cognitive function in healthy young people (Canter & Ernst, 2007). *Ginkgo biloba* (as EGB761) does not appear beneficial for the prevention of chemotherapy associated cognitive changes (Barton et al., 2013) or for the improvement of cognitive function in multiple sclerosis (Lovera et al., 2012).

Ginkgo's leaf extracts are used in Europe, both orally and intravenously, for the treatment of Alzheimer's dementia, multi-infarct dementia, peripheral vascular disease, and vertigo (Kaufmann, 2002; Li, Ma, Scherban, & Tam, 2002). Ginkgo's active ingredients are terpene trilactones (6%; specifically, ginkgolides and bilobalide) and flavanoid glycosides (24%), which are the bases for standardized leaf extracts. Ginkgo's mechanism of action is believed to be its in vitro antioxidative, antiplatelet, antihypoxic, antiedemic, hemorheological, and microcirculatory actions (Mahadevan & Park, 2008). It is more effective than beta-carotene and vitamin E as an oxidative scavenger and inhibitor of lipid peroxidation of cellular membranes (Pietschmann, Kuklinski, & Otterstein, 1992) and stimulates the release of nitric oxide (Chen, Salwinski, & Lee, 1997). Ginkgo is also a potent antagonist of platelet-activating factor (Engelsen, Nielson, & Winther, 2002) and thus inhibits platelet aggregation and promotes clot breakdown. Ginkgo in the CNS inhibits production of proinflammatory cytokines and upregulates anti-inflammatory cytokines (Jiao, Rui, Li, Yang, & Qiu, 2005). These properties may result in neuroprotective and ischemia reperfusion–protective effects (Oyama, Chikahisa, Ueha, Kanemaru, & Noda, 1996; Sener et al., 2005; Shen & Zhou, 1995).

Side effects with ginkgo are uncommon. They include gastrointestinal discomfort, headache, and dizziness. Because of its antiplatelet effect, however, it has been reported widely to have a risk of significant bleeding when used with anticoagulants and other antiplatelet agents (Bebbington, Kulkarni, & Roberts, 2005; Matthews, 1998; Rosenblatt & Mindel, 1997; Rowin & Lewis, 1996). The most recent studies on ginkgo and platelet activity in vivo do not support concerns for perioperative bleeding or potentiation of anticoagulant or antiplatelet drugs (Beckert, Concannon, Henry, Smith, & Puckett, 2007; Bone, 2008). At this time, most surgeons request that ginkgo be discontinued 10 days prior to surgery and not restarted until the surgical wound has healed sufficiently to allow for aspirin use.

St. John's Wort (Hypericum perforatum)

St. John's wort, one of the world's top-selling herbs, has been used for centuries in Europe as a sedative and as a balm for skin injuries. Since 1996, it has been widely promoted in the United States as a wonder drug for depression or as "nature's Prozac." Today, it is often used to treat mild to moderate depression, anxiety, and sleep disorders. A task force of the American Psychiatric Association has noted promising research results in depression and recommended further study (M. P. Freeman et al., 2010). One study with 100 postmenopausal women demonstrated significant reductions in hot flash duration and severity (Abdali, Khajehei, & Tavatabaee, 2010).

In vitro studies have shown that *Hypericum* extract inhibits the neuronal uptake of the neurotransmitters serotonin, noradrenaline, dopamine, gamma-aminobutyric acid (GABA), and L-glutamate (Müller, Rolli, Schafer, & Hafner, 1997). No in vivo monoamine oxidase (MAO)–inhibiting activity has been demonstrated with *Hypericum*.

Three significant reviews appeared in 2008 that demonstrated positive effects on depression for *Hypericum* (Carpenter, Crigger, Kugler, & Loya, 2008; Kasper et al., 2008; Linde, Berner, & Kriston, 2008). In the Cochrane review meta-analysis of 29 trials with 5,489 patients, 18 comparisons with placebo and 17 comparisons with prescription antidepressants were included. For nine large trials, the response-rate compared with placebo was 1.28 (95% CI [1.10, 1.49]), and for nine smaller trials, the response-rate ratio was 1.87 (95% CI [1.22, 2.87]). The review team concluded that St. John's wort extracts are superior to placebo and similarly effective as standard prescription antidepressants with fewer side effects (Linde et al., 2008). A 2016 systematic review of 35 studies with 6,994 patients demonstrated similar results, with St John's wort superior to placebo for mild and moderate depression and not significantly different than antidepressant medication. Fewer side effects were found with the St. John's wort group. A lack of research on severe depression and poor reporting of adverse side effects were noted as limitations (Apaydin et al., 2016).

There is no one active ingredient in St. John's wort. Bioactive components include the napthodianthones (hypericin and pseudohypericin) and the phloroglucinols (hyperforin and adhyperforin). Ginkgo also contains many flavonoids (Butterweck & Schmidt, 2007).

As previously noted in Exhibit 20.1, St. John's wort decreases the bioavailability of numerous agents. However, the most serious toxicity associated with it is the negative interactions with prescription drugs. St. John's wort is a potent inducer of both P-glycoprotein and cytochrome P450 (CYP) 3A4, the hepatic enzyme involved in the metabolism of more than 50% of all prescription drugs (Zhou & Lai, 2008). Significant interactions include anticancer agents (imatinib and irinotecan), anti-HIV drugs (indinavir, lamivudine, and nevirapine), anti-inflammatory drugs (ibuprofen and fexofenadine), antibiotics/antifungals (erythromycin and voriconazole), cardiac medications (digoxin, ivabradine, warfarin, verapamil, nifedipine, atorvastatin, pravastatin, and talinolol), CNS agents (amitriptyline, buspirone, phenytoin, methadone, midazolam, alprazolam, and sertraline), diabetes medications (tolbutamide and gliclazide), and immunosuppressants (cyclosporine and tacrolimus), as well as oral contraceptives, proton pump inhibitors, and theophylline (Di, Li, Xue, & Zhou, 2008). Hence, the use of St. John's wort can be life-threatening for people requiring prescription medications. Because of its long half-life, the herb should be discontinued at least 5 days prior to initiation of any of these medications, and close monitoring of drug levels may be indicated. Additional theoretical concerns include the risk of photosensitivity or the precipitation of a serotonergic crisis in interaction with other prescription antidepressants.

Recent Nursing Research in Medicinal Herbs

Research on the use of herbs for healing is an important area for nursing. Examples of recent nursing research in the use of medicinal herbs include effectiveness of Indian turmeric powder and honey for oral mucositis in cancer patients, with findings of a significantly positive difference between groups (Francis & Williams, 2014); effects of flaxseed on menopausal symptoms and quality of life. With findings of decreased menopausal symptoms and increased quality of life among women who used flaxseed for 3 months (Cetisli, Saruhan & Kivcak, 2015); and the effect of saw palmetto for symptom management during radiation therapy for men with prostate cancer. With results demonstrating safety at dosages up to 960 mg daily but no statistically significant results between groups for lower urinary tract symptoms, although results trended in a positive direction (Wyatt, Sikorskii, Safkhani, McVary & Herman, 2015).

Medicinal Mushrooms

In addition to a variety of medicinal herbs being used, a plant dietary supplement gaining ground in medicinal use, although outside the range of herbal therapy, is medicinal mushrooms. Many mushrooms contain biologically active polysaccharides in fruit bodies, cultured mycelium, and cultured broth. The chemical structure of the polysaccharides is thought to be associated with enhancing innate and cell-mediated immune responses and exhibit antitumor properties. Additional properties that medicinal mushrooms and fungi are thought to have include antioxidant, radical scavenging, cardiovascular, anti-hypercholesterolemic, detoxification, and antiviral, antibacterial, antiparasitic, and antifungal (Wasser 2014). There is still controversy on the use of mushrooms in Western medicine, with claims frequently outweighing the evidence (Money, 2016).

The NHIS survey found a significant increase in the use of fish oil, probiotics or prebiotics, and melatonin from 2007 to 2012. Conversely a decrease in the use of herbs such as echinacea, garlic, ginseng, *ginkgo biloba*, and saw palmetto was found from 2007 to 2012 (Clarke et al., 2015). As new plant therapies are promoted and researched, the medicinal herbs used by patients and consumers will continue to shift, making it challenging to stay abreast of what evidence and research is available. Ongoing herbal therapy research by scientists, nurses, and other healthcare professionals will be imperative.

CULTURAL APPLICATIONS

The practice of Western herbalism in medicine parallels that of Western pharmaceutical interventions. One herb with a defined pharmacological activity can be applied to a given patient with a given medical diagnosis. Successful treatment is understood as relief or eradication of the offending symptoms. Herbal medicines differ from pharmaceuticals in that—unlike plant-derived medications such as digoxin—single active agents are not identified, isolated, purified, and concentrated for human use. There is a presumed synergy of multiple bioactive components. Also, dosing is not as clearly identified. Rigorous scientific studies are thus much more difficult to conduct than for pharmaceuticals.

In sharp contrast to the North American experience, Asian herbal traditions use formulas containing multiple herbs that are customized for the patient and often for unmeasurable constitutional states and unquantifiable outcomes. Up to 12 ingredients can exist in these formulas. Ingredients can include plants, mushrooms, and minerals. In Chinese formulas, animal parts are often included.

Of particular interest may be Japan's Kampo tradition, as described in Sidebar 20.1. Today, in Japan, medical students are routinely taught to prescribe 148 ancient, multiherb formulas that are approved by Japan's equivalent of the FDA and covered by their national health plan. Approximately 70% of all physicians prescribe these multiherb formulas, including nearly 100% of Japanese gynecologists. Diagnosis is made by physical examination of the tongue, pulse, and abdomen. Diagnoses can be very subjective, such as *katakori* (literally, frozen shoulder, but patients have full range of motion) and *hiesho* (cold condition with normal body temperatures). There is no one-to-one correlation between a condition such as *hiesho* and a formula. Several formulas exist and are used for multiple conditions. The correct formula is based on the patient's history, physical examination, and response to initial treatment (Plotnikoff, Watanabe, & Yashiro, 2008).

SIDEBAR 20.1. KAMPO, JAPAN'S TRADITIONAL MEDICINE

Kenji Watanabe

Kampo, Japan's traditional medicine, is widely practiced, approved by the government's regulatory agencies, and covered by the national health plan. Unlike North American medical schools, Japanese medical students are taught to prescribe ancient, multiherb formulas. Both physicians and nurses are expected to know common uses and common side effects of these formulas.

Kampo literally means "way of the Han dynasty," the governmental period of ancient China from 220 BCE to 200 CE. During this time, many key medical texts were prepared. Japanese healers reinterpreted these to fit Japanese culture and historical experience. For this reason, Kampo today has many similarities to traditional Chinese medicine (TCM). However, there are several key points of differentiation. First, the Kampo physical examination focuses on the

(continued)

abdomen. Tongue and pulse diagnoses are considered, but the abdominal examination, termed *fukushin*, is prioritized. Second, although many formulas are shared, Kampo uses may be quite different. Third, Kampo diagnostic and therapeutic approaches are standardized and easily work with Western diagnoses and treatment plans. There is a robust scientific literature, especially in the basic sciences, to support prescription of rational herbal medicine.

Kampo herbal formulas are widely prescribed in both university and community hospitals across Japan. The Japanese Society of Oriental Medicine (JSOM) has annual meetings that attract many thousands of practitioners. Kampo is well understood in Japan.

Kampo's popularity and documented safety have promoted increasing international interest. As a result, JSOM has produced an introductory text in English. An excellent English translation of the works of revered Kampo master Keisetsu Otsuka has recently been published, and the International Society for Japanese Kampo Medicine (ISJKM) now holds international meetings in English (www.isjkm.com). Furthermore, in 2013, the journal *Evidence-Based Complementary & Alternative Medicine* hosted a special issue on the collaboration of Japanese Kampo medicine and Western medicine. In addition, the World Health Organization (WHO) is developing a common platform for Western medicine and traditional medicine via the *International Classification of Diseases* (*ICD*). Under the revision from *ICD-10* to *ICD-11* (currently *ICD-11* beta is on the web at https://icd.who.int/dev11/l-m/en), traditional Asian medicine, including Kampo, will be incorporated. This will enhance mutual communication between Western medicine and Kampo internationally.

Recent Articles of Interest to English-Speaking Audiences

Cameron, S., Reissenweber, H., & Watanabe, K. (2012). Asian medicine: Japan's paradigm [letter]. *Nature, 482*(7835), 35.

Gepshtein, Y., Plotnikitt, G. A., & Watanabe, K. (2008). Kampo in women's health: Japan's traditional approach to premenstrual symptoms. *Journal of Alternative Complementary Medicine, 14*(4), 427–435.

Hirose, T., Shinoda, Y., Yoshida, A., Kurimoto, M., Mori, K., Kawachi, Y, ... Sugiyama, T. (2016). Efficacy of kaiokanzoto in chronic constipation refractory to first-line laxatives. *Biomedical Reports, 5*(4), 497–500.

Ilto, A., Munakata, K., Imazu, Y., & Watanabe, K. (2012). First nationwide attitude survey of Japanese physicians on the use of traditional Japanese medicine (Kampo) in cancer treatment. Evidence-*Based Complementary & Alternative Medicine, 2012*(2012), 1–8. Article ID 957082.

Iwase, S., Yamaguchi, T., Miyajo, T., Terawaki, K., Inui, Q., & Uesono, Y. (2012). The clinical use of Kampo medicines (traditional Japanese herbal treatments) for controlling cancer patients' symptoms in Japan: A national cross-sectional survey. *BMC Complementary and Alternative Medicine, 12*, 222.

Kimata, Y., Ogawa, K., Okamoto, H., Chino, A., & Namiki, T. (2016). Efficacy of traditional (Kampo) medicine for treating chemotherapy-induced peripheral neuropathy: A retrospective case series study. *World Journal Clinical Cases, 4*(10), 310–317.

Kowago, K., Shindo, S., Inoue, H., Akasaka, J., Motohashi, S., Urabe, G., ... Ogino, H. (2016). The effect of hachimi-jin-gan (Ba wei di-huang-wan) on the quality of life of patients with peripheral arterial disease—A prospective study using Kampo medicine. *Annals of Vascular Diseases, 9*(4), 288–294.

(continued)

Mizoguchi, K., & Ikarashi, Y. (2017). Multiple psychopharmacological effects of the traditional Japanese Kampo medicine Yokukansan, and the brain regions it effects. *Frontiers in Pharmacology, 21*(8), 149.

Watanabe, K., Matsuura, K., Gao, P., Hottenbacher, L., Tokunaga, H., Nishimura, K., ... Witt, C. M. (2011). Traditional Japanese Kampo medicine: Clinical research between modernity and traditional medicine—the state of research and methodological suggestions for the future. Evidence-*Based Complementary* & Alternative *Medicine, 8*(1), 1–19.

FUTURE RESEARCH

Before even Western single-herb medicines can be more widely accepted by the conventional allopathic medical system, more randomized, double-blind, placebo-controlled trials are needed in the United States. The National Institutes of Health, National Center for Complementary and Integrative Health (NCCIH) has funded and will likely continue to fund promising clinical trials of herbal therapies. Understudied areas of research for herbal therapies include:

- Premenstrual and perimenopausal symptom management
- Prevention of chemotherapy side effects, including peripheral neuropathy
- Chronic pain
- Disabling fatigue
- Refractory insomnia

In addition, significant efforts are needed to identify the most promising herbal supports for radiation therapy, irritable bowel and inflammatory bowel, gastroparesis, as well as asthma and heart disease.

Western medicine has yet to explore the potential benefits from the world's many healing traditions that use customized combinations of herbs. The Kampo traditional medicines of Japan may be the best place to start, given the rigorous approach to safety, the strength of the published preclinical data, and the extent of use by mainstream health professionals. This study requires a new paradigm, one that accounts for potential synergy and counterbalancing activities of multiple ingredients. Although intriguing preliminary data exist for many dietary supplements, the historic paucity of funding mechanisms in these areas has meant that scientific support for the use of many commercial products lags significantly behind consumer marketing efforts.

The key message is this: Medicinal herbs for symptom management and well-being can be used by nursing for patients using evidenced-based literature and a holistic framework. Nursing has the opportunity and challenge to play a key role in the research, practice, and clinical use of plant therapies for symptom management and overall well-being.

WEBSITES AND OTHER RESOURCES

- American Botanical Council
  (www.herbalgram.org)
- American Nutraceutical Association
  (www.americanutra.com)

- Blumenthal, M., Goldberg, A., & Brinckmann, J. (Eds.). (2000). *Herbal medicine—The expanded Commission E Monographs.* Austin, TX: American Botanical Council.
- FDA Center for Food Safety and Applied Nutrition—a link to report adverse events (www.fda.gov/AboutFDA/CentersOffices/OfficeofFoods/CFSAN/ContactCFSAN/default.htm)
- *HerbalGram magazine*—published quarterly by the American Botanical Council and the Herb Research Foundation (www.herbalgram.org)
- Herb Research Foundation (www.herbs.org)
- Micromedex Alternative Medicine Database—an authoritative, full-text drug-information resource; includes alternative medicine and is one of the most comprehensive resources for herbal medicine. (www.library.ucsf.edu/db/micromedex.html)

REFERENCES

Abdali, K., Khajehei, M., & Tavatabaee, H. R. (2010). Effect of St. John's wort on severity, frequency and duration of hot flashes in premenopausal, perimenopausal and postmenopausal women: A randomized, double-blind, placebo controlled study. *Menopause, 17*(2), 326–331.

Ahmad, M., Saleem, S., Ahmad, A., Yousuf, S., Ansari, M. A., Khan, M. B., … Islam, F. (2005). Ginkgo biloba affords dose-dependent protection against 6-hydroxydopamine-induced parkinsonism in rats: Neurobehavioral, neuro-chemical and immunohistochemical evidence. *Journal of Neurochemistry, 93*, 94–104.

American Botanical Council. (2000). *Herbal medicine: Expanded Commission E monographs.* Austin, TX: American Botanical Council.

Apaydin, E. A., Maher, A. R., Shanman, R., Booth, M. S., Miles, J. N. V., Sorbero, M. E., & Hempel, S. (2016). A systematic review of St. John's wort for major depressive disorder. *Systematic Reviews, 5*(1), 148.

Archer, E. L., & Boyle, D. K. (2008). Herb and supplement use among the retail population of an independent, urban herb store. *Journal of Holistic Nursing, 26*, 27–35.

Arcury, T. A., Suerken, C. K., Brzywacz, J. G., Bell, R. A., Lang, W., & Quandt, S. A. (2006). Complementary and alternative medicine use among older adults: Ethnic variation. *Ethnic Diseases, 16*, 723–731.

Ardjomand-Woelkart, K., & Bauer, R. (2016). Review and assessment of medicinal safety data of orally used Echinacea preparations. *Planta Medica, 82*(1–2), 17–31.

Barnes, J., Anderson, L. A., Gibbons, S., & Phillipson, J. D. (2005). *Echinacea* species (*Echinacea angustifolica* [DC.] Hell., *Echinacea pallida* [Nutt.] Nutt., *Echinacea purpurea* [L.] Moench): A review of their chemistry, pharmacology and clinical properties. *Journal of Pharmacy and Pharmacology, 57*, 929–954.

Barnes, P. M., Bloom, B., & Nahin, R. (2008, December 10). Complementary and alternative medicine use among adults and children: United States, 2007. *National Health Statistics Report, 12*, 1–23.

Barnes, P. M., Powell-Griner, E., McFann, K., & Nahin, R. I. (2004). Complementary and alternative medicine use among adults: United States, 2002. *Advance Data, 343*, 1–19.

Barrett, B. (2003). Medicinal properties of echinacea: A critical review. *Phytomedicine, 10*, 66–86.

Barton, D. L., Burger, K., Novotny, P. J., Fitch, T. R., Kohli, S., Soori, G., … Loprinzi, C. L. (2013). The use of Ginkgo biloba for the prevention of chemotherapy-related cognitive dysfunction in women receiving adjuvant treatment for breast cancer, N00C9. *Support Care Cancer, 21*(4), 1185–1192.

Bebbington, A., Kulkarni, R., & Roberts, P. (2005). Ginkgo biloba: Persistent bleeding after total hip arthroplasty caused by herbal self-medication. *Journal of Arthroplasty, 20*, 125–126.

Beckert, B. W., Concannon, M. J., Henry, S. L., Smith, D. S., & Puckett, C. L. (2007). The effect of herbal medicines on platelet function: An in vivo experiment and review of the literature. *Plastic and Reconstructive Surgery, 120*, 2044–2050.

Birks, J., & Grimley Evans, J. (2007, April 18). Ginkgo biloba for cognitive impairment and dementia. *Cochrane Database of Systematic Reviews, 2*, CD003120. doi:10.1002/14651858. CD003120.pub2

Bone, K. M. (2008). Potential interaction of ginkgo biloba leaf with antiplatelet or anticoagulant drugs: What is the evidence? *Molecular Nutrition and Food Research, 52*, 764–771.

Borgelt, L. M., Franson, K. L., Nussbaum, A. M., & Wang, G. S. (2013). The pharmacologic and clinical effects of medical cannabis. *Pharmacotherapy, 33*(2), 195–209.

Bostwick, J. M. (2012). Blurred boundaries: The therapeutics and politics of medical marijuana. *Mayo Clinic Proceedings, 87*(2), 172–186.

Bostwick, J. M., Reisfield, G. M., & DuPont, R. L. (2013) Clinical decisions. Medicinal use of marijuana. *New England Journal of Medicine, 368*(9), 866–868.

Butterweck, V., & Schmidt, M. (2007). St. John's wort: Role of active compounds for its mechanism of action and efficacy. *Wiener medizinische Wochenschrift, 157*, 356–361.

Canter, P. H., & Ernst, E. (2007). Ginkgo biloba is not a smart drug: An updated systematic review of randomized clinical trials testing the nootropic effects of *G. biloba* extracts in healthy people. *Human Psychopharmacology, 22*, 265–278.

Carpenter, C., Crigger, N., Kugler, R., & Loya, A. (2008). *Hypericum* and nurses: A comprehensive literature review on the efficacy of St. John's wort in the treatment of depression. *Journal of Holistic Nursing, 26*, 200–207.

Cetisli, N. E., Saruhan, A., & Kivcak, B. (2015). The effects of flaxseed on menopausal symptoms and quality of life. *Holistic Nursing Practice, 29*(3), 151–157.

Chen, X., Salwinski, S., & Lee, T. J. (1997). Extracts of Ginkgo biloba and ginsenosides exert cerebral vasorelaxation via a nitric oxide pathway. *Clinical Experimental Pharmacology and Physiology, 24*, 958–959.

Cherniack, E. P., Ceron-Fuentes, J., Florez, H., Sandals, L., Rodriguez, O., & Palacios, J. C. (2008). Influence of race and ethnicity on alternative medicine as a self-treatment for common medical conditions in a population of multi-ethnic urban elderly. *Complementary Therapies in Clinical Practice, 14*, 116–123.

Clarke, T. C., Black, L. I., Stussman, B. J., Barnes, P. M., & Nahin, R. L. (2015). Trends in the use of complementary health approaches among adults: United States, 2002-2012, *National Health Statistics Reports, 79*, 1–16.

Crippa, J. A., Hallak, J. E., Machado-de-Sousa, J. P., Queiroz, R. H., Bergamaschi, M., Chagas, M. H., & Zuardi, A. W. (2013). Canabidiol for the treatment of cannabis withdrawal syndrome: A case report. *Journal of Clinical Pharmacology and Therapeutics, 38*(2), 162–164.

Di, Y. M., Li, C. G., Xue, C. C., & Zhou, S. F. (2008). Clinical drugs that interact with St. John's wort and implication in drug development. *Current Pharmacology Design, 14*, 1723–1742.

Engelsen, J., Nielson, J. D., & Winther, K. (2002). Effect of coenzyme Q10 and ginkgo biloba on warfarin dosage in stable, long-term warfarin treated outpatients: A randomized double blind placebo-crossover trial. *Thrombosis & Haemostatis, 87*(6), 1075–1076.

Erzigkeit, H. (1992). *SKT manual. A short cognitive performance test for assessing memory and attention. Concise version.* Castrop-Rauxel, Germany: Geromed.

Florence Nightingale Museum of London. (2016). Medicines & chest. Retrieved http://florence-nightingale-collections.co.uk/view/objects/asitem/items$0040:227

Francis, M., & Williams, S. (2014). Effectiveness of Indian turmeric powder with honey on complementary therapy in oral mucositis: A nursing perspective among cancer patients in Mysore. *Nursing Journal of India, 105*(6), 258–260.

Freeman, C., & Spelman, K. (2008). A critical evaluation of drug interactions with *Echinacea* spp. *Molecular Nutrition and Food Research, 52*, 789–798.

Freeman, M. P., Fava, M., Lake, J., Trivedi, M. H., Wisner, K. L., & Mischoulon, D. (2010). Complementary and alternative medicine in major depressive disorder: The American Psychiatric Association Task Force Report. *Journal of Clinical Psychiatry, 71*(6), 669–681.

Graham, R. E., Ahn, A. C., Davis, R. B., O'Connor, B. B., Eisenberg, D. M., & Phillips, R. S. (2005). Use of complementary and alternative medical therapies among racial and ethnic minority adults: Results from the 2002 National Health Interview Survey. *Journal of the National Medical Association, 97*, 535–545.

Haller, C. A., & Benowitz, N. L. (2000). Adverse cardiovascular and central nervous system events associated with dietary supplements containing ephedra alkaloids. *New England Journal of Medicine, 343*(25), 1833–1838.

Heinrich, M. (2015). Quality and safety of herbal medical products: Regulation and the need for quality assurance along the value chains. *British Journal of Clinical Pharmacology, 80*(1), 62–66.

Hermann, R., & von Richter, O. (2012). Clinical evidence of herbal drugs as perpetrators of pharmacokinetic drug interactions. *Planta Medica, 78*(13), 1458–1477.

Herrschaft, H., Nacu, A., Likhachev, S., Sholomov, I., Hoerr, R., & Schlaefke, S. (2012). Ginkgo biloba extract EGB761 in dementia with neuropsychiatric features: A randomized, placebo-controlled trial to confirm the efficacy and safety of a daily dose of 240 mg. *Journal of Psychiatric Research, 46*(6), 716–723.

Hofferberth, B. (1994). The efficacy of EGB761 in patients with senile dementia of the Alzheimer's type: A double-blind, placebo-controlled study on different levels of investigation. *Human Psychopharmacology, 9*, 215–222.

Huang, S. Y., Jeng, C., Kao, S. C., Yu, J. J., & Liu, D. Z. (2004). Improved haemorrheological properties by ginkgo biloba extract EGB761 in type 2 diabetes mellitus complicated with retinopathy. *Clinical Nutrition, 23*, 615–621.

Ilhan, A., Gurel, A., Armutcu, F., Kamisli, S., Iraz, M., Akyol, O., & Ozen, S. (2004). Ginkgo biloba prevents mobile phone-induced oxidative stress in rat brain. *Clinica Chimica Acta, 340*, 153–162.

Jawad, M., Schoop, R., Suter, A., Klein, P., & Eccles, R. (2012). Safety and efficacy profile of *Echinacea purpurea* to prevent common cold episodes: A randomized, double-blind, placebo-controlled trial. *Evidence-Based Complementary & Alternative Medicine, 2012*, 841315. doi:10.1155/2012/841315

Jiao, Y. B., Rui, Y. C., Li, T. J., Yang, P. Y., & Qiu, Y. (2005). Expression of pro-inflammatory and anti-inflammatory cytokines in brain of atherosclerotic rats and effects of ginkgo biloba extract. *Acta Pharmacologica Sinica, 26*, 835–839.

Kanowski, S., Herrmann, W. M., Stephan, K., Wierich, W., & Horr, R. (1996). Proof of efficacy of the ginkgo biloba extract Egb 761 in outpatients suffering from mild to moderate primary degenerative dementia of the Alzheimer's type of multi-infarct dementia. *Pharmacopsychiatry, 29*, 47–56.

Karsch-Völk, M., Barrett, B., Kiefer, D., Bauer, R., Ardjomand-Woelkart, K., & Linde, K. (2014). Echinacea for preventing and treating the common cold. *Cochrane Database of Systematic Reviews, 20*(2) CD000530.

Kasper, S., Gastpar, M., Müller, W. E., Volz, H. P., Dienel, A., Kieser, M., & Möller, H. J. (2008). Efficacy of St. John's wort extract WS 5570 in acute treatment of mild depression: A reanalysis of data from controlled clinical trials. *European Archives of Psychiatry and Clinical Neuroscience, 258*, 59–63.

Kaufmann, H. (2002). Treatment of patients with orthostatic hypotension and syncope. *Clinical Neuropharmacology, 25*(3), 133–141.

Kim, M. S., Lee, J. I., Lee, W. Y., & Kim, S. E. (2004). Neuroprotective effect of ginkgo biloba L. extract in a rat model of Parkinson's disease. *Phytotherapy Research, 18*, 663–666.

Kleijnen, J., & Knipschild, P. (1992). Ginkgo biloba for cerebral insufficiency. *British Journal of Pharmacology, 34*, 352.

LeBars, P. L., Katz, M. M., Berman, N., Itil, T. M., Freedman, A. M., & Schatzberg, A. F. (1997). A placebo-controlled, double-blind, randomized trial of an extract of ginkgo biloba for dementia. *Journal of the American Medical Association, 278*, 1327–1332.

Lee, A. N., & Werth, V. P. (2004). Activation of autoimmunity following use of immunostimulatory herbal supplements. *Archives of Dermatology, 140*, 723–727.

Lev-Ran, S., Le Foll, B., McKenzie, K., George, T. P., & Rehm, J. (2013). Cannabis use and cannabis use disorders among individuals with mental illness. *Comprehensive Psychiatry, 54*(6), 589–598.

Li, X. F., Ma, M., Scherban, K., & Tam, Y. K. (2002). Liquid chromatography-electrospray mass spectrometric studies of ginkgolides and bilobalide using simultaneous monitoring of proton, ammonium, and sodium adducts. *Analyst, 127,* 641–646.

Linde, K., Berner, M. M., & Kriston, L. (2008). St. John's wort for major depression. *Cochrane Database of Systematic Reviews, 4,* CD000448.

Lovera, J. F., Kim, E., Heriza, E., Fitzpatrick, M., Hunziker, J., Turner, A. P., … Bourdette, D. (2012). Ginkkgo biloba does not improve cognitive function in MS: A randomized placebo-controlled trial. *Neurology, 79*(12), 1278–1284.

Mahadevan, S., & Park, Y. (2008). Multifaceted therapeutic benefits of ginkgo biloba L.: Chemistry, efficacy, safety and uses. *Journal of Food Science, 73*(1), R14–R19.

Matthews, M. K., Jr. (1998). Association of ginkgo biloba with intracerebral hemorrhage. *Neurology, 50,* 1933–1934.

May, B. H., Lit, M., Xue, C. C., Yang, A. W., Zhang, A. L., Owens, M. D., & Story, D. F. (2009). Herbal medicine for dementia: A systematic review. *Phytotherapy Research, 23,* 447–459.

Mengs, U., Clare, C. B., & Poiley, J. A. (1991). Toxicity of *Echinacea purpurea.* Acute, subacute and genotoxicity studies. *Arzneimittel-Frosch, 41,* 1076–1081.

Miller, L. H., & Su, X. (2011) Artemisinin: Discovery from the Chinese herbal garden. *Cell, 146*(6), 855–858.

Money, N. (2016). Are mushrooms medicinal? *Fungal Biology, 120,* 449–453.

Müller, W. E., Rolli, M., Schafer, C., & Hafner, U. (1997). Effects of hypericum extract (L160) in biochemical models of antidepressant activity. *Pharmacopsychiatry, 30*(Suppl. 2), S102–S107.

Oyama, Y., Chikahisa, L., Ueha, T., Kanemaru, K., & Noda, K. (1996). Ginkgo biloba extract protects brain neurons against oxidative stress induced by hydrogen peroxide. *Brain Research, 712,* 349–352.

Pietschmann, A., Kuklinski, B., & Otterstein, A. (1992). Protection from UV-light-induced oxidative stress by nutritional radical scavengers. *Zeitschrift fur die Gesamte Innere Medizin und Ihre Grenzgebite, 47*(11), 518–522.

Pittler, M. H., & Ernst, E. (2005). Complementary therapies for peripheral artery disease: Systematic review. *Atherosclerosis, 18,* 1–7.

Plotnikoff, G. A, Watanabe, K., & Yashiro, F. (2008). Kampo: From old wisdom comes new knowledge. *HerbalGram, 78,* 46–56.

Rosenblatt, M., & Mindel, J. (1997). Spontaneous hyphema associated with ingestion of ginkgo biloba extract. *New England Journal of Medicine, 336,* 1108.

Rowin, J., & Lewis, S. L. (1996). Spontaneous bilateral subdural hematomas associated with chronic ginkgo biloba ingestion have also occurred. *Neurology, 46,* 1775–1776.

Senchina, D. S., McDann, D. A., Asp, J. M., Johnson, J. A., Cunnick, J. E., Kaiser, M. S., & Kohut, M. L. (2005). Changes in immunomodulatory properties of *Echinacea* spp. root infusions and tinctures stored at 4 degrees C for four days. *Clinica Chimica Acta, 355,* 67–82.

Sener, G., Sener, E., Sehirli, O., Ogune, A. V., Cetinel, S., Gedik, N., & Sakarcan, A. (2005). Ginkgo biloba extract ameliorates ischemia reperfusion-induced renal injury in rats. *Pharmacology Research, 52*(3), 216–222.

Shah, S. A., Sander, S., White, C. M., Rinaldi, M., & Coleman, C. I. (2007). Evaluation of echinacea for the prevention and treatment of the common cold: A meta-analysis. *Lancet Infectious Disease, 7,* 473–480.

Shen, J. G., & Zhou, D. Y. (1995). Efficiency of ginkgo biloba extract (Egb 761) in antioxidant protection against myocardial ischemia and re-perfusion injury. *Biochemical Molecular Biological Institute, 35,* 125–134.

Sikora, K. (1989). Complementary medicine and cancer treatment. *Practitioner, 233*(1476), 1285–1286.

U.S. Congress. (1994). *103rd Congress. Dietary Supplement Health and Education Act of 1994.* Pub. L. 103–417. 108 Stat/4325-4335. Washington, DC: Library of Congress.

U.S. Congress, House of Representatives, Committee on Government Reform. (1999, March 25). *Dietary Supplement Health and Education Act: Is the FDA trying to change the intent of Congress?* Washington, DC: U.S. Government Printing Office.

Walesiuk, A., Trofimiuk, E., & Braszko, J. J. (2005). Ginkgo biloba extract diminishes stress-induced memory deficits in rats. *Pharmacology Reporter, 57,* 176–187.

Ward, E., & Blumenthal, M. (2005). Americans confident in dietary supplements according to CRN survey. *HerbalGram, 66,* 64–65.

Wasser, S. P. (2014). Medicinal mushrooms science: Current perspectives, advances, evidences, and challenges. *Biomedical Journal, 37*(6), 345–356.

Wyatt, G. K., Sikorskii, A., Safikhani, A., McVary, K. T., & Herman, J. (2015). Saw palmetto for symptom management during radiation therapy for prostate cancer. *Journal of Pain and Symptom Management, 51*(6), 1046–1054.

Zhang, H. F., Huang, L. B., Zhong, Y. B., Zhou, Y. B., Wang, H. L., Zheng, G. Q., & Lin, Y. (2016). An overview of systematic reviews of *Ginkgo biloba* extracts for mild cognitive impairment and dementia. *Frontiers in Aging Neuroscience, 6*(8), 276.

Zhou, S. F., & Lai, X. (2008). An update on clinical drug interactions with the herbal antidepressant St. John's wort. *Current Drug Metabolism, 9*(5), 394–409.

Functional Foods and Nutraceuticals

MELISSA H. FRISVOLD

In the 21st century, the focus of the relationship between eating habits and health is changing from an emphasis on health maintenance through recommended dietary allowances of nutrients, vitamins, and minerals to an emphasis on the use of foods to provide better health, increase vitality, and aid in preventing disease and many chronic illnesses. The connection between food and health is not new. Indeed, the adage "Let food be your medicine and medicine your food" was adopted by Hippocrates (trans. 1932). Today, the philosophy that supports the paradigm of nutraceuticals as functional foods is once again at the forefront.

Nutraceuticals, because of their safety and potential nutritive and therapeutic effects, have received considerable attention (Shende, Desai, & Gaud, 2016). They provide a viable alternative to modern medicines and may be a useful tool in healthy living. Prescription drugs often have adverse effects that for some patients are difficult to tolerate. Some of the possible therapeutic benefits from nutraceuticals are antiobesity effects, immune enhancement, natural antioxidant protection, positive cardiovascular effects, antidiabetic properties, and anti-inflammatory effects (Pravin et al., 2016).

The United States is one of the largest consumers of nutraceuticals in the world. The U.S. nutraceutical market is expected to surpass $95 billion by 2022 (Wood, 2017). The vast array of nutraceutical products is staggering. Products range from single-ingredient nutrients such as calcium to drinks fortified with electrolytes and cereals fortified with iron (Haller, 2010). Many companies are using soy protein isolates in foods ranging from candy bars and salad dressings to infant formulas. Plant stanols and sterols are being added to margarine-like spreads in an effort to reduce total cholesterol and low-density lipoprotein (LDL) levels.

Coverage of all nutraceuticals is beyond the scope of this chapter. A plethora of functional foods have been developed recently. According to a consumer survey conducted by the Council for Responsible Nutrition (2016), more than 170 million Americans take dietary supplements. In the interest of brevity, several selected products are covered in depth in this chapter. Because the use of nutraceuticals is so prevalent and because their use may impact health and wellness, it is important that nurses know about them and their potential benefits and risks.

DEFINITION

According to Stephen DeFelice (1994), the Foundation for Innovation in Medicine coined the term *nutraceutical* in 1989 to give an identity to an area of health and medicine that held great promise. According to the foundation, a nutraceutical is any substance that may be considered a food or part of a food and provides health benefits. These products may range from dietary supplements, isolated nutrients, and herbal products to genetically engineered designer foods. The number and variety of nutraceuticals available in the United States are staggering; for example, many grocery stores carry cereals fortified with omega-3 fatty acids, ginseng-enriched sports drinks, dairy products with various strains of probiotics, and orange juice that contains added calcium. The intent of the Dietary Supplement Health and Education Act (DSHEA), passed in 1994, was to protect the rights of consumers to have access to dietary supplements (and thus nutraceuticals and functional foods) to promote good health (Food and Drug Administration [FDA], 2012). Under the provisions of the law, dietary supplement ingredients are exempt from drug regulations; thus, premarketing approval, including demonstration of benefit and safety, is not required (Haller, 2010).

Until recently, a formal definition in the United States did not exist for the term *functional foods*, which created a challenge for researchers and developers of these foods that wanted to sell them or educate the public about their products (Martirosyan & Singh, 2015). The following definition was accepted at a 2014 conference attended by representatives from the U.S. Department of Agriculture (USDA), the Functional Food Center (FFC), the Academic Society for Functional Foods and Bioactive Compounds (ASFFBC), and the Agricultural Research Service (ARS), to facilitate better communication among scientists, government officials, the public, and food experts. The accepted definition of functional foods is "natural or processed foods that contain known or unknown biologically-active compounds; which, in defined, effective non-toxic amounts, provide a clinically proven and documented health benefit for the prevention, management, or treatment of chronic disease" (Martirosyan & Singh, 2015, p. 215). The definition identifies the following key points about functional foods:

- Functional foods can be processed or natural.
- Functional foods contain known or unknown biologically active compounds.
- Functional foods must provide a clinically proven and documented health benefit.
- Functional foods that contain bioactive compounds must be consumed in effective nontoxic amounts (Martirosyan & Singh, 2015).

The Japanese, who were among the first to use functional foods, have highlighted three conditions that define a functional food:

- It is a food (not a capsule, tablet, or powder) derived from naturally occurring ingredients.
- It can and should be consumed as part of a daily diet.
- It has a particular function when ingested, serving to regulate a particular body process: enhancement of the biological defense mechanism, prevention

of a specific disease, recovery from a specific disease, control of physical and mental conditions, and slowing of the aging process (PA Consulting Group, 1990).

According to these definitions, unmodified whole foods such as fruits and vegetables represent the simplest form of a functional food. For example, broccoli, carrots, or tomatoes would be considered functional foods because they contain high levels of physiologically active components such as beta-carotene, lycopene, and sulforaphane. Modified foods, including those that have been fortified with nutrients or enhanced with phytochemicals, are also within the realm of functional foods.

SCIENTIFIC BASIS

During the past century, there have been many changes in the types of foods people eat, reflecting the application of scientific findings and technological innovations in the food industry. Although much research has been conducted on nutrition and health and disease, scientific exploration on the use of nutraceuticals has been more limited.

Interest in foodstuffs has generated investigation to link nutrient and food intake with improvements in health or prevention of disease. Studies in the epidemiological literature have been reviewed and suggest a possible association between a low consumption of fruits and vegetables and the incidence of certain diseases such as heart disease (He, Nowson, & MacGregor, 2006; He, Nowson, Lucas, & MacGregor, 2007, Wang et al., 2014), and a recent research article in the *Journal of the National Cancer Institute* (2013) suggests that vegetable consumption may reduce the risk of certain types of breast cancer (Rathner, 2013).

Much scientific study has been conducted on the role of the various products added to normal foods to enhance their ability to inhibit or prevent diseases. Many researchers regard dietary intake as the best means of acquiring necessary nutrients (Kottke, 1998). For example, the World Cancer Research Fund International/ American Institute for Cancer Research (2017) recommends the consumption of foods mostly of plant origin, which may protect against certain types of cancers. It is important to point out that these foods contain various micronutrients; therefore, it is difficult to tease out whether a certain element of the food alone is responsible for an identified protective effect. However, supplementation of nutrients is common.

Dietary Plant Stanols and Sterols

The cholesterol-lowering potential of dietary plant stanols and sterols has been known for many years (Plat et al., 2012). In fact, the use of plant stanols at a dose of 2 g daily is reported to be effective in lowering LDL cholesterol by 9% to 10% (Ras, Geleijnse, & Trautwein, 2014). Modification of plant stanols and sterols structurally enables them to be easily incorporated into fat-containing foods without losing their effectiveness in lowering cholesterol (Cater & Grundy, 1998). Dietary plant stanols and sterols inhibit the absorption of cholesterol in the small intestine, which in turn can lower LDL blood cholesterol (de Jong, Plat, & Mensink, 2003). Historically, plant stanols have been added to margarine-like products or yogurt drinks. Recently, a study by Laitinen, Gylling, Kaipiainen, Nissinen, and Simonen (2017) demonstrated that a chewable stanol ester capsule was also effective in lowering LDL cholesterol. It has been suggested that lifestyle modification, which includes dietary changes such as the inclusion of plant stanols and sterols, should be the primary treatment for lowering cholesterol (Turpeinen et al., 2012). Thus, functional foods might offer a safe and easily attainable method for decreasing heart disease risk (Turpeinen et al., 2012). A limited number of clinical trials also have demonstrated that a further reduction in LDL cholesterol may be achieved at doses as high as 9 g daily, but additional research is necessary before this can be recommended (Plat et al., 2012).

Plant sterols and their esters are generally recognized as safe (GRAS) food-grade substances, a designation indicating that there has been a history of safe intake of these products with no demonstrated harmful health effects found in the research (Wrick, 2005). Overall, the Nutrition Committee of the American Heart Association advises that stanols and sterol esters not be used as a preventive measure in the general population with normal cholesterol levels, in light of limited data regarding any potential risks. They may be used, however, for adults with hypercholesterolemia or adults requiring secondary prevention after an atherosclerotic event (Lichtenstein et al., 2006).

Glucosamine and Chondroitin Sulfate

Glucosamine, an amino sugar the body produces, and chondroitin sulfate, a complex carbohydrate found in and around cartilage cells, are natural substances (National Center for Complementary and Integrative Health, 2016a). Glucosamine and chondroitin sulfate are two separate products; however, they are often sold together to diminish the pain and stiffness of osteoarthritis. Historically, German physicians were reported to be the first to use glucosamine in 1969 to diminish pain and increase mobility in patients with osteoarthritis (Therapeutic Research Center [TRC], 2018a.). Most clinical research shows that taking glucosamine sulfate orally significantly improves symptoms of pain and functionality compared with placebo in patients with osteoarthritis of the knee (Natural Medicine, 2016). Meta-analyses by McAlindon et al. (2000) and by Towheed and Hochberg (1997) reviewed clinical trials of glucosamine and chondroitin in the treatment of osteoarthritis. McAlindon and colleagues included 13 double-blind, placebo-controlled trials of more than 4 weeks' duration, testing oral or parenteral glucosamine or chondroitin for the treatment of hip or knee arthritis. All 13 studies were classified as positive, demonstrating substantial benefits in treating arthritis when compared with placebo. Towheed and Hochberg reviewed nine randomized, controlled studies of glucosamine in osteoarthritis. Glucosamine was superior when compared with placebo in seven randomized trials. Two of the randomized trials compared glucosamine with ibuprofen. In these two trials, glucosamine was superior in one and equivalent in the other. A recent meta-analysis in 2010 concluded that compared with placebo, glucosamine, chondroitin, or the combination of these two products did not reduce joint pain (Wandel et al., 2010).

Coenzyme Q10

Coenzyme Q10 (CoQ10) is a compound made naturally in the body. It is used by cells to produce energy needed for cell growth and maintenance. It is also used by the body as an antioxidant. Tissue levels of CoQ10 decrease with age. It has been suggested that CoQ10 may stimulate the immune system and increase resistance to disease; however, there are no well-designed clinical trials to support this claim (National Cancer Institute, 2013). Cardiovascular health continues to be the main area of study for use with this compound. Several controlled trials of CoQ10 have been performed for the indication of congestive heart failure, and the results have been varied (Khatta et al., 2000). There have also been suggested benefits to health from CoQ10 for statin-associated myalgias (Caso, Kelly, McNurland, & Lawson, 2007). A meta-analysis (Banach et al., 2015) concluded that CoQ10 demonstrated no significant benefit in statin myopathy; however, two of the authors commented that there may be a benefit to continuing CoQ10 supplementation until larger studies are conducted because there are no known risks and there is some favorable anecdotal evidence for effectiveness (Saha & Whayne, 2016). A review article by Littarru and Tiano (2010) suggests that there may be some potential benefit from CoQ10 for fatigue and performance issues with exercise, for preeclampsia, and for decreased sperm count (Littarru & Tiano, 2010). Further research is needed to verify these claims. Other therapeutic claims attributed to CoQ10 involve hypertension, impaired immune status, adjuvant therapy for breast cancer, and various neurological disorders. As always, caution must be exercised when suggesting supplementation with any nutraceutical during pregnancy.

Probiotics

Probiotics are microorganism supplements intended to improve health or treat a certain disease. Probiotics are also called *friendly bacteria* and are available to consumers in the form of dietary supplements and foods (National Center for Complementary and Integrative Health, 2016b). Yogurt is an example of a probiotic food source. Probiotics also come in other forms such as tablets or capsules. They have not been approved by the FDA for any indication. Although the exact mechanism of action of these microbes is unclear, several have been proposed: lowering of intestinal pH and inhibition of pathogenic bacteria, physical or chemical prevention of colonization of pathogenic bacteria, and induction or enhancement of an immune response (Anonymous, 2013). The focus of research and the most promising results continue to be in disorders associated with the gastrointestinal tract. Based on the results of a few randomized controlled clinical trials, probiotics may be useful for treating *Clostridium difficile* (Johnson et al., 2012) and diarrhea, which is associated with antibiotic use (Kligler & Cohrssen, 2008). Probiotics have also been studied for potential use in women with bacterial vaginosis, vulvovaginal candidiasis, and urinary tract infections. The results have been conflicting. There is some evidence to support the use of probiotics for symptomatic and asymptomatic bacterial vaginosis but no evidence to support their use for vulvovaginal candidiasis (Jurden, Buchanan, Kelsberg, & Safranek, 2012). A study by Heczko et al. (2015) demonstrated that in women with recurrent bacterial vaginosis, a probiotic supplementation lengthened remission and clinical outcomes by increasing *Lactobacillus* counts and maintaining a low vaginal PH.

Further studies are necessary because some of the initial work demonstrated some promise, but these studies should focus on specific strains of probiotics. Finally, according to the TRC (2018b) on probiotics, there is grade A evidence for (i.e., strong evidence to support) the use of probiotics for diarrhea and atopic dermatitis. There is grade B evidence to support probiotic use for immune enhancement, ulcerative colitis, dental caries, cirrhosis, and sinusitis. It is important to note that there are many different strains of probiotics, and they are not all recommended for treatment of various health conditions; therefore, each condition should be carefully researched before recommendations for use are made.

INTERVENTION

Many people are using nutraceuticals. Hence, it is important that nurses include assessment of nutraceutical use when they obtain the health history of the patient. Exhibit 21.1 presents guidelines for nurses to use in assessing patients. Reputable websites for information about foods and nutraceuticals appear at the end of this chapter. Patients should be encouraged to be open about their use of nutraceuticals as part of communicating their preferences and efforts toward good health. Likewise, the response of health providers should be open and nonjudgmental, despite the potential need to counsel changes or discontinuance of a nutraceutical based on the evidence or knowledge of the provider. The expertise of professionals of other disciplines may be called on as well, through referral or consultation, to ensure that the patient receives up-to-date information from the latest evidence regarding safety and efficacy of any foods or products used.

Exhibit 21.1. Guidelines: Nutraceutical Assessment Guide for Nurses

- Screen for nutraceutical use as a routine part of the health assessment interview process. Because surgical complications can arise from nutritional supplement use, their dosage is often discontinued a few weeks before surgery.
- Acquire a working knowledge of functional foods and nutraceuticals that includes benefits/risks, costs, and possible drug interactions.
- Develop effective communication strategies to ensure that all members of a patient's healthcare team are aware of any nutraceutical use.
- Explore the reasons for the use of nutritional supplements and functional foods. Can the same benefits be achieved by using another product that is safer or less expensive?
- Consider the unique healthcare needs of various populations. It is important that pregnant women, children, older adults, and populations with certain medical conditions discuss any nutritional supplementation use with their healthcare provider prior to initiation.
- Provide educational resources for patients that are easy to access, timely, evidence based, and easy to understand.
- Remember to consult with and refer patients to nutritionists—knowledgeable and accessible resources in this promising and rapidly changing area of health and wellness.

Measurement of Outcomes

Outcomes of therapy can be assessed in a number of ways, depending on the nutraceutical and the intent of the therapy. For example, blood levels of the nutrient or effect on the target organ (e.g., bone density, with the use of calcium) could be monitored over time. Also, it is important that potential side effects of the therapy be evaluated in periodic physical assessments and comprehensive histories. Positive or negative changes in subjective health, energy, and symptoms, or those subsequent to changes in nutraceutical use, can also be assessed in individuals as data for tolerance as part of cost–benefit evaluation. Good teaching of nutraceutical principles, intended purpose, and doses and effects of functional foods will result in informed use by clients and greater awareness of intended and adverse effects.

PRECAUTIONS

It is of paramount importance that nutraceutical use be assessed as part of the health history and nutritional assessment. Safe use, including safe dosage, drug interactions, and side effects, must be carefully considered. MEDLINE offers a system for checking interactions among commonly used nutraceuticals and prescription drugs (MEDLINE, 2017).

A consistent concern cited in the literature is the lack of regulation of nutraceuticals. Dietary supplements fall under the jurisdiction of the FDA but do not have the same regulations as food and drug products. According to the Dietary Supplement Health and Education Act (DSHEA), the manufacturer is responsible for ensuring that a product is safe before it is marketed, and once the supplement reaches the market, the FDA is responsible to take action if issues with the product arise (FDA, 2012).

One safety mechanism in place to ensure the production of quality products for consumers is a voluntary dietary supplement verification program through the U.S. Pharmacopeial Convention (USP). If a product contains the USP-verified mark on its label, it demonstrates that the item has been tested and audited as a supplement that meets certain criteria for declared potency and amount, that it does not contain harmful levels of contaminants, and that it meets the FDA's good manufacturing practices (U.S. Pharmacopeial Convention, 2013).

USES

Nutraceuticals have been used to promote health and to prevent and treat illness. Nutraceuticals can be used to target deficiencies, establish optimal nutritional balance, or treat diseases. Because heart disease, cancer, and stroke are leading causes of death in the United States, greater access to nutraceuticals that have been shown to improve risk-factor profiles is desirable. Furthermore, people in the United States and worldwide could benefit from nutraceuticals when deficiencies of specific nutrients are noted.

Children and Adolescents

Nutraceuticals and functional foods may also play an important role in the health of children and adolescents. Except for probiotic use, there is a paucity of research in the literature related to nutraceuticals. More randomized clinical trials would be beneficial.

Probiotics may be useful in preventing antibiotic-associated diarrhea (AAD) in children. Antibiotics are often prescribed to children; however, these agents alter the microbial balance within the gastrointestinal tract and may cause diarrhea. The Cochrane IBD Group concluded that there is moderate evidence to support the use of probiotics in the treatment of AAD (Goldenberg et al., 2015).

Heart disease, once thought to be a disease of aging, is now recognized as starting in childhood. One recommended approach to this problem is through dietary interventions that treat dyslipidemia with a low-fat diet supplemented with water-soluble fiber, plant stanols, and plant sterols in children older than age 6 with familial hypercholesterolemia (Kwiterovich, 2008; Gylling et al., 2014).

In 2001, the American Academy of Pediatrics (AAP) published a landmark survey of its members that looked at the beliefs and use of complementary and alternative therapies (CAM) in their respective practices. Based on the findings of this survey, in 2002, the AAP developed a task force to educate families, patients, and physicians about complementary therapies. One outcome of this task force was the recommendation to research the use of CAM therapies in the pediatric population. It is important to recognize that many families are using nutraceuticals such as nutritional supplements or functional foods with their children. It is estimated that 31% of children use dietary supplements (Bailey et al., 2013). Most supplements used by children are provided by parents independently of discussions with or recommendations from their child's healthcare provider. In a study on CAM use in teenagers, it was found that among teenagers who use CAM, 75% use herbal products and other nutritional supplements (Kemper, Vohra, & Walls, 2008).

Women's Health and Nutritional Needs

Throughout the life span, women have unique nutritional needs that place them at risk for nutrition-related diseases and conditions. Nutrition has been shown to have a significant influence on the risk of chronic disease and on the maintenance of optimal health status. A balanced diet is a key component of women's health. Foods such as iron-fortified cereals, and calcium-fortified cereals and juices, may be necessary to meet daily requirements. Although food should be the first choice in meeting such needs, nutritional supplementation may be necessary (Academy of Nutrition and Dietetics, 2014). Following are some examples of increased nutritional needs across the life span of women:

- An increase in calcium during pregnancy and menopause is necessary.
- Folic acid requirements increase during pregnancy to prevent neural tube defects.
- Iron needs increase during menstruation and pregnancy.

It is also important to remember that intake of certain nutrients above a certain level can be teratogenic (e.g., too much vitamin A in the first trimester of pregnancy), and because many foods are often enriched with vitamins and minerals, it is possible to consume too much.

CULTURAL APPLICATIONS

The influence of culture on both the use and acceptance of functional foods is an important consideration. Food is connected to one's identity, culture, and social context (Nordstrom, Coff, Jonsson, Nordenfelt, & Gorman, 2013). A functional food may be more accepted if it is seen as consistent with traditional consumption (Wansink, 2002). A study by Mullie et al. (2009) found a correlation between culture and the intake of functional foods. For example, soy is widely used in Asian cultures and is considered to be a traditional food source, with customary soy intake being estimated at 30 to 50 g per day (Cornwell, Cohick, & Raskin, 2004). Hence, the use of soy as a nutraceutical may be more widely and easily accepted by someone in an Asian culture because this food is already so widely used. In addition, how food itself is viewed within the context of culture may have a strong influence on the use of nutraceuticals and functional foods. The use of nutraceuticals in Eastern Europe is described in Sidebar 21.1.

SIDEBAR 21.1. NUTRACEUTICALS IN RUSSIA

Natalia Haire

Russia has a long history and great tradition of herbal medicine. Back in Ancient Rus (the ancient ancestors of Russians), there were healers and wise men who knew the secrets of herbs and their influence on the human body. They would harvest medicinal plants and create recipes to cure various health conditions. Many Russian traditions, beliefs, and stories passed through the generations and were represented in Russian fairy tales. There would always be a character who made herbal potions, and healers and sorceresses who would use their knowledge to heal or poison people using herbal medicine.

In Russia today, dietary supplements can be quite expensive, and often the general population is not able to afford supplements; therefore, people mostly resort to herbs and phytotherapy. Russia has a rich folk tradition of herbal healing. In fact, today, a majority of Russian people prefer to use such "grandmother" recipes to heal themselves, despite the availability of modern medicinal approaches. Doctors and medical professionals study herbs and their applications while in medical school. They use this knowledge and offer treatment using herbal preparations as adjuncts, or alternatives, to modern medicine when appropriate. Typically, medical providers do not prescribe herbal preparations to patients. They may suggest herb use only if scientific data are available to support its effectiveness. There are phytotherapists who specialize in herbal medicine. Nowadays, herbal centers are quite popular in Russia. Herbal centers provide education and services for healthy living, preventive treatment, and adjunct therapy to Western medicine.

(continued)

> Georgia is one of the Russian provinces known for human longevity. Many of its residents are active and healthy past 100 years of age. They say that the quality of their drinking water and consumption of traditional yogurt, red wine, and teas made of a high-altitude herb known as "golden root," contribute to healthy and long life.
>
> Today, herbs and supplements are used widely among Russian people. The older generations prefer grandmother recipes and natural supplements for self-healing, whereas younger generations strive for healthy living and choose natural products and supplements. Herbal centers, phytotherapists, nutritional supplements, and healthy food options are heavily advertised today in Russia.

FUTURE RESEARCH

Although nutraceuticals have a long-standing historical use, increased interest in these substances to promote health, prevent disease, and treat specific medical conditions is reflected in heightened attention to nutritional science and growing consumption. A consistent theme throughout this chapter has been the need for more research in this area. The book *Complementary and Alternative Medicine in the United States* (Institute of Medicine, 2005) summarizes succinctly what the goal for research in this arena should be: "In terms of medical therapies, a commitment to public welfare is the obligation to generate and provide to health care practitioners, policy makers, and the public access to the best information available on the efficacy of CAM therapies" (p. 169). Consistent with this sentiment, and because there is so much interest and hope in this area, interdisciplinary research teams may explore the following questions:

- Which of the current nutraceuticals should be incorporated in a normal diet on a regular basis to promote health?
- Are nutraceuticals cost-effective?
- What are the side effects associated with short- and long-term use of specific nutraceuticals?
- Can we increase research in the use of nutraceuticals in the pediatric population?
- What are innovative ways to educate healthcare providers about nutraceuticals?
- Can we discover more effective methods to educate the U.S. healthcare consumer about the benefits and risks of nutraceuticals?
- How does culture affect the use of functional foods?

ACKNOWLEDGMENT

The author wishes to acknowledge and thank Bridget Doyle for her contributions to this chapter in a previous edition.

WEBSITES

Reputable websites for information about foods and nutraceuticals include the following:

- Academy of Nutrition and Dietetics
  (www.eatright.org)
- American Nutraceutical Association
  (www.ana-jana.org)
- International Food Information Council Foundation
  (www.foodinsight.org)
- Mayo Clinic
  (www.mayoclinic.org)
- National Institutes of Health—National Center for Complementary and Integrative Health
  (https://nccih.nih.gov)
- National Institutes of Health—National Library of Medicine
  (www.nlm.nih.gov)
- National Institutes of Health—Office of Dietary Supplements
  (dietary-supplements.info.nih.gov)
- Natural Medicines Comprehensive Database
  (www.naturaldatabase.com)
- U.S. Department of Agriculture—Food and Nutrition Information Center
  (www.nal.usda.gov)
- U.S. Department of Health and Human Services—Office of Disease Prevention and Health Promotion
  (www.healthfinder.gov)
- U.S. Food and Drug Administration—Center for Food Safety and Applied Nutrition
  (www.fda.gov/aboutfda/centersoffices/officeoffoods/cfsan)

REFERENCES

Academy of Nutrition and Dietetics (2014). Healthy eating for women. Retrieved from http://www.eatright.org/resource/food/nutrition/dietary-guidelines-and-myplate/healthy-eating-for-women

American Academy of Pediatrics. (2001). *Periodic Survey #49: Complementary and alternative medicine (CAM) therapies in pediatric practices.* Retrieved May 25, 2005, from http://www.aap.org/research/periodicsurvey/ps49bex.htm

Anonymous. (2013). Probiotics revisited [review]. *The Medical Letter on Drugs & Therapeutics,* 55(1407), 3–4.

Bailey, R. L., Gahche, J. J., Thomas, P. R., & Dwyer, J. T. (2013). Why children use dietary supplements. *Pediatric Research, 74,* 737–741.

Banach, M., Serban, C., Sahebkar, A., Ursoniu, S., Rysz, J., Muntner, P., … Mikhailidis, D. P. (2015). Effects of coenzyme Q10 on statin-induced myopathy: a meta-analysis of randomized controlled trials. *Mayo Clinic Proceedings, 90,* 24–34. doi:10.1016/j.mayocp.2014.08.021

Caso, G., Kelly, P., McNurland, M. A., & Lawson, W. E. (2007). Effect of coenzyme q10 on myopathic symptoms in patients treated with asthma. *American Journal of Cardiology, 99*(10), 1409.

Cater, N. B., & Grundy, S. M. (1998). Lowering serum cholesterol with plant sterols and stanols: Historical perspectives. In T. T. Nguyen (Ed.), *New developments in the dietary management of high cholesterol* (Postgraduate Medicine Special Report, pp. 6–14). Minneapolis, MN: McGraw-Hill.

Cornwell, T., Cohick, W., & Raskin, I. (2004). Dietary phytoestrogens and health. *Phytochemistry, 65*, 995–1016.

Council for Responsible Nutrition. (2016). *The 2016 CRN Consumer Survey on Dietary Supplements.* Retrieved from https://www.crnusa.org/resources/crn-2016-annual-survey-dietary-supplements

de Jong, A., Plat, J., & Mensink, R. P. (2003). Metabolic effects of plant sterols and stanols [review]. *Journal of Nutritional Biochemistry, 14*(7), 362–369.

DeFelice, S. L. (1994). *What is a true nutraceutical and what is the nature & size of the U.S. nutraceutical market?* The Foundation for Innovation in Medicine. Retrieved from http://www.fimdefelice.org/p2462.html

Food and Drug Administration. (2012). *Dietary supplement.* Retrieved from http://www.fda.gov/food/dietarysupplements

Goldenberg, J. Z., Lytven, L., Steurich, J., Parkin, P., Mahunt, S., & Johnston, B. C. (2015). Probiotics for the prevention of pediatric antibiotic associated diarrhea. *Cochrane Database of Systematic Reviews, 12*, CD004827.

Gylling, H., Plat, J., Turley, S., Ginsberg, H. N., Ellegard, L., Jessup, W., … Riccardi, G. (2014). Plant sterols and plant stanols in the management of dyslipidaemia and prevention of cardiovascular disease. *Atherosclerosis, 232*(2), 346–360. doi:10.1016/jatherosclerosis.2013.11043

Haller, C. A. (2010). Nutraceuticals: Has there been any progress? *Clinical Pharmacology & Therapeutics, 87*(2), 137–141.

He, F. J., Nowson, C. A., Lucas, M., & MacGregor, G. A. (2007). Increased consumption of fruit and vegetables is related to a reduced risk of coronary heart disease: Meta-analysis of cohort studies. *Journal of Hypertension, 21*(9), 717–728.

He, F. J., Nowson, C. A., & MacGregor, G. A. (2006). Fruit and vegetable consumption and stroke: Meta-analysis of cohort studies. *Lancet 367*, 320–326.

Heczko, P. B., Tomusiak, A., Adamski, P., Jakimiuk, A. J., Stefanski, G., Mikolajczyk-Cichonska, A., … Strus, M. (2015). Supplementation of standard antibiotic therapy with oral probiotics for bacterial vaginosis and aerobic vaginitis: A randomized, double-blind, placebo-controlled trial. *BMC Women's Health, 15*, 115. doi:10.1186/s12905-015-0246-6

Hippocrates. (1932). *Hippocrates* (W. H. S. Jones, Trans.). Cambridge, MA: Harvard University Press.

Institute of Medicine. (2005). *Complementary and alternative medicine in the United States.* Washington, DC: National Academies Press.

Johnson, S., Maziade, P. J., McFarland, L. V., Trick, W., Donskey, C., Currie, B., … Goldstein, E. J. (2012). Is primary prevention of *Clostridium difficile* infection possible with specific probiotics? *International Journal of Infectious Diseases, 16*, e786–e792.

Jurden, L., Buchanan, M., Kelsberg, G., & Safranek, S. (2012). Can probiotics safely prevent recurrent vaginitis? *Journal of Family Practice, 61*, 357–358.

Kemper, K. J., Vohra, S., & Walls, R. (2008). The use of complementary and alternative medicine in pediatrics. *Pediatrics, 122*(6), 1374–1386.

Khatta, M., Alexander, B. S., Krichten, C. M., Fisher, M. L., Freudenberger, R., Robinson, S. W., & Gottlieb, S. S. (2000). The effect of coenzyme Q10 in patients with congestive heart failure. *Annals of Internal Medicine, 132*(8), 636–640.

Kligler, B., & Cohrssen, A. (2008). Probiotics. *Complementary & Alternative Medicine, 78*(9), 1073–1078.

Kottke, M. K. (1998). Scientific and regulatory aspects of nutraceutical products in the United States. *Drug Development and Industrial Pharmacy, 24*(12), 1177–1195.

Kwiterovich, P. (2008). Recognition and management of dyslipidemia in children and adolescents. *Journal of Clinical Endocrinology & Metabolism, 93*(11), 4200–4209.

Laitinen, K., Gylling, H., Kaipiainen, L., Nissinen, M. J., & Simonen, P. (2017). Cholesterol lowering efficacy of plant stanol ester in a new type of product matrix, a chewable dietary supplement. *Journal of Functional Foods, 30*, 119–124.

Lichtenstein, A. H., Appel, L. J., Brands, M., Carnethon, M., Daniels, S., Franch, H. A., ... Wylie-Rosett, J. (2006). AHA scientific statement diet and lifestyle recommendations revision 2006: A scientific statement from the American Heart Association Nutrition Committee. *Circulation*, *114*, 82–96. doi:10.1161/CIRCULATIONAHA.106.17615103

Littarru, G. P., & Tiano, L. (2010). Clinical aspects of coenzyme Q10: An update. *Nutrition*, *26*, 250–254.

Martirosyan, D. M., & Singh, J. (2015). A new definition of functional food by FFC: What makes a new definition unique? *Functional Foods in Health and Disease*, *5*(6), 209–223.

McAlindon, T. E., LaValley, M. P., Gulin, J. P., & Felson, D. T. (2000). Glucosamine and chondroitin for treatment of osteoarthritis: A systematic quality assessment and meta-analysis. *Journal of the American Medical Association*, *283*(11), 1483–1484.

MEDLINE. (2017). *Drugs, herbs and supplements*. Retrieved from http://www.nlm.nih.gov/medlineplus/druginformation.html

Mullie, P., Guelinckx, I., Clarys, P., Degrave, E., Hulens, M., & Vansant, G., (2009). Cultural, socioeconomic and nutritional determinants of functional food consumption patterns. *European Journal of Clinical Nutrition*, *63*, 1290–1296.

National Cancer Institute. (2013). *Coenzyme Q10: Questions and answers, cancer facts*. Retrieved from http://www.cancer.gov/cancertopics/pdq/cam/coenzymeQ10/patient/page2

National Center for Complementary and Integrative Health. (2016a). *Glucosamine and chondroitin*. Retrieved from http://nccih.nih.gov

National Center for Complementary and Integrative Health. (2016b). *Probiotics*. Retrieved from www.nccih.nih.gov

Natural Medicine. (2016). Glucosamine sulfate. Retrieved from https://naturalmedicinestherapeuticresearchcom.proxy1.athensams.net/databases/food,herbssupplements/professional.aspx?productid=807#effectiveness

Nordstrom, K., Coff, C., Jonsson, H., Nordenfelt, L., & Gorman, U. (2013). Food and health: individual, cultural or scientific matters? *Genes & Nutrition*, *8*(4), 357–363. doi:10.1007/s12263-013-0336-8

PA Consulting Group. (1990). *Functional foods: A new global added value market?* London, UK: Author.

Plat, J., Mackay, D., Baumgartner, S., Clifton, P. M., Gylling, H., & Jones, P. J. J. (2012). Progress and prospective of plant sterol and plant stanol research: Report of the Maastricht meeting. *Atherosclerosis*, *225*, 521–533.

Ras, R. T., Geleijnse, J. M., & Trautwein, E. A. (2014). LDL-cholesterol-lowering effect of plant sterols and stanols across different dose ranges: A meta-analysis of randomised controlled studies. *British Journal of Nutrition*, *112*, 214–219.

Rathner, Z. (2013). Fruit and vegetable intake is associated with lower risk of ER- breast cancer [First published online January 24, 2013]. *Journal of the National Cancer Institute*. doi:10.1093/jnci/djt009

Saha, S. P., & Whayne, T. F. (2016). Coenzyme Q-10 in human health: Supporting evidence? *Southern Medical Journal*, *109*(1), 17–21.

Shende, P., Desai, D., & Gaud, R. S. (2016). Nutraceuticals an imperative to wellness. *Research and Reviews: Journal of Pharmacy and Pharmaceutical Sciences*, *5*, 69–74.

Therapeutic Research Center. (2018a). *Herbs/supplements/glucosamine*. Retrieved from https://naturalmedicines.therapeuticresearch.com

Therapeutic Research Center. (2018b). *Probiotics*. Retrieved from https://naturalmedicines.therapeuticresearch.com

Towheed, T. E., & Hochberg, M. C. (1997). A systematic review of randomized controlled trials of pharmacological therapy in osteoarthritis of the hip. *Journal of Rheumatology*, *24*, 349–357.

Turpeinen, A. M., Ikonen, M., Kivimäki, A. S., Kautiainen, H., Vapaatalo, H., & Korpela, R. (2012). A spread containing bioactive milk peptides Ile–Pro–Pro and Val–Pro Pro, and plant sterols has antihypertensive and cholesterol-lowering effects. *Food and Function*, *3*, 621–627.

U.S. Pharmacopeial Convention. (2013). *USP verified dietary supplements*. Retrieved from http://www.usp.org/print/usp-verification-services/usp-verified-dietary-supplements/verification-process

Wandel, S., Juni, P., Tendal, B., Nuesch, E., Villiger, P. M., Welton, N. J., & Reichenbach, S. (2010). Effects of glucosamine, chondroitin, or placebo in patients with osteoarthritis of hip or knee: Network meta-analysis. *British Medical Journal, 341*, c4675. doi:10.1136/bmj.c4675

Wang, X., Ouyang, Y., Liu, J., Zhu, M., Zhao, G., Bao, W., & Hu, F. B. (2014). Fruit and vegetable consumption and mortality from all causes, cardiovascular disease, and cancer: Systematic review and dose-response meta-analysis of prospective cohort studies. *British Medical Journal, 349*, g4490. doi:10.1136/bmj.g4490

Wansink, B. (2002). Changing habits on the home front: Lost lessons from World War II research. *Journal of Public Policy Marketing, 21*, 90–99.

Wood, L. (2017). United States nutraceuticals market 2017: Prospects, trend analysis, market size and forecasts up to 2022 research and markets. *Research and Markets. Business Wire.* Retrieved from https://www.businesswire.com/news/home/20170306005891/en/United-States-Nutraceuticals-Market-2017-Prospects-Trend

World Cancer Research Fund International. (2017). *Our cancer prevention recommendation—Plant foods.* Retrieved from http://www.wcrf.org/int/research-we-fund/cancer-prevention-recommendations/plant-foods

Wrick, K. L. (2005). The impact of regulations in the business of nutraceuticals in the United States: Yesterday, today and tomorrow. In C. M. Hasler (Ed.), *Regulation of functional foods & nutraceuticals: A global perspective* (pp. 3–36). Hoboken, NJ: Wiley-Blackwell.

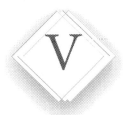

Energy Therapies

The National Center for Complementary and Integrative Health (NCCIH, 2016) does not specify a distinct category for energy therapies but places them within Mind and Body Practices. The diverse therapies included in Section V reveal nurses' interest in and use of energy therapies. The body of research on energy therapies continues to grow since the early work by Krieger (1979) and others begun in the 1970s. A number of these therapies have organizations that have developed training programs and certification programs for practitioners.

The concept of energy and its use is universal. Most cultures have a word to describe energy: *qi* (pronounced *chee*) is a basic element of traditional Chinese medicine (TCM); *ki* is the Japanese word for energy; in India it is *prana*; the Dakota word for energy is *ton*; and the Sioux word is *waken*. Scientists and consumers express some skepticism about the efficacy of energy therapies because of the difficulty in determining how energy works and how the effects can be measured. As technology evolves, new ways to detect what has previously seemed invisible are being discovered.

Two types of energy are sometimes distinguished: veritable (measurable) and putative (yet to be measured). Light therapy (Chapter 22) is a veritable type. Putative therapies include healing touch (Chapter 23) and Reiki (Chapter 24). Much of TCM is based on the flow of energy throughout the body on meridians. Acupressure (Chapter 25) and reflexology (Chapter 26) are based on the flow of energy through meridians identified in TCM.

Healing touch encompasses a group of therapies used by nurses around the world. These techniques may or may not involve actual physical touching of the body. The nurse (or other therapist) seeks to bring energy into the patient or to balance energy within the person. Reiki, an energy therapy originating in Japan, is becoming more widely used in the United States.

Light therapy has been used to prevent or treat seasonal affective disorder, which is more common in northern climates. Intuitively we know the importance of light as our spirits are lifted by sunshine, especially after many days of dreary weather.

Although difficulties are encountered in the measurement of outcomes from many of the energy therapies, intuitively many people recognize the existence of energy forces and their impact on health promotion and healing.

REFERENCES

Krieger, D. (1979). *The therapeutic touch: How to use your hands to help or to heal.* New York, NY: Simon & Schuster.

National Center for Complementary and Integrative Health. (2016). NCCIH facts-at-a-glance and mission. Retrieved from https://nccih.nih.gov/about/ataglance

22

Light Therapy

NILOUFAR NIAKOSARI HADIDI

This chapter provides a definition and overview of light therapy—its history, cultural applications, and scientific basis. It details the use of light therapy to treat seasonal affective disorders (SADs) and identifies other health conditions for which light therapy could be beneficial. Readers are introduced to techniques that could be used by nurses educated in its practice, along with precautions for its use. Recommendations for future research are likewise provided.

DEFINITION

Light therapy is defined as daily exposure to full-spectrum or bright light as a standard treatment for SAD as well as nonseasonal depression (Kuiper, McLean, Fritz, Lampe, & Malhi, 2013). This needs to be differentiated from phototherapy, which is used to treat conditions such as hyperbilirubinemia and psoriasis (Lam, 1998). This chapter focuses on the description and use of light therapy in the treatment of SAD.

SAD is a mood disorder that occurs more frequently in the dark winter months and disappears spontaneously in spring. However, it has been found to occur with less frequency in summer and can occur repeatedly year after year. According to the *Diagnostic and Statistical Manual of Mental Disorders*, fifth edition (*DSM-5*; American Psychiatric Association, 2013), criteria for diagnosing SAD include at least two years of (a) depression that begins and ends during a specific season each year, (b) no depression episode during the season that individual usually feels normal, and (c) a greater number of seasons with depression than seasons without depression (American Psychiatric Association, 2013). SAD has variations of winter and summer seasons (Haggarty et al., 2002; Kasof, 2009; Øyane, Ursin, Pallesen, Holsten, & Bjorvatn, 2008), although the prevalence rates of winter SAD appears to be much higher than those of summer SAD (Magnusson, 2000).

These seasonal episodes may take the form of major depressive or bipolar disorders. Many symptoms of SAD are similar to symptoms of nonseasonal depressive episodes: low mood (often without prominent diurnal variation), loss of interest, anhedonia, anergia, poor motivation, low libido, anxiety, irritability, and social withdrawal (Eagles, 2004). More than half of patients with SAD experience an increase in sleep duration with poor quality. Furthermore, approximately the same numbers of patients experience increases in appetite and weight gain and have cravings for carbohydrates and chocolate (Eagles, 2004). Symptoms often start in autumn and winter, peak from December to February, and then subside during spring and summer.

The prevalence rates of SAD have been estimated to be between 1% and 10% in the general population, with symptoms present for approximately 40% of the year; these patients experience significant morbidity and impairment in psychosocial function (Meesters & Gordijn, 2016). In the United States, the prevalence is 1% in Florida, whereas it is 9% in Alaska (Horowitz, 2008); it seems to be related to latitude. SAD is reported to occur four times as often in men than women, with age of onset between 18 and 30 years of age (Rosenthal, 2012). The exact causes of SAD are unknown; however, research has demonstrated that reduced sunlight may disrupt the circadian rhythm that is responsible for the body's internal clock (Edery, 2000). The disruption of this cycle may lead to depression.

History of Light Therapy

Since the beginning of time, people have realized the healing power of light. The history of light therapy goes back to ancient Egypt, where sunlight was used for medical treatments. Healing temples were built with colored crystals affixed on the surface of stone walls so that they were aligned with the sun's rays. People would lie down on benches and their bodies would be immersed in pure or colored lights (Curtis-King, 2008). Later, Hippocrates described the use of sunlight to cure various medical disorders. Although ancient Romans and Arab physicians had no scientific explanation for light therapy at the time, they knew that the healing power of light was helpful for medical treatments (Curtis-King, 2008).

In 1980, Dr. A. J. Lewy and colleagues at the National Institute of Mental Health (NIMH) conducted studies showing that high-intensity light affects melatonin release by the pineal gland in the brain (Lewy, Kern, Rosenthal, & Wehr, 1982). Since then, research has confirmed the impact of light therapy on seasonal depression. Researchers discovered that specialized bright light (20 times brighter than normal indoor light) was the most effective treatment for winter depression (Kripke, 1998a). Furthermore, research is confirming that this light is effective in improving the symptoms of nonseasonal depression as well (Kripke, 1998b). In fact, a systematic review of 62 reports on the efficacy of light therapy on nonseasonal depression found it to be effective and an excellent criterion to include in the treatment of nonseasonal depression (Even, Schroder, Friedman, & Rouillon, 2008). Light therapy has been reported to have a 70% positive response (Miller, 2005).

A more recent systematic review of eight studies of SAD and two studies of nonseasonal depression concluded that although there were methodological problems with the reviewed studies, bright light therapy is considered to be effective for the treatment of SAD (Mårtensson, Pettersson, Berglund, & Ekselius, 2015). Furthermore, a meta-analysis of 10 studies involving 458 patients indicated that bright light therapy of ≥5,000 lux for ≥30 minutes with antidepressants is more effective than antidepressants alone (Penders et al., 2016).

SCIENTIFIC BASIS

Research has demonstrated that individuals with SAD are positively affected by light (Mårtensson et al., 2015; Penders et al., 2016), sometimes as immediately as after even one light therapy session (Reeves et al., 2012). Light plays an important role in the secretion of melatonin, as well as serotonin.

Melatonin is a natural hormone produced by the pineal gland, a pea-sized structure located at the center of the brain. Melatonin synthesis is stimulated by darkness. When light enters the retina, it stimulates the hypothalamus and inhibits the pineal gland from converting serotonin to melatonin (Miller, 2005). It is important to note that the impact of melatonin on circadian rhythms is compromised by cardiovascular and neurodegenerative diseases, as well as aging (Altun & Ugur-Altun, 2007). Studies suggest that administering melatonin supplements at night may help individuals with disrupted circadian rhythms. In a recent meta-analysis of 19 studies involving 1,683 subjects, melatonin demonstrated significant efficacy independent of dose or duration (Ferracioli-Oda, Qawasmi, & Bloch, 2013).

INTERVENTION

The recommended device for provision of light therapy is a fluorescent light box that produces light intensities of greater than 2,500 lux (Westrin & Lam, 2007). Lux is a unit of illumination intensity that corrects for the photopic spectral sensitivity of the human eye. To better understand the concept of lux, indoor evening room light is usually less than 100 lux, whereas a brightly lit office is less than 500 lux. In contrast, outdoor light is much brighter: A cloudy, gray winter day is around 4,000 lux, and a sunny day can be 50,000 lux to 100,000 lux or more (Westrin & Lam, 2007). The most effective dose has been reported to be 10,000 lux for 30 minutes daily; lower intensities (i.e., 2,500 lux) can also be effective; however, they require longer durations of 2 to 3 hours (Terman & Terman, 2005). In a study of 83 women and 25 men who received either one week ($n = 42$) or two weeks ($n = 66$) of light therapy, there was no difference on depression outcome (Knapen, Van de Werken, Gordijn, & Meesters, 2014).

Technique

Broad-spectrum white light from fluorescent lamps in which ultraviolet (UV) and infrared (IR) light are used should be filtered because these wavelengths are potentially damaging to the eyes (Howland, 2009). Although some studies indicate that bright light therapy does not benefit nondepressed individuals without a history of SAD (Avery et al., 2001; Kasper et al., 1989), one study reported improved mood and vitality more than 1 month after using 1 hour of bright light exposure daily in healthy individuals. This effect was enhanced by the addition of physical exercise to light exposure (Partonen & Lönnqvist, 2000).

It is recommended that patients diagnosed with SAD start light therapy in the fall and continue until symptoms are resolved in the spring or summer (Kurlansik & Ibay, 2012). Light must enter the eyes for light therapy to be effective in the treatment of depressive conditions; however, the person should not be looking at the light directly. The result of several clinical trials has led to the recommended dose of 10,000 lux for 30 minutes soon after awakening in the morning (Terman & Terman, 2005).

The light enters the eye and is transmitted with nerve impulses to the pineal gland, which controls melatonin secretion. Patients often report relief of depressive symptoms in 3 to 4 days. The time of day is also an important consideration in light therapy. Often, light therapy is administered in the early morning on arising. Using a pooled clustering technique of 332 patients from 14 research centers across 5 years, Terman et al. (1989) concluded that early morning exposure was more effective in reducing depression than when administered at other times of the day. However, the exact timing of light therapy shown to be effective may differ between individuals based on individual timing of sleep and activity ranging from evening types to morning types (Meesters & Gordijn, 2016).

Whereas the exact mechanism of light therapy is unknown but believed to be through an ocular process, extraocular transcranial phototransduction in mammals results in changes in reproductive cycles and increased serotonin levels in the brain (Campbell, Murphy, & Suhner, 2001). Based on this information, Timonen et al. (2012) have hypothesized that light therapy may be effective if delivered in methods other than through eye mediation. They conducted a pilot study of 22 physically healthy patients with SAD in whom light therapy (6.0–8.5 lumens) was administered via earplugs in bilateral ear canals for 8 to 12 minutes per session 5 days a week for 4 weeks. This study was conducted during the darkest part of the year in Finland. A total of 77% of the subjects experienced full remission of SAD symptoms (Timonen et al., 2012). Some 92% achieved at least a 50% reduction in self-reported anxiety symptoms. The preliminary results of this pilot study challenge the existing model of the mechanism of action of light therapy, warranting further exploration.

It is often recommended that individuals with SAD exercise outdoors during daylight as much as possible (Eagles, 2004). Social contact should be continued, and it is helpful to sufferers of SAD if family and friends have some knowledge of this condition and what to expect.

Studies have demonstrated, however, that only 12% to 41% of patients with SAD continue to use light therapy, even after they have had successful use of the therapy in a previous winter (Rohan, Roecklein, Lacy, & Vacek, 2009; Schwartz, Brown, Wehr, & Rosenthal, 1996). Roecklein, Schumacher, Miller, and Ernecoff (2012) found that continued use of light therapy was more likely to occur if patients were confident that they would use the therapy even if it was inconvenient and if they had family and friends who were supportive of adherence to the therapy. This would suggest that if a provider enhances the behavioral change of therapy use through engaging family support and improving self-efficacy, patient adherence to light therapy may improve, increasing the likelihood of ongoing symptom relief.

Light Therapy or Antidepressant?

The more individuals have visible symptoms of SAD, characterized by hypersomnia or excessive daytime sleepiness, carbohydrate carving, and weight gain, the more they would benefit from light therapy rather than from antidepressants (Eagles, 2004). Furthermore, people often have a preference for natural light therapy over pharmacological antidepressants (Eagles, 2004).

The use of light therapy for non-SAD and bipolar disorder has been reported in the literature. In a study on the impact of light therapy as an adjuvant treatment to antidepressants, the investigators randomized 30 bipolar and depressed patients into either the treatment group receiving antidepressant and light therapy or the control group receiving antidepressant and placebo. The result indicated that there was a significant improvement (p <.05) in mood in the treatment group, with individuals receiving light therapy and antidepressant showing faster response (Benedetti et al., 2003). Similarly, in a randomized clinical trial of 122 patients receiving 8 weeks of light therapy (10,000 lux early morning for 30 minutes), antidepressant, combination, or sham-placebo (i.e., inactive negative ion generator that emits an audible quiet hum plus a placebo pill) showed that both light therapy alone and the combination of light therapy with antidepressant treatment was significantly better in regard to depression outcome than the sham-placebo group (Lam et al., 2016).

Measurement of Outcomes

Several clinical placebo-controlled studies have used light therapy to treat SAD. These studies confirm that light is not only as effective as other methods, but it also causes no long-term side effects. A meta-analysis of randomized controlled trials of bright light therapy for the treatment of SAD suggests that light therapy is effective, with effect sizes equivalent to those of antidepressant pharmacology trials for SAD (Golden et al., 2005). However, the authors indicated that most of the studies meeting their selection criteria for meta-analysis did not meet the recognized criteria for rigorous clinical trials.

Studies on use of light therapy as a preventive measure for SAD suggest that a brief course of light therapy at the onset of symptoms is sufficient to prevent relapse for the rest of the winter (Westrin & Lam, 2007)

Another meta-analysis of the literature (work published between January 1975 and July 2003) on phototherapy (either bright light or dawn simulation) suggested that bright light therapy is an effective treatment for SAD. Dawn simulation involves using a program that mimics natural springtime. The strategy is to set the time of sunrise signal earlier than outdoors in winter by using a relatively dim light, gradually increasing the light over 90 minutes from 0.001 to 300 lux while the patient sleeps with eyes dark-adapted (Terman & Terman, 2005). In their 6-year study comparing bright light, dawn simulation, and brief light pulse compared with a control group receiving high- and low-density negative air ionization while asleep, the investigators concluded that after 3 weeks of treatment, all three conditions were more effective than in the control group (Terman & Terman, 2006).

PRECAUTIONS AND SIDE EFFECTS

Bright-light therapy is generally considered safe. However, it may be associated with some side effects, including eye strain, headache, nausea, and agitation (Kanerva et al., 2012). These side effects usually subside spontaneously, so patients are not required to discontinue light therapy (Terman & Terman, 2005).

Adverse effects associated with light therapy are often attributed partially to factors such as parameters of light exposure, timing, dose (e.g., intensity, duration), and method of exposure (e.g., diffused, direct, focused). For example, if morning light is timed too early, patients experience premature awakening, with difficulty falling sleep again. If, on the other hand, evening light is scheduled too late, patients experience initial insomnia and hyperactivity (Terman & Terman, 2005). The major contradictions for the use of light therapy are existing eye disease, migraine headaches (if elicited by light), phototoxic medication use, and history of mania (Emens & Burgess, 2015). In rare cases, mania in bipolar patients has been observed after bright light therapy (Pail et al., 2011; Terman & Terman 2005). An ophthalmological examination is often recommended for these high-risk patients before starting light therapy.

It is possible to buy a light-therapy box over the counter without a physician's prescription; however, one must know that not all light-therapy boxes being sold have been tested for safety and effectiveness. That is why it is crucial to consult with one's healthcare provider before buying one.

It is important to keep in mind that light therapy should be considered adjunctive therapy for patients with any diagnosable depressive or mood disorders. Primary assessment and treatment for these types of disorders should always be done by psychiatric professionals to ensure appropriate comprehensive treatment.

USES

In addition to the use of light therapy for SAD, other uses of light therapy have been reported. These include, for example, the treatment of chronic depression, antepartum depression, premenstrual depression, and sleep–wake cycle issues (Pail et al., 2011). Other uses of light therapy are for subsyndromal SAD (similar to SAD, except that patients do not meet the criteria for major depressive disorder), antepartum and postpartum major depressive disorder, premenstrual dysphoric disorder, bulimia nervosa, and attention deficit disorder (Terman & Terman, 2005).

Light therapy for the treatment of sleep problems in older adults has been suggested by several studies. As humans age, sleep patterns change; most commonly, with advancing age, adults have difficulty falling and staying asleep, have early-morning awakenings, and have difficulty falling back to sleep (Montgomery & Dennis, 2002). Severe sleep disturbances may lead to depression and cognitive impairments (Ford & Kamerow, 1989). Lack of sleep can impair memory, disrupt metabolism, and hasten death (Davenport, 2002). In a study of 16 men and women between the ages of 62 and 81 who had sleep disturbance and who were exposed to bright light therapy, Campbell, Dawson, and Anderson (1993) found substantial positive changes in sleep quality as a result of light therapy use. Waking time within sleep was reduced by an hour, and sleep efficiency improved from 77.5% to 90% without altering time spent in bed. A recent systematic review of 53 studies of 1,154 subjects with Alzheimer's disease and dementia showed that light therapy was effective for the treatment of sleep problems in general (van Maanen, Meijer, van der Heijden, & Oort, 2016).

A Committee on Chronotherapeutics that had been formed by the International Society for Affective Disorders concluded that light therapy is effective for the treatment of patients with SADs, as well as those with major depressive disorders (Wirz-Justice et al., 2005). Thus, light therapy can be provided as an adjunctive therapy or as an alternative therapy for patients who are unwilling or unable to take antidepressants (Dallaspezia et al., 2012; Martiny et al., 2012; Wirz-Justice et al., 2005). Antepartum and perinatal depression is a common condition requiring judicious intervention to treat the mother while minimizing any potential risks to the unborn child or nursing infant. Light therapy can be a nonpharmacological approach for improving depressive symptoms in the pregnant or nursing mother with no known risk to the fetus or infant (Crowley & Youngstedt, 2012; Wirz-Justice et al., 2011).

Age-Related Implications

Light therapy may be an effective therapy for improving sleep patterns of individuals with dementia (Mishima et al., 2007; Skjerve, Bjorvatn, & Holsten, 2004). To determine whether high-intensity ambient light in public areas of long-term care facilities would improve sleep patterns and circadian rhythms of individuals with dementia, Sloane et al. (2007) conducted a study in geriatric units on 66 older adults with dementia. Results suggested that bright light had a modest but measurable salutary effect on sleep in this population. Furthermore, the investigators concluded that ambient light might be preferable to stationary devices such as light boxes for older people with dementia in long-term care settings.

Light therapy has been shown to be effective in additional older populations. Seniors living in long-term care facilities had improved cognitive function indicators as well as improvement in anxiety scores, when receiving light therapy (Royer et al., 2012). Furthermore, 89 patients older than the age of 60 with major depressive disorders demonstrated improved mood, increased sleep efficiency, and a steeper rise of evening melatonin when exposed to 3 weeks of bright light therapy (Lieverse et al., 2011). In a quasiexperimental study, 34 older adults living in a long-term care facility sat in front of a 10,000-lux light box 30 minutes in the morning, three times a week for 4 weeks, compared with 31 older adults receiving routine care. The results showed significant reductions in depression and sleep problems in the light therapy groups compared with the control group (Wu, Sung, Lee, & Smith, 2015).

It is important to note that, because of age-related changes of clouding of the lens and ocular media and cataract formation, exposure to blue and white light can cause discomfort in some cases (Reme, Rol, Grothmann, Kaase, & Terman, 1996).

CULTURAL APPLICATIONS

The ancient Chinese knew of the healing power of natural light. The Chinese principles of feng shui are based not only on the principle of the right placement of certain natural elements, but also on the use of light to bring a sense of balance and harmony to life with good "chi" or "life-giving energy" (Curtis-King, 2008).

Light has long been used in health and creating healing environments for aesthetic and practical reasons in countries around the world. Well-used light in the ambient environment can boost mood and well-being. The "built" environment can capitalize on natural light. The use of light in architecture in Iran is described in Sidebar 22.1.

SIDEBAR 22.1.   USE OF LIGHT AS AN ARCHITECTURAL ASSET IN IRAN

Mansour Hadidi

Light (fire) was one of the four sacred elements in ancient Persia; the other three were Water, Earth (soil), and Air (wind). Zoroastrians (followers of the Persian prophet Zoroaster) believed that fire must never be extinguished in the temple. Zoroaster is thought to have lived in eastern Persia (today's Iran) in 600 BCE. Zoroastrians (Persians) probably were the first to introduce the idea of binary powers (as opposed to the Greeks who believed in multiple gods and goddesses). Ahura Mazda was the god of light and goodness; Angra Mainyu was the god of darkness and "evil spirit," who at the end, was believed to be defeated by goodness. The words ahura and mazda mean "light" and "wisdom," respectively.

Iran is a light-rich country, located between the 25° north at its southernmost and 39° north at its northernmost latitude. There is a broad range of temperatures, climate and elevations, and water and desert areas, with some regions seeing no rain for half the year. Due to its global position, sunlight is a beautiful asset of the country. The elevation in mountainous regions also contributes to the intensity and effects of sunlight. The climate is temperate, and there is plentiful sunshine on most days, especially in the arid desert areas.

Architects in Iran, even from early times, have understood the importance of light in the design and construction of buildings. Natural light, plentiful in Iran, plays an important role in the illumination of buildings. The beauty of natural light can be observed in homes, workspaces, hotels, hospitals, schools, mosques, and other buildings. Exposure to light can be uplifting and energizing. It can improve mood and vitality with potential effects on human productivity. Early morning exposure has wakening effects and can be more effective.

Stained glass was used to soften the light where the heat from light was excessive. Architects used a balance between light and heat. Another approach was using indirect light. For example, in areas close to the desert, small patios were designed to bring in light while preventing direct sunshine and heat as a result. An important consideration is the direction of windows in buildings. Although southern exposures are the most popular for daytime living areas (such as the living and family rooms) because they receive the highest amount of natural light during the day, northern windows are best for bedrooms and spaces that are used at night.

With the advent of electricity, air-conditioning, and heating appliances, architects had more freedom to design buildings with other factors in mind. For example, although architects were aware that light could add to the beauty and illumination of a building, the view of the vista's surroundings became a higher priority. In old structures, reticular stone panels were often used to prevent excessive heat from sunshine. However, in modern buildings, large glass windows mostly cover the façade.

FUTURE RESEARCH

Future research should focus on mechanisms of action and response mediators of light therapy and light therapy as a preventive strategy for SAD, as well as for other conditions such as non-SAD, bipolar disorder, premenopausal syndrome, and premenstrual depression. It is also important to determine the outcomes of light therapy compared to more traditional treatments such as medications for major depressive disorders in large randomized clinical trials.

Successful preliminary studies have focused on the impact of melatonin in the treatment of severe postoperative delirium unresponsive to antipsychotics or benzodiazepines (Hanania & Kitain, 2002). It would be interesting to investigate whether light therapy would have a similar impact on reducing the incidence or severity of postoperative delirium.

REFERENCES

Altun, A., & Ugur-Altun, B. (2007). Melatonin: Therapeutic and clinical utilization. *International Journal of Clinical Practice*, *61*(5), 835–845.

American Psychiatric Association. (2013). *Diagnostic and statistical manual of mental disorders* (5th ed.). Arlington, VA: American Psychiatric Publishing.

Avery, D. H., Eder, D. N., Bolte, M. A., Hellekson, C. J., Dunner, D. L., Vitiello, M. V., & Prinz, P. N. (2001). Dawn simulation and bright light in the treatment of SAD: A controlled study. *Biological Psychiatry*, *50*(3), 205–216.

Benedetti, F., Colombo, C., Pontiggia, A., Bernasconi, A., Florita, M., & Smeraldi, E. (2003). Morning light treatment hastens the antidepressant effect of citalopram: A placebo-controlled trial. *Journal of Clinical Psychiatry*, *64*(6), 648–653.

Campbell, S. S., Dawson, D., & Anderson, M. W. (1993). Alleviation of sleep maintenance insomnia with timed exposure to bright light. *Journal of American Geriatrics Society*, *41*(8), 829–836.

Campbell, S. S., Murphy, P. J., & Suhner, A. G. (2001). Extraocular phototransduction and circadian timing systems in vertebrates. *Chronobiology International*, *18*, 137–172.

Crowley, S. K., & Youngstedt, S. D. (2012). Efficacy of light therapy for perinatal depression: A review. *Journal of Physiological Anthropology*, *31*, 15. doi:10.1186/1880-6805-31-15

Curtis-King, L. (2008). The healing power of incoherent polarized light. *Light and Colour*, *144*, 24–26.

Dallaspezia, S., Benedetti, F., Colombo, C., Barbini, B., Fulgosi, M. C., Garinelli, C., & Smeraldi, E. (2012). Optimized light therapy for non-seasonal major depressive disorder. *Journal of Affective Disorders*, *138*(3), 337–342.

Davenport, R. J. (2002). Up all night. *Science of Aging Knowledge Environment*, *30*, 104. Retrieved from http://sageke.sciencemag.org/cgi/content/abstract/sageke;2002/30/nw104

Eagles, J. M. (2004). Light therapy and the management of winter depression. *Advances in Psychiatric Treatment*, *10*, 233–240.

Edery, I. (2000). Circadian rhythms in a nutshell. *Physiological Genomics*, *3*, 59–74.

Emens, J. S., & Burgess, H. J. (2015). Effect of light and melatonin and other melatonin receptor agonists on human circadian physiology. *Sleep Medicine Clinic*, *10*(4), 435–453.

Even, C., Schroder, C. M., Friedman, S., & Rouillon, F. (2008). Efficacy of light therapy in non-seasonal depression: A systematic review. *Journal of Affective Disorders*, *108*(1), 11–24.

Ferracioli-Oda, E., Qawasmi, A., & Bloch, M. H. (2013). Meta-analysis: Melatonin for the treatment of primary sleep disorders. *PLOS ONE*, *8*(5), e63773.

Ford, D. E., & Kamerow, D. B. (1989). Epidemiologic study of sleep disturbances and psychiatric disorders. *Journal of the American Medical Association*, *262*, 1479–1484.

Golden, R. N., Gaynes, B. N., Ekstrom, R. D., Hamer, R. M., Jacobsen, F. M., Suppes, T., ... Nemeroff, C. B. (2005). The efficacy of light therapy in the treatment of mood disorders: A review and meta-analysis of the evidence. *American Journal of Psychiatry, 162*(4), 656–662.

Haggarty, J. M., Cernovsky, Z., Husni, M., Minor, K., Kermeen, P., & Merskey, H. (2002). Seasonal affective disorder in an Arctic community. *Acta Psychiatrica Scandinavica, 105*(5), 378–384.

Hanania, M., & Kitain, E. (2002). Melatonin for treatment and prevention of postoperative delirium. *Anesthesia and Analgesia, 94,* 338–339.

Horowitz, S. (2008). Shedding light on seasonal affective disorder. *Alternative and Complementary Therapies, 14*(6), 282–287. doi:10.1089/act.2008.14608

Howland, R. H. (2009). An overview of seasonal affective disorder and its treatment options. *Physician and Sportsmedicine, 37*(4), 104.

Kanerva, N., Kronholm, E., Partonen, T., Ovaskainen, M. L., Kaartinen, N. E., Konttinen, H., ... Männistö, S. (2012). Tendency toward eveningness is associated with unhealthy dietary habits. *Chronobiology International, 29,* 920–927.

Kasof, J. (2009). Cultural variation in seasonal depression: Cross-national differences in winter versus summer patterns of seasonal affective disorder. *Journal of Affective Disorders, 115*(1), 79–86.

Kasper, S., Rogers, S. L., Yancey, A., Schulz, P. M., Skwerer, R. G., & Rosenthal, N. E. (1989). Phototherapy in individuals with and without subsyndromal seasonal affective disorder. *Archives of General Psychiatry, 46*(9), 837.

Knapen, S. E., Van de Werken, M., Gordijn, M. C. M., & Meesters, Y. (2014). The duration of light treatment and therapy outcome in seasonal affective disorder. *Journal of Affective Disorders, 166,* 343–346.

Kripke, D. F. (1998a). Light therapy and depression. *Journal of Affective Disorders, 62*(3), 221–223.

Kripke, D. F. (1998b). Light treatment for non-seasonal major depression: Are we ready? In R. W. Lam (Ed.), *Seasonal affective disorder and beyond* (pp. 159–172). Washington, DC: American Psychiatric Publishing.

Kuiper, S., McLean, L., Fritz, K., Lampe, L., & Malhi, G. S. (2013). Getting depression clinical practice guidelines right: Time for change? *Acta Psychiatrica Scandinavica, 128*(444), 24–30.

Kurlansik, S. L., & Ibay, A. D. (2012). Seasonal affective disorder. *American Family Physician, 86*(11), 1037–1041.

Lam, R. W. (Ed.). (1998). *Seasonal affective disorder and beyond: Light treatment for SAD and non-SAD conditions.* Washington, DC: American Psychiatric Publishing.

Lam, R. W., Levitt, A. J., Levitan, R. D., Michalak, E. E., Cheung, A. H., Morehouse, R., ... Tam, E. M. (2016). Efficacy of bright light treatment, fluoxetine, and the combination in patients with nonseasonal major depressive disorder: A randomized clinical trial. *JAMA Psychiatry, 73*(1), 56–63.

Lewy, A. J., Kern, H. A., Rosenthal, N. E., & Wehr, T. A. (1982). Bright artificial light treatment of a manic-depressive patient with a seasonal mood cycle. *American Journal of Psychiatry, 139,* 1496–1498.

Lieverse, R., Van Someren, E. J. W., Nielen, M. M. A., Uitdehaag, B. M. J., Smit, J. H., & Hoogendijk, W. J. G. (2011). Bright light treatment in elderly patients with nonseasonal major depressive disorders: A randomized, placebo-controlled trial. *Archives of General Psychiatry, 68*(1), 61–70.

Magnusson, A. (2000). An overview of epidemiological studies on seasonal affective disorder. *Acta Psychiatrica Scandinavica, 101*(3), 176–184.

Mårtensson, B., Pettersson, A., Berglund, L., & Ekselius, L. (2015). Bright white light therapy in depression: A critical review of the evidence. *Journal of Affective Disorders, 182,* 1–7.

Martiny, K., Refsgaard, E., Lund, V., Lunde, M., Sorensen, L., Thougaard, B., ... Bech, P. (2012). A 9-week randomized trial comparing a chronotherapeutic intervention (wake and light therapy) to exercise in major depressive disorder patients treated with duloxetine. *Journal of Clinical Psychiatry, 73*(9), 1234–1242.

Meesters, Y., & Gordijn, M. C. (2016). Seasonal affective disorder, winter type: Current insights and treatment options. *Psychology Research and Behavior Management, 9,* 317.

Miller, A. L. (2005). Epidemiology, etiology, and natural treatment of seasonal affective disorder. *Alternative Medicine Review: A Journal of Clinical Therapeutics, 10*(1), 5–13.

Mishima, K., Okawa, M., Hishikawa, Y., Hozumi, S., Hori, H., & Takahashi, K. (2007). Morning bright light therapy for sleep and behavior disorders in elderly patients with dementia. *Acta Psychiatrica Scandinavica, 89*(1), 1–7.

Montgomery, P., & Dennis, J. A. (2002). Bright light therapy for sleep problems in adults aged 60+. *Cochrane Database of Systematic Reviews, 2002*(2), CD003403. doi:10.1002/14651858. CD003403

Øyane, N. M., Ursin, R., Pallesen, S., Holsten, F., & Bjorvatn, B. (2008). Self-reported seasonality is associated with complaints of sleep problems and deficient sleep duration: The Hordaland Health Study. *Journal of Sleep Research, 17*(1), 63–72.

Pail, G., Huf, W., Pjrek, E., Winker, D., Willeit, M., Praschak-Rieder, N., & Kasper, S. (2011). Bright light therapy in the treatment of mood disorders. *Neuropsychobiology, 64*(3), 152–162.

Partonen, T., & Lönnqvist, J. (2000). Bright light improves vitality and alleviates distress in healthy people. *Journal of Affective Disorders, 57*, 55–61.

Penders, T. M., Stanciu, C. N., Schoemann, A. M., Ninan, P. T., Bloch, R., & Saeed, S. A. (2016). Bright light therapy as augmentation of pharmacotherapy for treatment of depression: A systematic review and meta-analysis. *Primary Care Companion for CNS Disorders, 18*(5). doi:10.4088/PCC.15r01906

Reeves, G. M., Nijjar, G. V., Langenberg, P., Johnson, M. A., Khabazghazvini, B., Sleemi, A., ... Postolache, T. T. (2012). Improvement in depression scores after 1 hour of light therapy treatment in patients with seasonal affective disorder. *Journal of Nervous and Mental Disease, 200*(1), 51–55.

Reme, C. E., Rol, P., Grothmann, K., Kaase, H., & Terman, M. (1996). Bright light therapy in focus: Lamp emission spectra and ocular safety. *International Journal of Technology Assessment in Health Care, 4*, 403–413.

Roecklein, K. A., Schumacher, J. A., Miller, M. A., & Ernecoff, N. C. (2012). Cognitive and behavioral predictors of light therapy use. *PLOS ONE, 7*(6), e39275.

Rohan, K. J., Roecklein, K. A., Lacy, T. J., & Vacek, P. M. (2009). Winter depression recurrence one year after cognitive–behavioral therapy, light therapy, or combination treatment. *Behavioral Therapy, 40*, 225–238.

Rosenthal, N. (2012). What is seasonal affective disorder? Answers from the doctor who first described the condition. Retrieved from http://www.normanrosenthal.com/ seasonal-affective-disorder

Royer, M., Ballentine, N. H., Eslinger, P. J., Houser, K., Mistrick, R., Behr, R., & Rakos, K. (2012). Light therapy for seniors in long term care. *Journal of American Medical Directors Association, 13*(2), 100–102.

Schwartz, P. J., Brown, C., Wehr, T. A., & Rosenthal, N. E. (1996). Winter seasonal affective disorder: A follow up study of the first 59 patients of the National Institute of Mental Health seasonal studies program. *American Journal of Psychiatry, 153*, 1028–1036.

Skjerve, A., Bjorvatn, B., & Holsten, F. (2004). Light therapy for behavioural and psychological symptoms of dementia. *International Journal of Geriatric Psychiatry, 19*(6), 516–522.

Sloane, P. D., Williams, C. S., Mitchell, C. M., Preisser, J. S., Wood, W., Barrick, A. L., ... Zimmerman, S. (2007). High-intensity environmental light in dementia: Effect on sleep and activity. *Journal of the American Geriatrics Society, 55*(10), 1524–1533.

Terman, M., & Terman, J. (2006). Controlled trial of naturalistic dawn simulation and negative air ionization for seasonal affective disorder. *American Journal of Psychiatry, 163*(12), 2126–2133.

Terman, M., & Terman, J. S. (2005). Light therapy for seasonal and nonseasonal depression: Efficacy, protocol, safety and side effects. *CNS Spectrums, 10*(8), 647.

Terman, M., Terman, J. S., Quitkin, F. M., McGrath, P. J., Stewart, J. W., & Rafferty, B. (1989). Light therapy for seasonal affective disorder. A review of efficacy. *Neuropsychopharmacology, 2*(1), 1–22.

Timonen, M., Nissila, J., Liettu, A., Jokelainen, J., Jurvelin, H., Aunio, A., ... Takala, T. (2012). Can transcranial brain-targeted bright light treatment via ear canals be effective in relieving symptoms in seasonal affective disorder? A pilot study. *Medical Hypotheses, 78*(4), 511–515.

van Maanen, A., Meijer, A. M., van der Heijden, K. B., & Oort, F. J. (2016). The effects of light therapy on sleep problems: A systematic review and meta-analysis. *Sleep Medicine Reviews, 29*, 52–62.

Westrin, A., & Lam, R. W. (2007). Seasonal affective disorder: A clinical update. *Annals of Clinical Psychiatry, 19*(4), 239–246.

Wirz-Justice, A., Bader, A., Frison, U., Stieglitz, R. D., Alder, J., Bitzer, J., … Riecher-Rossler, A. (2011). A randomized, double-blind, placebo-controlled study of light therapy for antepartum depression. *Journal of Clinical Psychiatry, 72*(7), 986–993.

Wirz-Justice, A., Benedetti, F., Berger, M., Lam, R. W., Martiny, K., Terman, M., & Wu, J. C. (2005). Chronotherapeutics (light and wake therapy) in affective disorders. *Psychological Medicine, 35*(7), 939–944.

Wu, M. C., Sung, H. C., Lee, W. L., & Smith, G. D. (2015). The effects of light therapy on depression and sleep disruption in older adults in a long-term care facility. *International Journal of Nursing Practice, 21*(5), 653–659.

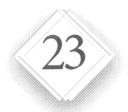

Healing Touch

Alexa W. Umbreit and Lauren Johnson

All cultures, both ancient and modern, have developed some form of touch therapy as part of people's desire to heal and care for one another. The oldest written evidence of the use of touch to enhance healing comes from Asia more than 5,000 years ago (Jackson & Latini, 2016; Krieger, 1979). This therapeutic use of the hands has been passed on from generation to generation as a tool for healing. However, philosophical and cultural differences have influenced the way touch has been used throughout the world. The Eastern viewpoint has based its touch-healing practices on energy channels (meridians), energy fields (auras), and energy centers (chakras). Expert practitioners in energetic touch therapies use their hands to influence this flow of energy to promote balance and healing. The Western viewpoint focuses on physiological changes that occur at the cellular level from touch therapies that are believed to influence healing. A blending of both Eastern and Western techniques has led to an explosion of a wide variety of touch therapies (Jackson & Latini, 2016). Nursing has used touch throughout its history and today's nurses are integrating many touch techniques into their practice. One of these therapies is Healing Touch (HT), "a nurturing, holistic, and integrative biofield therapy that facilitates health and healing and is taught in universities, medical and nursing schools, and other settings internationally" (Healing Beyond Borders, 2017a).

DEFINITION

HT is a type of therapy that works in harmony with and is complementary to standard medical care. HT uses gentle touch to balance physical, mental, and emotional well-being, as well as energy-based techniques to influence and support the human biofield, within the body (energy centers) and surrounding the body (energy fields), supporting the body's natural ability to heal (Healing Beyond Borders, 2017b; Healing Touch Program, 2017a). HT is classified as an integrative health mind and body therapy by the National Institutes of Health, National Center for Complementary and Integrative Health (NCCIH, 2016). Based on a holistic view of health and illness, HT focuses on creating an energetic balance of the whole body at the physical, emotional, mental, and spiritual levels rather than on dysfunctional parts of the body. Through this process of balancing the energy system and therefore opening energy blockages, an environment is created that is conducive to self-healing. Through the interaction of the energy fields between practitioner and client, the use of the HT practitioner's hands, an intention focusing on the client's highest good, and a centering process, noninvasive HT techniques specific for the client's needs are used to create this energetic balance (Umbreit, 2000). Krieger (1979) describes the centering process as a meditation in which one eliminates all distractions and concentrates on that place of quietude within which one can feel truly integrated, unified, and focused. Finding this "place of quietude within" is achieved by many through deep belly breathing, prayer, meditation, or any other technique that slows one down, calms the mind, and accesses a deeper spirit of compassion and strength. To be centered is to be fully present with another person or situation and engaged with heart and mind, deeper feelings, and thoughts. The centered state of mind is maintained throughout the HT treatment.

Umbreit (2000) describes the role of the HT practitioner as observation, assessment, and repatterning of the client's energy field, which is disrupted when there is disease, illness, psychological stressors, and pain. Practitioners describe these disruptions in the energy field as blockages, leaks, imbalances, or congestion. The goal of the HT practitioner is to open these blockages, seal the leaks, rebalance the energy field to symmetry, and release congestion.

HT evolved from the pioneering work of the therapeutic touch (TT) community that was started in 1970 by a nurse, Dr. Dolores Krieger, and Dora Kunz, a natural intuitive healer, who assisted many physicians with perplexing patient cases. Together they established TT, described as a "contemporary interpretation of several ancient healing practices ... [consisting of learning] skills for consciously directing or sensitively modulating human energies" (Krieger, 1993, p. 11). The practice is based on the assumption that humans are complex energy fields that are imbalanced with disease; the practitioner uses her hands as "sensors" to smooth, repattern, or boost areas that need attention to restore balance or the integrity of body, mind, and spirit (Therapeutic Touch, 2017). In healthcare, TT philosophy, practice, and research have become the bases for many newer energetic modalities, including HT.

The HT curriculum, started in 1989 and endorsed by the American Holistic Nurses Association (AHNA), involves a formal educational program that teaches techniques, including interventions described by Joy (1979) and Bailey (1984), concepts presented by Bruyere (1989) and Brennan (1986), and original techniques developed by the founder of HT, Janet Mentgen, and other healers (Healing Beyond Borders, 2017c). The six-level HT educational curriculum in energy-based practice moves from beginning to advanced practice, certification, and instructor level. Advanced practice requires at least 100 hours of workshop instruction plus a 1-year rigorous and comprehensive course of study involving an extensive reading program and education on a wide variety of complementary therapies. In addition, there is work on case studies, mentoring, ethics, client–practitioner relationships, development of higher sense perception, establishment of a practice, and integration of activities within the health community. Emphasis is based on self-care and development of the student (Healing Beyond Borders, 2017d; Wardell, Kagel, & Anselme, 2014a). After this, students may apply for certification. Instructor status requires more education and mentoring. The HT coursework is open to registered nurses, body-oriented therapists, psychotherapists, licensed healthcare professionals, and individuals who desire an in-depth understanding and practice of healing work using touch and energy-based concepts (Anselme, Kagel, & O'Neill, 2014; Healing Beyond Borders, 2017e; Healing Touch Program, 2017b).

SCIENTIFIC BASIS

The nursing profession has long been described as dedicated to the art and science of human caring. Rogers (1990), Watson (1985), and Thornton (2013) have written extensively about caring as a central quality of the nursing profession, along with nursing's concern for the promotion of health and well-being, taking into account the individual's constant interaction with the environment. It was this concern that led nurse-theorist Rogers to develop her concepts of the nature of individuals and the environment as energy fields in constant interplay, which affects the health of human beings (Eschiti, 2014). Rogers's theoretical framework postulates that all living things are composed of energy, and there is a continual exchange of energy among them as they strive toward the goal of balance and universal order. Using the hands, intention, and centering, the HT practitioner assesses the client's energy field and helps direct it to a more open, symmetrical pattern that enhances the client's ability to self-heal. The nursing diagnosis used for HT and other biofield therapies is defined as an "Imbalanced Energy Field [state in which a] disruption of the flow of energy surrounding a person's being results in a disharmony of the body, mind, and/ or spirit" (American Holistic Nurses Association, 2017; Carpenito, 2013, p. 252).

The concept of energy systems as part of the human interactive environment and healing has been part of many cultures for centuries. It is believed by traditional societies that a life force is involved in the interchange between humans and their surroundings. This life force is called by many names in different cultures: Chinese, *qi*; Japanese, *ki*; Greek, *pneuma*; Tibetan, *lung*; Native American, *oki, orenda, ton*; Hindu, *prana*; and Western, *biofield* (Shields & Wilson, 2016), to name a few. The common principle is that an imbalance in this energy force can result in illness.

Although we are able to measure or evaluate some of the effects of energy-based healing interactions on illness and symptoms, it is still not clear how biofield/energy field modalities, including HT, influence the energy patterns of a recipient or how recipients use the energy to enhance their self-healing processes. Schwartz (2007) states that present-day physicists continue to further analyze Einstein's premise that everything is energy and organized in energy fields. Experts in the fields of physics, engineering, biology, and physiology continue to conduct research in this area of energy exchange in an attempt to explain what occurs during an energetic interaction (Feinstein & Eden, 2008; Forbes, Rust, & Becker, 2004; Oschman, 2016b). Current studies of photon emission could provide evidence that enhances the assessment of health and the impact of different types of interventions. These studies help explain how photonic energy exchanges occur between practitioners' hands and diseased body tissues (Ives et al., 2014; Oschman, 2016a). The growing study of psychoneuroimmunology suggests a more integrative body system and the existence of extensive two-way communication between the brain and body (Anderson, 2016). Increased understanding and study of these communication pathways may help better explain the relaxation response and the physiological effects of mind–body therapies, including HT. Scientists are learning more about the relaxation response and seeking to explain the clinical benefits of mind–body practices such as yoga and meditation (Bhasin et al., 2013). With our expanding knowledge of the role of inflammation in acute and chronic health conditions, researchers are investigating cellular mechanisms associated with inflammation and the physiological effect of biofield therapies such as massage and HT (Kiang, Ives, & Jonas, 2005).

Oschman (2008) reports that various energy therapies stimulate tissue healing by the production of pulsating electromagnetic fields that induce currents to flow within the body's tissue. It is proposed that these currents are generated via the heartbeat and move throughout the circulatory system and the "living matrix," which Oschman (2008) describes as an informational nervous system of the body where electron movement occurs, producing these waves. He states that the heart generates the body's largest electromagnetic field, which can be measured in the space around the body using the superconducting quantum interference device (SQUID). The SQUID has been used to measure the biomagnetic fields emanating from the hands of energy field practitioners who use TT, qigong, yoga, and meditation. It has been found that low electromagnetic frequencies (a coherent pattern) can be emitted from a trained energy healer's hands at a rate needed for tissue healing, which has the possibility to convert a stalled healing process to active repair by restoring coherence to the tissue (Oschman, 2008).

Other instruments have been invented to directly measure the human energy field (e.g., Kirlian photography, gaseous discharge visualization, and polycontrast interference), but these instruments are not consistently accurate (Duerden, 2004). Eschiti (2007) states, "until science is able to provide accurate, direct measurement of the human energy field, research will need to be conducted by measuring possible effects on the field in an indirect manner" (p. 10).

It is unknown precisely how symptoms are managed by HT interventions. What have been observed are changes in outcomes being measured in nursing research. It may be postulated that because biofields are in constant interaction within and outside the physical body, internal mechanisms are stimulated by this movement of energy (Umbreit, 2000). However, any explanations given for energy healing remain theoretical because of limited experimental data and difficulty using traditional scientific analysis because paradoxical findings often coexist (Engebretson & Wardell, 2002). There continues to be much to learn and understand about the human biofield, the effects of energy therapies on the biofield, and ways and reasons that these effects occur.

Systematic reviews of studies and randomized controlled trials (RCTs) and a synthesis of best evidence focusing on biofield therapies, including HT, describe studies of medium quality overall. The reviews suggest moderate to strong evidence that HT reduces pain per self-report for those with pain (Anderson & Taylor, 2011; Hammerschlag, Marx, & Aickin, 2014; Jain & Mills, 2010; Umbreit, 2000). Studies specific to HT interventions have focused on managing the symptoms of pain, anxiety, nausea, and stress; decreasing the side effects of cancer treatments; promoting faster postprocedural recovery; reducing the length of hospital stay and readmissions; improving mood or health-related quality of life; examining effects on complications; improving mental health, including posttraumatic stress disorder (PTSD); using HT with the older adult to manage pain and improve appetite, sleep, behavior patterns, and functional abilities; increasing relaxation; supporting immune function; and promoting a sense of well-being (Bulbrook, 2000; Cook, Guerrerio, & Slater, 2004; Dowd, Kolcaba, Steiner, & Fashinpaur, 2007; FitzHenry et al., 2014; Geddes, 2002; Hardwick, 2012; Jain, McMahon, et al., 2012; Jain, Pavlik, et al.,

2012; Krucoff et al., 2001, 2005; Lu, Hart, Lutgendorf, Oh, & Silverman, 2016; Lu, Hart, Lutgendorf, Oh, & Schilling, 2013; Lu, Hart, Lutgendorf, & Perkhounkova, 2013; Lutgendorf et al., 2014; MacIntyre et al., 2008; Maville, Bowen, & Benham, 2008; Megel, Anderson, Lu, & Strybol, 2012; Post-White et al., 2003; Scandrett-Hibdon, Hardy, & Mentgen, 1999; Seskevich, Crater, Lane, & Krucoff, 2004; Silva, 1996; Wang & Hermann, 2006; Wardell, 2000; Wardell, Rintala, & Tan, 2008; Wardell & Weymouth, 2004; Wilkinson et al., 2002).

In pediatrics, several small research studies have been completed (Cone, Gottschlich, Khoury, Simakajornboon, & Kagan, 2014; Kemper, Fletcher, Hamilton, & McLean, 2012; McDonough-Means, Edde, & Bell, 2009; Speel, 2012; Verret, 2000; Wong, Ghiasuddin, Kimata, & Patelesio, 2012; Zimmer, Bogenschutz, Meier, & Rolf, 2009) that examine various outcomes.

A proposed model of how HT may promote positive changes in client symptoms follows. A trained HT practitioner uses the hands to assess, sense or evaluate the client's biofield. The practitioner then sends coherent energy waves from provider hands to the client that in turn affects the incoherent energy patterns that cause disease or imbalance in the client's energy field and body. Due to a resonant effect, the incoherent energy pattern shifts to a healthier, coherent pattern affecting the client's circulatory, endocrine, and nervous systems, and/or other unidentified mechanisms, promoting positive client responses with the potential to restore optimal health. The HT practitioner moves and repatterns a client's energy field, promoting a more open and symmetric pattern to enhance the client's perceived sense of well-being. This movement of energy may stimulate physiological, neurochemical, and psychological changes that promote positive effects on pain, anxiety, wound healing, immune system function, depression, and sense of well-being.

INTERVENTION

Techniques

Nearly 30 techniques are taught in the HT curriculum, from the simple to the complex. The HT practitioner determines which to use after an assessment of the client's expressed needs, symptoms, and results of an energy field hand scan. These strategies range from localized to full-body techniques. Table 23.1 lists several basic techniques, along with indications and brief descriptions of the procedures. These techniques, which treat a wide range of client symptoms, should be practiced in a supervised setting with an instructor before working with a client. Most of the HT techniques involve two basic types of hand gestures (called *magnetic passes*) that are described in terms of "hands in motion" (used to clear congestion or density from the energy field) or "hands still" (used to reestablish energy flow and balance; Anselme et al., 2014). In the hands-in-motion gestures, the hands make gentle brushing or combing motions, usually downward and outward, to remove congested energy from the field. The hands remain relaxed, palms facing downward toward the patient, between 1 and 6 inches above the skin or clothing. The hand strokes may be slow and sweeping or short and rapid. In the hands-still position, the practitioner holds hands over an area of the client's body for 1 to several minutes, either lightly touching the skin or just above it. The practitioner uses "intent" to facilitate a transfer of energy to the specific body part of the client from a "universal source" of energy, with the practitioner as the conduit of this energy.

Table 23.1   Basic Healing Touch Techniques

Techniques	Indications	Brief Description of Procedure
Full body		
Basic HT sequence	Influences the human energy field Used for: promoting relaxation; reducing pain; lowering anxiety, tension, and stress; facilitating wound healing; promoting restoration of the body; promoting a sense of well-being	1. Assess client's energy field with a hand scan over the body. 2. Use magnetic passes in client's energy field (hands in motion and/or hands still) to move congestion and density from the field. 3. Reassess client's energy field with hand scan to determine the effects of intervention. 4. Ground the client to the present moment and to connection to the earth.
Magnetic clearing	Clears the body of congestion and emotional debris in the field Used for: history of drug use; postanesthesia; reducing pain; clearing out toxins; posttrauma; systemic disease; after breathing polluted air; history of smoking; environmental sensitivities; emotional clearing and release of unresolved feelings (e.g., anger, fear, worry, tension); easing nausea; chemotherapy or radiation; and kidney dialysis	1. Assess client's energy field with a hand scan over the body. 2. Place hands 12–18 inches above the top of client's head with fingers spread, relaxed, and curled, thumbs touching or close together. 3. Move hands very slowly in long continuous raking motions over the body from above the head to off the toes, 1–6 inches above the body, each sweep taking about 30 seconds (work the middle of the body first, followed by each side). 4. Repeat procedure 30 times, which takes about 15 minutes. 5. Reassess client's energy field with hand scan to determine effects of intervention. 6. Ground the client to the present moment and to connection to the earth.

(continued)

Table 23.1 Basic Healing Touch Techniques (*continued*)

Techniques	Indications	Brief Description of Procedure
Full body		
Chakra connection (Joy, 1979)	Connects, opens, and balances the energy centers (chakras), enhancing the flow of energy throughout the body. Used for: balancing; before and after medical–surgical procedures; promoting relaxation; diminishing pain; easing anxiety; postchemotherapy or radiation; general well-being	1. Assess client's energy field with a hand scan over the body. 2. Place hands on or over the minor energy centers (chakras) on the extremities and the major energy centers (chakras) on the trunk in a defined sequential manner, holding each area for at least 1 minute. 3. Reassess client's energy field with hand scan to determine effects of intervention. 4. Ground the client to the present moment and to connection to the earth.
Chakra spread	Opens the energy centers (chakras), producing a deep clearing of energy blocks Used for: physical or emotional pain; before and after medical procedures/ surgery; severe stress reactions; terminal illness; stress; assisting in coping with various life transitions	1. Assess client's energy field with a hand scan over the body. 2. Hold the client's feet then hands, one by one, in a gentle embrace for at least 1 minute. 3. Place hands (palms up) above each energy center (chakra), moving the hands slowly downward toward the chakra, then spreading the hands outward as far as possible; motion is repeated three times for each energy center, moving from the upper to the lower chakras. 4. Repeat entire sequence two times. 5. Reassess client's energy field with hand scan to determine effects of intervention. 6. End treatment with holding the client's hand and heart center (procedure is done in silence and takes 10–15 minutes; is used very carefully by experienced practitioners for special needs and sacred moments in healing).

(continued)

Table 23.1 Basic Healing Touch Techniques (*continued*)

Techniques	Indications	Brief Description of Procedure
Localized		
Energetic ultrasound	Breaks up congestion, energy patterns, and blockages Used for: easing pain; assists in stopping internal bleeding and bruising, sealing lacerations, healing fractures, and joint injuries; eye or ear issues; accelerating healing; tumors; swelling; inserting intravenous catheters, helping to bring blood vessels to skin surface; stimulating return of bowel motility after surgery	1. Hand scan client's localized area to assess energy field. 2. Hold the thumb and first and second fingers together, directing energy from the palm down the fingers. 3. Imagine a beam of light coming from the fingers of one hand into the client's body. 4. Place opposite hand behind the body part being worked on. 5. Move the hand in any direction over the affected part, continuously moving for 3–5 minutes. 6. Repeat hand scan to determine the effect of intervention.
Energetic laser	Cuts, seals, and breaks up congestion in the energy field Used for: relieving pain; stopping bleeding from a laceration; assisting in wound repair; fractured bones; joint injuries and surgeries; tumors; eye and ear problems	1. Hand scan client's localized area to assess energy field. 2. Hold one or more fingers still and pointed toward the problem area. 3. Use for a few seconds to a minute. 4. Repeat hand scan to determine effect of intervention.
Mind clearing	Promotes mental clarity, peace, and calm Used for: quieting the mind; promoting clarity in thinking and facilitating insights; for deep relaxation; deepening intuition; promoting sleep	1. Hold fingertips or palms on designated parts of the neck and head, holding each part 1–3 minutes. 2. Gently massage mandibular joint. 3. End with light sweeping touches across the forehead and cheeks three times and a gentle hold around the jaw.

(continued)

Table 23.1   Basic Healing Touch Techniques *(continued)*

Techniques	Indications	Brief Description of Procedure
Localized		
Pain drain	Drains pain or energy congestion Used for: acute or chronic pain	1. Place left hand on area of pain or energy congestion and right hand downward away from body. 2. Siphon off congested energy from painful area through left hand and out right hand. 3. Place right hand on painful or congested area and place left hand upward in the air to bring in healing energy from the universal energy field (each position is generally held 3–5 minutes).
Wound sealing	Repairs energy field tears or leaks that occur from physical trauma Used for: ongoing pain at the site of surgery, trauma, wounds, after childbirth; after radiation; clients who may report extreme fatigue	1. Hand scan body above a scar or injury to determine whether any leaks of energy are felt coming from the site (may feel like a column of cool air). 2. Move hands over the area, gathering energy. 3. Bring gathered energy down to the client's skin over the injury and hold for 1 minute with hands. 4. Rescan the area to determine that the energy field feels evenly symmetrical over the entire body.

Note: Each technique begins with determining the client's specific need for HT and obtaining client permission. Mutual goals are set. This is followed by the practitioner centering, physically and psychologically, and setting the intention for the client's highest good. Assessment of energy-field disturbances are determined. Each technique ends with evaluating the energy field and the client's experience and asking for feedback.

Source: Adapted from Anselme, L., Kagel, S., & O'Neill, M. (Eds.). (2014). *HTI healing touch certificate program level 1 student handbook* (2nd ed.). Lakewood, CO: Healing Touch International; Hover-Kramer, D. (2002). *Healing touch: A guidebook for practitioners* (2nd ed.). Albany, NY: Delmar.

Although several HT techniques can be done with the client in a seated position, most are done while the client is lying down and fully dressed in the most relaxed state possible to promote a more profound effect. The practitioner briefly describes HT and the procedure plan, invites the client to ask any questions at any time, and receives permission to do the treatment and to touch the client. HT therapists use the principles of holistic communication, which calls forth the full use of self in interacting with another. Thornton and Mariano (2016) describe this as the acknowledgement of "the infinite and sacred nature of Being; the use of centering, grounding, intention, and intuition; and caring, healing, [and] transcendent presence" (p. 477) as key elements. They also state "Holistic communication invites us to engage our higher Self as we meet another in that transcendent space where profound healing occurs" (p. 477). Both practitioner and client are enriched and nurtured during this process.

Measurement of Outcomes

HT outcomes that have been measured include:

- Patient satisfaction
- Anxiety and stress reduction
- Improved mood and reduced fatigue and nausea
- Pain reduction
- Improved sense of well-being
- Reduction in PTSD, and hostility and cynicism in post-deployed active military
- Decrease in depression
- Positive changes in blood pressure (BP), blood glucose, and salivary immunoglobulin A
- Decreased length of hospitalization and adverse periprocedural outcomes after cardiac procedures
- Diminished agitation levels in dementia patients
- Improved behaviors of patients with Alzheimer's disease
- Improved functional status for patients with mobility issues
- Stress recovery in a neonatal intensive care unit
- Improved health-related quality of life
- Preservation of natural killer cell activity
- Improved sleep quality and quantity in pediatric burn patients

Outcomes measured must reflect the specific client need and presenting symptoms, and the particular HT technique used. Instruments, scales, and data that have been used to measure/evaluate outcomes include:

- Patient satisfaction self-report tools
- Pain, anxiety, and nausea scales
- Measures of posttraumatic stress effects
- Hostility, agitation, and depression scales
- Clinical biophysical data such as BP, oxygen saturation, polysomnographic data, and immune function indicators
- Recovery measures
- Physical functional measures
- Degree of learning
- Health-related quality of life indices

It is difficult to determine whether the outcome of the HT intervention is due solely to the treatment or to other factors as well. The effect of the practitioner's presence has always been considered a confounding variable affecting client outcome, but this is also true in many nursing interventions.

PRECAUTIONS

Precautions to be aware of when using HT techniques include the following:

- The energy fields of infants, children, older people, the extremely ill, and the dying are sensitive to energy work, so treatments should be gentle and time limited.
- Gentle energy treatments are also required for pregnant women because the energy field also includes the fetus.
- Energy work with a cancer patient should be focused on balancing the whole field rather than concentrating on a particular area.
- The effect of medications and chemicals in the body may be enhanced with energy work, so one must be alert to the possibility of side effects and sensitivity reactions to these substances.

It is recommended that experienced practitioners work with clients in the above situations. However, to help develop a knowledgeable practice, a student or an apprentice in HT can provide treatments in these situations if supervised by a mentor (Umbreit, 2000). HT is not considered a curative treatment and must always be used with conventional medical care. However, practitioners and clients have reported that clients have experienced a sense of healing at a more holistic level of mind, body, and spirit, even if a cure is not possible. Umbreit (2000) reports anecdotal comments from clients that include feeling "wonderful," "relaxed," "peaceful," "in a meditative state," "warm," "soothed," "safe," "reassured," "more balanced," "mellow," "happier with life," "as if all my tension was melting," and a "sense of inner peace." Slater (2009) states, "After a session, most people experience a sense of relaxation, lessened stress, increased energy, and other signs of increased vitality" (p. 664). Because HT is a noninvasive intervention, these clients' responses have enormous implications for improving quality of life in their striving toward wellness.

USES

HT interventions have been used with all age groups, from the neonate to the older adult. Besides the general curriculum for learning HT, there are also classes available for specifically working with pregnant women, infants, and children (Kluny, 2017). Models of delivering services range from volunteer to staff-provided programs. HT is being used within diverse healthcare facilities: hospitals, long-term-care facilities, private practices, hospices, outpatient clinics, home care, communities, church-related health and spiritual ministry departments, and spas (Healing Beyond Borders, 2017e; Kagel & Anselme, 2014). The HT curriculum is considered a CE offering but has also been integrated into community college and university systems in both traditional allied health training and advanced training for holistic health professionals (Kagel & Anselme, 2014).

HT studies have shown positive results in the following clinical situations:

- Reduction of anxiety and stress
- Promotion of relaxation
- Reduction in acute and chronic pain
- Promotion of postoperative recovery
- Aid in preparation for medical treatments and procedures
- Improvement of cancer treatment side effects
- Reduction in symptoms of depression
- Promotion of a sense of well-being
- Reduction in agitation levels
- Improvement of PTSD symptoms
- Improvement in quality of life physically, emotionally, relationally, and spiritually

Table 23.2 lists several research studies that have supported the use of HT interventions in some of these clinical situations. There are some studies not published in peer-reviewed medical, nursing, or psychology journals, but information can be accessed through Healing Beyond Border's research section (www.healingbeyond-borders.org) or Healing Touch Program's website (www.healingtouchprogram.com). The research continues to be controversial because the exact mechanism of action

Table 23.2   Selected Research Studies Using Healing Touch Interventions (1996–2016)

Uses	Selected Sources
Anxiety/stress reduction	Dubrey (2012a); Gehlhaart and Dail (2000); Guevara, Silva, and Menidas (2012); Taylor (2001); Wilkinson et al. (2002)
Pediatrics: Promotion of sleep and relaxation/relief of anxiety, stress, pain, depression, fatigue, spasticity	Cone, Gottschlich, Khoury, Simakajornboon, and Kagan (2014); Kemper, Fletcher, Hamilton, and McLean (2012); McDonough-Means, Edde, Bell (2009); Speel (2012); Verret (2000); Wong, Ghiasuddin, Kimata, and Patelesio (2012); Zimmer, Bogenschutz, Meier, and Rolf (2009)
Acute and chronic pain reduction	Cordes, Proffitt, and Roth (2012); Darbonne (2012); Diener (2001); Hardwick (2012); Hjersted-Smith and Jones (2012); Kiley (2012); Lu et al., (2013b); Merritt and Randall (2012); Protzman (2012); Slater (2012); Wardell (2000); Wardell, Rintala, and Tan (2008); Welcher and Kish (2001); Weymouth and Sandberg-Lewis (2000)
Promotion of postoperative recovery	Anderson et al., (2015); Laffey and Neizgoda (2012); MacIntyre et al. (2008); Silva (1996)

(continued)

Table 23.2 Selected Research Studies Using Healing Touch Interventions (1996–2016) (*continued*)

Uses	Selected Sources
Aid in medical procedures/ treatments	Seskevich et al. (2004)
Improvement of cancer treatment side effects and general well-being in cancer patients	Cook et al. (2004); Danhauer, Tooze, Holder, Miller, and Jesse (2008); FitzHenry et al., (2014); Jain, Pavlik, et al., (2012); Lu, Hart, Lutgendorf, Oh, and Silverman (2016); Lutgendorf et al., (2014); Post-White et al. (2003); Rexilius, Mundt, Megel, and Agrawal (2002); Turner (2012)
Mental health	Dubrey (2012b); Van Aken (2012)
Older adults	Decker, Wardell, and Cron (2012); Gehlhaart and Dail (2000); Lu et al., (2013a); Ostuni and Pietro (2012); Wang and Hermann (2006)
PTSD	Guevara et al. (2012); Jain, McMahon, et al. (2012)
Personal growth and transformation; spiritual meaning and awareness	Wardell (2001); Ziembroski, Gilbert, Bossarte, and Guldbery (2003)

PTSD, post-traumatic stress disorder

cannot be seen or easily explained in our Western view of what constitutes sound scientific research, and few double-blind studies have been done in this area. Until a reliable and easily available tool is developed to measure changes in the energy system, objective measurement of changes in the flow of an energy field is not possible. However, skilled practitioners do report a change in clients' energy fields that they perceive through the use of their senses, most commonly through touch.

CULTURAL APPLICATIONS

HT is being taught and practiced in 37 countries around the world, including impoverished communities with few economic resources; people in more countries continue to request HT education each year. The richness of HT is that it lends itself to flowing to and across continents and cultures, maintaining standardization, yet appropriately adapting to the culture and available resources (Van Aken, 2012). HT students are able to use their skills in their communities: hospitals, clinics, homes, rural areas, villages, and places where healthcare may be limited and living conditions very difficult. Even in impoverished places of the world, where strife, abject poverty, and hidden hopelessness pervade daily life, learning and practicing HT has helped empower people to address their serious social and public health issues by decreasing their suffering, especially where women and children are marginalized (Starke, 2008). HT has offered tools to address difficult situations and ways to work in the absence of medications (Goff, 2007).

Frost (2014) reported on her HT experiences in South Africa, teaching caregivers of people suffering and dying of AIDS and some of the millions of orphaned children in Africa. Many live in desperately inadequate settlement camps, and the caregivers were so appreciative to learn the basic HT technique to use as part of the care to support their ill patients. Frost also writes about helping to set up a HT clinic for women and children of the "first peoples" from the Kalahari Desert region. The clinic space was a large tree with spreading shade limbs with a few mismatched chairs. Techniques taught addressed the women's main complaints of headaches and body pain; after the classes, they reported easing of pain, feeling relaxed, and feeling good.

Kagel's (2014) experiences after being invited to teach HT in several varied and marginalized locations around Ecuador posed many cultural challenges that with patience, creativity, and finding of needed resources, were met graciously. Some of her students spoke Spanish, some Quichua (a local dialect), often in the same class, so one or two translators were needed. Many students did not read, so the translator created pictorial references easily distributed to the students to support their future practice. Kagel reports that teaching in Ecuador was very different than in the United States. Community leaders controlled the scheduling of classes in Ecuador, and all HT classes had to be approved by government officials after interviews, explanations of the work, and intended benefits to the community were presented. Once approved, officials set the days and times of the classes; classes had to start after work (3 p.m.) and finish before dark "so that the women would not 'disappear' walking home. Women were given a day off during the weekend to cook, wash clothes in the open air laundry tubs, care for their families, and be ready for the new work week" (p. 54). Kagel goes on to share her story in Sidebar 23.1. Sidebar 23.2 details the experiences of accessing energy healing therapies, in general, in France.

SIDEBAR 23.1 HEALING TOUCH IN ECUADOR

Sue Kagel

We were escorted in and out of dangerous communities, teaching in churches, community buildings, and in one situation, the second floor of a small police department. Our classrooms often had no heat or bedding. We were creative and used whatever was available. One room had only chairs, so we taught techniques for chair use, a few used gym mats or thin mattresses on the floor and we worked kneeling. In another class, I demonstrated techniques sitting on the floor with one of our teen volunteers lying on the cold linoleum floor. A church setting had desks and benches, so we pushed them together to create space for people to recline and used chairs. Roosters crowed, kids ran in and out, babies cried, nursed, and slept, rooftops rattled and flapped in the wind. We held the energy for the class and stayed in flexible, loving, healing presence.

In one location, the class swelled the second day as excited students brought their family members and friends. Rather than moving to the next technique sequences, we brought the new members up to speed and advanced the students at the same time. They were so grateful to have new tools to use, as medical care was scarce.

Several communities were located on the mountainside, so pain-relief techniques for legs and shoulders were taught to address the problems incurred

(continued)

from carrying huge loads up and down steep slopes. Techniques to address the problems of family and domestic violence issues were also taught. At the lower altitudes, headaches and dehydration from the heat were addressed at the people's request. For the day-care workers, we focused on heart-centered presence, energetic balancing, pain management, and calming techniques for the children rather than corporal punishment. All classes needed to be short and focused. Class sizes changed unexpectedly, so constant adjustments had to be made. Those we served noted decreased emotional stress, relief of physical symptoms, and a decrease of aggressive, violent behaviors in families who took the Healing Touch classes. Grounding, centering, body awareness, and breathing became tools used in community gatherings and individually to continue supporting their well-being.

SIDEBAR 23.2 ENERGY HEALING IN FRANCE

Chris Lepoutre

Energy healing is not a part of the occidental (Western) healthcare system in France. It would be highly unusual for a physician to request that an energy healer work with a patient. Patients or their family may ask an energy healer to visit a patient in the hospital, but this request is not made by the hospital staff.

Being an energy healer is not freely shared with others. Some see energy healers as witches. If it is known that you are an energy healer, you may be shunned. In the Judeo-Christian culture, energy healers are often viewed as the hand of the devil. A Catholic priest, who was using energy healing, was told by his bishop to end this activity or resign.

However, many people go to energy healers for therapy, although it is an underground activity. Some physicians may informally advise a person to go for healing to an energy healer, but this is never a formal referral. More often it is a nurse who will whisper about the therapy to the patient or family. This is particularly true for some specific illnesses such as shingles or burns.

It is not uncommon for a person who has had energy healing to share his or her experience with friends. The person may recommend this therapy to friends for the treatment of specific health issues through word of mouth. In these cases, sessions are typically paid for with cash as an "underground" economy.

There is no formal well-publicized education program for energy healing in France. Information on 2-day education sessions can be found on the Internet. At the end of the 2-day course, the person receives a certificate. However, there is no government recognition for preparation in healing touch.

As an indication that interest in and use of energy healing is growing in France, some energy healers have recently begun to open offices to provide this therapy. However, these are viewed as stores and not as a medical business.

FUTURE RESEARCH

Research studies and anecdotal cases in HT offer promising, yet certainly not conclusive data on the positive outcomes from this complementary therapy. Qualitative responses from clients have been especially important in helping guide the direction of the research and may provide insight into the phenomenon of energy exchange in the future. Some of the problems encountered in nursing research include insufficient funding to support the work, multiple variables that are hard to control in a clinical setting versus a laboratory setting, and the use of small sample sizes that can be easily affected by highly variable data and sampling error.

There is the additional difficulty of testing the efficacy of an energy-based therapy in which the energy exchange between practitioner and client cannot be seen by most people, but is only observed as subjective responses from clients. The whole conceptual framework of energy fields and energy exchange does not fit the cause–effect model that Western science is focused on. Rogers's theory (1990) speaks about energy changing, exchanging, and patterning, one moment in time never replicating itself. The focus is on nature's restoring universal order and balance, and restoring energy balance is the goal of HT. This is an area of research that obviously will require a multidisciplinary effort by Western and Eastern medicine, quantum physics, biology, psychology, philosophy, spirituality, and nursing. Outcome studies, as well as studies of mechanism, will help support the development and understanding of the phenomenon of energy exchange. Mediating factors may contribute to decrease in pain intensity, anxiety reduction, acceleration of healing, immune system enhancement, diminished depression, and increased sense of well-being. More studies that measure some of these mediating mechanisms are recommended.

The choice of valid instruments for measuring outcomes is critical in HT studies. Results can be skewed in either direction if the instruments are not reliable. However, to obtain subject cooperation when working with those who are ill, measurement instruments must be easy to use and not burdensome to patients who are already facing difficulties.

Other challenges to be controlled in conducting HT research studies include the experience of the HT practitioner, the phenomenon of the caregiver's presence, the type of HT treatment modality chosen, the duration and number of treatments, the time when the treatment is done, the time when measurements are done, and long-term effects of HT. There is a wide range of skill levels of HT practitioners from novice to certified practitioner and comparable skill level is important in planning a research study. It is important to note that "the deepest and longest lasting healing will be at the hands of a healer who has the greatest breadth and depth of training, practice, and personal healing" (Slater, 2009, p. 649). The phenomenon of presence of the HT practitioner may also affect the outcome of the research and needs to be controlled in the study design. Because many HT interventions can be used, a research study needs to be consistent in the type of therapy chosen. The challenge with duration and number of treatments is that, under normal circumstances, an HT intervention is not used for a prescribed length of time or number of treatments. The work is done until the practitioner intuitively determines that it is time to stop or that no more treatments are needed. Research could restrict this professional decision-making process. Choosing when to give a HT treatment, when to measure outcomes and ascertaining how long the outcome may last continue to be challenging. Experienced HT practitioners must have input into determining these timelines by observing patterns they may typically see in their own professional practice.

In summary, there continues to be some criticism within the scientific community of current energy/biofield therapy research pointing to study quality and limitations such as small subject numbers, controls for placebo effect, possible Hawthorne effect, and nonblinding of participants. The effects of HT interventions have been supported by a limited number of rigorous research studies. Some reports are from anecdotes or case studies in a variety of clinical situations with all age groups and states of illness or wellness (Scandrett-Hibdon, Hardy, & Mentgen, 1999; Wardell, Kagel, & Anselme, 2014b) and from studies that unfortunately were missing some vital information, which led to problems with both internal and external validity (Wardell & Weymouth, 2004). Researchers can design future studies that demonstrate added rigor and overcome some of these limitations. For example, by adding mock groups, it is possible to reduce the placebo effect. Goals of future HT research include increasing the number of studies and RCTs that are replicable and that have larger numbers of participants using standardized, reliable, and valid instruments. In addition, investigators can conduct studies that help determine the optimal amount, techniques, or protocol of HT to alleviate various symptoms and conditions.

The next steps for research must build on the studies already completed. Replication of studies would help strengthen the validity of HT. The following are questions related to specific areas to build on:

- Is HT equally effective in acute versus chronic pain? How long and how frequent do treatments need to be for the client to report a decrease in pain? How long does this improvement last?
- How is postoperative recovery affected by administering HT (pain relief, wound healing, restoring of bowel function, ease of physical activity, length of stay in the hospital)?
- Does HT have a positive effect on degenerative diseases such as arthritis, multiple sclerosis, fibromyalgia, stroke, immune deficiency disorders, chronic lung conditions, other inflammatory-based diseases, and cancer?
- Does HT assist in managing the side effects of treatments in cancer patients?
- What are the psychological and spiritual benefits reported by HT recipients?
- What is the impact of HT as a complement to help eliminate PTSD and depression in our military and others who have experienced trauma?
- What tools are effective in measuring a change in energy in the recipient before and after HT or an exchange of energy between practitioner and recipient?
- Does HT reduce medical costs for pharmaceuticals, hospital stays, and clinic time?

In the quest to examine the impact of HT scientifically, care must be taken to not to be too quick to dismiss the overwhelming positive client feedback from its clinical application. Creativity is necessary in conducting research of this phenomenon that cannot be seen by the naked eye, but is so often felt by the human spirit.

WEBSITES

Information on HT

- American Holistic Nurses Association (AHNA)
  (www.ahna.org)
- Healing Beyond Borders (HBB), formerly Healing Touch International, Inc.
  (www.healingbeyondborders.org)
- Healing Touch Program (HTP)
  (www.healingtouchprogram.com)
- Consciousness and Healing Initiative
  (www.CHI.is)
- Healing Touch for Babies
  (www.healingtouchforbabies.com)
- You Tube: Introduction to Healing Touch with Sue Kagel, RN, BSN, CHTP/I, HNC
  (www.youtube.com/watch?v=HhrMiMlWx4E)

HBB International Affiliate HT Organizations

- Australian Foundation for Healing Touch Inc.
  (healingtouch.org.au)
- Healing Touch Canada Inc.
  (healingtouchcanada.net)
- Healing Touch Association of Canada
  (htac-jm.org)
- Healing Touch Sweden
  (healingtouch.se)
- Healing Touch Netherlands
  (healingtouch.nl)
- Healing Touch New Zealand Inc.
  (healingtouchnz.com)
- Healing Touch Peru
  (prosh-promoviendosaludholistica.blogspot.com)

Information on Therapeutic Touch

- Therapeutic Touch International Association
  (www.therapeutictouch.org)

REFERENCES

American Holistic Nurses Association. (2017). NANDA-I vote approves imbalanced energy field nursing diagnoses. *American Nurses Holistic Association Newsletter, 15*(4), 1.

Anderson, J. G. (2016, October). *A deep dive into psychoneuroimmunology.* Paper presented at the Healing Beyond Borders Conference, Colorado Springs, CO.

Anderson, J. G., Suchicital, L., Lang, M., Kukic, A., Mangione, L., Swengros, D., … Friesen, M.A. (2015). The effects of healing touch on pain, nausea and anxiety following bariatric surgery: A pilot study. *Journal of Science and Healing, 1*(3), 208–216.

Anderson, J. G., & Taylor, A. G. (2011). Effects of healing touch in clinical practice. *Journal of Holistic Nursing, 29*(3), 221–228.

Anselme, L., Kagel, S., & O'Neill, M. (Eds.). (2014). *HTI healing touch certificate program level 1 student handbook* (2nd ed.). Lakewood, CO: Healing Touch International.

Bailey, A. (1984). *Esoteric healing*. Albany, NY: Lucis Trust.

Bhasin, M. K., Dusek, J. A., Chang, B. H., Joseph, M. G., Denninger, J. W., Fricchione, G. L., ... Libermann, T. A. (2013). Relaxation response induces temporal transcriptome changes in energy metabolism, insulin secretion and inflammatory pathways. *PLOS ONE, 8*(5), e62817.

Brennan, B. (1986). *Hands of light*. New York, NY: Bantam.

Bruyere, R. L. (1989). *Wheels of light*. New York, NY: Simon & Schuster.

Bulbrook, M. J. (2000). *Healing stories to inspire, teach and heal*. Carrboro: North Carolina Center for Healing Touch.

Carpenito, L. J. (2013). *Nursing diagnosis: Application to clinical practice* (14th ed., pp. 252–255). Philadelphia, PA: Lippincott Williams & Wilkins.

Cook, C., Guerrerio, J., & Slater, V. (2004). Healing touch and quality of life in women receiving radiation treatment for cancer: A randomized controlled trial. *Alternative Therapies, 10*(3), 34–41.

Cone, L., Gottschlich, M. M., Khoury, J., Simakajornboon, N., & Kagan, R. J. (2014). The effect of healing touch on sleep patterns of pediatric burn patients: A prospective pilot study. *Journal of Sleep Disorders: Treatments and Care, 3*(2), 1–6. Retrieved from doi:10.4172/2325-9639.1000136

Cordes, P., Proffitt, C., & Roth, J. (2012). The effect of healing touch therapy on the pain and joint mobility experienced by patients with total knee replacements. In M. Megel, J. G. Anderson, D. Lu, & N. Strybol (Eds.), *Healing touch research survey* (14th ed., pp. 67–68). Lakewood, CO: Healing Touch International.

Danhauer, S. C., Tooze, J. A., Holder, P., Miller, C., & Jesse, M. T. (2008). Healing touch as a supportive intervention for adult acute leukemia patients: A pilot investigation of effects on distress and treatment-related symptoms. *Journal of the Society for Integrative Oncology, 6*(3), 89–97.

Darbonne, M. (2012). The effects of healing touch modalities on patients with chronic pain. In M. Megel, J. G. Anderson, D. Lu, & N. Strybol (Eds.), *Healing touch research survey* (14th ed., pp. 76–77). Lakewood, CO: Healing Touch International.

Decker, S., Wardell, D. W., & Cron, S. G. (2012). Using a healing touch intervention in older adults with persistent pain: A feasibility study. *Journal of Holistic Nursing, 30*(3), 205–213.

Diener, D. (2001). A pilot study of the effect of chakra connection and magnetic unruffle on perception of pain in people with fibromyalgia. *Healing Touch Newsletter: Research Edition, 1*(3), 7–8.

Dowd, T., Kolcaba, K., Steiner, R., & Fashinpaur, D. (2007). Comparison of a healing touch, coaching, and a combined intervention on comfort and stress in younger college students. *Holistic Nursing Practice, 21*(4), 194–202.

Dubrey, R. (2012a). A quality assurance project on the effectiveness of healing touch treatments as perceived by patients at the wellness institute. In M. Megel, J. G. Anderson, D. Lu, & N. Strybol (Eds.), *Healing touch research survey* (14th ed., p. 89). Lakewood, CO: Healing Touch International.

Dubrey, R. (2012b). The effect of healing touch on in-patients going through stage 1 recovery from alcoholism. In M. Megel, J. G. Anderson, D. Lu, & N. Strybol (Eds.), *Healing touch research survey* (14th ed., pp. 105–106). Lakewood, CO: Healing Touch International.

Duerden, T. (2004). An aura of confusion. Part 2: The aided eye—"Imaging the aura?" *Complementary Therapies in Nurse Midwifery, 10*, 116–123.

Engebretson, J., & Wardell, D. W. (2002). Experience of a Reiki session. *Alternative Therapies, 8*(2), 48–53.

Eschiti, V. (2007). Healing touch: A low-tech intervention in high-tech settings. *Dimensions of Critical Care Nursing, 26*(1), 9–14.

Eschiti, V. (2014). Martha Rogers: The science of unitary human beings in foundational aspects of healing work. In D. Wardell, S. Kagel, & L. Anselme (Eds.), *Healing touch: Enhancing life through energy therapy* (pp. 76–68). Bloomington, IN: iUniverse LLC.

Feinstein, D., & Eden, D. (2008). Six pillars of energy medicine: Clinical strengths of a complementary paradigm. *Alternative Therapies, 14*(1), 44–54.

FitzHenry, F., Wells, N., Slater, V., Dietrich, M. S., Wisawatapnimit, P., & Chakravarthy, A. B. (2014). A randomized placebo-controlled pilot study of the impact of healing touch on fatigue in breast cancer patients undergoing radiation therapy. *Integrated Cancer Therapies, 13*(2), 105–113.

Forbes, M. A., Rust, R., & Becker, G. J. (2004). Surface electromyography (EMG) as a measurement for biofield research: Results from a single case study. *Journal of Alternative & Complementary Medicine, 10*(4), 617–626.

Frost, M. (2014). South Africa. In D. Wardell, S. Kagel, & L. Anselme (Eds.), *Healing touch: Enhancing life through energy therapy* (pp. 57–61). Bloomington, IN: iUniverse LLC.

Geddes, N. (2002). Research related to healing touch. In D. Hover-Kramer (Ed.), *Healing touch: A guidebook for practitioners* (2nd ed., pp. 24–40). Albany, NY: Delmar.

Gehlhaart, C., & Dail, P. (2000). Effectiveness of healing touch and therapeutic touch on elderly residents of long term care facilities on reducing pain and anxiety level. *Healing Touch Newsletter, 0*(3), 8.

Goff, R. (2007). Carrying light into South Africa. *Healing Touch International, Inc. Quarterly Newsletter, 1*, 6–7.

Guevara, E., Silva, C., & Menidas, N., (2012). The effect of healing touch therapy on post-traumatic stress disorder (PTSD) symptoms on domestic violence abused Mexican women. In M. Megel, J. G. Anderson, D. Lu, & N. Strybol (Eds.), *Healing touch research survey* (14th ed., pp. 106–107). Lakewood, CO: Healing Touch International.

Hammerschlag, R., Marx, B. L., & Aickin, M. (2014). Nontouch biofield therapy: A systematic review of human randomized controlled trials reporting use of only nonphysical contact treatment. *Journal of Alternative and Complementary Medicine, 20*(12), 881–892.

Hardwick, M. E. (2012). Nursing intervention using healing touch in bilateral total knee arthroplasty. In M. Megel, J. G. Anderson, D. Lu, & N. Strybol (Eds.), *Healing touch research survey* (14th ed., p. 68). Lakewood, CO: Healing Touch International.

Healing Beyond Borders. (2017a). *Vision and Mmission.* Retrieved from http://www.healingbeyondborders.org

Healing Beyond Borders. (2017b). *About: What is healing touch?* Retrieved from http://www.healingbeyondborders.org

Healing Beyond Borders. (2017c). *About: How was the curriculum developed?* Retrieved from http://www.healingbeyondborders.org

Healing Beyond Borders. (2017d). *Scope of practice.* Retrieved from http://www.healingbeyondborders.org

Healing Beyond Borders. (2017e). *About: Where is healing touch used?* Retrieved from http://www.healingbeyondborders.org

Healing Touch Program. (2017a). *What is healing touch?* Retrieved from http://www.healingtouchprogram.com

Healing Touch Program. (2017b). *Who can practice healing touch?* Retrieved from http://www.healingtouchprogram.com

Hjersted-Smith, C., & Jones, S. (2012). The effects of healing touch on pain and anxiety with end stage liver disease. In M. Megel, J. G. Anderson, D. Lu, & N. Strybol (Eds.), *Healing touch research survey* (14th ed., pp. 83–84). Lakewood, CO: Healing Touch International.

Hover-Kramer, D. (2002). *Healing touch: A guidebook for practitioners* (2nd ed.). Albany, NY: Delmar.

Ives, J. A., van Wijk, E. P. A., Bat, N., Crawford, C., Walter, A., Jonas, W. B., ... van der Greef, J. (2014). Ultraweak photon emission as a non-invasive health assessment: A systematic review. *PLOS ONE, 9*(2), e87401. doi:10.1371/journal.pone.0087401

Jackson, C., & Latini, C. (2016). Touch & hand mediated therapies. In B. Dossey & L. Keegan (Eds.), *Holistic nursing: A handbook for practice* (7th ed., pp. 299–319). Burlington, MA: Jones & Bartlett.

Jain, S., McMahon, G. F., Hasen, P., Kozub, M. P., Porter, V., King, R., & Guarneri, E. M. (2012). Healing touch with guided imagery for PTSD in returning active duty military: A randomized controlled trial. *Military Medicine, 177*(9), 1015–1021.

Jain, S., & Mills, P. J. (2010). Biofield therapies: Helpful or full of hype? A best evidence synthesis. *International Journal of Behavioral Medicine, 17*(1), 1–16. doi:10.1007/s12529-009-062-4

Jain, S., Pavlik, D., Distefan, J., Bruyere, R. L., Acer, J., Garcia, R., ... Mills, P. J. (2012). Complementary medicine for fatigue and cortisol variability in breast cancer survivors. *Cancer, 118*, 777–787.

Joy, B. (1979). *Joy's way.* New York, NY: G. P. Putnam's Sons.

Kagel, S. (2014). Ecuador. In D. Wardell, S. Kagel, & L. Anselme (Eds.), *Healing touch: Enhancing life through energy therapy* (pp. 53–57). Bloomington, IN: iUniverse LLC.

Kagel, S., & Anselme, L. (2014). Integrating from self to family, community, & the world. In D. Wardell, S. Kagel, & L. Anselme (Eds.), *Healing touch: Enhancing life through energy therapy* (pp. 332–335). Bloomington, IN: iUniverse LLC.

Kemper, K., Fletcher, N., Hamilton, C., & McLean, T. (2012). Impact of healing touch on pediatric oncology outpatients: A pilot study. In M. Megel, J. G. Anderson, D. Lu, & N. Strybol (Eds.), *Healing touch research survey* (14th ed., pp. 19–20). Lakewood, CO: Healing Touch International.

Kiang, J. G., Ives, J. A., & Jonas, W. B. (2005). External bioenergy-induced increases in intracellular free calcium concentrations are mediated by Na^+/Ca^{2+} exchanger and L-type calcium channel. *Molecular and Cellular Biochemistry, 271*, 51–59.

Kiley, S. (2012). The evaluation of healing touch for headache pain. In M. Megel, J. G. Anderson, D. Lu, & N. Strybol (Eds.), *Healing touch research survey* (14th ed., p. 78). Lakewood, CO: Healing Touch International.

Kluny, R. (2017). *Healing touch for babies.* Retrieved from htttp://www.healingtouchforbabies.com

Krieger, D. (1979). *The therapeutic touch: How to use your hands to help or to heal.* New York, NY: Simon & Schuster.

Krieger, D. (1993). *Accepting your power to heal.* Santa Fe, NM: Bear & Co.

Krucoff, M., Crater, S., Gallup, D., Blankenship, J., Cuffe, M., Guarneri, M., ... Lee, K. (2005). Music, imagery, touch, and prayer as adjuncts to interventional cardiac care: The monitoring and actualization of noetic trainings (MANTRA) II randomized study. *Lancet, 366*(9481), 211–217.

Krucoff, M., Crater, S., Green, C., Massa, A., Seskevich, J., Lane, J., ... Koenig, H. (2001). Integrative noetic therapies as adjuncts to percutaneous intervention during unstable coronary syndromes: Monitoring and actualization of noetic training (MANTRA) feasibility pilot. *American Heart Journal, 142*(5), 760–769.

Laffey, E., & Neizgoda, J. (2012). Wound care and complementary medicine: The impact of healing touch. A case study. In M. Megel, J. G. Anderson, D. Lu, & N. Strybol (Eds.), *Healing touch research survey* (14th ed., pp. 101–102). Lakewood, CO: Healing Touch International.

Lu, D. F., Hart, L. K., Lutgendorf, S. K., Oh, H., & Schilling, M. (2013). Slowing progression of early stages of AD with alternative therapies: A feasibility study. *Geriatric Nursing, 34*(6):457–464.

Lu, D. F., Hart, L. K., Lutgendorf, S. K., Oh, H., & Silverman, M. (2016). Effects of healing touch and relaxation therapy on adult patients undergoing hematopoietic stem cell transplant: A feasibility study. *Cancer Nursing, 39*(3), E1–E11.

Lu, D. F, Hart, L. K., Lutgendorf, S. K., & Perkhounkova, Y. (2013). The effect of healing touch on the pain and mobility of persons with osteoarthritis: A feasibility study. *Geriatric Nursing, 34*(4), 314–322.

Lutgendorf, S. K., Mullen-Houser, E., Russell, D., DeGeest, K., Jacobson, G., Hart, L., ... Lubaroff, D. M. (2014). Preservation of immune function in cervical cancer patients during chemoradiation using a novel integrative approach. *Brain, Behavior and Immunity, 24*(8), 1231–1240.

MacIntyre, B., Hamilton, J., Fricke, T., Ma, W., Mehle, S., & Michel, M. (2008). The efficacy of healing touch in coronary artery bypass surgery recovery: A randomized clinical trial. *Alternative Therapies in Healing and Medicine, 14*(4), 24–32.

Maville, J., Bowen, J., & Benham, G. (2008). Effect of healing touch on stress perception and biological correlates. *Holistic Nursing Practice, 22*(2), 103–110.

McDonough-Means, S. I., Edde, E. L., & Bell, I. R. (2009). Healing touch shows potential stress mitigation in ill neonates [Abstract]. *Journal of Developmental and Behavioral Pediatrics, 30*(6). doi:10.1097/DBP.0b013e3181c77898

Megel, M. E., Anderson, J. G., Lu, D., & Strybol, N. (2012). *Healing touch research survey* (14th ed.). Lakewood, CO: Healing Touch International.

Merritt, P., & Randall, D. (2012). The effect of healing touch and other forms of energy work on cancer pain. In M. Megel, J. G. Anderson, D. Lu, & N. Strybol (Eds.), *Healing touch research survey* (14th ed., p. 24). Lakewood, CO: Healing Touch International.

National Center for Complementary and Integrative Health. (2016, June). *Complementary, alternative, or integrative health: What's in a name?* Retrieved from htttp://www.nccih.nih.gov

Oschman, J. (2008, September). *Validating the heart's work.* Paper presented at the Healing Touch International Conference, Milwaukee, WI.

Oschman, J. (2016a, October). *Scientific basis of energy medicine.* Paper presented at the Healing Beyond Borders Conference, Colorado Springs, CO.

Oschman, J. L. (2016b). *Energy medicine: The scientific basis* (2nd ed.). New York, NY: Elsevier.

Ostuni, E., & Pietro, M. J. (2012). Effects of healing touch on nursing home residents in later stages of Alzheimer's. In M. Megel, J. G. Anderson, D. Lu, & N. Strybol (Eds.), *Healing touch research survey* (14th ed., pp. 47–48). Lakewood, CO: Healing Touch International.

Post-White, J., Kinney, M. E., Savik, K., Gau, J. B., Wilcox, C., & Lerner, I. (2003). Therapeutic massage and healing touch improve symptoms in cancer. *Integrative Cancer Therapies, 2*(4), 332–344.

Protzman, L. (2012). The effect of healing touch on pain and relaxation. In M. Megel, J. G. Anderson, D. Lu, & N. Strybol (Eds.), *Healing touch research survey* (14th ed., p. 81). Lakewood, CO: Healing Touch International.

Rexilius, S., Mundt, C., Megel, M., & Agrawal, S. (2002). Therapeutic effects of healing touch and massage therapy on caregivers of autologous hematopoietic stem cell transplant patients. *Oncology Nursing Forum, 29*(3), 1–14.

Rogers, M. (1990). Nursing: Science of unitary, irreducible, human beings: Update 1990. In E. A. M. Barrett (Ed.), *Vision of Rogers' science-based nursing* (pp. 5–11). New York, NY: National League for Nursing.

Scandrett-Hibdon, S., Hardy, C., & Mentgen, J. (1999). *Energetic patterns: Healing touch case studies* (Vol. 1). Lakewood, CO: Colorado Center for Healing Touch.

Schwartz, G. E. (2007). *The energy healing experiments.* New York, NY: Atria Books.

Seskevich, J., Crater, S., Lane, J., & Krucoff, M. (2004). Beneficial effects of noetic therapies on mood before percutaneous intervention for unstable coronary symptoms. *Nursing Research, 53*(2), 116–121.

Shields, D., & Wilson, D. (2016). Energy healing. In B. Dossey & L. Keegan (Eds.), *Holistic nursing: A handbook for practice* (7th ed., pp. 187–220). Burlington, MA: Jones & Bartlett.

Silva, C. (1996). The effects of relaxation touch on the recovery level of postanesthesia abdominal hysterectomy patients. *Alternative Therapies, 2*(4), 94.

Slater, V. (2009). Energy healing. In B. Dossey & L. Keegan (Eds.), *Holistic nursing: A handbook for practice* (5th ed., pp. 647–673). Sudbury, MA: Jones & Bartlett.

Slater, V. (2012). Safety, elements, and effects of healing touch on chronic non-malignant abdominal pain. In M. Megel, J. G. Anderson, D. Lu, & N. Strybol (Eds.), *Healing touch research survey* (14th ed., pp. 84–85). Lakewood, CO: Healing Touch International.

Speel, L. (2012). A pilot study on the effect of healing touch–mind cleaning and magnetic unruffling on high school students with mental and physical disabilities. In M. Megel, J. G. Anderson, D. Lu, & N. Strybol (Eds.), *Healing touch research survey* (14th ed., pp. 96–98). Lakewood, CO: Healing Touch International.

Starke, B. A. (2008, July). Presence in Nepal. *Energy Magazine, 25*, 11–14.

Taylor, B. (2001). The effect of healing touch on the coping ability, self esteem, and general health of undergraduate nursing students. *Complementary Therapies in Nursing and Midwifery, 7*(1), 34–42.

Therapeutic Touch International Association. (2017). *What is therapeutic touch?* Retrieved from www.therapeutictouch.org

Thornton, L. (2013). *Whole person caring.* Indianapolis, IN: Sigma Tau International.

Thornton, L., & Mariano, C. (2016). Evolving from therapeutic to holistic communication. In B. Dossey & L. Keegan (Eds.), *Holistic nursing: A handbook for practice* (7th ed., p. 477). Burlington, MA: Jones & Bartlett.

Turner, K. (2012). Preliminary data analysis of the healing touch partners program. In M. Megel, J. G. Anderson, D. Lu, & N. Strybol (Eds.), *Healing touch research survey* (14th ed., pp. 27–29). Lakewood, CO: Healing Touch International.

Umbreit, A. (2000). Healing touch: Applications in the acute care setting. *AACN Clinical Issues, 11*(1), 105–119.

Van Aken, R. (2012). The experiential process of healing touch for people with moderate depression. In M. Megel, J. G. Anderson, D. Lu, & N. Strybol (Eds.), *Healing Touch Research Survey* (14th ed., pp. 108–109). Lakewood, CO: Healing Touch International.

Verret, P. (2000). Healing touch as a relaxation intervention in children with spasticity. *Healing Touch Newsletter: Research Edition, 0*(3), 6–7.

Wang, K., & Hermann, C. (2006). Pilot study to test the effectiveness of healing touch on agitation levels in people with dementia. *Geriatric Nursing, 27*(1), 42–40.

Wardell, D. (2000). The trauma release technique: How it is taught and experienced in healing touch. *Alternative and Complementary Therapies, 6*(1), 20–27.

Wardell, D. (2001). Spirituality of healing touch participants. *Journal of Holistic Nursing, 19*(1), 71–86.

Wardell, D., Kagel, S., & Anselme, L. (2014a). History of healing touch education & certification. In D. Wardell, S. Kagel, & L. Anselme (Eds.), *Healing touch: Enhancing life through energy therapy* (pp. 63–67). Bloomington, IN: iUniverse LLC.

Wardell, D., Kagel, S., & Anselme, L. (2014b). Healing touch through the life continuum: Clinical application; Healing touch for specific health care issues. In D. Wardell, S. Kagel, & L. Anselme (Eds.), *Healing touch: Enhancing life through energy therapy* (pp. 211–308). Bloomington, IN: iUniverse LLC.

Wardell, D. W., Rintala, D., & Tan, G. (2008). Study descriptions of healing touch with veterans experiencing chronic neuropathic pain from spinal cord injury. *Explore: The Journal of Science & Healing, 4*(3), 187–195.

Wardell, D. W., & Weymouth, K. F. (2004). Review of studies of healing touch. *Journal of Nursing Scholarship, 36*(2), 147–154.

Watson, J. (1985). *Nursing: The philosophy and science of caring.* Boulder, CO: Associated University Press.

Welcher, B., & Kish, J. (2001). Reducing pain and anxiety through healing touch. *Healing Touch Newsletter, 1*(3), 19

Weymouth, K., & Sandberg-Lewis, S. (2000). Comparing the efficacy of healing touch and chiropractic adjustment in treating chronic low back pain: A pilot study. *Healing Touch Newsletter, 00*(3), 7–8.

Wilkinson, D., Knox, P., Chatman, J., Johnson, T., Barbour, N., Myles, Y., & Reel, A. (2002). The clinical effectiveness of healing touch. *Journal of Alternative and Complementary Medicine, 8*(1), 33–47.

Wong, J., Ghiasuddin, A., Kimata, C., & Patelesio, B. (2012). The psychosocial and hematological impact of healing touch on pediatric oncology patients: A randomized, prospective intervention study. In M. Megel, J. G. Anderson, D. Lu, & N. Strybol (Eds.), *Healing touch research survey* (14th ed., pp. 30–37). Lakewood, CO: Healing Touch International.

Ziembroski, J., Gilbert, N., Bossarte, R., & Guldbery, G. (2003). Healing touch and hospice care: Examining outcomes at the end of life. *Alternative and Complementary Therapies, 9*(3), 146–151.

Zimmer, M. H., Bogenschutz, L., Meier, M. E., & Rolf, W. G. (2009). Effect of healing touch on children's pain and comfort in the postoperative period [Abstract]. *Alternative Therapies in Health and Medicine, 15*(3), S186.

Reiki

Debbie Ringdahl

The Reiki principles:

- Just for today, I will live in the attitude of gratitude.
- Just for today, I will not worry.
- Just for today, I will not be angry.
- Just for today, I will do my work honestly.
- Just for today, I will show love and respect for every living being. (Miles, 2006)

Reiki is an energy-healing method that can be used as an integrative therapy for a broad range of acute and chronic health problems. Increasingly, it is gaining acceptance as an adjunct to the management of chronic conditions: pain management, oncology, hospice and palliative care, and stress reduction. In 2017, the Center for Reiki Research identified 76 hospitals, medical clinics, and hospice programs where Reiki was offered as part of the standard practice. It is possible that the number of hospitals using Reiki is underreported. For instance, this author notes that only one of six area healthcare facilities using Reiki in the metropolitan Minneapolis—St. Paul is listed, suggesting a greater usage of Reiki than these numbers indicate. According to the American Hospital Association, in 2007, 15% of, or over 800 American, hospitals offered Reiki as part of hospital services (Center for Reiki Research, 2017b).

The 2010 Complementary and Alternative Medicine Survey of Hospitals (Ananth, 2011) reported that Reiki and therapeutic touch (TT) were offered in 21% of inpatient settings surveyed. A 2007 national survey found that 1.2 million adults and 161,000 children received one or more energy-healing sessions such as Reiki in the previous year (Barnes, Bloom, & Nahin, 2008). (The 2012 National Health Interview Survey did not collect data on energy therapies but focused on dietary supplements, deep breathing, meditation, chiropractic or osteopathic manipulation, yoga, tai chi, and qigong.)

According to the National Center for Complementary and Integrative Health (NCCIH, 2017a), Reiki falls into the subgroup of mind and body practices, a diverse group of modalities or techniques that can be practiced or taught by a trained practitioner or teacher. The NCCIH defines *Reiki* as "a *complementary health approach* in which practitioners place their hands lightly on or just above a person, with the goal of facilitating the person's own healing response." (NCCIH, 2017). Reiki, TT, and Healing Touch (HT) are all therapies that are used to support the healing process. Although each has its own history, techniques, and practice standards, they share many similarities. All three traditions include the fundamental assumption that a universal life force sustains all living organisms (Ringdahl, 2014), that human beings have an energetic and spiritual dimension that is a part of the healing process, and that positive energetic influences exist in human interactions (Engebretson & Wardell, 2012).The focus is on balancing the total energies of a person and stimulating the body's own natural healing ability, rather than on the treating specific physical diseases (Hover-Kramer, 2011b; Ringdahl; 2014; Senderovich et al., 2016). The common thread that exists among these modalities lies in their capacity to reduce stress, promote relaxation, and mitigate pain. All three of these energy practices have been introduced into clinical care over the past few decades, representing a renewed interest in the therapeutic use of intentional touch in clinical practice. An additional important consideration is the high safety profile that exists with energy-healing practices. In their exploration of the use of Reiki in a dialysis unit, Ferraresi et al. (2013) suggest that healthcare providers should consider not only efficacy, but also side effects, availability, cost, and patient request when evaluating Reiki (and other integrative modalities) for pain management.

A Reiki practitioner does not need to be prepared as a healthcare practitioner; however, nurses, physical therapists, massage therapists, and physicians who practice Reiki may have greater access and acceptability within the healthcare system in performing hands-on treatments. In addition, Reiki practice by nurses supports a high-touch practice model in a high-tech practice environment. The Institute of Medicine (IOM) 2009 Summit on Integrative Medicine and the Health of the Public identified that empathy and compassion enhanced care and improved outcomes with grade A evidence (IOM, 2010). Although this evidence is not specific to physical touch, research suggests that recipients of touch therapies frequently experience an integration of mind, body, and spirit that promotes feelings of wellbeing (Engebretson & Wardell, 2012). Watson's conceptualization of the reciprocal nature of caring also supports the value of Reiki touch in providing nursing care (Watson, 2011).

In addition to Reiki's origins as an oral tradition, political and cultural events. Reiki began with an oral tradition and relied on practitioners to pass on the method developed by the founder, Usui. Reiki historians generally agree that its roots may stem from hands-on healing techniques that were used in Tibet or India more than 2,000 years ago. Reiki emerged in modern times around 1900 through the work of a Japanese businessman and practitioner of Tendai Buddhism, Mikao Usui (Miles, 2006). Usui had a transformative experience that resulted in the development of Reiki and this resulted in the precise format he established for administering Reiki. One of Dr. Usui's students, Chujiro Hayashi, wrote down the hand positions and suggested ways of using them for various ailments (Rand, 2000). Hawayo Takata is credited with the spread of Reiki in the Americas and Europe. Reiki is now practiced throughout North and South America, Europe, New Zealand, Australia, and other parts of the world (Oschman, 2016), including Japan.

In recent years, several additional branches of Reiki have developed: Karuna Reiki, Holy Fire Reiki (ICRT, 2017b), Seichem Reiki (Reiki and Seichem Association, 2017), and Temari Reiki (Townsend, 2013). There are currently no uniform standards in Reiki education, either at the national or international level. Because of the noninvasive nature of the treatments, this does not present problems in Reiki hands-on practice but may contribute to variable levels of professionalism among practitioners. This lack of standardization may also pose problems when working to develop practice standards for integration of Reiki into the conventional healthcare system.

DEFINITION

The word *Reiki* is composed of two Japanese words—*rei* and *ki*. *Rei* is usually translated as "universal," although some authors suggest that it also has a deeper connotation of "all-knowing spiritual consciousness." *Ki* refers to the life force energy that flows throughout all living things, known in certain other parts of the world as *chi*, *prana*, or *mana*. When *ki* energy is unrestricted, there is thought to be less susceptibility to illness or imbalances of mind, body, or spirit (Rand, 2000). In its combined form, the word *Reiki* is taken to mean "spiritually guided life force" energy or "universal life force energy."

The mind–body component of Reiki healing is evidenced in the underlying belief that the deepest level of healing occurs through the spirit. The emphasis is on healing, not cure, which is believed to occur by Reiki energy connecting individuals to their own innate spiritual wisdom and "highest good." Reiki is considered a nondirective healing tradition: Reiki energy flows through, but is not directed by, the practitioner, leaving the healing component to the individual receiving the treatment. Reiki is not only a healing technique, but also a philosophy of living that acknowledges mind–body–spirit unity and human connectedness to all things.

The ability to practice Reiki is transmitted in stages directly from teacher to student via initiations called *attunements*. This attunement process differentiates Reiki from other hands-on healing methods. During attunements, teachers open the students' energy channels by using specific visual symbols that were revealed to Dr. Usui. There are three degrees of attunement preparatory to achieving the status of Master Teacher, at which stage the practitioner is considered fully open to the flow of universal life force energy. By tradition, the Usui Reiki symbols and their Japanese names are confidential. This arises from the sacred nature of the techniques rather than from proprietary motives; the symbols are believed not to convey Reiki energy if used by noninitiates.

Level I Reiki is taught as a hands-on technique that includes basic information about Reiki history, application, principles, and hand positions. At level II, students are taught symbols that allow the transfer of energy through space and time, also known as *absentee* or *distance healing*. The higher vibration of energy available at level II is considered to work at a deeper level of healing and with greater intuitive awareness. Level III, or the mastery level, was traditionally achieved through an apprenticeship with a Reiki master and includes more in-depth study of Reiki practice and teaching. Increasingly, the mastery level is achieved through 3- to 5-day workshops. At all levels, Reiki skill develops through years of committed practice.

SCIENTIFIC BASIS

Biofield science is an emerging field of study that views energy as a part of a complex system that has the capacity to influence the whole system. According to Rubik, Muehsam, Hammerschlag, and Jain (2015), "The biofield or biological field, a complex organizing energy field engaged in the generation, maintenance, and regulation of biological homeodynamics, is a useful concept that provides the rudiments of a scientific foundation for energy medicine and thereby advances the research and practice of it" (p. 8). Reiki as an energy-healing tradition is consistent with a human biofield modality. Biofield theory suggests that complex interactions involving energy-healing modalities may be mediated by forces and processes yet to be discovered and understood. As other examples in science and medicine have revealed, theories once viewed as implausible over time become accepted through research and science (Kafatos et al., 2015).

Researchers have attempted to study the biological effects of biofields on biomolecules, in vitro cells, bacteria, plants, and animals, as well as the clinical effects on hemoglobin, immune functioning, and wound healing (Movaffaghi & Farsi, 2009). There is increasing evidence that living systems are sensitive to bioinformation and that biofield therapies can influence diverse cellular and biological systems (Bowden, Goddard, & Gruzelier, 2010). The notion that cellular and molecular changes occur within the energy spectrum of biofields is congruent with the view that subtle energy shifts may manifest as a physiological cause or effect and also play a role in intercellular and intracellular communication (Movaffaghi & Farsi, 2009). Morse and Beem (2011) reported a case with an increase in absolute neutrophil count following Reiki, resulting in toleration of interferon and subsequent clearance of hepatitis C virus.

There have also been studies focused on identifying the physical properties of biofields to determine potential mechanisms of action (Movaffaghi & Farsi, 2009). An emerging body of evidence confirms the existence of energy fields and suggests new ways of measuring energy, although these are not specific to Reiki. Traditional electrical measurements such as electrocardiograms and electroencephalograms can now be supplemented by biomagnetic field mapping to obtain more accurate information about the human condition. Electromagnetic information has been used to both diagnose and treat disease (Oschman, 2016).

Studies conducted to ascertain the impact of biofields on Reiki practitioners has been inconclusive. Baldwin, Rand, and Schwartz (2013) used a superconducting quantum interference device (SQUID) to measure the electromagnetic field from the hands and heart of three Reiki masters and four volunteers using Reiki on the self and were unable to demonstrate consistent high-intensity magnetic fields. Superconducting quantum interference devices have been used to show the effect of disease on the magnetic field of the body, and pulsating magnetic fields have been used to improve healing (Oschman, 2016). Recent advances in bioelectromagnetics suggest that disturbances in the electromagnetic parts of the biofield can significantly impact health processes (Muehsam, Chevalier, Barsotti, & Gurfein, 2015).

A Reiki session commonly puts the recipient's body into a state of relaxation, presumably by downregulating autonomic nervous system tone, which lowers blood pressure and relieves tension and anxiety (Meland, 2009). Mackay, Hansen, and McFarlane (2004) concluded that Reiki has some effect on the autonomic nervous system by comparing heart rate, cardiac vagal tone, blood pressure, cardiac sensitivity to baroreceptors, and breathing activity among three groups of subjects: those resting, receiving Reiki, or receiving placebo Reiki. Friedman, Burg, Miles, Lee, and Lampert (2010) found an increase in high-frequency heart rate variability in patients recovering from acute coronary syndrome who received Reiki compared with those listening to music or resting. Kerr, Wasserman and Moore (2007) theorized that sensory reorganization is the mechanism for pain and stress reduction that occurs with touch-healing therapies. To date, the strongest support for the measurable physiological effect of Reiki was demonstrated in an animal model (Baldwin, Wagers, & Schwartz, 2008).

Methodological problems, which hinder the interpretation of results, have been identified in a number of studies. Although case studies and anecdotal examples have been relatively consistent in reporting positive responses to Reiki treatments, they do not represent the scientific rigor that is demanded within an evidence-based healthcare system. Efforts to strengthen research design and mitigate the confounding effects of human touch have led to the development of sham or placebo Reiki (Mansour, Beuche, Laing, Leis, & Nurse, 1999), now frequently incorporated into randomized controlled trials (RCTs).

Rogers's Science of Unitary Human Beings has been used as a theoretical framework for understanding the experience of Reiki. This theory connects scientific principles of energy as matter to the human energy field and energetic interconnections that occur in the environment (Ring, 2009). These concepts are similar to those of experts who suggest that rather than identifying the unique characteristics of each subtle energy field, we should view biofield theory as a unifying concept for understanding the wide range of forces that influence health and well-being on the physical, emotional, social, and spiritual levels (Kreitzer & Saper, 2015).

INTERVENTION

The Reiki practitioner acts as a conduit for this healing-intended energy to the self or others. In this section, we discuss the parameters used by Reiki practitioners, specific guidelines for conducting a Reiki session, and physiological and psychological effectiveness.

Technique

A level I Reiki practitioner uses a series of 12 to 15 hand positions for a full session and six to seven hand positions for a seated session (see Exhibit 24.1). A level II Reiki practitioner also uses hand positions but may use various Reiki symbols to focus the *ki* energy or perform distance healings. If touch is contraindicated for any reason, the hands can be held 1 to 4 inches above the body. A full Reiki session usually lasts 45 to 90 minutes, and a seated session usually lasts 15 to 20 minutes. Reiki practitioners, especially if they are nurses working in a clinical setting, often do not have the luxury of providing a full session. At such times, shorter and more targeted treatments may be offered for specific purposes. In *The Original Reiki Handbook of Dr. Mikao Usui* (Petter, 1999), the use of particular hand positions is recommended for addressing specific health problems. Although Reiki practitioners often provide Reiki sessions to individuals with specific health problems, Reiki practice is not intended to treat a health condition but rather support balance restoration.

Exhibit 24.1 Reiki Seated Session

(Each hand position is held for approximately 2–3 minutes)

1. General approach: Use touch therapy competencies: apply hands for approximately 2–3 minutes of light touch in each hand position; vary positions and duration based on individual needs
2. Hands on shoulders (introduction to light touch)
3. One hand on forehead, one hand on upper nape of neck
4. One hand on chest, other hand on upper back
5. One hand around each ankle
6. Hands on shoulders (conclusion to light touch)

One of the hallmarks of Reiki practice is its relative simplicity. In Mikao Usui's words, "Everyone can learn and practice Reiki" (Lubeck, Petter, & Rand, 2001). Reiki energy flows through the hands without using cognitive, emotional, or spiritual skills. The attunement process provides access to the energy without requiring ongoing practice or conscious intention. This makes Reiki particularly easy to learn and simple to use. Potter (2003) compared her experience with TT after receiving a level I attunement. She found that her work became less directive and the effort to stay centered was no longer a concern.

Guidelines for a Hands-On Reiki Session

The recipient may sit or lie down, and either method is suitable for Reiki practice. Because Reiki tends to be very relaxing, it is often preferable to lie down, but a seated session may be more practical if a table or bed is not available. Patients typically remain clothed. A massage table or hospital bed for a full session is ideal, providing comfort for both patient and practitioner. After practitioners center themselves and establish the intent to heal with Reiki, the energy flows automatically from their hands without cognitive effort. The hands rest gently on the person's body, with the fingers touching so that each hand functions as a unit. Reiki can also be provided with the hands 2 to 3 inches off the body. The sequence of hand positions may vary but generally includes all seven major chakras and the endocrine glands. The success of a Reiki treatment does not depend on the use of certain hand positions, for the *ki* energy goes where it is needed.

In clinical practice, four basic principles of physical touch should be considered: (a) Ask permission to touch, (b) provide basic information about what you will be doing, (c) describe anticipated benefits and range of outcomes, and (d) ensure the right to decline or discontinue receiving physical touch. Standards of practice have been developed by several professional Reiki organizations and include ethics related to intention, healing environment, healing principles, and the nondiagnostic nature of the work (International Association of Reiki Professionals [IARP], 2017; ICRT, 2017a). The American Holistic Nursing Association and American Nurses Association (2013) developed scope and standards of practice for holistic nursing, but these are not specific to any one integrative therapy. In the book *Creating Healing Relationships: Professional Standards for Energy Therapy*

Exhibit 24.2 Reiki Practice Competencies

- Ask permission to touch before any encounter.
- Provide basic information about what you will be doing, including use of light touch, basic hand positions, and length of session.
- Describe the areas of the body you will be touching and what sensations the patient may experience. Ask whether there are areas they would prefer not to be touched.
- Describe anticipated benefits and range of outcomes.
- Let them know you will stop at any time. Ask whether they prefer to be wakened if they fall asleep.
- Create an environment that promotes feelings of safety. If possible, ensure privacy. In a hospital setting, consider putting a sign on the door asking to not be disturbed.
- Clearly communicate that Reiki practice is not diagnostic or used to treat specific disease conditions.

Practitioners, Hover-Kramer (2011a) describes parameters for level of competence, record keeping, professional responsibility, boundaries, confidentiality, marketing, and informed consent. Although Reiki is not considered a religious practice, some believe that a spiritual consent form should be used to protect individual cultural, spiritual, and religious beliefs/practices (Arvonio, 2014). General competencies for Reiki practice are provided in Exhibit 24.2.

In an effort to provide guidelines to ensure safety and protection of the public using integrative therapies, a diverse group of complementary and alternative providers, healthcare providers, ethicists, legal consultants, health policy specialists, and consumers developed ethical guidelines for boundaries of touch in the practice of complementary medicine (Schiff et al., 2010). They provided guiding principles and ethical rules addressing behavior and language regarding inappropriate touch and exposure, as well as right of the client to discontinue treatment.

As more healthcare institutions offer complementary therapies, policies and guidelines must be developed that provide standards for implementation. Reiki practice at a Magnet®-designated facility in Pennsylvania requires evidence of competency in practice and adherence to written hospital policy when administering Reiki (Kryak & Vitale, 2011). A protocol for Reiki use in the operating room was developed at a hospital in New Hampshire following a request to have a Reiki practitioner be present during surgery (Sawyer, 1998). This author developed a Reiki protocol for use by nurses providing care to chemotherapy patients (Ringdahl, 2008). A. Vitale (2014) provides an outline for starting a Reiki program in a healthcare facility using a business model approach; she discusses institutional congruence, business plan development, and Reiki program start-up.

Measurement of Outcomes

Recipients' subjective feelings during a Reiki session are not considered indications of effectiveness. Patients may feel sensations similar to those of the practitioner, but they may also feel nothing. Sensations may include heat, cold, numbness, involuntary muscle twitching, heaviness, buoyancy, trembling, throbbing, static electricity, tingling, color, and heightened or decreased awareness of sound (Engebretson & Wardell, 2002). It is not uncommon for clients to fall asleep during a treatment, with reports of increased relaxation, peacefulness, and reconnection to their center. These subjective feelings are supported in research studies that demonstrate physiological and psychological evidence of stress reduction following a Reiki session (Bowden et al., 2010; Bukowski, 2015; Caitlin & Taylor-Ford, 2011).

Reiki research outcomes are focused primarily on reducing stress and pain, increasing relaxation and an overall sense of well-being, particularly in the area of chronic disease and pain management. Application of Reiki for anxiety and/or pain management among patients with cancer, undergoing rehabilitation, and recovering from surgery has been the focus of several studies and literature reviews (Anderson & Taylor, 2012; Birocco et al., 2012; Demir, Can, & Celek, 2013; Fleisher et al., 2014; Hulse, Stuart-Shor, & Russo, 2010; Marcus, Blazek-O'Neill, & Kopar, 2012; Midilli & Eser, 2015; Midilli & Gunduzoglu, 2016; Notte, Fazzini, & Mooney, 2016; Potter, 2013).

Achieving institutional approval for Reiki use requires both evidence of safety and effectiveness and the development of policies or clinical guidelines. Five systematic reviews on Reiki research representing 24 studies and nine RCTs resulted in the following: Four studies demonstrated pain reduction, two studies showed decreased depression and anxiety, and one study showed decreased fatigue and quality of life among cancer patients (Jain & Mills, 2010; vander-Vaart, Gijsen, de Wildt, & Koren, 2009). A literature review of randomized trials with effect size calculations examined seven studies and found that the majority achieved statistical significance or near-significance for pain and/or anxiety (Thrane & Cohen, 2014). A literature review examining the effects of energy healing on pain found that use of energy healing (Reiki, TT, and HT) either decreased the amount of pain medications or increased the time span between doses of narcotic analgesics (Fazzino, Griffin, McNulty, & Fitzpatrick, 2010). The variation in populations and outcomes measured serves to reinforce the notion that Reiki may have application among populations with diverse health needs. This author served as coinvestigator in a study testing the feasibility, acceptability, and safety of Reiki touch for premature infants (Duckett, 2008), a new area of Reiki application.

Physiological outcome measures examined in other studies involving touch, such as hematological tests, blood pressure and heart rate, bioelectric measures, wound-healing rate, inhibition of harmful microorganisms, and body temperature changes, are also appropriate for Reiki. Psychological measures, including perceived pain, cognitive function, memory, and levels of anxiety, depression, or hostility, are equally important.

Although both hands-on and distance healing are forms of energy healing, the presence of touch has the capacity to confound the research results, as all touch may have some healing properties. An overview of the scientific evidence on distant healing therapies identified both methodological limitations and positive outcomes meriting further study (Hammerschlag, Marx, & Aickin, 2014; Radin, Schlitz, & Bauer, 2015).

A Cochrane review conducted to evaluate the efficacy of Reiki for depression and anxiety described the results of three RCTs (Joyce & Herbison, 2015); none had sufficient evidence to demonstrate a positive or negative effect on anxiety and depression. It has also been speculated that energy-healing impacts outcomes in a way that is difficult to measure. "The phenomenon of energy has a qualitative nature and can never be completely knowable, measurable, or ultimately predictable" (Todaro-Franceschi, 2009, p. 135). Many research models are not complex enough to capture the subjective experience of a Reiki session. Using a qualitative research design, Engebretson and Wardell found that participants had a diverse and descriptive language that accompanied their experience, creating a more complete picture of the subjective experience of a Reiki session (Engebretson & Wardell, 2002). A secondary qualitative analysis of this data validated the taxonomy of spiritual experiences that emerged during a Reiki session (Engebretson & Wardell, 2012). Using a qualitative approach to describe Reiki experiences in women who have cancer, Kirshbaum, Stead, and Bartys (2016) demonstrated that Reiki had multiple positive effects that could significantly impact quality of life for this population.

PRECAUTIONS

No serious adverse effects of Reiki treatments have been published. Some patients, however, may experience emotional release that may be uncomfortable or disturbing. Therefore, practitioners must be prepared to provide assistance and appropriate referrals if emotional distress persists. Moreover, some individuals may dislike being touched. Practitioners can avoid this discomfort by assessing the person's level of comfort with touch and taking into account gender and cultural considerations. Few patients who are fully informed object to the therapy; this is true even among vulnerable populations such as victims of torture (Kennedy, 2001) or those with long-term mental health problems (Collinge, Wentworth, & Sabo, 2005), in whom responses to Reiki have been favorable.

USES

An increasing body of literature supports the use of Reiki as a stress-reduction and relaxation technique. Therapies that contribute to a relaxation response have the potential for enhancing overall well-being and reducing the physiological effects of stress. The range of potential practical applications with patients is broad and depends on the setting. Reiki has been used for preoperative and postoperative patients; in oncology, hospice, and palliative care; for pain management, rehabilitation and long-term care; for stress and anxiety reduction; for self-care and stress reduction for healthcare providers; and for pediatric symptom management. In addition, this author has anecdotal evidence and experience working with nursing students who practice Reiki in a variety of specialty settings, including pediatric and adult bone marrow transplant units, labor and delivery suites, emergency departments, chemotherapy infusion units, chemical dependency inpatient units, Huntington's chorea units, and veteran's health facilities.

Energy touch therapies are considered to be within the scope of nursing practice and touch is recognized in the Nursing Interventions Classification (NIC) Code (Bulechek, Butcher, Dochterman, & Wagner, 2012). In the past 15 years, many professional organizations and state boards of nursing have developed statements that provide parameters for integrative therapy use by nurses, reinforcing the notion that integrative nursing care is often accompanied by the use of specific complementary modalities. Several authors have documented the effective use of Reiki in the direct provision of nursing care (Ringdahl, 2008; Ringdahl & Voss, 2016). A qualitative research study conducted to provide a theoretical construct for Reiki concluded that Reiki was congruent with nursing modalities (Ring, 2009). Bremner, Bennett, and Chambers (2014) described a project designed to introduce nursing students to a more holistic care model through engagement in a nurse-managed community clinic by assessing need and evaluating Reiki outcomes.

Increased evidence of efficacy and support for integrative nursing practice supports a shift to greater nursing engagement in Reiki practice, including informal application in all clinical encounters (Natale, 2010). The common theme described in many Reiki programs is the benefit of Reiki for pain relief, stress and anxiety reduction, and promoting relaxation (Hahn, Reilly, & Buchanan, 2014).

Within hospitals, the introduction of Reiki into patient care has been initiated primarily through volunteers (Fleisher et al., 2014; Hahn et al. (2014); however, increasingly, there is support for embedding these modalities into direct care through educational programs for healthcare providers (Clark, 2013; Kryak & Vitale, 2011; Ringdahl, 2008). Access to Reiki within a hospital setting may also exist through an integrative health team that provides a variety of services through a nurse and physician referral system that includes Reiki. Ambulatory care models for integrative therapies exist primarily through contracting with complementary and alternative medicine (CAM) practitioners to provide specific services. These services may exist within an integrative care clinic that has a specialty focus, such as oncology or women's health. Exhibit 24.3 provides a list of populations/settings in which Reiki has been used. In a biomedical treatment setting, Reiki is best seen as a complementary healing modality, whereas in other circumstances it can either be used alone or with other approaches.

Several recent studies have been conducted on the use of Reiki with children, focusing on symptom management (Bukowski & Berardi, 2014; Kundu, Lin, Oron, & Doorenbos, 2014; Thrane, Maurer, Ren, Danford, & Cohen, 2016). The use of Reiki among parent caregivers has potential for mitigating parental stress by reducing their child's stress. A recent pilot program demonstrated that teaching Reiki to caregivers of hospitalized pediatric patients improved patient comfort, provided relaxation, reduced pain and assisted the caregivers in becoming active participants in their child's care. A participation rate of 94.4% was achieved by offering shorter and more frequent classes, as well as adapting classes to take place in their child's room (Kundu, Dolan-Oves, Dimmers, Towle, & Doorenbos, 2013). A similar format was used by the author in offering a Reiki class to parents of children on a pediatric bone marrow transplant unit, demonstrating that Reiki has capacity to reduce stress for both child and caregivers in the hospital and during recovery at home (see Exhibit 24.4). Another pilot study using Reiki for symptom management for children receiving palliative care showed a decrease in pain, anxiety, heart, and respiratory rates following two Reiki sessions received at home (Thrane et al., 2016). A case report of a 9-year old girl with a history of several chronic conditions demonstrated that twice-weekly Reiki sessions over a period of

Exhibit 24.3 Applications for Reiki in Clinical Settings

Application	Reference
Perioperative and procedural support	Ferraresi et al. (2013); Hulse et al. (2010); Midilli and Eser (2015); Midilli and Gunduzoglu (2016); Notte et al. (2016); Toms (2011); VanderVaart et al. (2011)
Hospice and palliative care	Burden, Herron-Marx, and Clifford (2005); Hemming and Maher (2005)
Supporting oncology patients	Anderson and Taylor (2012); Birocco et al. (2012); Bossi, Ott, and DeCristofaro (2008); Caitlin and Taylor-Ford (2011); Coakley and Barron (2012); Demir et al. (2013); DiScipio (2016); Kirshbaum et al. (2016); Marcus et al. (2012); Potter (2013)
Pain management	Fazzino et al. (2010); Gillispie, Gillipsie, and Stevens (2007); Lee, Pittler, and Ernst (2008); Park, McCaffrey, Dunn, and Goodman, (2011)
Decreasing depression and/or anxiety and stress levels	Shore (2004); Thrane and Cohen (2014)
Enhancing immune function	Bowden et al. (2010)
Long-term care and rehabilitation	Crawford, Leaver, and Mahoney (2006); Meland (2009); Richeson et al. (2010); Swann, (2009)
Improving hematological measures	Morse and Beem (2011)
Cardiovascular disease management	Anderson and Taylor (2011)
Fibromyalgia	Assefi, Bogart, Goldberg, and Buchwald (2008)
Self-care and stress reduction for healthcare providers	Bukowski (2015); Cuneo et al. (2011); Natale (2010); Rosada, Rubik, Mainguy, Plummer, and Mehl-Medrona (2015)
Pediatric use	Bukowski and Berardi (2014); Kundu et al. (2014); Thrane et al. (2016).
Reiki training programs	Clark (2013); Fleisher et al. (2014); Hahn et al. (2014); Kundu et al. (2013); Ringdahl and Voss (2016); A. Vitale (2014).
Nursing education	Bremner et al. (2014); Clark (2013)

Exhibit 24.4 Teaching Reiki to Parents in a Pediatric Bone Marrow Transplant Unit

Following a comprehensive needs assessment, a pilot program was designed to teach the parent/family caregivers of pediatric bone marrow transplant patients how to practice Reiki. Reiki was selected because the integrative nurse clinician identified significant symptom relief when using Reiki on these patients and the parents identified that learning relaxation techniques would be the most helpful additional support provided during their child's hospitalization. The Reiki curriculum was redesigned to meet the unique needs of this group. Many significant outcomes were achieved: (a) It was readily apparent that each attendee experienced an internal shift in personal well-being throughout the 3 weeks. (b) Many parents reported using Reiki on themselves for their own stress management and to aid in falling asleep. (c) Furthermore, the intervention seemed to give parents permission to take time for themselves but also provided a meaningful way to connect with their child (Ringdahl & Voss, 2016).

---

6 weeks reduced stress in both mother and child and improved the child's sleep (Bukowski & Berardi, 2014).

Self-Treatment and Practitioner Benefits

One of the more unique features of Reiki therapy is its capacity for self-use. Reiki practitioners can place their hands on the head, abdomen, chest, or other areas of the body, reducing pain and/or increasing a sense of relaxation. A recent study conducted among college students demonstrated that after 20 weeks of performing self-reiki twice a week, there was a significant reduction in stress levels (Bukowski, 2015). The concepts of empowerment and self-treatment have particular value when considering chronic health problems. For some Reiki practitioners, teaching level I Reiki provides the clients with a greater sense of control over some of their health problems, including pain management and stress reduction. This author teaches levels I and II to patients with a variety of health problems, including fibromyalgia, mood disorders, cancer, and neurological problems such as advanced amyotrophic lateral sclerosis (ALS). Clients with physical limitations may gain particular benefits from learning level II, or distance healing.

In addition, those using Reiki receive the benefits of the therapies while performing them on patients. Reiki practitioners report feeling energized, relaxed, and/or more centered after performing a Reiki treatment. Research on Reiki use by nurses has demonstrated positive effects on the practitioner, including greater job satisfaction and increase in caring behaviors (Brathovde, 2006). The increased sense of well-being that occurs when giving and receiving Reiki may influence the patient–nurse relationship and create a less stressful work environment.

Reiki may also be used for healthcare provider self-care, with the potential for reducing stress. Several research studies have shown beneficial effects of Reiki for nurses and other healthcare providers in positively influencing well-being, quality of care, stress reduction (Cuneo et al., 2011), and burnout.

CULTURAL APPLICATIONS

Energy and touch therapies are found in the health traditions of most cultures. Like Reiki, *johre* originated in Japan. It is a spirituality-based energy modality that aims to release negativity from the individual's spiritual self (Brooks, Schwartz, Reece, & Nangle, 2006). *Anagami* healing practices include massage, bonesetting, and curing of sprains (Joshi, 2004).

Although healthcare workers may find that some of the energy and healing practices used in non-Western cultures differ greatly from Western health practices and even from the more frequently used complementary therapies, respecting the person's belief in these practices is important in the healing process.

Sidebar 24.1 details the current use of Reiki in Japan, the country in which the therapy originated.

FUTURE RESEARCH

The trajectory of Reiki research has enjoyed a significant acceleration within the past 15 years and researchers are developing more improved methodology and research designs. The Center for Reiki Research website and The Touchstone Process provide a clearinghouse for disseminating current Reiki research information for practitioners and researchers. The Touchstone Project has a process for systematically analyzing published, peer-reviewed studies of Reiki and has results from 69 studies accessible online, with the majority of

SIDEBAR 24.1 REIKI PRACTICE IN JAPAN

Ikuko Ebihara

Reiki was started in Japan by Dr. Mikao Usui. The practice was forgotten after World War II until it was imported back from abroad in the 1990s. The traditional Usui Reiki has been regaining popularity in Japan since then, but acceptance has been slow.

People in Japan find Reiki practitioners and masters by word of mouth and Internet search. The common reason for seeking Reiki practice is to restore mind and body balance; it is not for seeking remedies for physical discomfort. Reiki does not have any national standards; it is not recognized as a medical or physiotherapeutic practice.

There are numerous traditional medicines in Japan, but only a limited number of therapies are nationally recognized. Judo therapies, acupuncture, and moxibustion are examples of nationally recognized practices; they have national certification systems. Insurance and reimbursement are available for such therapies; however, even though they are reimbursable, they are not usually provided at hospitals. Western medicine and Japanese traditional medicines are governed by different regulations. Patients may visit both care providers. In Japan, as in most Western countries, Western and alternative practices are rarely provided by the same healthcare organizations.

studies conducted since 2010 (Center for Reiki Research, 2017). Analysis of these studies has generated data supporting Reiki as a noninvasive tool for healing at the physical and nonphysical levels, particularly in alleviating pain, depression, and anxiety.

However, most published research on Reiki has been conducted with small, nonrandom convenience samples, raising questions about the validity and generalizability of findings. Outcomes for touch therapies such as Reiki are typically not disease specific and establishing an appropriate time frame for detecting effect is variable (Engebretson & Wardell, 2007). Further experiments are required with greater numbers of subjects to provide the statistical power necessary for meaningful interpretation (Baldwin et al., 2010).

New models of research that enlarge the definition of outcomes need to be explored. Clinical evaluation of Reiki represents a challenge using current standards of assessment. Combining subjective and physiological measures in such research studies will allow broader assessment of the effects of Reiki. Because the goals of Reiki may be broader than symptom relief and include concepts of physiological and psychological balance, qualitative studies that can address values and meaning are also important, as evidenced in the research by Engebretson and Wardell (2002).

Forgues (2009) reviewed key methodological issues that exist in energy-based therapy (EBT) research studies, including the challenges in verification of effectiveness and use of appropriate research methodology. There remains ongoing debate among researchers about whether the current scientific research model works with EBT research and whether all therapies should be held to the same standard. RCTs are considered the current gold standard of research, and EBT integration into clinical practice requires this level of rigorous research. An analysis grid was developed by Forgues (2009) to assess methodological quality, EBT specificity, and treatment effectiveness.

A. T. Vitale (2007) identified limitations in research design and the use of linear research methods as problematic in conducting Reiki research. Current outcome measures may not accurately reflect or measure all aspects of a Reiki treatment. Lack of standardization in Reiki practice also impacts reliability and validity. Some research studies do not identify all components of the Reiki intervention used, including length of treatment, type of treatment, or level/training of the Reiki practitioner. There is a need to develop research designs that consider subtler and longer lasting outcomes than those that have typically been used. If energy treatment works on a different level from the conventional medical model, the results may not be as dramatic and may require larger groups and a longer treatment period to show a positive outcome. Little research has explored the spiritual dimension of Reiki practice, and yet recipients of a Reiki session often describe feelings associated with spiritual well-being (Engebretson & Wardell, 2012).

Within a clinical setting, Reiki practice has potential for (a) reducing stress and anxiety, (b) promoting health and well-being, (c) promoting trust, (d) potentiating drug therapy, (e) reducing medication use and medication side effects, and (f) reducing recovery time. Reiki may have particular application for people suffering from chronic physical and mental health conditions. There is also the potential for reducing stress and burnout and promoting positive well-being and competency among both formal and informal caregivers. Only a few of these areas of Reiki practice have been explored in the research literature.

Suggested questions for future research include:

- What are the physiological and/or psychological effects of Reiki treatments for specific conditions when used alone or with other therapies?
- What is the best way to use Reiki in providing stress reduction for healthcare providers?
- Is the traditional gold standard of RCTs appropriate for evaluating Reiki?
- What populations would most benefit from learning Reiki as a stress-reduction strategy?
- How can Reiki be incorporated into nursing clinical practice?

WEBSITES

Additional information about Reiki can be obtained from the following websites.

- Center for Reiki Research
  (www.centerforreikiresearch.org)
- International Association of Reiki Professionals (IARP)
  (www.iarp.org)
- International Center for Reiki Training (ICRT)
  (www.reiki.org)
- Reiki online module, Taking Charge of Your Health, University of Minnesota Center for Spirituality and Healing
  (www.takingcharge.csh.umn.edu/explore-healing-practices/reiki)
- The Touchstone Process
  (www.centerforreikiresearch.org/RRTouchstone.aspx)

REFERENCES

American Holistic Nurses Association & American Nurses Association. (2013). *Holistic nursing: Scope and standards of practice* (2nd ed.). Silver Spring, MD. Retrieved from http://Nursebooks.org

Ananth, S. (2011). *2010 complementary and alternative medicine survey of hospitals.* Alexandria, VA: Samueli Institute.

Anderson, J. G., & Taylor, A. G. (2011). Biofield therapies in cardiovascular disease management: A brief review. *Holistic Nursing Practice, 25*(4), 199–204.

Anderson, J. G., & Taylor, A. G. (2012). Biofield therapies and cancer pain. *Clinical Journal of Oncology Nursing, 16*(1), 43–48.

Arvonio, M. (2014). Cultural competency, autonomy, and spiritual conflicts related to. Reiki/CAM therapies: Should patients be informed? *Linacre Quarterly, 81*(1), 47–56.

Assefi, N., Bogart, A., Goldberg, J., & Buchwald, D. (2008). Reiki for the treatment of fibromyalgia: A randomized controlled trial. *Journal of Alternative and Complementary Medicine, 14*(9), 1115–1122.

Baldwin, A. L., Rand, W. L., & Schwartz, G. E. (2013). Practicing Reiki does not appear to routinely produce high-intensity electromagnetic fields from the heart or hands of Reiki practitioners. *Journal of Alternative and Complementary Medicine, 19*(6), 518–526.

Baldwin, A. L., Vitale, A., Brownell, D., Scicisnski, J., Kearns, M., & Rand, W. (2010). The Touchstone Process: An ongoing critical evaluation of Reiki in the scientific literature. *Holistic Nursing Practice, 24*(5), 260–276.

Baldwin, A. L., Wagers, C., & Schwartz, G. E. (2008). Reiki improves heart rate homeostasis in laboratory rats. *Journal of Alternative and Complementary Medicine, 14*(4), 417–422.

Barnes, P. M., Bloom, B., & Nahin, R. (2008). Complementary and alternative medicine use among adults and children, United States, 2007. *CDC National Health Statistics Reports, 12*, 1–23.

Birocco, N., Guillame, C., Storto, S., Ritorto, G., Catino, C., Gir, N., … Ciuffreda, L. (2012). The effects of Reiki therapy on pain and anxiety in patients attending a day oncology and infusion services unit. *American Journal of Hospice and Palliative Care, 29*(4), 290–294.

Bossi, L. M., Ott, M. J., & DeCristofaro, S. (2008). Reiki as a clinical intervention in oncology nursing practice. *Clinical Journal of Oncology Nursing, 12*(3), 489–494.

Bowden, D., Goddard, L., & Gruzelier, J. (2010). A randomised controlled single-blind trial of the effects of Reiki and positive imagery on well-being and salivary cortisol. *Brain Research Bulletin, 81*, 66–72.

Bowden, D., Goddard, L., & Gruzelier, J. (2011) A randomised controlled single-blind trial of the efficacy of Reiki at benefitting mood and well-being. *Evidence-Based Complementary & Alternative Medicine, 381862*, 1–8.

Brathovde, A. (2006). A pilot study: Reiki for self-care and healthcare providers. *Holistic Nursing Practice, 20*(2), 95–101.

Bremner, M., Bennett, D., & Chambers, D. (2014). Integrating Reiki and community-engaged scholarship: An interdisciplinary educational innovation. *Journal of Nursing Education, 53*(9), 541–543.

Brooks, A. J., Schwartz, G., Reece, K., & Nangle, G. (2006). The effect of Johrei healing on substance abuse recovery: A pilot study. *Journal of Alternative and Complementary Medicine, 12*, 625–631.

Bukowski, E. (2015). The use of self-reiki for stress reduction and relaxation. *Journal of Integrative Medicine, 13*(5), 336–340.

Bukowski, E., & Berardi, B. (2014). Reiki brief report: Using Reiki to reduce stress levels in a nine-year-old child. *Explore: The Journal of Science & Healing, 10*(4), 253–255.

Bulechek, G., Butcher, H., Dochterman, J. M., & Wagner, C. (2012). *Nursing Interventions Classification (NIC)* (6th ed.). St. Louis, MO: Mosby.

Burden, B., Herron-Marx, S., & Clifford, C. (2005). The increasing use of Reiki as a complementary therapy in specialist palliative care. *International Journal of Palliative Care Nursing, 11*(5), 248–253.

Caitlin, A., & Taylor-Ford, R. L. (2011). Investigation of standard care versus sham Reiki placebo versus actual Reiki therapy to enhance comfort and well-being in a chemotherapy infusion center. *Oncology Nursing Forum, 38*(3), E212–E220.

Center for Reiki Research. (2017a). Retrieved from http://www.centerforreikiresearch.org

Center for Reiki Research. (2017b). *Reiki in hospitals.* Retrieved from http://www.centerforreikiresearch.org/HospitalList.aspx

Center for Reiki Research. (2017c). *Reiki research study summaries.* Retrieved from http://www.centerforreikiresearch.org/RRSummariesHome.aspx

Clark, C. (2013). An integral nursing education experience: Outcomes from a BSN Reiki course. *Holistic Nursing Practice, 27*(1), 13–22.

Coakley, A. B., & Barron, A. M. (2012). Energy therapies in oncology nursing. *Seminars in Oncology Nursing, 28*(1), 55–63.

Collinge, W., Wentworth, R., & Sabo, S. (2005). Integrating complementary therapies into community mental health practice: An exploration. *Journal of Alternative and Complementary Medicine, 11*, 569–574.

Crawford, S. E., Leaver, V. W., & Mahoney, S. D. (2006). Using Reiki to decrease memory and behavior problems in cognitive impairment and mild Alzheimer's disease. *Journal of Alternative and Complementary Medicine, 12*(9), 911–913.

Cuneo, C., Cooper, M., Drew, C., Naoum-Heffernan, C., Sherman, T., & Walz, K. (2011). The effect of Reiki on work-related stress of the registered nurse. *Journal of Holistic Nursing, 29*(1), 33–43.

Demir, M., Can, G., & Celek, E. (2013). Effect of Reiki on symptom management in oncology. *Asian Pacific Journal of Cancer Prevention, 16*(12), 4859–4862.

Diaz-Rodriquez, L., Arroyo-Morales, M., Cantarero-Villanueva, I., Fernandez-Lao, C., Polley, M., & Fernandez-de-las-Penas, C. (2011). The application of Reiki in nurses diagnosed with burnout syndrome has beneficial effects on concentration of salivary IgA and blood pressure. *Latin American Journal of Nursing, 19*(5), 1132–1138.

DiScipio, W. (2016). Perceived relaxation as a function of restorative yoga combined with Reiki for cancer survivors. *Complementary Therapies in Clinical Practice, 24*, 116–122.

Duckett, L. (2008). *Testing feasibility, acceptability, and safety of Reiki touch for premature infants.* Minneapolis: University of Minnesota IRB application.

Engebretson, J., & Wardell, D. (2002). Experience of a Reiki session. *Alternative Therapies, 8*(2), 48–53.

Engebretson, J., & Wardell, D. (2007). Energy-based modalities. *Nursing Clinics of North America, 42*, 243–259.

Engebretson, J., & Wardell, D. W. (2012). Energy therapies: Focus on spirituality. *Explore: The Journal of Science & Healing, 8*(6), 353–359.

Fazzino, D., Griffin, M., McNulty, R., & Fitzpatrick, J. (2010). Energy healing and pain: A review of the literature. *Holistic Nursing Practice, 24*(2), 79–88.

Ferraresi, M., Clari, R., Moro, I., Banino, E., Boero, E., Crosio, A., ... Piccoli, G. (2013). Reiki and related therapies in the dialysis ward: An evidence-based and ethical discussion to debate if these complementary and alternative medicines are welcomed or banned. *BMC Nephrology, 14*, 129.

Fleisher, K. A, Mackenzie. E. R, Frankel, E. S., Seluzicki C., Casarett, D., & Mao, J. J. (2014). Integrative Reiki for cancer patients: A program evaluation. *Integrative Cancer Therapies, 13*(1), 62–67.

Forgues, E. (2009). Methodological issues pertaining to the evaluation of energy-based therapies, avenues for a methodological guide. *Journal of Complementary and Integrative Medicine, 6*(1), 1–17.

Friedman, R. S. C., Burg, N. M., Miles, P., Lee, F., & Lampert, R. (2010). Effects of Reiki on autonomic activity after acute coronary syndrome. *Journal of the American College of Cardiology, 56*, 995–996.

Gillipsie, E., Gillipsie, B., & Stevens, M. (2007). Painful diabetic neuropathy: Impact of an alternative approach. *Diabetes Care, 30*, 999–1001.

Hahn, J., Reilly, P., & Buchanan, T. (2014). Development of a hospital Reiki training program: Training volunteers to provide Reiki to patients, families, and staff in the acute care setting. *Dimensions of Critical Care Nursing, 33*(1), 15–21.

Hammerschlag, R., Marx, B., & Aickin, M. (2014). Nontouch biofield therapy: A systematic review of human randomized controlled trials reporting use of only nonphysical contact treatment. *Journal of Alternative and Complementary Medicine, 20*(12), 881–892.

Hemming, L., & Maher, D. (2005). Complementary therapies in palliative care: A summary of current evidence. *British Journal of Community Nursing, 10*(10), 448–452.

Hover-Kramer, D. (2011a). *Creating healing relationships: Professional standards for energy therapy practitioners.* Santa Rosa, CA: Energy Psychology Press.

Hover-Kramer, D. (2011b). *Healing touch: Essential energy medicine for yourself and others.* Loiusville, CO Sounds True Publishing.

Hulse, R. S., Stuart-Shor, E. M., & Russo, J. (2010). Endoscopic procedure with a modified Reiki intervention. *Journal of Gastroenterology Nursing, 33*(1), 20–26.

Institute of Medicine. (2010). *Integrative medicine and the health of the public: A summary of the February 2009 summit.* Washington, DC: National Academies Press.

International Association of Reiki Professionals. (2017). *Code of ethics for Reiki practitioners and Reiki master teachers.* Retrieved from https://iarp.org/iarp-code-ethics/

International Center for Reiki Training. (2017a). *ICRT Reiki membership code of ethics.* Retrieved from https://www.Reikimembership.com/Code_of_Ethics.aspx

International Center for Reiki Training. (2017b). *What is the history of Reiki?* Retrieved from http://www.reiki.org/FAQ/HistoryOfReiki.html

Jain, S., & Mills, P. J. (2010). Biofield therapies: Helpful or full of hype? A best evidence synthesis. *International Journal of Behavioral Medicine, 17*, 1–16.

Joshi, V. (2004). Human spiritual agency in angami healing. Part 1. Divinational healers. *Anthropology and Medicine, 11*, 269–291.

Joyce, J., & Herbison, G. P. (2015) Reiki for depression and anxiety. *Cochrane Database of Systematic Reviews.* doi:10.1002/14651858.CD006833.pub2

Kafatos, M. C., Chevalier, G., Chopra, D., Hubacher, J., Kak, S., & Theise, N. (2015). Biofield science: Current physics perspectives. *Global Advances in Health and Medicine, Biofield Special Issue, 4*(Suppl.), 25–34.

Kennedy, P. (2001). Working with survivors of torture in Sarajevo with Reiki. *Complementary Therapies in Nursing and Midwifery, 7*(1), 4–7.

Kerr, C. E., Wasserman, R. H., & Moore, C. I. (2007). Cortical dynamics as a therapeutic mechanism for touch healing. *Journal of Alternative Complementary Medicine, 13*(1), 59–66.

Kirshbaum, M., Stead, M., & Bartys, S. (2016). An exploratory study of Reiki experiences in women who have cancer. *International Journal of Palliative Care Nursing, 22*(4), 166–172.

Kreitzer, M. J., & Saper, R. (2015). Exploring the biofield. *Global Advances in Health and Medicine, Biofield Special Issue, 4*(Suppl.), 3–4.

Kryak, E., & Vitale, A. (2011). Reiki and its journey into a hospital setting. *Holistic Nursing Practice, 25*(5), 238–245.

Kundu, A., Dolan-Oves, R., Dimmers, M. A., Towle, C. B., & Doorenbos A. Z. (2013). Reiki training for caregivers of hospitalized pediatric patients: A pilot program. *Complementary Therapies in Clinical Practice, 19*(1), 50–54.

Kundu, A., Lin, Y., Oron, A., & Doorenbos, A. (2014). Reiki therapy for postoperative oral pain in pediatric patients: Pilot data from a double-blind, randomized clinical trial. *Complementary Therapies in Clinical Practice, 20*, 21–15.

Lee, M. S., Pittler, M. H., & Ernst, E. (2008). Effects of Reiki in clinical practice: A systematic review of randomized control trials. *International Journal of Clinical Practice, 62*(6), 947–954.

Lubeck, W., Petter, F., & Rand, W. (2001). *The spirit of Reiki: The complete handbook of the Reiki system*. Twin Lakes, WI: Lotus Press.

Mackay, N., Hansen, S., & McFarlane, X. O. (2004). Autonomic nervous system changes during Reiki treatment: A preliminary study. *Journal of Alternative and Complementary Medicine, 10*(6), 1077–1081.

Mansour, A. A., Beuche, M., Laing, G., Leis, A., & Nurse, J. (1999). A study to test the effectiveness of placebo Reiki standardization procedures developed for a planned Reiki efficacy study. *Journal of Alternative and Complementary Medicine, 5*(2), 153–164.

Marcus, D., Blazek-O'Neill, B., & Kopar, J. (2012). Symptom improvement: Reported after receiving Reiki at cancer infusion center. *American Journal of Hospice, 30*(2), 216–217.

Meland, B. (2009). Effects of Reiki on pain and anxiety in the elderly diagnosed with dementia: A series of case reports. *Alternative Therapies, 15*(4), 56–57.

Midilli, T., & Eser, I. (2015). Effects of Reiki on post-cesarean delivery pain, anxiety, and hemodynamic parameters: A randomized, controlled clinical trial. *Pain Management Nursing, 16*(3), 388–399.

Midilli, T., & Gunduzoglu, C. (2016) Effects of Reiki on pain and vital signs when applied to the incision area of the body after cesarean section surgery: A single-blinded, randomized, double-controlled study. *Holistic Nursing Practice, 30*(6), 368–378.

Miles, P. (2006). *Reiki: A comprehensive guide*. New York, NY: Jeremy P. Tarcher/Penguin.

Morse, M. L., & Beem, L. A. W. (2011). Benefits of Reiki therapy for a severely neutropenic patient with associated influences on a true random number generator. *Journal of Alternative and Complementary Medicine, 17*(12), 1180–1190.

Movaffaghi, Z., & Farsi, M. (2009). Biofield therapies: Biophysical basis and biological regulations? *Complementary Therapies in Clinical Practice, 15*, 35–37.

Muehsam, D., Chevalier, G., Barsotti, T., & Gurfein, B. (2015). An overview of biofield devices. *Global Advances in Health and Medicine, 4*(Suppl.), 52–57.

Natale, G. W. (2010). Reconnecting to nursing through Reiki. *Creative Nursing, 16*(4), 171–176.

National Center for Complementary and Integrative Health. (2017a). *Reiki: In depth*. Retrieved from https://nccih.nih.gov/health/reiki/introduction.htm

National Center for Complementary and Integrative Health. (2017b). *Complementary, alternative, or integrative health: What's in a name?* Retrieved from https://nccih.nih.gov/sites/What's_In_A_Name-06-16-2016.pdf

Notte, B., Fazzini, C., & Mooney, R. (2016). Reiki's effect on patients with total knee arthroscopy: A pilot study. *Nursing, 46*(2), 17–23.

Oschman, J. (2016). *Energy medicine: The scientific basis* (2nd ed.). New York, NY: Elsevier.

Park, J., McCaffrey, R., Dunn, D., & Goodman, R. (2011). Managing osteoarthritis: Comparisons of chair yoga, Reiki, and education (pilot study). *Holistic Nursing Practice, 25*(6), 316–326.

Petter, F. (1999). *The original Reiki handbook of Dr. Mikao Usui.* Twin Lakes, WI: Lotus Press.

Potter, P. (2003). What are the distinctions between Reiki and therapeutic touch? *Clinical Journal of Oncology Nursing, 7*(1), 89–91.

Potter, P. (2013). Energy therapies in advanced practice oncology: An evidence-informed practice approach. *Journal of the Advanced Practitioner in Oncology, 4*(3), 139–151.

Radin, D., Schlitz, M., & Baur, C. (2015). Distant healing intention therapies: An overview of the scientific evidence. *Global Advances in Health and Medicine, 4*(Suppl.), 67–71.

Rand, W. (2000). *Reiki, the healing touch: First and second degree manual.* Southfield, MI: Vision.

Reiki and Seichem Association. (2017). *What is Seichem?* Retrieved from http://reikiseichem.org/WhatIsSeichem.php

Richeson, N., Spross, J., Lutz, K., & Peng, C. (2010). Effects of Reiki on anxiety, depression, pain, and physiological factors in community-dwelling older adults. *Research in Gerontological Nursing, 3*(3), 187–199.

Ring, M. E. (2009). Reiki and changes in pattern manifestation. *Nursing Science Quarterly, 22*(3), 250–258.

Ringdahl, D. (2008). *Implementation of a hospital-based Reiki program* (Unpublished University of Minnesota DNP project). Minneapolis: University of Minnesota.

Ringdahl, D. (2014). Reiki. In R. Lindquist, M. Snyder, & M. F. Tracy, (Eds.), *Complementary and alternative therapies in nursing* (7th ed., pp. 419–439). New York, NY: Springer Publishing.

Ringdahl, D., & Voss, M. (2016). *Teaching Reiki to caregivers of children receiving bone marrow transplants.* (Unpublished University of Minnesota DNP project). Minneapolis: University of Minnesota.

Rosada, R. M, Rubik, B., Mainguy, B., Plummer, J., & Mehl Madrona L. (2015). Reiki reduces burnout among community mental health clinicians. *Journal of Alternative and Complementary Medicine, 8,* 489–495.

Rubik, B., Muehsam, D., Hammerschlag, R., & Jain, S. (2015). Biofield science and healing: History, terminology, and concepts. *Global Advances in Health and Medicine, Biofield Special Issue,* 8–15.

Sawyer, J. (1998). The first Reiki practitioner in our OR. *AORN Journal, 67*(3), 674–676.

Schiff, E., Ben-Arye, E., Shilo, M., Levy, M., Schachter, L., Weitchner, N., ... Stone, J. (2010). Development of ethical rules for boundaries of touch in complementary medicine–Outcomes of a Delphi process. *Complementary Therapies in Clinical Practice, 16,* 194–197.

Senderovich, H., Ip, M. L., Berall, A., Karuza, J., Gordon, M., Binns, M., ... Dunal, L. (2016). Therapeutic Touch in a geriatric palliative care unit—A retrospective review. *Complementary Therapies in Clinical Practice, 24,* 134–138.

Shore, A. G. (2004). Long term effects of energetic healing on symptoms of psychological depression and self-perceived stress. *Alternative Therapies, 10*(3), 42–48.

Swann, J. (2009). An introduction to Reiki as an alternative therapy in care homes. *Nursing & Residential Care, 11*(1), 31–34.

Thrane., S. & Cohen, S. (2014). Effect of Reiki therapy on pain and anxiety in adults: An in-depth literature review of randomized trials with effect size calculations. *Pain Management Nursing, 15*(4), 897–908.

Thrane, S., Maurer, S., Ren, D., Danford, C., & Cohen, S. (2016). Reiki therapy for symptom management in children receiving palliative care: A pilot study. *American Journal of Hospice and Palliative Medicine, 34*(4), 373–379.

Todaro-Franceschi, V. (2009). Energy: A bridging concept for nursing science. *Nursing Science Quarterly, 14*(2), 132–140.

Toms, R. (2011). Reiki therapy: A nursing intervention for critical care. *Critical Care Nursing Quarterly, 34*(3), 213–217.

Townsend, J.S. (2013). Temari Reiki: A new hands-off approach to traditional Reiki. *International Journal of Nursing Practice, 19*(Suppl. 2), 34–38.

vanderVaart, S., Berger, H., Tam, C., Goh, Y. H., Gijsen, V., de Wildt, S. N., ... Koren, G. (2011). The effect of distant Reiki on pain in women after elective Caesarean section: A double-blinded randomized controlled trial. *BMJ Open:* 1, e000021. doi:1136/bmjopen-2010-000021 vanderVaart, S., Gijsen, V. M., de Wildt S. N., & Koren, G. (2009). A systematic review of the therapeutic effects of Reiki. *Journal of Alternative and Complementary Medicine, 15*(11), 1157–1169.

Vitale, A. (2014). Initiating a Reiki or CAM program in a healthcare organization—Developing a business plan. *Holistic Nursing Practice, 28*(6), 376–380.

Vitale, A. T. (2007). An integrative review of Reiki touch therapy research. *Holistic Nursing Practice, 21*(4), 167–179.

Watson, J. (2011). *Nursing: Human science and human care* (2nd ed.). Boston, MA: Jones & Bartlett.

Acupressure

PAMELA WEISS-FARNAN

Touch has been central to the practice of nursing since its inception. This chapter describes a form of touch—and its application in nursing care—known in traditional Chinese medicine (TCM) as *acupressure*. This method of treatment is common in many cultures. As Dossey, Keegan, and Guzzetta (2000) note, "All cultures have demonstrated that some form of rubbing, pressing, massaging or holding are [*sic*] natural manifestations of the desire to heal and care for one another" (p. 615). Acupressure is also integral to the practice of shiatsu, *tui na*, *tsubo*, and *jin shin jiyutsu*.

DEFINITIONS

To assist the reader, the following definitions are provided:

- *Acupressure:* An "ancient healing art that uses the fingers to press certain points on the body to stimulate the body's self-curative abilities" (Gach, 1990, p. 3).
- *Acupuncture:* The term *acupuncture* describes a family of procedures involving the stimulation of points on the body using a variety of techniques. The acupuncture technique that has been most often studied scientifically involves penetrating the skin with thin, solid, metallic needles that are manipulated by the hands or by electrical stimulation. Practiced in China and other Asian countries for thousands of years, acupuncture is one of the key components of TCM (National Center for Complementary and Integrative Health [NCCIH], 2017).
- *Auricular acupuncture:* A microacupuncture technique similar to reflexology in which points in the ear are stimulated with pressure that stimulates the central nervous system through the cranial nerves/spinal nerves on the auricle of the ear (Fan et al., 2016).
- *Jin shin jyutsu:* A physiophilosophy that involves the application of the hands for gently balancing the flow of life energy in the body; more generally, it is the awakening to awareness of complete harmony within the self and the universe (Lamke, Catlin, & Mason-Chadd, 2014).

- *Meridians*: Human energy pathways that connect the various acupressure and acupuncture points and the internal organs (www.acupuncture.com).
- *Qi:* The force that animates and controls the observable functions of living beings (acufinder.com, 2018).
- *Shiatsu:* This term means "finger pressure" in Japanese; in practice a practitioner uses touch, comfortable pressure, and manipulative techniques to adjust the body's physical structure and balance its energy flow (www.shiatsu .com).

Traditional Chinese Medicine

TCM is an ancient system of health developed more than 3,000 years ago in Asia. This system is based on the concept that qi flows throughout the body and that balance of yin and yang forces represents health and well-being. As Kaptchuk (1983) describes it:

> This system of care is based on ancient texts and is the result of a continuous process of critical thinking, as well as extensive clinical observation and testing. It represents a thorough formulation and reformulation of material by respected clinicians and theoreticians. It is also, however, rooted in the philosophy, logic and sensibility, and habits of a civilization entirely foreign to our own. It has therefore developed its own perception of the body and health and disease. (p. 2)

The focus of care within this system is to restore balance in the body. To do so, yin and yang must be balanced. Yin aspects are associated with cold, passivity, interiority, and decreases. Yang aspects are associated with warmth, activity, external forces, and increases. Yin and yang are always in relation to each other (Kaptchuk, 1983). According to this conceptualization, they are in continuous flux, and there is always yin within yang and yang within yin.

Unschuld (1999) reflects that TCM theory is a mixture of beliefs that pathogenic influences from the outside combine with the lack of balance or harmony within the person and result in illness. TCM is also concerned with the concept of qi. Qi flows in the body through specific pathways identified as meridians or channels. If the qi is blocked or diminished, a person experiences pain or illness.

There are 12 bilateral meridians and eight extra meridians. All meridians have an exterior and an interior pathway and are named according to the organ system. Located on the meridians are specific points. In the 12 major meridians, the points are bilateral and in the West are called *acupuncture points*. This nomenclature implies that the points are designated for needle insertion and does not fully reflect the TCM concept of the point.

Acupuncture points are also used for acupressure. The points do not have a corresponding anatomical structure but are described by their location relative to other anatomical landmarks. This contributes to the skepticism of many Western-trained scientists about their existence. In Chinese, the name of the point usually is descriptive of its function or location. Mistranslation over the years has often limited the importance of the anatomical basis for the nomenclature of points and the apparent knowledge of anatomy of Chinese scholars (Schnorrenberger, 1996).

There are 365 (Kaptchuk, 1983) to 700 (Yang, 2006) major points on the meridians. Yang (2006) stated that 108 points could be stimulated using the fingers. In a traditionally formulated TCM treatment plan, whether the modality is needles or pressure, the points are combined to achieve maximal benefit for the patient. Rarely is only one point used. There are also points that should not be stimulated, especially during pregnancy, which are referred to as *forbidden points*. These points according to Betts and Budd (2011) are LI4, SP6, GB21, BL32, BL60, and BL67.

SCIENTIFIC BASIS

Western medicine is the dominant system of healthcare in the United States. It is characterized by hospitals; clinics; pharmaceutical resources; and a workforce of physicians, nurses, specialized therapists, and various support service personnel. There are many differences between Western medicine and TCM that become more evident as nurses seek to add TCM modalities to their practice. Western medicine emphasizes disease, causal agents, and treatments that are designed to control or destroy the cause of disease (Kaptchuk, 1983). Once a causal agent or mechanism is identified, treatment plans are developed that focus on the agent or mechanism as a consistent factor in all human manifestations of the disease. In Western journals, almost all studies using the modality of acupuncture and acupressure emphasize the specific effects of needling one point known to address a specific symptom. Medical researchers are eager to find the mechanism by which acupuncture alleviates the symptoms.

Some mechanisms of action of acupuncture and/or acupressure have been suggested through Western medical research. As research has expanded into the mechanism, other researchers have hypothesized that the therapeutic effects produced by stimulation of the points with needles or with pressure may be due to the following:

- Local effects, including activation of the diffuse, noxious, inhibitory response that is induced with an immediate suppression of pain transmission
- Conduction of electromagnetic signals that may start the flow of pain-killing biochemicals, such as endorphins, and of immune system cells to specific sites in the body that are injured or vulnerable to disease
- Activation of opioid systems, which also reduces pain
- Changes in brain chemistry, sensation, and involuntary responses by changing the release of neurotransmitters and neurohormones in a health-promoting way (Huang et al., 2012; Liang, Chen, & Cooper, 2012)
- Changes in the response of the fascia, producing a relaxation effect (Cheng, 2009, 2014; Dale, 1997; Han, 2003; Kawakita, 2014; Lund & Lundeberg, 2016; MacPherson et al., 2016; Takeshige, 1989; Wu, 1995; Wu, Zhou, & Zhou, 1994)
- Patient expectations, reassurance from the practitioner, or noninsertive physiological stimulation (Cherkin et al., 2009)

The scientific research into an underlying mechanism demonstrates one of the differences between Western medicine and the TCM system. The focus in TCM is the imbalance in the patient, and the causality is always multifactorial. The function of the points is described in terms of TCM diagnosis. For example, Western medicine research has focused on pericardium 6, or *nei guan*, for the treatment of nausea. In English its name means "inner border gate." Lade (1986) describes the point:

> The name refers to the point's role as the gateway or connecting point of the triple burner channel and the yin-linking vessel. Inner refers to the palmar aspect of the forearm and to the point's location on the yin channel. The actions of this point are: to regulate and tonify the heart, transform heart phlegm, facilitate qi flow, regulate the yin-linking vessel and clear heart fire, redirect rebellious qi downward, expand and relax the chest and benefit the diaphragm. The indications for use of the point are: asthma, bronchitis, pertussis, hiccups, vomiting, diaphragmatic spasms, intercostal neuralgia, chest fullness, and pain and dyspnea. (pp. 196, 197)

Whereas Western medicine focuses on the treatment of nausea for this point, the TCM paradigm suggests multiple uses. In TCM theory, nausea is considered rebellious qi (qi that flows in the wrong direction). Nausea and vomiting are examples of this. *Nei guan* (pericardium 6) is used as one of the points in the treatment of a patient with nausea. In TCM theory, nausea is considered one of the external manifestations of the imbalance; however, in an authentic TCM treatment, a practitioner would evaluate the imbalances that set up the manifestation and treat the underlying condition. Therefore, a combination of points to treat nausea would be used, possibly including other primary points for antiemesis (Hoo, 1997): Stomach 36 on the stomach meridian located on the knee, Ren 12 on the ren/conception meridian located on the upper abdomen, or the Spleen 4 on the spleen meridian located on the foot. Application of multiple acupoints may be more effective for the treatment of nausea; however, in Western medicine, the focus on finding the single active point or the mechanism creates an almost insurmountable challenge to the fullest application of the therapy.

In 1997, the National Institutes of Health [NIH] held the first consensus conference on acupuncture. The conference members concluded that:

> Acupuncture is effective in the treatment of adult nausea and vomiting in chemotherapy and probably pregnancy and in postoperative dental pain. The conference members stated there is an indication that acupuncture may be helpful in the treatment of addiction, stroke rehabilitation, headache, menstrual cramps, tennis elbow, fibromyalgia, myofascial pain, osteoarthritis, low back pain, carpal tunnel syndrome, and asthma, in which acupuncture may be useful as an adjunct treatment or an acceptable alternative or be included in a comprehensive management program. (NIH, 1997)

Since that original statement, the conditions that can be treated successfully have expanded in number. The NCCIH (2016) has remained cautious about endorsing completely the broad list from the WHO (Chmielnicki, 2014–2017); however, it has funded research in numerous areas.

Research evidence underlying the use of the point called *nei guan* (pericardium 6) for nausea is reviewed in the text that follows. This NIH statement was the springboard for increasing the number of studies completed for the treatment of nausea and vomiting that includes the use of devices to apply pressure or stimulation to pericardium 6. These devices included an elastic bracelet with a pressure button called a Sea-Band or an electrical stimulation device called a ReliefBand.[1]

In recent years, the research focusing on the effectiveness of pericardium 6 for the treatment of nausea and vomiting have increased. Table 25.1 demonstrates that studies continue to find conflicting results about the effectiveness of using pericardium 6 for the treatment of nausea and vomiting from any condition. Meta-analyses published by the Cochrane Collaborative conclude that the use of acupressure for the treatment of a number of symptoms may be useful but more rigorous trials are required (Griffiths et al., 2012; Lee & Frazier, 2011; Robinson, Lorenc, & Liao, 2011). In later reviews, the quality of the articles and the reviews remained problematic when effect sizes were examined and when criteria were applied for the reporting of clinical trials according to Standards for Reporting Interventions in Clinical Trials of Acupuncture (STRICTA; Au et al., 2015).

Table 25.2 presents a brief overview of recent studies examining the use of acupressure in a variety of patients. The conditions included in the table include such things as insomnia, post-operative and cancer-related nausea and vomiting, pain of dysmenorrhea, labor and delivery, and pain experienced in other settings, as well as anxiety, insomnia, and symptoms associated with traumatic brain injury (TBI). A variety of pressure-related modalities were used in these studies to assess their efficacy in providing relief. Numerous studies were done outside of the United States, where the cultural barriers about the use of this ancient type of medicine are lower because the use of acupressure is an accepted part of the cultural health practices.

Pediatric patients have not been studied extensively using acupressure as an intervention; however, in the framework of TCM, children are considered sensitive to any type of energy and may enjoy the same benefits that are found in adult populations. Acupressure is less invasive than other treatments and may be more acceptable to pediatric patients.

Table 25.1 Sample of Studies Using P6 for Nausea

Author	Condition	Modality	Conclusion
Molassiotis et al. (2013)	Chemotherapy-related acute and delayed nausea	Sea-Bands on Ps6	No statistically significant decrease in nausea episodes, but nausea experience was less troubling to patients.
Suh (2012)	Chemotherapy-induced nausea and vomiting in patients with breast cancer	Three treatment groups: control, acupressure on P6 only, or nurse-led counseling and acupressure on P6	Synergistic effects of nurse counseling and use of acupressure was effective in reducing chemotherapy-induced nausea.

(continued)

Table 25.1   Sample of Studies Using P6 for Nausea (*continued*)

Author	Condition	Modality	Conclusion
Allais et al. (2012)	Migraine-associated nausea	Application of Sea-Band at P6	Application of Sea-Bands was effective in controlling nausea when applied with a migraine.
Alessandrini, Napolitano, Micarelli, de Padova, and Bruno (2012)	Vertigo	Comparison of two groups with acupressure on P6 and one group with incorrect acupressure point	Sea-Bands improved neurovegetative symptoms in patients with spontaneous and provoked vertigo.
Hsiung, Chang, and Yeh (2015)	Postoperative pain and nausea and vomiting for patients who had gastric cancer	Acupressure stimulation of *nei guan* (P6) and Zusanli (ST36)	Acupressure can improve comfort of patients by alleviating pain and decreasing time until first flatus.
Genç and Tan (2015)	Chemotherapy-induced, nausea, vomiting, and anxiety in breast cancer patients	Acupressure at P6	Mean scores on vomiting, retching, and anxiety were lowered after application of pressure at P6
Avc, Ovayolu, and Ouayolu (2016)	Nausea and vomiting with patients with acute myeloblastic leukemia	One group of patients using finger pressure and one group using Sea-Bands	Severity of nausea and vomiting was reduced in Sea-Band group.

Table 25.2   Evidence of Effective Selected Uses of Acupuncture/Acupressure

Author	Condition	Modality	Conclusion
Robinson et al. (2011)	Pain (low back, dysmenorrhea, labor); postoperative nausea and vomiting	Acupressure (finger pressure on points) and Sea-Bands	Meta-analysis of nine shiatsu and 71 acupressure studies. Most studies have small sample sizes, but efficacy is highest in conditions noted.
McFadden et al. (2011)	Traumatic brain injury	Acupressure: one group received 40-minute acupressure treatments twice per week	Patients who received acupressure had significant improvement on measures of fatigue, cognition, short-term memory, and hand–eye coordination.
Carotenuto, Galla, Parisi, Rocella, and Esposito (2013)	Psychophysiological insomnia in adolescents	Sea-Bands at Heart 7 on the wrist	There was a significant increase in measures of sleep duration and reduction of wake after sleep.
Song et al. (2014)	Allergic disease, nausea, and vomiting in cancer, pain of dysmenorrhea, and stress/fatigue	Self-administered acupressure for symptom management	Acupressure shows promise for alleviating symptoms. More rigorous study designs are needed.
Au et al. (2015)	Anxiety	Acupressure at Heart 7 and Yintang	Meta-analysis of 39 studies, seven RCTs. All studies reported the positive effect of acupressure on relieving pretreatment stress on individuals.

(continued)

Table 25.2   Evidence of Effective Selected Uses of Acupuncture/
Acupressure (*continued*)

Author	Condition	Modality	Conclusion
Levett, Smith, Dahlen, and Bensoussan (2014)	Pain management in labor and delivery	Various method of interventions (needles, pressure)	Meta-analysis concluded that outcome measures and methods did not reflect question being asked.
Pak, Micalos, Maria, and Lord (2015)	Pain management in patients requiring paramedic interventions	Acupoint stimulation with fingers and hands on GV20 and LI4.	Paramedics could use alternative therapies, including acupressure, to control pain.

RCTs, randomized controlled trials.

The number of studies continues to increase, but the methodological problems persist. This may result from funding issues or remaining skepticism about a simple intervention improving health and well-being. However, the growing concern over pharmacological interventions and the motivation for nurses to provide innovative and easily implemented treatments provide the incentive for nurses to consider incorporating acupressure techniques into their practices. Acupressure techniques are easily learned, are minimally invasive, and have a salutary positive impact on patient outcomes.

INTERVENTION

A TCM practitioner would follow a multistep diagnostic process to choose the correct points to stimulate. Nurses can use a Western, symptom-based system of determining the points that will provide relief for the patient's suffering. The nurse will also be able to teach the patient and the family to implement acupressure techniques to assist the patient in reducing symptoms and stimulating the body's own healing strengths.

Guidelines for Use

Nurses can incorporate acupressure into the care of patients by using some common points that have specific actions to relieve common symptoms. The nurse can treat the patient with acupressure or teach the patient or family members to use acupressure as part of a care plan.

Prior to touching patients, the nurse must assess their readiness to be touched. Shames and Keegan (2000) recommend the following assessment of patients:

- Perception of mind–body situation
- Pathophysiological problems that may require referral

- History of psychological disorders
- Cultural beliefs about touch
- Previous experience with body therapies (p. 264)

Each point is located using an anatomical marker. Many books describe point locations. The standard measure is the *cun*, which is different for each individual. One *cun* for a particular patient is defined as the "width of the interphalangeal joint of the patient's thumb" or as "the distance between the two radial ends of the flexor creases of a flexed middle finger of the patient. Two cun is the width of the index finger, the middle finger, and the ring finger" (Hoo, 1997).

Stimulating the Point

Several different types of techniques are used to stimulate the points, according to Gach (1990):

- *Firm stationary pressure*—using the thumbs, fingers, palms, sides of hands, or knuckles
- *Slow motion kneading*—using the thumbs and fingers with the heels of the hands to squeeze large muscle groups
- *Brisk rubbing*—using friction to stimulate the blood and lymph
- *Quick tapping*—using the fingertips to stimulate muscles on unprotected areas of the body such as the face (p. 9)

Evaluating Acupressure's Effect

Gach (1990) has developed guidelines for assessing results. The elements of the assessment include:

- Identifying the problems being addressed with acupressure
- Identifying the points being used for the treatment
- Determining the length of time for the acupressure
- Identifying what makes the condition worse (e.g., standing, cold weather, menstruation, constipation, lack of exercise, stress, traveling, other variables)
- Describing the changes experienced by the patient after 3 days and after 1 week of treatment
- Describing the changes in the condition and overall feeling of well-being (p. 13)

USES

There are many uses for acupressure. Some conditions for which it has been used are shown in Table 25.2.

Nausea

Point: Pericardium 6 (P6; *Nei Guan*, "Inner Gate")

Location: Pericardium 6 is located on the inner aspect of the wrist 2 *cun* (units) proximal to the transverse crease of the wrist between the tendons

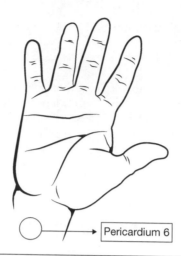

Figure 25.1   Pressure point Pericardium 6. This point has multiple functions and is one of the most important points

of the palmaris longus and flexor carpi radialis muscles (Lade, 1986). The patient should place the middle three fingers (index, middle, and ring fingers) on the opposite hand that is palm upward. The point under the ring finger between the two tendons is pericardium 6 (see Figure 25.1).

Functions: Its functions were outlined previously in the discussion on the research on this point.

Method of Stimulation: The point can be stimulated using firm pressure either with a rotating pattern with the thumb or the static pressure of a Sea-Band.

Indications in Nursing: This point can be used for the treatment of nausea in many situations, but research, as cited previously, has focused on postoperative nausea, the nausea of pregnancy, and the nausea accompanying chemotherapy.

Pain and Gastrointestinal Disorders

Point: Large Intestine 4 (LI4; *Hoku,* "Joining the Valley")

Location: This point is on the back of the hand halfway between the junction of the first and second metacarpal bones, which form a depression or valley when the thumb is abducted (Lade, 1986). There are two ways to locate this point easily. The patient holds the hand with the thumb touching the index finger; when the hand is held at eye level, the highest mound at the base of the thumb and index finger is the location of LI4. Alternately, the nurse instructs the patient to place the thumb of one hand in the web between the thumb and index finger of the opposite hand. The patient should match the first crease on the thumb of one hand to the web of the other and then rotate the thumb to touch the fleshy area between the index finger and the thumb. The point is where the tip of the thumb touches the area between the thumb and the index finger.

Functions: This point has multiple functions and is one of the most important points of the body. It alleviates pain, tones qi, and generates protective qi (in Western medicine this would be considered an immune system–building function); moistens the large intestine and in so doing relieves diarrhea or constipation; clears the nose; regulates the lungs in asthma, bronchitis, or the common cold; and expedites labor. This point is contraindicated in pregnancy because of the latter function (Lade, 1986, pp. 40–41).

Method of Stimulation: Firm pressure can be applied on this point with a rotating thumb massage technique. This point is often sensitive and the patient reports a feeling of discomfort. This is normal and not indicative of a problem.

Indications in Nursing: This point will relieve any pain in the body. In addition, individuals with diarrhea or constipation may feel relief because stimulating the point balances the gastrointestinal functions. This point can be used to induce labor and, coupled with its pain-relieving effect, may be helpful.

PRECAUTIONS

There are overall guidelines and precautions carefully outlined by Gach (1990) in his book *Acupressure Potent Points*:

- Never press any area in an abrupt, forceful, or jarring way. Apply finger pressure in a slow, rhythmic manner to enable layers of tissues and the internal organs to respond (p. 11).
- Use abdominal points cautiously, especially if the patient is ill. Avoid the abdominal area altogether if the patient has a life-threatening disease, especially intestinal cancer, tuberculosis, or leukemia. Avoid the abdominal area during pregnancy (pp. 11–12).
- During pregnancy, strong stimulation of certain points should be avoided: LI4 (fourth point on the large intestine meridian), K3 (third point on the kidney meridian), and SP6 (sixth point on the spleen meridian). Each of these points may have an effect on the pregnancy (p. 192).
- Lymph areas such as the groin, the area of the throat just below the ears, and the outer breast near the armpits are very sensitive. Touch these areas lightly (p. 12).
- Do not work directly on a serious burn, ulcer, or area of infection.
- Do not work directly on a newly formed scar. New surgical or other wounds should not be touched directly. Continuous holding on the periphery of the injury will stimulate the injury to heal (p. 12).
- After an acupressure treatment, tolerance to cold is lowered and the energy of the body is focused on healing, so advise the patient to wear warm clothes and keep out of drafts (p. 12).
- Use acupressure cautiously in individuals with a new acute or serious illness (p. 12).
- Acupressure is not a sole treatment for cancer, contagious skin disease, or sexually transmitted disease (pp. 11–12).
- Brisk rubbing, deep pressure, or kneading should not be used for patients with heart disease, cancer, or high blood pressure (p. 9).

CULTURAL APPLICATIONS

Nurses work with patients from differing cultural backgrounds. Multiple cultures throughout the world use manual therapies to either promote or maintain health or to treat illness. Although the therapies are part of the indigenous healing methods used by different groups of people, they are classified as complementary and alternative medicine (CAM) in the United States. However, within many cultures, individuals and families treat manual therapies as mainstream and integral to their health practices. Such remains the case in mainland China. The contemporary use of acupressure in northern China is described in Sidebar 25.1.

Folk and indigenous healing practices are common not only for the people of Asian origin (Chinese, Thai, Cambodian, Vietnamese, and Japanese), but also for almost every other culture. The practices include massage: pressure, rubbing, stretching, and pulling the skin, with and without herbal preparations, oils, or poultices. For example, many indigenous practices are focused on preparing for childbirth. To illustrate, in Oaxaca (a Mexican state), a practice called *sobada* massage is used as a diagnostic tool for gestational age, for relieving the aches and pain of pregnancy and delivery, and then stimulating the baby immediately after birth. In India, infant massage with various oils is a regular practice, and recent research has confirmed that massage with coconut oil enhances the baby's weight gain (Sankaranarayanan, 2005).

Although Western-trained nurses may not understand how different cultural groups incorporate skin massage and rubbing and may misinterpret what they may observe, it is important for them to allow the family to express the types of practices they use as part of their routine caring for each other and their children (Davis, 2000). Struthers (2008) emphasized that there is a "need for nurses and other healthcare

---

SIDEBAR 25.1 ACUPRESSURE AND ITS INTERNATIONAL APPEAL

Fang Yu

On a weekend in April 2017, I was showing off our renowned Mall of America to my nephew, a Beijing native who came to the United States for high school. While searching for a restaurant for lunch, our eyes were caught by the Chinese language art of a massage parlor which boasts its foundation in acupressure. I instantly traveled down memory lane to similar acupressure-based massage parlors I had seen and visited in Washington, DC; New Orleans; and cities in mainland China. Acupressure is a practice of the traditional Chinese medicine (TCM) that has been used to heal diseases for more than 3,000 years. The massage industry in China have boosted acupressure onto new heights and into a national sensation in the past three decades. As I stood in front of the massage parlor inside the Mall of America, it dawned on me that acupressure has truly transcended borders and come to life in the United States and around the world. At that moment, I felt a deep connection to my Chinese root and culture.

(continued)

In China, as elsewhere, the wide use of acupressure is founded in its unique features of accessibility and ease of use. It does not require any medical facilities, equipment, or devices and is easy to learn and do by anyone. Early healers had found that certain techniques of rubbing and pressing could relieve symptoms such as hemorrhage, pain, and swelling. The acupressure points used in a treatment may or may not be in the same area of the body where the targeted symptom manifests. The selection and effectiveness of the acupressure points are grounded in how they stimulate the channels and collaterals to bring about relief by rebalancing yin and yang, as well as qi (life energy in TCM) and blood. Fingers used for rubbing and pressing can be a single finger (often thumb or middle finger), double fingers (two thumbs, two middle fingers, one thumb and one middle finger, or one thumb and one index finger), or multiple fingers.

Acupressure has gained an unthinkable popularity and momentum in modern China. Prior to the economic reform in 1978, acupressure was used widely for the treatments of common ailments and diseases, especially in rural regions where there was a significant shortage of doctors and limited access to healthcare. Many practitioners learned from their parents and local elders to use acupressure to treat back pain, headache, stomach pain, and bi zheng (painful obstruction syndrome). The economic reform has drastically changed China in so many ways. One result is the drive to pursue longevity, well-being, and health; this provided an impetus for Chinese businessmen to develop business models grounded in TCM. The acupressure-based massage parlors claim their effectiveness on promoting wellness, correcting suboptimal health states, preventing diseases, and treating ailments. They are popular and affordable places for the public to relax and socialize. The latest statistics suggest that acupressure-based massage parlors dot the streets of Shanghai every 1,500 feet. The parlors use cheap labor: often migrant farmers and laid-off city dwellers with limited education. The workers typically received targeted on-the-job training from their employers, and the quality of training vary considerably across parlors.

As we were standing in front of the massage parlor, my nephew asked if he could go in and get a massage. I chuckled because I consider my trips to China incomplete if I had not visited an acupressure-based massage parlor. Maybe for Chinese who visit abroad, an international trip would also be incomplete if they did not get a home-style massage, like my nephew.

providers to become knowledgeable regarding traditional indigenous healthcare that their clients may be receiving—to foster open communication" (p. 74). What the practices are called varies from one cultural group to another, but each uses skin stimulation as part of health routines and family bonding.

FUTURE RESEARCH

There are many areas of research in which the methods of TCM and the underlying theory are being tested using the research techniques of Western medicine. Research questions about the usefulness of acupressure strategies can be posed in many areas of nursing, including their use for palliative care, rehabilitation nursing, support of women in labor, and health-promotion and disease-prevention programs.

Gach and Henning (2004) has expanded his self-care manuals to include trauma, stress, and common emotional imbalances.

Acupressure is used by millions of people around the world. Incorporating this technique into nursing care plans will unite us in the commonality we share—the desire to relieve human suffering.

WEBSITES

Accupressure.com

(www.acupressure.com)

This is the website of Dr. Michael Reed Gach, who has written extensively on acupressure. (A list of his publications appears on the website.) It includes a list of online courses that will yield certification in acupressure interventions. Point locations for treatment based on symptoms or Western medical diagnosis is also available at this site.

Acupuncture and Acupressure for Pregnancy and Childbirth

(acupuncture.rhizome.net.nz)

This website, maintained by of Debra Betts (2018), provides details on the use of acupressure in pregnancy and childbirth. She offers multiple brochures for patients and practitioners in numerous languages.

NOTE

Bands to stimulate Pericardium 6 (P6) are provided by multiple companies. A Google search yields over 400,000 sources. Most devices are expandable wristbands with a button or a magnetic closure that places pressure on P6. A few of the models also provide an electric stimulation that provides a more intense treatment. All of the products are available as over-the-counter products and do not require a physician's order.

REFERENCES

Acufinder.com. (2017). *The definition of* "Qi." Retrieved from https://www.acufinder.com/Acupuncture+Information/Detail/The+Definition+of+Qi+

Alessandrini, M., Napolitano, B., Micarelli, A., de Padova, A., & Bruno, E. (2012). P6 acupressure effectiveness on acute vertiginous patients: A double blind randomized study. *Journal of Alternative and Complementary Medicine, 18*(12), 1121–1126. doi:10.1089/acm.2011.0384

Allais, G. R., Rolando, S., Gabellari, I. C., Burzio, C., Airola, G., Borgogno, P., ... Benedetto, C. (2012). Acupressure in the control of migraine-associated nausea. *Neurological Sciences, 33*(Suppl. 1), S207–S210.

Au, D. W. H., Tsang, H. W. H., Ling, P. P. M., Leung, C. H. T., Ip, P. K., & Cheung W. M. (2015). Effects of acupressure on anxiety: A systematic review and meta-analysis. *Acupuncture in Medicine, 22*(3), 10720–2014. doi:10.1136/acupmed-2014-010720

Avc, H., Ovayolu, N., & Ovayolu, Ö. (2016). Effect of acupressure on nausea-vomiting in patients with acute myeloblastic leukemia. *Holistic Nursing Practice, 30*(5), 257–62. Retrieved from https://www.ncbi.nlm.nih.gov/pubmed/27501207

Betts, D. (2018). *Acupuncture and acupressure for pregnancy and childbirth.* Retrieved from https://acupuncture.rhizome.net.nz/download-booklet

Betts, D., & Budd, D. (2011). Forbidden points in pregnancy: Historical wisdom? *Acupuncture in Medicine, 29,* 137–139. doi:10.1136/aim.2010.003814

Carotenuto, M., Galla, B., Parisi L., Rocella, M., & Esposito, M. (2013). Acupressure therapy for insomnia in adolescents: A polysomnographic study. *Neuropsychiatric Disease and Treatment, 9,* 157–162. Retrieved from https://iris.unipa.it/retrieve/handle/10447/97928/126792/NDT-41892-acupressure-therapy-for-the-insomnia-in-adolescents--a-polys_012413%5B1%5D%20(1).pdf

Cheng, K. J. (2009). Neuroanatomical basis of acupuncture treatment for some common illnesses. *Acupuncture in Medicine, 27*(2), 61–64. doi:10.1136/aim.2009.000455

Cheng, K. J. (2014). Neurobiological mechanisms of acupuncture for some common illnesses: A clinician's perspective. *Journal of Acupuncture and Meridian Studies, 7*(3), 105–114. Retrieved from http://www.jams-kpi.com/article/S2005-2901(13)00174-X/fulltext#sec2.4

Cherkin, D. C., Sherman, K. J., Avins, A. L., Erro, J. H., Ichikawa, L., Barolow, W. E., … Deyo, R. A. (2009). A randomized trial comparing acupuncture, simulated acupuncture, and usual care for chronic low back pain. *Archives of Internal Medicine, 169*(9), 858–866.

Chmielnicki, B. World Health Organization. (2014–2017). *Evidence based acupuncture: WHO official position.* Retrieved from http://www.evidencebasedacupuncture.org/who-official-position

Dale, R. (1997). Demythologizing acupuncture. Part 1: The scientific mechanisms and the clinical uses. *Alternative and Complementary Therapies Journal, 3*(2), 125–131.

Davis, R. (2000). Cultural health care or child abuse? The Southeast Asian practice of cao gio. *Journal of the Academy of Nurse Practitioners, 3*(2), 125–131.

Dossey, B. M., Keegan, L., & Guzzetta, C. E. (2000). *Holistic nursing: A handbook for practice.* Gaithersburg, MD: Aspen.

Fan, S. (2016). *Auricular acupuncture.* Retrieved from http://acupuncturewellnessfan.com/therapy/acupuncture-in-dc-va-md/auricular-acupuncture-in-dc-va-md

Gach, M. R. (1990). *Acupressure's potent points: A guide to self-care for common ailments.* New York, NY: Random House. https://www.penguinrandomhouse.com/books/57326/acupressures-potent-points-by-michael-reed-gach/9780553349702/

Gach, M. R., & Henning, B. A. (2004). *Acupressure: A self-care guide for trauma, stress, and common emotional imbalances.* New York, NY: Bantam Books.

Geng, F., & Tan, M. (2015). The effect of acupressure application on chemotherapy-induced nausea, vomiting, and anxiety in patients with breast cancer. *Palliative & Supportive Care, 13*(2), 275–284. doi:10.1017/S1478951514000248

Griffiths, J. D., Gyte, G. M. L., Paranjothy, S., Brown, H. C., Broughton, H. K., & … Thomas, J. (2012). Interventions for preventing nausea and vomiting in women undergoing regional anesthesia for caesarean section. *Cochrane Database of Systematic Reviews, 9,* CD007579. doi:10.1002/14651858.CD007579.pub2

Han, J-S. (2003). Acupuncture: Neuropeptide release produced by electrical stimulation of different frequencies. *Trends in Neuroscience, 26*(1), 17–22.

Hoo, J. J. (1997). Acupressure for hyperemesis gravidarum. *American Journal of Obstetrics and Gynecology, 176*(6), 1395–1396. doi:10.1016/s0002-9378(97)70369-7

Hsiung, W.-T., Chang, Y.-C., & Yeh, M.-L. (2015). Acupressure improves the postoperative comfort of gastric cancer patients: A randomized controlled trial. *Complementary Therapies in Medicine, 23*(3), 339–346. doi:10.1016/j.ctim.2015.03.010

Huang, W., Pach, D., Napadow, V., Park, K., Long, X., Neumann, J., … Fleckenstein, J. (2012). Characterizing acupuncture stimuli using brain imaging with fMRI—a systematic review and meta-analysis of the literature. *Deutsche Zeitschrift für Akupunktur, 55*(3), 26–28. doi:10.1016/j.dza.2012.08.008

Kawakita, K., & Okada, K. (2014). Acupuncture therapy: Mechanism of action, efficacy, and safety: A potential intervention for psychogenic disorders? *Biopsychosocial Medicine, 8,* 4. doi:10.1186/1751-0759-8-4. Retrieved from https://www.ncbi.nlm.nih.gov/pmc/articles/PMC3996195/

Lade, A. (1986). *Images and functions.* Seattle, WA: Eastland.

Lamke, D., Catlin, A., & Mason-Chadd, M. (2014). "Not just a theory": The relationship between Jin Shin Jyutsu® self-care training for nurses and stress, physical health, emotional health, and caring efficacy. *Journal of Holistic Nursing, 32*(4), 278–289. doi:10.1177/0898010114531906

Lee, E. J., & Frazier, S. K. (2011). The efficacy of Acupressure for symptom management: A systematic review. *Journal of Pain and Symptom Management, 42*(4), 589–603. doi:10.1016/j.jpainsymman.2011.01.007

Levett, K. M., Smith, C. A., Dahlen, H. G., & Bensoussan, A. (2014). Acupuncture and acupressure for pain management in labour and birth: A critical narrative review of current systematic review evidence. *Complementary Therapies in Medicine, 22*(3), 523–540. doi:10.1016/j.ctim.2014.03.011

Liang, F., Chen, R., & Cooper, E. L. (2012). Neuroendocrine mechanisms of acupuncture. *Evidence-Based Complementary & Alternative Medicine, 2012*, 1–2. doi:10.1155/2012/792793

Lund, I., & Lundeberg, T. (2016, December 15). *Mechanisms of acupuncture.* Science Direct Elsevier, Research Gate. Retrieved from https://www.researchgate.net/publication/311505128_Mechanisms_of_Acupuncture

MacPherson, H., Hammerschlag, R., Coeytaux, R. R., Davis, R. T., Harris, R. E., & Kong, J.-T., Wayne, P. M. (2016). Unanticipated insights into biomedicine from the study of acupuncture. *Journal of Alternative and Complementary Medicine, 22*(2), 101–107. doi:10.1089/acm.2015.0184

McFadden, K. L., Healy, K. M., Dettmann, M. L., Kaye, J. T., Ito, T. A., & Hernández, T. D. (2011). Acupressure as a non-pharmacological intervention for traumatic brain injury (TBI). *Journal of Neurotrauma, 28*(1), 21–34. doi:10.1089/neu.2010.1515

Molassiotis, A., Russell, W., Hughes, J., Breckons, M., Lloyd-Williams, M., Richardson, J., … Ryder, W. (2013). The effectiveness and cost-effectiveness of acupressure for the control and management of chemotherapy-related acute and delayed nausea: Assessment of nausea in chemotherapy research (aNCHoR), a randomised controlled trial. *Health Technology Assessment, 17*(26), 1–114. doi:10.3310/hta17260

National Center for Complementary and Integrative Health. (2017). Acupuncture. Retrieved from https://nccih.nih.gov/health/acupuncture

National Center for Complementary and Integrative Health. (2016, September 1). Acupuncture: In depth. Retrieved from https://nccih.nih.gov/health/acupuncture/introduction#hed3

National Institutes of Health. (1997). NIH Consensus Development Conference Statement. Acupuncture. Retrieved from http://consensus.nih.gov/1997/1997Acupuncture107html.htm

Pak, S. C., Micalos, P. S., Maria, S. J., & Lord, B. (2015). Nonpharmacological interventions for pain management in paramedicine and the emergency setting: A review of the literature. *Evidence-Based Complementary & Alternative Medicine, 2015*, 1–8. doi:10.1155/2015/873039

Robinson, N., Lorenc, A., & Liao, X. (2011). The evidence for Shiatsu: A systematic review of Shiatsu and acupressure. *BMC Complementary and Alternative Medicine, 11*, 88. doi:10.1186/1472-6882-11-88

Sankaranarayanan, K. M. (2005). Oil massage in neonates: An open randomized controlled study of coconut versus mineral oil. *Indian Pediatric, 42*(9), 877–884.

Schnorrenberger, C. C. (1996). Morphological foundations for acupuncture: An anatomical nomenclature of acupuncture structures. *Acupuncture in Medicine, 14*(2), 89–103.

Shames, K., & Keegan, L. (2000). Touch: Connecting with the healing power in 2000. In B. Dossey, L. Keegan, & C. E. Guzzetta (Eds.), *Holistic nursing: A handbook for practice* (3rd ed., pp. 613–635). Gaithersburg, MD: Aspen.

Song, H. J., Seo, H.-J., Lee, H., Son, H., Choi, S. M., & Lee, S. (2015). Effect of self-acupressure for symptom management: A systematic review. *Complementary Therapies in Medicine, 23*(1), 68–78. doi:10.1016/j.ctim.2014.11.002

Struthers, R. (2008). The experience of being an Anishinabe man healer: Ancient healing in the modern world. *Journal of Cultural Diversity, 15*(2), 70–75.

Suh, E. E. (2012). The effects of P6 acupressure and nurse-provided counseling on chemotherapy-induced nausea and vomiting in patients with breast cancer. *Oncology Nursing Forum, 39*(1), E1–E9. doi:10.1188/12.onf.e1-e9

Takeshige, C. (1989). Mechanism of acupuncture analgesia based on animal experiments: Scientific bases of acupuncture. Berlin, Germany: Springer-Verlag.

Unschuld, P. U. (1999). The past 1000 years of Chinese medicine. *Lancet, 354,* SIV9. doi:10.1016/s0140-6736(99)90352-5

Wu, B. (1995). Effect of acupuncture on the regulation of cell-mediated immunity in patients with malignant tumors [in Chinese]. *Zhen Ci Yan Jiu, 20*(3), 67–71.

Wu, B., Zhou, R. X., & Zhou, M. S. (1994). Effect of acupuncture on interleukin-2 level and NK cell immunoactivity of peripheral blood of malignant tumor patients [in Chinese]. *Zhongguo Zhong Xi Yi Jie He Za Zhi, 14*(9), 537–539.

Yang, J-M. (2006). *Chinese quigong massage* (2nd ed.). Boston, MA: Jang's Martial Arts Academy (YMAA) Publication Center, Inc.

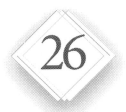

Reflexology

THÓRA JENNÝ GUNNARSDÓTTIR

Reflexology is a complex complementary alternative therapy used for symptom management and for increased well-being. In reflexology, the whole body has been mapped out in the hands and in the feet and can be manipulated directly using specific massage techniques. The corresponding areas on the feet are easier to locate because they cover a larger area and are more specific, rendering them easier to work on than the hands. In this chapter, the focus is on reflexology of the feet. Reflexology shares the philosophical base of holism congruent with nursing. As such, it provides the nurse with an important tool to provide healing to patients, and it has been shown to positively affect some symptoms. Reflexology can be used as a prime tool to provide caring and presence; it is a way to show compassion, in addition to doing something that may help a patient to become more whole and feel better. Although there is much growth in research on the effects of reflexology, the scientific basis behind this therapy needs to be further established.

DEFINITION

Reflexology is defined as a science concerning the principle that reflex areas in the feet and hands correspond to all the glands, organs, and parts of the body. Stimulating these reflexes properly can help many health problems in a natural way, a type of preventive maintenance (International Institute of Reflexology, 2016). The International Institute asserts that its purpose is not to treat or diagnose for any specific medical disorder, but to promote better health and well-being. The National Center for Complementary and Integrative Health (NCCIH) defines reflexology as a practice in which different amounts of pressure are applied to specific points on the feet or hands. These points are believed to match certain other parts of the body (NCCIH, 2016).

Reflexology is a specific pressure technique that works on precise reflex points of the feet that correspond to other body parts as depicted in Figure 26.1. Different definitions have been put forth, but they all convey that the basic principle behind reflexology: The extremities are connected to all other parts and internal organs of the human body, and there is a relationship between organs, systems, and processes.

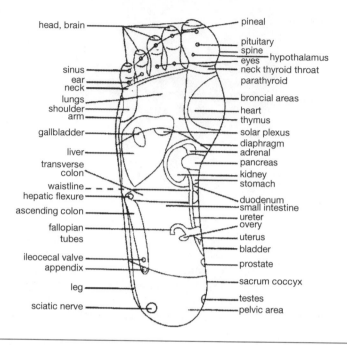

Figure 26.1   Relationship of body parts with reflexology points on the foot.

Source: Andrews, S., & Dempsey, B. (2007). Foot reflexology map, dummies. Hoboken, NJ: John Wiley and Sons, Inc. Retrieved from https://www.wiley.com/en-us/Acupressure+and+Reflexology+For+Dummiesp-9780470139424

Therefore, by using specific pressure techniques on the foot or hand it may be possible to affect the whole body. The left foot/hand represents the left side of the body and the right foot/hand represents the right side of the body.

SCIENTIFIC BASIS

The foundations of reflexology can be traced to two different theories or schools of thought documented in the reflexology literature. The first theory originated in traditional Chinese medicine (TCM) and the second one in a Western technique known as *zone therapy.*

Traditional Chinese Medicine

The idea that the whole body can be represented in its parts is not new. For example, tongue diagnosis has been documented in China for at least 2,000 years. The whole body is also represented in the iris of the eye, the face, and the ear (Maciocia, 2005). Reflexology is congruent with the principle of organ representation from TCM: *The whole represents itself in the parts* (Kaptchuk, 2000). This means that the feet can be viewed as a microcosm of the body, as a kind of holographic image in which all organs, glands, and other body parts are mirrored on the soles.

TCM posits that there are invisible energy pathways, or meridians, within the body, that carry energy called *qi*, which is the vital energy behind all processes.

All organs are interconnected with one another by a meridian network system and, to maintain health, energy needs to be flowing in balance. Factors impeding the free circulation of qi are divided into categories of "excess" and "deficiency." *Excess* refers to the presence of something that is "too much" for the individual to handle—too much food to digest, too much waste to eliminate, and so forth. *Deficiency* refers to the absence or relative insufficiency of one or more aspects of the life energies necessary for sustaining health and well-being. A deficiency or excess of life energy can allow outside factors to overwhelm the individual, thus inducing pathology, and leading to pain and illness (Maciocia, 2005).

In a healthy person with energy in balance, the feet feel soft when palpated and should have the same texture in every area. When an area is felt to be "empty" or is lacking in texture when palpated, it is an indication of deficiency in the energy of that particular organ or area in the body. If an area feels stiff and hard in texture when palpated, it indicates an excess of energy. A lack of energy found in one area means that some other area has too much energy because the energy must be in balance. On empty areas, it is necessary to slowly build aggressive pressure to increase the energy flow, and more vigorous, light but firm pressure is applied on the area that has too much energy to direct the flow out and away from it. In that way, reflexology redirects excess energy from one area into another where there is an apparent deficiency so as to supplement a deficiency or to "sedate" an excess pattern.

Zone Therapy

The second theory, often referred to as *zone therapy*, originated in the West. At the beginning of the 20th century, Dr. William Fitzgerald found that pressure applied to some parts of the feet induced anesthesia in specific parts of one's body. He then determined that the entire body and all its organs were "laid out" in a certain configuration on the soles of the feet. He divided the body into 10 longitudinal zones, running from the top of the head to the toes and proposed that parts of the body within a certain zone were linked with one another hence the name "zone" therapy.

An American therapist, Eunice Ingham, is credited with establishing reflexology in its present form (Ingham, 1984). She used the zones as a guiding map but began to chart the feet according to where pressure would produce distinct effects in the body. She developed a map of the entire body on the feet and called the areas *reflexes*. Her proposition was that when the bloodstream becomes blocked with waste materials or excess acid, calcium deposits start to form in the nerve endings, impeding the normal circulation of the blood and creating an imbalance in the various parts of the body, depending on where the blockage is. She believed that by using the specific pressure of reflexology, the calcium deposits on the feet can be detected as "gritty areas," which may feel painful when touched. Ingham describes these as "particles of frost" or "crystal blocks" when examined under a microscope. The pressure and massage techniques taught in reflexology are designed to dissipate these formations and break down their crystalline structures. The corresponding area connected with this particular nerve ending receives an added supply of blood. In this way, the circulatory and lymphatic systems are stimulated, thus encouraging the release and removal of toxins, and the body starts to heal itself. Other theories have been considered in the literature but are not detailed in this chapter.

INTERVENTION

The patient should lie comfortably, covered in a blanket, somewhat higher than the chair in which the reflexologist sits, and has pillows under the knees and the head to induce relaxation. In addition, the patient is barefoot and in a comfortable position, with any tight clothes loosened so as to not hinder circulation. Then the patient is assessed continuously for tolerance of the amount of pressure applied. The pressure needs to be firm enough to activate the body's healing potentials but must also be tolerable to the patient. Sensitivity varies in each individual, and the feet usually become more sensitive with subsequent treatments. Each area is worked, finishing the toe area on the one foot and then treating the toe area on the other, and so on, going from one foot to the other.

Although it is emphasized that reflexology is to be applied to the feet as a whole, it is important to work specifically on several systems of the body. These specific systems are, for example, the digestive system to increase proper elimination, the lymphatic system to increase the clearance of waste materials, the bladder and kidneys to increase urine and energy flow (the kidneys are one source of qi), the solar plexus (where feelings and emotions are stored) to increase relaxation, all internal glands to stimulate their respective functions, and the lungs to increase oxygen consumption. By using reflexology on these body systems, the reflexologist is both increasing circulation and elimination and affecting the flow of qi, because all organs are interconnected with each other by meridians.

There is still ambiguity regarding the mechanism behind the action of reflexology, but it has certainly been shown to have profound physiological effects, which may be partly attributed to the relaxation derived from the therapeutic interaction and the impact of touch. Reflexology sessions can be improved by other elements such as aromatherapy, peaceful music, and good environment.

Techniques

Learning reflexology requires specific training, although its application is quite easy, and it can be applied in many circumstances. There are several techniques used, depending on what area of the feet is worked on. One hand is used to support the foot while the fingers and the thumb of the other are used to massage the skin. A period of 45 minutes to 1 hour is estimated to be enough time to perform reflexology on both feet and allows for extra time for work on specific areas that need further care. At the end of each session, the client is encouraged to relax for several minutes. There are some standard pressure techniques for working on the reflexes of the feet. The two techniques described here are *thumb walking* and *hook and back up* (Kunz & Kunz, 2003). Other grips are used depending on which area one is working on. It is important to not forget any area and to finish one area before starting the next one (see Exhibit 26.1).

Measurement of Outcomes

The philosophy behind reflexology states that it affects the body as whole, but based on the literature, more studies have measured physiological or psychological outcomes of reflexology than its overall effects. It is important to measure the effect of reflexology over a number of sessions to gain insight into its overall benefits.

Exhibit 26.1   Reflexology Techniques

Thumb Walking

The goal of the thumb-walking technique is to apply a constant, steady pressure to the surface of the foot or the hand:

1. With the other hand (holding hand) stretch the sole of the foot. Rest your working thumb on the sole and your fingers on the top of the foot. Drop your wrist to create leverage, which exerts pressure with the thumb.

2. Bend and unbend the thumb's first joint, moving it forward a little bit at a time. When your working hand feels stretched, reposition it and continue walking it forward. Take a little step forward with each unbend. The goal is to work with a small area in each step to create a feeling of constant, steady pressure. Always walk in a forward direction, not backward. Keep your thumb slightly cocked as you work to prevent overextending it.

Hook and Backup

The hook-and-backup technique is used to work a specific point rather than to cover a larger area. It is a relatively stationary technique, with only small movements of the working thumb involved. To avoid digging your fingernail into the flesh, apply pressure using more of the flat of the thumb:

1. Support and protect the area to be worked with holding hand. The hand wraps around the area while the thumb and fingers hold it in place. Place the fingers of the working hand over those of the holding hand.

2. Place the working thumb in the center of the area to be worked. Hook and backup, using the edge of the thumb.

Source: Adapted from Kunz B., & Kunz, K. (2003). *Reflexology: Health at your fingertips.* New York, NY: DK Publishing.

PRECAUTIONS

Reports from people have indicated reflexology to be a largely pleasant experience, leaving them both calm and relaxed. However, many do not like to have their feet touched, so approval from the patient is needed before starting. Before starting reflexology, the condition of the feet must be examined for swelling, color, ulcerations, toe deformities, and odor. The physical condition of the person is also very important; hence, the health history is reviewed. If there is a problem regarding the blood flow to the limbs because of diabetes, neurological diseases, or arteriosclerosis, the therapist must be careful about the pressure of the massage. Older adults may need special precautions because of concerns such as restricted movement, incontinence, arthritis, and aching joints. When dealing with such conditions, it may be better to consider the person's comfort and feel of the touch as the primary goals.

Some symptoms of adverse effects after undergoing complementary therapy are often referred to as *healing crisis*. Healing crises are said to happen frequently during and immediately following treatment as localized or distal pain, perspiration or shivering, and changes in the heart rate, respiration, or temperature.

This phenomenon is also described as a cleansing process because the treatment is believed to activate the body's healing power, where accumulated waste products and toxins, which have often lain dormant in the body, are then released into the bloodstream. In one study of the effects of reflexology on fibromyalgia syndrome, the participants were specifically observed and asked about healing crises as part of the reflexology treatment (Gunnarsdottir & Jonsdottir, 2010). The participants, six women who were given 10 reflexology treatments, described several symptoms as healing crisis: Headaches, increased thirst, increased pain, increased urination, more frequent bowel movements, aggravated skin conditions, increased perspiration, fatigue, feverishness, dizziness, exhaustion, and increased energy. These symptoms appeared during the early stages and lasted for a day or two each time. Because of reports of such reactions, reflexologists may need to be very careful when performing reflexology on people who are seriously ill (e.g., cancer patients), as they may not tolerate healing crises. It is also important to explain to people what can be expected after a treatment.

A group of researchers in England have been looking at the effects of reflexology on the hemodynamic system. A recent study on the effects of reflexology on arterial compliance found that it had no significant effect on heart rate, blood pressure, or augmentation index in healthy individuals (Rollinson, Jones, Scott, Megson, & Leslie, 2016). Another study on healthy individuals demonstrated that reflexology applied to the upper part of the left foot may have a modest specific effect on the cardiac index (Jones, Thomson, Lauder, Howie, & Leslie, 2012). They also looked at patients with chronic heart failure and found that reflexology seems to have no immediate hemodynamic effects (Jones, Thomson, Lauder, Howie, & Leslie, 2013).

USES

Research testing the effects of reflexology is limited and includes studies of many approaches to practices of reflexology. Some conditions for which it has been used are listed in Exhibit 26.2. Although most of these studies are fairly new, many of them base the findings on limited numbers of subjects and weak research designs.

A case study design was used to test the effects of reflexology on six cases of women with fibromyalgia (Gunnarsdottir & Peden-McAlpine, 2010). Each participant had 10 sessions of reflexology over 10 weeks. Data were collected by observation, interviews, and diaries and then analyzed within each case and across cases. The findings showed that symptoms of pain in multiple areas started to localize and decrease in severity. The areas that responded best were the head, shoulders, neck, and arms.

A three-group randomized controlled design was used to compare the effects of aromatherapy massage, reflexology, and control conditions on pain and fatigue of rheumatoid arthritis patients (Metin & Ozdemir, 2016). Although reflexology and massage decreased both pain and fatigue, reflexology was more effective.

Subjective reports in studies of reflexology are few but indicate that the experience is mostly positive, producing relaxing, calming, and comforting effects. Patients receiving reflexology frequently experience relaxation as a benefit (Dyer, Thomas, Sandsund, & Shaw, 2013; Johns, Blake, & Sinclair, 2010) and feel more energy and sense of well-being (Gunnarsdottir & Jonsdottir,

---

Exhibit 26.2   Uses of Reflexology

- Improve quality of life for women with breast cancer (Sharp et al., 2010)
- Improve constipation in women (Woodward, Norton, & Barriball, 2010)
- Promote relaxation in people with Parkinson's disease (Johns, Blake, & Sinclair, 2010)
- Improve symptoms of fibromyalgia (Gunnarsdottir & Peden-McAlpine, 2010)
- Decrease low back pain (Eghbali, Safari, Nazari, & Abdoli, 2012)
  - Affect hemodynamic variables (Jones, Thomson, Irvine, & Leslie, 2013)
- Increase relaxation and well-being in adult outpatient oncology (Dye et al., 2013)
- Improve premenstrual syndrome and dysmenorrhea (Kim & Cho, 2002)
- Increase sleep quality postpartum (Manjuri & Latheef, 2016) and during the menopausal period (Asltoghiri & Ghodsi, 2012)
- Have positive effect during labor (Hanjani, Tourzani, & Shoghi, 2015)
- Decrease fatigue in women with multiple sclerosis (Nazari, Shahreza, Shaygannejad, & Valiai, 2015)
- Decrease menopausal period problems (Gozuyesil & Baser, 2016)
- Decrease fatigue and pain in patients with rheumatoid arthritis in a rheumatoid clinic (Metin & Ozdemir, 2016)
- Improve sleep and fatigue in hemodialysis patients (Unal & Akpinar, 2016)

2010; Woodward, Norton, & Barriball, 2010). Patients have also commented on how reflexology can create space for them to talk about their worries and concerns, which is an important part of the therapy as whole (Mackereth, Booth, Hillier, & Caress, 2009).

One systematic review of the effect of reflexology on physiological and bio-chemical outcomes shows that positive effects can be attributed to the treatment, specifically a reduction in stress parameters (McCullough, Liddle, Sinclair, Close, & Hughes, 2014). Other systematic reviews of the effect of reflexology have been conducted (Ernst, Posadzki, & Lee, 2011; Kim, Kang, & Ernst, 2010; Wang, Tsai, Lee, Chang, & Yang, 2008). Their findings suggest that the effectiveness of reflexology as treatment is currently not based on evidence from independent, high-quality clinical trials. There may be several reasons for limited scientific evidence of reflexology's effects (Gunnarsdottir & Peden-Mc-Alpine, 2010). The methods used in the studies differ and are often not adequately explained. The length and frequency of sessions are different, and the principle behind reflexology states that it can affect the body as a whole. It is important to measure the effect of reflexology over a number of sessions to gain insight into its overall benefits. There may also be problems with localizations of reflexology points. One researcher, a nurse, Jenny Jones, has looked specifically at the localization of the heart point and did a survey among members of the Association of Reflexologists in the United Kingdom (Jones, Thomson, Lauder, & Leslie, 2012). The findings showed lack of clarity and consistency regarding the indication of reflexology for cardiac patients and inconsistencies in reflexology teaching literature and marked inconsistencies in the heart point placement.

Reflexology in Scandinavia

As a part of a larger study on use of healthcare services in Iceland, the scope of the use of complementary and alternative medicine (CAM) providers was assessed (Helgadottir, Vilhjalmsson, & Gunnarsdottir, 2010). A sample of 1,532 Icelandic adults, between ages 18 and 75, responded to a survey, yielding a 60% response rate. Almost 32% of the respondents had visited a CAM provider in the previous 12 months, an estimated increase of 5% since 1998. The most common therapy was massage; however, visits to reflexologists were ranked second, with 4.3% use, which shows it is quite widespread.

Reflexology is quite popular in Scandinavia (Hansen et al., 2005). The most frequent use is in Denmark, where it is practiced both in private clinics and in health communities; it was one of the most frequently used complementary therapy in Denmark (Kjøller & Rasmussen, 2002). Reflexology in Denmark is further described in Sidebar 26.1. In Norway, reflexology ranked number four in popularity (Hansen et al., 2005), and in Sweden it ranks sixth (Stockholm County Council, 2001) among complementary therapies. Although these findings are based on rather old studies, reflexology is known by the author to be still quite popular.

CULTURAL APPLICATIONS

The roots of reflexology are embedded in ancient history, when pressure therapies were recognized as preventive and therapeutic. Evidence indicates that therapeutic foot massage has been practiced throughout history by a variety of cultures. The oldest documentation depicting the practice of reflexology was unearthed in Egypt and dated around 2500 to 2330 BCE. The use of reflex pressure applied to the feet

---

SIDEBAR 26.1   REFLEXOLOGY IN DENMARK

Leila Eriksen

Reflexology is the second most used complementary therapy in Denmark. It is practiced both in private clinics and in health communities. A number of private insurance companies support reflexology treatments. Danish reflexologists have 300 hours of education in, for example, anatomy and physiology, besides the theoretical and practical education. More than one in five people in Denmark have used reflexology. However, it is unknown why particular age groups seek reflexology and what specific issues they seek to address. A national survey was completed by 490 Danish reflexologists that included data from 2,368 clients. The data showed that a majority of reflexology clients request treatment for muscle pain (44%). Other problems include stomach pain/digestive problems, headache/migraine, fatigue, and hormonal problems. One in five clients (22%) chooses to have reflexology on their own initiative. In another survey (unpublished study, Leila Eriksen), it was shown that 26 of 58 (approximately 45%) Danish children with cancer have used reflexology.

as a healing therapy has been practiced by the North American native peoples for generations.

As discussed earlier in the chapter, there are different perspectives on the effects of reflexology in Eastern and Western cultures. The TCM energy channels are one of the main concepts in reflexology and acupuncture; in both therapies, energy is channeled throughout the body. Energy is channeled through the meridians and through the zones in reflexology. Both practices assert that diseases are caused by blockages in energy channels. In acupuncture/acupressure, energy is stimulated or sedated with needles/finger pressure. Six meridians are present in the feet, where they either end or begin. The other ends of the meridians going from or to the feet start or end in the fingers. Therefore, the meridians in the upper and lower parts of the body are connected.

Reflexology on the whole foot is also done on the acupuncture points there and can help clear congestions in the meridians. It can also be used purposively, as it may be very helpful to push, press, or massage these points to increase energy in the meridians. Such stimulation is helpful in increasing energy movement along the meridians and in the organs to which they are connected. In this way, the use of reflexology is based more on energy and assessment and movement of energy throughout the body. Zone therapy as developed by Eunice Ingham is mostly practiced in Europe and the United States.

Reflexology, reflex zone therapy, and *reflexotherapy* are all terms that refer to the current use of the treatment. Distinctions are apparently due to scientific, philosophical, and political differences of opinion between authorities.

Numerous schools of reflexology have been established throughout the world. Interestingly, there seems to be much interest in the use and research of reflexology in countries such as Malaysia, Thailand, India, Iran, and Turkey, as evident by a growing number of studies on reflexology from these countries.

FUTURE RESEARCH

In the pursuit of greater integration of complementary therapies into conventional healthcare, it is inevitable that reflexology will evolve and will need to be adapted to meet the needs of the system in which it finds itself. Practitioners need to be critical and acknowledge the value of research and inquiry in this process. The scientific basis for reflexology is growing, and promising results of its use for some symptoms are beginning to emerge, but more rigorous research is needed if reflexology is to be used effectively by nurses in healthcare settings. In a summary article of the current practice of reflexology, it is argued that qualitative research may assist in understanding the impact of the context and the process of reflexology intervention (Embong, Soh, Ming, & Wong, 2015). Nurses are in a primary position to conduct research on reflexology because their holistic background is in tune with the philosophies behind reflexology. The principle behind reflexology states that it can affect the body as a whole. However, it is not clear how these holistic changes come about. Some questions for future research are:

1. What are the specific effects of reflexology, and how do these effects compare with other complementary therapies? How can these specific effects be captured in research?
2. What is the mechanism underlying the effects of reflexology?

There is an urgent need to explore the experience of having reflexology to try to gain more information about what takes place during sessions and how the framework from which it is derived and delivered supports the intervention.

WEBSITES

International Institute of Reflexology

(www.reflexology-usa.net)

This is the only school licensed to teach the Original Ingham Method. Reflexology has grown to international proportions under the able direction of Ingham's nephew Dwight Byers, today's leading authority. The school also has branches around the world.

International Council of Reflexologists

(www.icr-reflexology.org)

Established in Toronto, it holds an international conference on reflexology every other year.

Association of Reflexologists in the United Kingdom

(www.aor.org.uk)

This is a good resource that includes a list of worldwide reflexology organizations, as well as interactive information on reflexology products and practice.

RiEN

(www.carecam.dk; click on the English flag for the English language)

RiEN is a network of reflexology associations and providers, representing 20 countries and 20,000 reflexologists around Europe; this network has been active in different research and consultation regarding research in this area.

REFERENCES

Asltoghiri, M., & Ghodsi, Z. (2012). The effects of reflexology on sleep disorder in menopausal women. *Procedia—Social and Behavioral Sciences, 31,* 242–246.

Dyer, J., Thomas, K., Sandsund, C., & Shaw, C. (2013). Is reflexology as effective as aromatherapy massage for symptom relief in an adult outpatient oncology population? *Complementary Therapies in Clinical Practice, 19,* 139–146.

Eghbali, M., Safari, R., Nazari, F., & Abdoli, S. (2012). The effects of reflexology on chronic low back pain intensity in nurses employed in hospitals affiliated with Isfahan University of Medical Sciences. *Iranian Journal of Nursing and Midwifery Research, 17*(3), 239–243.

Embong, N. H., Soh, Y. C., Ming, L. C., & Wong, T. W. (2015). Revisiting reflexology: Concept, evidence, current practice, and practitioner training. *Journal of Traditional and Complementary Medicine, 5,* 197–206.

Ernst, E., Posadzki, M., & Lee, M. S. (2011). Reflexology: An update of a systematic review of randomized clinical trials. *Maturitas, 68,* 116–120.

Gozuyesil, E., & Baser, M. (2016). The effect of foot reflexology applied to women aged between 40 and 60 on vasomotor complaints and quality of life. *Complementary Therapies in Clinical Practice, 24*, 78–85.

Gunnarsdottir, T. J., & Jonsdottir, H. (2010). Healing crisis in reflexology: Becoming worse before becoming better. *Complementary Therapies in Clinical Practice, 16*, 239–243.

Gunnarsdottir, T. J., & Peden-McAlpine, C. (2010). Effects of reflexology on fibromyalgia symptoms: A multiple case study. *Complementary Therapies in Clinical Practice, 16*, 167–172.

Hanjani, S. M., Tourzani, Z. M., & Shoghi, M. (2015). The effect of foot reflexology on anxiety, pain, and outcomes of the labor in primigravida women. *Acta Medica Iranica, 53*(8), 507–511.

Hansen, B., Grimsgaard, S., Launsø, L., Fønnebø, V., Falkenberg, T., & Rasmussen, N. K. (2005). Use of complementary and alternative medicine in the Scandinavian countries. *Scandinavian Journal of Primary Health Care, 23*, 57–62.

Helgadottir, B., Vilhjalmsson, R., & Gunnarsdottir, T. J. (2010). Notkun óhefðbundinnar heilbrigðisþjónustu á Íslandi. [Use of complementary and alternative therapies in Iceland]. *The Icelandic Medical Journal, 96*, 269–275.

Ingham, E. D. (1984). *Stories the feet can tell thru reflexology/Stories the feet have told thru reflexology.* Saint Petersburg, FL: Ingham Publishing.

International Institute of Reflexology. (2016). *Facts about reflexology.* Retrieved from http://www.reflexology-usa.net/facts.htm

Johns, C., Blake, D., & Sinclair, A. (2010). Can reflexology maintain or improve the well-being of people with Parkinson's disease? *Complementary Therapies in Clinical Practice, 16*, 96–100.

Jones, J., Thomson, P., Lauder, W., Howie, K., & Leslie, S. J. (2012). Reflexology has an acute (immediate) haemodynamic effect in healthy volunteers: A double-blind randomized controlled trial. *Complementary Therapies in Clinical Practice, 18*, 204–211.

Jones, J., Thomson, P., Lauder, W., Howie, K., & Leslie, S. J. (2013). Reflexology has no immediate haemodynamic effect in patients with chronic heart failure: A double blind randomized controlled trial. *Complementary Therapies in Clinical Practice, 19*, 133–138.

Jones, J., Thomson, P., Lauder, W., & Leslie, S. J. (2012). Reported treatment strategies for reflexology in cardiac patients and inconsistencies in the location of the heart reflex point: An online survey. *Complementary Therapies in Clinical Practice, 18*, 145–150.

Jones, J., Thomson, P., Irvine, K., & Leslie, S. J. (2013). Is there a specific hemodynamic effect in reflexology? A systematic review of randomized controlled trials. *The Journal of Alternative and Complementary Medicine, 19*(4), 319–328.

Kaptchuk, T. J. (2000). *The web that has no weaver: Understanding Chinese medicine.* Chicago, IL: Contemporary Books.

Kim, J., Kang, J. W., & Ernst, E. (2010). Reflexology for the symptomatic treatment of breast cancer: A systematic review. *Integrative Cancer Therapies, 9*(4), 326–330.

Kim, Y. H., & Cho, S. H. (2002). The effect of foot reflexology on premenstrual syndrome and dysmenorrhea in female college students. *Korean Journal of Women's Health, 8*(2), 212–221.

Kjøller, M. & Rasmussen, N. K. (2002). *Sundhed og Sygelighed in Danmark 2000 – og udviklingen siden 1987. [Health and Morbidity in Denmark 2000 – and development since 1987].* Copenhagen, Denmark: National Institute of Public Health.

Kunz, K., & Kunz, B. (2003). *Reflexology: Health at your fingertips.* New York, NY: DK Publishing.

Maciocia, G. (2005). *The foundations of Chinese medicine* (2nd ed.). London, UK: Elsevier.

Mackereth, P. A., Booth, K., Hillier, V. F., & Caress, A. (2009). What do people talk about during reflexology? Analysis of worries and concerns expressed during sessions for patients with multiple sclerosis. *Complementary Therapies in Clinical Practice, 15*, 85–90.

Manjuri, A. E., & Latheef, F. (2016). Effectiveness of foot reflexology vs back massage on quality of sleep among post cesarean mothers. *International Journal of Pharma and Bio Sciences, 7*(2), 558–562.

McCullough, J. E. M., Liddle, S. D., Sinclair, M., Close, C., & Hughes, C. M. (2014). The physiological and biochemical outcomes associated with a reflexology treatment: A systematic review. *Evidence-Based Complementary & Alternative Medicine, 2014*, 1–16.

Metin, Z. G., & Ozdemir, L. (2016). The effects of aromatherapy massage and reflexology on pain and fatigue in patients with rheumatoid arthritis: A randomized controlled trial. *Pain Management Nursing, 17*(2), 140–149.

National Center for Complementary and Integrative Health. (2016). *Reflexology*. Retrieved from http://nccam.nih.gov/health/reflexology

Nazari, F., Shahreza, M. S., Shaygannejad, V., & Valiani, M. (2015). Comparing the effects of reflexology and relaxation on fatigue in women with multiple sclerosis. *Iran Journal of Nursing and Midwifery Research, 20*(2), 200–204.

Rollinson, K., Jones, J., Scott, N., Megson, I. L., & Leslie, S. J. (2016). The acute (immediate) effects of reflexology on arterial compliance in healthy volunteers: A randomized study. *Complementary Therapies in Clinical Practice, 22*, 16–20.

Sharp, D. M., Walker, M. B., Chaturvedi, A., Upadhyay, S., Hamid, A., Walker, A. A., … Walker, L. G. (2010). A randomized, controlled trial of the psychological effects of reflexology in early breast cancer. *European Journal of Cancer, 46*, 312–322.

Stockholm County Council. (2001). Stockholmare och den komplementära medicine. Hälso och sjukvårdsnämden [Stockholmers and complementary medicine. County health service]. Stockholm, Sweden: Author.

Wang, M., Tsai, P., Lee, P., Chang, W., & Yang, C. (2008). The efficacy of reflexology: A systematic review. *Journal of Advanced Nursing, 62*(5), 512–520.

Woodward, S., Norton, C., & Barriball, K. (2010). A pilot study of the effectiveness of reflexology in treating idiopathic constipation in women. *Complementary Therapies in Clinical Practice, 16*, 41–46.

Unal, K. S., & Akpinar, R. B. (2016). The effect of foot reflexology and back massage on hemodialysis patients' fatigue and sleep quality. *Complementary Therapies in Clinical Practice, 24*, 139–144.

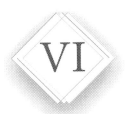

Education, Practice, Research, and Personal Use

The new title for the center that focuses on complementary therapies in the National Institutes of Health (NIH) conveys that these therapies are becoming an integral part of Western health: National Center for Complementary and Integrative Health (NCCIH). Complementary therapies have moved from the periphery of conventional healthcare to being integrated into the fabric of education (Chapter 27), practice (Chapter 28), research (Chapter 29), and personal health and self-care regimens (Chapter 30). Nurses have been instrumental in this integration. Although great strides have been made, continuing efforts are necessary if holistic health care is to be available to all people.

Use of complementary therapies in practice settings has been increasing, largely because of the public's demand for these treatments (NCCIH, 2016). Whether these are well-known therapies, such as music, chiropractic care, and yoga, or ones that seem quite foreign to many, such as the Alexander technique and smudging ceremonies, health systems are looking very different from the way they were 50 or even 25 years ago. As health professions integrate content on complementary therapies into program curricula, healthcare systems continue to reflect a more holistic care. A particular need is for healthcare workers to gain knowledge about the health practices of indigenous people.

Concerns about the safety and efficacy of many of the complementary therapies continue. Funding for research on complementary therapies by NCCIH has increased, thus providing a greater basis for evidence-based practice. Other NIH institutes are also funding research on complementary therapies and on increasing their inclusion in health curricula. Not only is the increase in research important, but reviews and meta-analyses of studies on specific procedures provide invaluable assistance to practitioners, educators, and researchers. New methods of inquiry and measurements for outcomes are needed for numerous therapies, particularly those practiced in non-Western and indigenous cultures.

Guidelines for the use of complementary treatments have been developed by professional organizations such as the American Holistic Nurses Association and the Oncology Nurses Association and address safety in the use of complementary therapies. In addition, many state BONs have delineated guidance for the use of complementary therapies within nursing practice.

As noted in Chapter 27, professional nursing education organizations have specifications for content on complementary therapies that should be incorporated into the various curricula. If these are to be truly implemented, many more pre-pared faculty members are needed to teach nursing students, both at the basic and the graduate levels. Faculty are also at the forefront in conducting research on com-plementary therapies.

Not only in the United States but across the globe, greater attention is being given to the integration of complementary therapies into healthcare. As has been noted numerous times in this text, the mobility of individuals globally for travel, for education, or as immigrants and refugees is requiring that nurses and other health professionals become more conversant about the wide diversity in healthcare prac-tices and are used around the world. Nurses, as caring, competent professionals, have the opportunity and challenge to be leaders in these efforts.

Parting words by the editors can be found in Chapter 31. In this final chapter, we share our reflections regarding trajectories of change and anticipations related to how complementary and alternative therapy use will be expanded. We consider a bright future for the use of complementary therapies in integrative care models and the impact that this will have on nursing education and practice, as well as patient outcomes and satisfaction. Future challenges to be overcome by the profes-sion and exciting opportunities for leadership and change are outlined, as we share our dreams and visions for a preferred future.

REFERENCES

National Center for Complementary Therapies and Integrative Health. (2016). *Complementary, alternative, or integrative health: What's in a name?* [NCCIH Pub No. D347]. Washington, DC: Author. Retrieved from https://nccih.nih.gov/health/integrative-health

Integrating Complementary Therapies Into Education

Carie A. Braun

Nursing curricula must constantly evolve to improve patient care quality and keep pace with the ever-changing healthcare environment. Significant changes surrounding nurse educators include increased globalization, technological advancements, health policy and economics, and increased patient care complexity (Hegarty, Walsh, Condon, & Sweeney, 2009; Solomon et al., 2016). Salmon (2010) notes, however, that, despite constant change, integrative health is fundamentally connected to the past, present, and future of nursing education, research, and practice.

The impact of globalization has heightened the need to seamlessly integrate complementary and alternative therapies into holistic patient care. This is primarily due to the proliferative use of complementary and alternative therapies by the public, safety issues with combining conventional and alternative modalities, cultural competence and the emphasis on patient-centered care, and increasing evidence of the positive impact of integrative healthcare systems on healthcare outcomes (Moore, 2010; Schultz, Chao, & McGinnis, 2009). These influences have permeated the practice of nursing and, as a result, the licensing examination has evolved to emphasize holistic care and integrative health, which includes a basic knowledge of complementary therapies. The NCLEX-RN®, a reflection of actual nursing practice and an important indicator of nursing program quality, has expected knowledge of complementary therapies for entry-level RNs since 2004 (Stratton, Benn, Lie, Zeller, & Nedrow, 2007). The detailed test plan for the NCLEX-RN in 2016 continues to require the knowledge of health promotion and maintenance, including the safe integration of complementary therapies into the patient's plan of care.

Other documents guiding nursing curricula have been equally influential. The American Association of Colleges of Nursing (AACN) specifically identified baccalaureate generalist practice to include a beginning understanding of complementary and alternative modalities (AACN, 2008). For graduate education, the *AACN Essentials of Master's Education for Nursing* (AACN, 2011) required master's-level nurses to deliver healthcare services within integrated care systems. Similarly, the

AACN Essentials of Doctoral Education for Advanced Practice Nursing (AACN, 2006) directed Doctor of Nursing Practice (DNP) programs to prepare graduates to synthesize concepts related to clinical prevention and population health, including psychosocial dimensions and cultural diversity. The report by the Institute of Medicine (IOM, 2011) on the future of nursing affirmed that nurses should practice to the full extent of their education and should achieve higher levels of knowledge to promote quality patient-centered care.

The initial discourse in the 1990s about whether or not complementary therapies *should* be taught in nursing and other healthcare programs has now been replaced with a pervasive discussion and debate about *what* should be included and *how* to deepen the integration of complementary therapies within a holistic patient-care paradigm (Cutshall et al., 2010; Little, 2013; Van Sant-Smith, 2015). The challenge for nurse educators is to promote professional nursing education that remains socially responsive and flexible (Salmon, 2010).

DEFINING COMPLEMENTARY THERAPY CORE COMPETENCIES

A universally accepted list of complementary therapy core competencies for nursing has yet to be developed. However, the close alignment of nursing with holistic and integrative healthcare provides solid justification for moving forward. Booth-LaForce et al. (2010), Chlan and Halcón (2003), and Kreitzer, Mann, and Lumpkin (2008) have advocated for an integrated curriculum grounded in holistic, patient-centered care beginning at the baccalaureate level. These authors have suggested several core competencies, including

- Awareness and assessment of therapies and practices
- Evaluation of the evidence base underlying therapies and practices
- Skill development in therapies and practices
- Self-awareness and self-care
- Awareness of the theoretical basis underlying therapies and practices

These competencies are evident in the scope and standards for practicing nurses. The American Nurses Association (ANA, 2015), in the book *Nursing: Scope and Standards of Practice*, third edition, spells out the practice parameters and responsibilities for all RNs in the United States. The practice standards of assessment, diagnosis, outcome identification, planning, implementation, and evaluation allow for an individualized plan of care that is sensitive to diverse healthcare practices for all patients. The professional performance standards of quality of practice, practice evaluation, education, collegiality, collaboration, ethics, research, resource utilization, and leadership commit nurses constantly to improve knowledge, skills, and competencies appropriate to the nursing role.

The ANA's *Nursing: Scope and Standards of Practice* (ANA, 2015) indicates that nurses must be knowledgeable about and sensitive to a range of health practices so that holistic nursing care can be provided. The document does not identify specific therapies that nurses may or may not incorporate into nursing practice. Specific therapies, which are within the realm of nursing given the appropriate training, are outlined in the *Nursing Interventions Classification* (Bulechek, Butcher,

Dochterman, & Wagner, 2013) and include acupressure, animal-assisted therapy, aromatherapy, art therapy, biofeedback, massage, music therapy, self-hypnosis facilitation, and therapeutic touch. Although the knowledge base for many complementary therapies may be part of the educational program, performance proficiency is often not achieved during an undergraduate or even graduate nursing education. Therefore, even though nurses *can* perform these therapies, they *should* perform them only with the appropriate training and certification.

Complementary therapy education expectations are also evident in various board of nursing (BON) documents within the states and territories of the United States that regulate nursing practice to ensure patient safety. Of the 53 BONs surveyed in 2001, 47% had statements or positions that included specific complementary therapies or examples of these practices, 13% had them under discussion, and 40% had not formally addressed the topic but did not necessarily discourage these practices (Sparber, 2001). Although this survey has not been repeated, the percentage of BONs with formal position statements is likely on the rise. BONs are increasingly aware of and supportive of the integration of complementary therapies into nursing practice, and they are continuously clarifying what is within the scope of nursing practice and identifying basic education and competencies required for nursing practice. The American Holistic Nurses Association (AHNA) provides a resource for finding a state's position on holistic nursing practice at http://www.ahna.org/Resources. For example, the Minnesota Board of Nursing reaffirmed in 2010 a *Statement of Accountability for Utilization of Integrative Therapies in Nursing Practice*. An excerpt from this statement is as follows

> Complementary and alternative practices and integrative therapies may address health needs by promoting comfort, healing and well-being, and may be adjunctive or primary interventions in nursing care. The Board believes the utilization of integrative therapies and alternative healthcare practices within the practice of nursing should be consistent with the consumer expectation for public safety, without undue regulation or restriction on the integrative therapies desired by consumers. (p. 1)

Because the interpretation of the nursing scope of practice can vary based on the different state or territorial BONs, nurses must be aware of their own state's position regarding complementary therapies, must have the documented knowledge and competencies to perform the therapy, and must adhere to licensure and credentialing regulations.

Internationally, similar nursing regulatory agencies have articulated the role of the RN and/or advanced practice nurse in understanding and practicing complementary therapies. For example, the Government of Western Australia's Community Midwifery Program (2015) has published a standard protocol for use of complementary therapies in midwifery practice. The guidelines indicate, "Only midwives who have undertaken postregistration educational qualifications in specialized techniques and modalities of the recognized complementary and alternative medicine (CAM) should administer or advise pregnant women" (p. 1). Selection and verification of the educational program in the specific complementary therapy is the responsibility of the midwife.

Specialty organizations have also weighed in on the debate about which complementary therapies nurses can and should perform. The AHNA and the ANA have jointly developed the *Scope and Standards of Practice for Holistic Nursing* (2013), which includes a core curriculum and certification for an integrative healthcare practice infused with the principles of complementary and alternative therapies and competencies consistent with holistic nursing practice. The certification, although not required in most prelicensure or advanced practice educational programs, offers important insights as to the expectations of certification in holistic nursing practice.

Increasingly, nursing programs are becoming more attentive to the role of complementary therapies in patient health. Multiple authors have suggested specific content applicable to the undergraduate and graduate nursing curriculum (Cuellar, Cahill, Ford, & Aycock, 2003; Gaster, Unterborn, Scott, & Schneeweiss, 2007; Kreitzer et al., 2008; Lee et al., 2007). The following is a compilation of suggested student learning outcomes that address the necessary dimensions for educating students within general nursing practice:

- Describe the prevalence and patterns of complementary therapy use by the public.
- Compare and contrast the underlying principles and beliefs in Western belief systems and alternative health belief systems.
- Communicate effectively with patients and families about complementary and alternative therapies.
- Critique the scientific evidence available for the most commonly used complementary and alternative therapies.
- Identify reputable sources of information to support continued learning about complementary and alternative therapies.
- Explore the roles, training, and credentialing of complementary and alternative therapy practitioners.
- Reflect on and improve self-care measures and wellness to incorporate complementary therapies for self, where applicable.

CURRENT STATE OF COMPLEMENTARY THERAPIES IN NURSING EDUCATION

Koithan (2015) recognized that the integration of complementary therapies in nursing education requires little or no shift in philosophical paradigm because issues such as wellness, prevention, and holistic health have long been at the core of nursing practice. There is ample evidence to suggest that nursing education programs, albeit inconsistently, are already attending to the knowledge base needed and to the understanding of the role of complementary therapies in healthcare. For example, multiple studies have confirmed that nursing faculty and students believe that complementary therapies must be integrated into the nursing curriculum and that nurses must be prepared to advise patients regarding best practices in integrative healthcare (Al-Rukban et al., 2012; Avino, 2011; Cutshall et al., 2010; Geisler, Cheung, Johnson Steinhagen, Neubeck, & Brueggeman, 2015; Halcón, Chlan, Kreitzer, & Leonard, 2003; Kim, Erlen, Kim, & Sok, 2006; Nedrow, Istvan et al., 2007; Poreddi et al., 2016; Yildirim et al., 2010). A few of these studies also determined that nursing students, on graduation, did not feel prepared to integrate complementary therapies and that more education was desired (Kim et al., 2006;

Poreddi et al., 2016; Topuz, Uysal, & Yilmaz, 2015; Yildirim et al., 2010). Avino (2011) reported that students were open to the health benefits of complementary therapies, although they did not want to be overwhelmed with information or trained to personally provide each therapy.

Dutta et al. (2003), Fenton and Morris (2003), and Richardson (2003) sampled nursing schools across the United States to determine the extent to which the schools integrated complementary and alternative modalities into their curricula. For all three studies, a large percentage already included complementary therapies in the curriculum (49%–85%), and almost all of the programs were planning to incorporate additional complementary therapies in the future. The same appears to be true for family nurse practitioner programs (Burman, 2003). Very few of the responding schools had a separate required course on complementary therapies (11%–15%), whereas most offered a separate elective course (37%–84%) and approximately one third offered a continuing education option. The most commonly included therapies were spirituality/prayer/meditation, relaxation, guided imagery, herbals, acupuncture, massage, and therapeutic touch.

Internationally, nursing education programs are also addressing the need to integrate complementary therapies. Sok, Erlen, and Kim (2004) reported that more than 10 universities in the United Kingdom offered students full-time degree programs in complementary and alternative therapies, such as osteopathy, chiropractic medicine, herbal medicines, acupuncture, and homeopathy. Hon et al. (2006) reported that the regulatory body for nursing in Hong Kong now requires the nursing curriculum to contain 20 hours devoted to traditional Chinese medicine (TCM). Similarly, Yeh and Chung (2007) investigated the current and expected levels of competence in TCM that baccalaureate nurses should possess in Taiwan. In Korea, one college of nursing science now has a 1-year program that leads to a certificate in complementary and alternative therapies for clinical nurses and researchers (Sok et al., 2004). At one large university in Turkey, the majority of nursing and midwifery students (93.5%) had personal experience with complementary and alternative therapies, with knowledge of the therapies coming from the school (60%) (Camurdan & Gül, 2013). To contrast these efforts, only 13% of nursing colleges in Saudi Arabia introduced complementary therapies briefly within a course. None of the respondents reported having a dedicated complementary therapies course, continuing education related to complementary therapies, or faculty interest/expertise in complementary therapies (Al-Rukban et al., 2012). The authors of this study indicated that the interest in complementary therapies was just beginning and further integration was underway.

FACULTY QUALIFICATIONS AND DEVELOPMENT

Although the majority of nursing programs in the United States and throughout the world integrate complementary therapies in some way, the greatest challenges have included finding qualified faculty, an already crowded curriculum, lack of definition for "best practices" in integrative care, and sustainability of complementary therapy content within the curriculum (Avino, 2011; Lee et al., 2007). In one study, the top three therapies for which additional training was desired by faculty included nutritional supplements, herbal medicine, and massage (Avino, 2011). In another survey, greater knowledge was desired in TCM, qigong, Ayurveda, and energy modulation (Cutshall et al., 2010). Avino (2011) also found that the preferred pedagogy for undergraduate nursing students was direct active learning and the least preferred was through online modules. Studies are yet to be published on the use of simulation in integrative healthcare situations.

Stratton et al. (2007) identified essential faculty development needed to facilitate learning in integrative healthcare. First and foremost, a critical mass of knowledgeable faculty is essential to the successful integration and sustainability of complementary therapies into a nursing curriculum. Viewing complementary therapy information through the lens of evidence-based practice can facilitate acceptance and provide an opportunity for faculty to become more familiar with complementary therapy principles and research (Stratton et al., 2007). Faculty development requires time and resources, access to scholarly writings, reference and research resources, reassigned time, consultations, collaboration, continuing education, and support. Ideally, continuing-education workshops or conferences should be structured using a collaborative approach representing the varying perspectives of complementary and alternative therapy practitioners. Encouraging and supporting faculty research in the area of complementary therapies is another mechanism of generating a team of qualified faculty.

IMPLEMENTATION MODELS

Integrative Curricula

Significant changes have occurred within the National Institutes of Health in the past 3 years with regard to complementary and alternative therapy education. The mission of the National Center for Complementary and Integrative Health (NCCIH. 2017), formerly the National Center for Complementary and Alternative Medicine (NCCAM), is to "define, through rigorous scientific investigation, the usefulness and safety of complementary and integrative interventions and to provide the public with research-based information to guide health-care decision making." Among the nine major divisions of the Center, the Office of Communications and Public Liaison handles activities pertaining to implementing integrative healthcare education and outreach initiatives.

The CAM Education Program, started in 2000 by the NCCAM, is now completed, but the impact continues. This project was designed to incorporate CAM information into the curricula of selected health profession schools (Pearson & Chesney, 2007) and has been influential in providing models for integrating complementary and alternative therapies into healthcare education (Nedrow, Istvan, et al., 2007). The 72-member Consortium for Academic Health Centers for Integrative Medicine (www.imconsortium.org) coordinates integrative health systems, including integrative education, research, policy, and patient care. The mission of the consortium is to advance integrative healthcare within academic institutions.

A significant example of postbaccalaureate education, stemming from the CAM Education Project, is found at https://cam.georgetown.edu/about-the-program. Georgetown University's (Washington, DC) CAM-MS Program in Physiology is a 30-credit-hour graduate degree developed to prepare integrative healthcare practitioners and scientists and to encourage graduates to pursue future doctoral research in complementary therapies. The program graduated nine students enrolled in its first class in 2004, and since then, the CAM program has expanded to include a capped class of 30 physiology students every year.

At least four programs in the CAM Education Project created integrative curricula in nursing. The School of Nursing at the University of Minnesota and the Center for Spirituality and Healing revised curricula to incorporate complementary and alternative therapies into baccalaureate, master's, and doctoral programs (Halcón, Leonard, Snyder, Garwick, & Kreitzer, 2001). The curricular revisions strengthened didactic and experiential learning to encompass complementary therapies theory and research, supported interdisciplinary courses as part of the graduate minor in complementary therapies and healing practices, and incorporated self-care concepts. These programs have continued and expanded (www.csh.umn.edu/education/focus-areas/integrative-nursing). The University of Minnesota offers an Integrative Health and Healing specialty within the Doctor of Nursing Practice (DNP) program to "prepare graduates to developing integrative approaches to health promotion, disease prevention and chronic disease management and encourage such practices throughout healthcare systems" (www .nursing.umn.edu/degrees-programs/doctor-nursing-practice/post-baccalaureate/ integrative-health-and-healing).

At Rush University (Chicago) all students in the undergraduate and graduate programs (including an entry-level generalist master's and advanced specialty practice) were exposed to complementary therapy through required courses such as pharmacology, health assessment, nutrition, research, and community health nursing. This project started in 2001. Curricular competencies were outlined for assessment, therapy indications and contraindications, safety, evidence-based practice, and collaboration. Much of the coursework was designed through web-based modules for use in the curriculum and as continuing-education offerings.

The University of Washington School of Nursing (Seattle), in partnership with Bastyr University (Kenmore, WA; San Diego, CA), provided faculty development on complementary therapies through a summer educational program (Booth-LaForce et al., 2010; Fenton & Morris, 2003; Nedrow, Heitkemper, et al., 2007). Faculty used what they learned to support the integration of complementary therapies throughout the nursing curriculum. As a result of this implementation project, about half of faculty incorporated complementary therapy content in class, and more than half indicated that their complementary therapy knowledge increased a moderate or great extent. A higher number of students (70%) indicated that their knowledge of complementary therapies improved, with intended self-reported competencies increased throughout the grant period.

Nursing programs throughout the world are implementing integrative educational models to build the complementary therapy knowledge base of generalist nurses. Helms (2006) proposed a sustainable model in which every course included complementary therapy content, with course objectives reflective of complementary and alternative therapy integration in patient care. For example, healthcare system or policy courses included the history of and philosophical basis for complementary and alternative therapies and health systems. Health assessment courses included history taking inclusive of complementary and alternative therapies. Pharmacology courses were a logical placement for herbal medicines, essential oils, and homeopathic preparations. Nutrition courses added dietary/biologically based therapies. Psychiatric nursing courses emphasized cognitive behavioral therapy or meditation. And nursing research courses included all aspects of complementary therapy efficacy through the lens of evidence-based practice. In addition, the use of simulation, which emphasizes integrative healthcare would be an important addition to nursing curricula.

Major and Minor Fields of Study

Following the lead of the CAM Education Project, colleges and universities throughout the United States are offering major or minor studies in integrative health, nursing, medicine, and other disciplines from the bachelor's degree to the doctorate. Sofhauser (2002) described the development of a 15-credit minor in complementary health at the Indiana University, South Bend. This program continues to enroll students today. The University of Arizona provides a BS program in integrative health, which "provides a foundation in integrative health, a holistic approach to wellness that focuses on the mind, body and spirit" (https://nursingandhealth.asu.edu/integrative-health). Multiple examples of integrative health majors or minors are available to students interested in complementary and alternative therapies.

Course in Complementary Therapies

Another potential approach for learning about complementary and alternative therapies is through specific courses. Groft and Kalischuk (2005) described a 13-week, 3-hour-per-session undergraduate elective course on health and healing. Students explored a range of complementary and alternative therapies commonly used by patients. The course was determined to be highly effective in aiding students' understanding of healing and wholeness. More recently, van der Reit, Francis, and Levett-Jones (2011) implemented and evaluated an elective course for undergraduate students that included a study tour to Thailand, where students learned the techniques of Thai massage and other complementary therapies. The course was positively evaluated and also improved global health awareness.

Experiential Learning

Active learning is recommended for any students interested in complementary therapies. Chlan, Halcón, Kreitzer, and Leonard (2005) studied the influence of skills laboratory practice on nursing student confidence levels in performing select complementary therapy skills. Student confidence in the performance of the five therapies (hand massage, imagery, music interventions, reflexology, and breathing/mindfulness) increased after the session. The greatest increases in confidence were seen with hand massage, reflexology, and imagery. This study demonstrated the immense value of bringing practical application of CAM into undergraduate nursing education. Similarly, Adler (2009) and Cook and Robinson (2006) implemented an intensive massage therapy experience to promote nursing student competence. The majority of student participants indicated that the experience was valuable in their development as nurses by contributing to the nurse–patient relationship and holism in patient care. Clinical experiences have also been described that allow students to participate through assessment and observation of the application of Reiki (Bremner, Bennett, & Chambers, 2014). Application of therapies has also been introduced through student research projects. Johnson (2014) studied the use of aromatherapy to decrease test anxiety in nursing students, with positive results.

Continuing-Education Offerings

For practicing nurses, effective continuing-education opportunities are needed to advance knowledge and skills in complementary therapies. The AHNA has endorsed several continuing-education modules and certification programs that promote holistic nursing practice. Nurse practitioners responding to one survey indicated complementary therapy continuing education needed to include information on scientific principles, evidence of efficacy, potential interactions with conventional medicine, and pharmacology. The preferred mechanism for advancing this knowledge was online continuing nursing education (67%), conferences (60%), workshops (60%), and newsletters (51%) (Patterson, Kaczorowski, Arthur, Smith, & Mills, 2003). The NCCIH also offers online continuing-education modules across a range of integrative therapy topics. Many online and conference opportunities can assist practicing nurses in improving complementary therapy knowledge and skills (see the website list at the end of this chapter).

FACILITATING AND EVALUATING STUDENT LEARNING

Active and creative pedagogies are needed to facilitate student learning and support effective teaching of complementary therapies. Swanson et al. (2012) reported that online case-based modules were an effective method of teaching graduate nursing students about the clinical issues surrounding complementary and alternative therapies. According to Lee et al. (2007), CAM Education Project schools used a variety of instructional delivery strategies to help students learn about complementary therapies, including classroom-based programs, online modules, and experiential learning. These authors also recognized that personal reflection and self-care are critical components of student learning. At the course level, traditional student learning evaluation methods, such as written papers, examinations, and other projects, were used along with explorative methods, such as through interviews, focus groups, and 1-minute feedback papers, to gain course evaluation information for course improvement (Stratton et al., 2007). Stratton et al. (2007) noted:

> In the absence of a single, established set of approved CAM education or competency standards, an array of curricula exist. Consequently, the approaches to evaluating student learning were equally diverse and involved the development and refinement of assessment tools to measure a wide variety of attitudes, beliefs, motivations, knowledge bases, and skills. (p. 959)

CONCLUSIONS

Lindeman (2000) predicted that the future of nursing education would include "greater diversity in clinical experiences to provide contact with people from different cultures, ethnic groups, economic levels, and with alternatives to [W]estern medicine" (p. 11). This certainly has been the case. Nursing education bears a significant responsibility in the movement toward integrative health. Koithan (2015) describes what this looks like for student nurses:

> In adopting this principle, our care becomes individualized, tailored, and meaningful. We do not recommend therapies, whether biomedical, mind–body, or manipulative, that a person cannot afford or access. We do not ask the impossible of our clients or their families. We consider the full ramifications of our interventions on the ecological (environmental) and social (communities and organizations) systems within which we exist. As such, our practice becomes sustainable and moral, one that is mindful and respectful of the complexities of life. We listen more and talk less, recognizing that personal wisdom may be just as important as professional knowledge as together we identify and strengthen resources (biopsychosocial–spiritual) that restore and replenish and ultimately support the emergence of health and well-being. (p. 194)

Although Dossey (2013) recognized that the paradigm of nursing education has shifted from a disease-focused to a more holistic approach that integrates patient-centered health practices, it is only through thoughtful reflection on the current curricula, adherence to the scope and standards of practice for nurses, and attention to educational and healthcare influences that can we continue to move forward.

Karin Gerber, a nurse educator from South Africa, details the inclusion of complementary therapies within the curriculum at Nelson Mandela Metropolitan University (NMMU). Content from an interview is found in Sidebar 27.1.

SIDEBAR 27.1 INTEGRATION OF TRADITIONAL HEALERS WITH NURSING EDUCATION IN SOUTH AFRICA

Karin Gerber

Throughout the world, nurse educators are responding to the need to integrate complementary and traditional healing into nursing curricula, including South Africa, the "Rainbow Nation," where health practices are as diverse as the people. In an interview with two nurse educators from Nelson Mandela Metropolitan University (NMMU), located in Port Elizabeth, South Africa, it was affirmed that traditional African healing practices are presented to the nursing students alongside Western modalities. The nurse educators teach students to be open to various methods of healing but to always seek best practices in their nursing care. The nursing program is science oriented but inclusive of a broad view of therapies based on patient and family preferences. Of particular note is the collaboration of nursing education with traditional healers within the Nguni and Xhosa societies of South Africa: the diviner (*sangoma* or *amagqirha*) and the herbalist (*inyanga* or *ixwele*).

The diviners and herbalists are highly respected and serve approximately 60% of the people of South Africa. Traditional healers in South Africa greatly outnumber Western-medicine doctors at a rate of 8:1 (Truter, 2007). The distinction between the two types of healers is often blurred; however, in general,

(continued)

the herbalist is concerned with medicines made from plants and animals, and the diviner is a spiritualist, using divination for healing purposes. Herbalists make use of more than 3,000 botanical, zoological, and mineral products to bring healing (van Wyk, van Oudtshoorn, & Gericke, 1999). These products are used as a bath-water or steaming preparation, ingested (often with a goal to induce vomiting) or inserted as an enema, are placed into incisions in the skin, or inhaled nasally (van Wyk et al., 1999). The diviner, through ancestral channeling, prayer, purification, throwing of the bones, use of incense, dream interpretation, or animal sacrifice with a goal of appeasing the spirits, seeks to establish a positive relationship and restitution between the ill person and the spirits causing the illness (Campbell, 1998). The Traditional Health Practitioners Act of 2007 (Republic of South Africa, Government Gazette, 2008) legally recognizes diviners, herbalists, traditional surgeons, and traditional birth attendants as traditional health practitioners. Western-medicine providers continue to study the efficacy of the herbal remedies used, including those for HIV/AIDS, pneumonia, and diarrhea, all major causes of death in South Africa.

Clearly, public acceptance and use of traditional healers has a major influence on the integration of course content at NMMU. The nurse educators noted that each of the nursing courses has relevant content related to traditional healing, and students often talk about their own personal experiences with the healing modalities. Students are made aware of the risks of the various healing practices because some are known to be toxic, particularly to the kidneys, causing patients to require dialysis. Students are taught how to work together with traditional healers in situations where traditional healing and Western medicine are complementary, such as in the induction of labor. Nurse educators also work with students in the communities to promote optimal health in areas where ritualistic cutting in initiations or as part of traditional healing has led to high rates of infection and mortality. Overall, there is a conscientious effort to help students understand what is helpful and what can be harmful and how to intervene to promote optimal patient care.

References

Campbell, S. (1998). *Called to heal*. Twin Lakes, WI: Lotus Press.

Republic of South Africa, Government Gazette. (2008, January 10). *Traditional Healers Act of 2007 (511 No. 42)*. Retrieved from http://www.info.gov.za/view/DownloadFileAction?id=77788

Truter, I. (2007). African traditional healers: Cultural and religious beliefs intertwined in a holistic way. *South Africa Pharmaceutical Journal, 74*, 56–60.

van Wyk, B., van Oudtshoorn, B., & Gericke, N. (1999). *Medicinal plants of South Africa*. Pretoria, South Africa: Briza.

WEBSITES

There is an abundance of reputable resources to facilitate effective teaching and student learning in the area of complementary and alternative therapies. A beginning list follows:

- American Holistic Nurses Association-Educational Resources (www.ahna.org/Resources)

- Center Institute for Research and Education in Integrative Medicine (www.healthandhealingny.org/professionals/nurse.asp)
- CINAHL: Cumulative Index to Nursing & Allied Health Literature (www.ebscohost.com/academic/cinahl-plus-with-full-text)
- Consortium for Academic Health Centers for Integrative Medicine (www.imconsortium.org)
- National Center for Complementary and Integrative Health-Online Continuing Education Series (https://nccih.nih.gov/training/videolectures)

REFERENCES

Adler, P. (2009). Teaching massage to nursing students of geriatrics through active learning. *Journal of Holistic Nursing, 27*, 51–56.

Al-Rukban, M., AlBedah, A., Khalil, M., El-Olemy, A., Khalil, A., & Alrasheid, M. (2012). Status of complementary and alternative medicine in the curricula of health colleges in Saudi Arabia. *Complementary Therapies in Medicine, 20*, 334–339.

American Association of Colleges of Nursing. (2006). *The essentials of doctoral education for advanced practice nursing.* Retrieved from http://www.aacnnursing.org/Portals/42/Publications/DNPEssentials.pdf

American Association of Colleges of Nursing. (2008). *The essentials of baccalaureate education for professional nursing practice.* Retrieved from http://www.aacnnursing.org/Portals/42/Publications/BaccEssentials08.pdf

American Association of Colleges of Nursing. (2011). *The essentials of master's education for nursing.* Retrieved from http://www.aacnnursing.org/Portals/42/Publications/MastersEssentials11.pdf

American Holistic Nurses Association & American Nurses Association. (2013). *Holistic nursing: Scope and standards of practice.* Silver Spring, MD: Author.

American Nurses Association. (2015). *Nursing: Scope and standards of practice* (3rd ed.). Washington, DC: American Nurses Association.

Avino, K. (2011). Knowledge, attitudes, and practices of nursing faculty and students related to complementary and alternative medicine. *Holistic Nursing Practice, 25*, 280–288.

Booth-LaForce, C., Scott, C., Heitkemper, M., Cornman, J., Lan, M., Bond, E., & Swanson, K. (2010). Complementary and alternative (CAM) attitudes and competencies of nursing students and faculty: Results of integrating CAM into the nursing curriculum. *Journal of Professional Nursing, 26*, 293–300.

Bremner, M., Bennett, D., & Chambers, D. (2014). Integrating Reiki and community-engaged scholarship: An interdisciplinary educational intervention. *Journal of Nursing Education, 53*, 541–543.

Bulechek, G., Butcher, H., Dochterman, J., & Wagner, C. (Eds.). (2013). *Nursing interventions classification (NIC)* (6th ed.). St. Louis, MO: Elsevier.

Burman, M. (2003). Complementary and alternative medicine: Core competencies for family nurse practitioners. *Journal of Nursing Education, 42*, 28–34.

Camurdan, C., & Gül, A. (2013). Complementary and alternative medicine use among nursing and midwifery students in Turkey. *Nurse Education in Practice, 13*, 350–354.

Chlan, L., & Halcón, L. (2003). Developing an integrated baccalaureate nursing education program: Infusing complementary/alternative therapies into critical care curricula. *Critical Care Nursing Clinics of North America, 15*, 373–379.

Chlan, L., Halcón, L., Kreitzer, M., & Leonard, B. (2005). Influence of an experiential education session on nursing students' confidence levels in performing selected complementary therapy skills. *Complementary Health Practice Review, 10*, 189–201.

Cook, N., & Robinson, J. (2006). Effectiveness and value of massage skills training during pre-registration nurse education. *Nurse Education Today, 26*, 555–563.

Cuellar, N., Cahill, B., Ford, J., & Aycock, T. (2003). The development of an educational workshop on complementary and alternative medicine: What every nurse should know. *Journal of Continuing Education in Nursing, 34*, 128–135.

Cutshall, S., Derscheid, D., Miers, A., Ruegg, S., Schroeder, B., Tucker, S., & Wentworth, L. (2010). Knowledge, attitudes, and use of complementary and alternative therapies among clinical nurse specialists in an academic medical center. *Clinical Nurse Specialist, 24*, 125–131.

Dossey, B. (2013). Integral and holistic nursing: Local to global. In B. Dossey & L. Keegan (Eds.), *Holistic nursing: A handbook for practice* (6th ed., pp. 3–58). Burlington, MA: Jones & Bartlett.

Dutta, A., Dutta, A., Bwayo, S., Xue, Z., Akiyode, O., Ayuk-Egbe, P., . . . Clarke-Tasker, V. (2003). Complementary and alternative medicine instruction in nursing curricula. *Journal of National Black Nurses Association, 14*, 30–33.

Fenton, M., & Morris, D. (2003). The integration of holistic nursing practices and complementary and alternative modalities into curricula of schools of nursing. *Alternative Therapies, 9*, 62–67.

Gaster, B., Unterborn, J., Scott, R., & Schneeweiss, R. (2007). What should students learn about complementary and alternative medicine? *Academic Medicine, 82*, 934–938.

Geisler, C., Cheung, C., Johnson Steinhagen, S., Neubeck, P., & Brueggeman, A. (2015). Nurse practitioner knowledge, use, and referral of complementary/alternative therapies. *Journal of the American Association of Nurse Practitioners, 27*, 380–388.

Government of Western Australia Department of Health. (2015). *Standard protocols: Use of complementary therapies*. Retrieved from http://www.health.wa.gov.au

Groft, J., & Kalischuk, R. (2005). Nursing students learn about complementary and alternative health care practices. *Complementary Health Practice Review, 10*, 133–146.

Halcón, L., Chlan, L., Kreitzer, M., & Leonard, B. (2003). Complementary therapies and healing practices: Faculty/student beliefs and attitudes and the implications for nursing education. *Journal of Professional Nursing, 19*, 387–397.

Halcón, L., Leonard, B., Snyder, M., Garwick, A., & Kreitzer, M. (2001). Incorporating alternative and complementary health practices within university-based nursing education. *Complementary Health Practice Review, 6*, 127–135.

Hegarty, J., Walsh, F., Condon, C., & Sweeney, J. (2009). The undergraduate education of nurses: Looking to the future. *International Journal of Nursing Education Scholarship, 6*(1), 1–11.

Helms, J. (2006). Complementary and alternative therapies: A new frontier for nursing education? *Journal of Nursing Education, 45*, 117–123.

Hon, K., Twinn, S., Leung, T., Thompson, D., Wong, Y., & Fok, T. (2006). Chinese nursing students' attitudes toward traditional Chinese medicine. *Journal of Nursing Education, 45*, 182–185.

Institute of Medicine (IOM). (2011). *The future of nursing: Leading change, advancing health*. Retrieved from https://www.nap.edu/read/12956/chapter/1#iii

Johnson, C. (2014). Effect of aromatherapy on cognitive test anxiety among nursing students. *Alternative and Complementary Therapies, 20*, 84–87.

Kim, S., Erlen, J., Kim, K., & Sok, S. (2006). Nursing students' and faculty members' knowledge of, experience with, and attitudes towards complementary and alternative therapies. *Journal of Nursing Education, 45*, 375–378.

Koithan, M. (2015). The promise of integrative nursing. *Creative Nursing, 21*, 193–199.

Kreitzer, M., Mann, D., & Lumpkin, M. (2008). CAM competencies for the health professions. *Complementary Health Practice Review, 13*, 63–72.

Lee, M., Benn, R., Wimstatt, L., Cornman, J., Hedgecock, J., Gerick, S., . . . Haramati, A. (2007). Integrating complementary and alternative medicine instruction into health professions education: Organizational and instructional strategies. *Academic Medicine, 82*, 939–945.

Lindeman, C. (2000). The future of nursing education. *Journal of Nursing Education, 39*, 5–12.

Little, C. (2013). Integrative health care: Implications for nursing practice and education. *British Journal of Nursing, 22*, 1160–1164.

Minnesota Board of Nursing. (2010). *Statement of accountability for utilization of integrative therapies in nursing practice*. Retrieved from https://mn.gov/boards/assets/Integrative_Therapies_Stmt_acsbl_12-2017_tcm21-37140.pdf

Moore, K. (2010). Rationale for complementary and alternative medicine in nursing school curriculum. *Journal of Alternative and Complementary Medicine, 16*, 611–12.

National Center for Complementary and Integrative Health (NCCIH). (2017). *About NCCIH*. Retrieved from https://nccih.nih.gov/about

Nedrow, A., Heitkemper, M., Frenkel, M., Mann, D., Wayne, P., & Hughes, E. (2007). Collaborations between allopathic and complementary and alternative medicine health professionals: Four initiatives. *Academic Medicine, 82*, 962–966.

Nedrow, A., Istvan, J., Haas, M., Barrett, R., Salveson, C., Moore, G., …Keenan, E. (2007). Implications for education in complementary and alternative medicine: A survey of entry attitudes in students at five health professional schools. *Journal of Alternative and Complementary Medicine, 13*, 381–386.

Patterson, C., Kaczorowski, J., Arthur, H., Smith, K., & Mills, D. (2003). Complementary therapy practice: Defining the role of advanced nurse practitioners. *Journal of Clinical Nursing, 12*, 816–823.

Pearson, N., & Chesney, M. (2007). The CAM education program of the National Center for Complementary and Alternative Medicine: An overview. *Academic Medicine, 82*, 921–926.

Poreddi, V., Thiyagarajan, S., Swamy, P., Gandhi, S., Thimmaiah, R., & BadaMath, S. (2016). Nursing student attitudes and understanding of complementary and alternative therapies: An Indian perspective. *Nursing Education Perspectives, 37*, 32–37.

Richardson, S. (2003). Complementary health and healing in nursing education. *Journal of Holistic Nursing, 21*, 20–35.

Salmon, M. (2010). The commons: Nursing education, societal relevance, and going it together. *Alternative Therapies in Health and Medicine, 16*(5), 18.

Schultz, A., Chao, S., & McGinnis, M. (2009). *Integrative medicine and the health of the public: A summary of the 2009 summit.* Institute of Medicine: Washington, DC: National Academies Press.

Sofhauser, C. (2002). Development of a minor in complementary health. *Nurse Educator, 27*, 118–122.

Sok, S., Erlen, J., & Kim, K. (2004). Complementary and alternative therapies in nursing curricula: A new direction for nurse educators. *Journal of Nursing Education, 43*, 401–405.

Solomon, D., Singleton, K., Zhiyuan, S., Zell, K., Vriezen, K., & Albert, N. (2016). Multicenter study of nursing role complexity on environmental stressors and emotional exhaustion. *Applied Nursing Research, 30*, 52–57.

Sparber, A. (2001). State boards of nursing and scope of practice of registered nurses performing complementary therapies. *Online Journal of Issues in Nursing, 6.* Retrieved from http://www .nursingworld.org/MainMenuCategories/ANAMarketplace/ANAPeriodicals/OJIN/Tableof Contents/Volume62001/No3Sept01/ArticlePreviousTopic/CmplementaryTherapiesReport.html

Stratton, T., Benn, R., Lie, D., Zeller, J., & Nedrow, A. (2007). Evaluating CAM education in health professions programs. *Academic Medicine, 82*, 956–961.

Swanson, B., Zeller, J., Keithley, J., Fung, S., Johnson, A., Suhayda, R., … Downie, P. (2012). Case-based online modules to teach graduate-level nursing students about complementary and alternative medical therapies. *Journal of Professional Nursing, 28*, 125–129.

Topuz, S., Uysal, G., & Yilmaz, A. (2015). Knowledge and opinions of nursing students regarding complementary and alternative medicine for cancer patients. *International Journal of Caring Sciences, 8*, 656–664.

van der Reit, P., Francis, L., & Levett-Jones, T. (2011). Complementary therapies in healthcare: Design, implementation, and evaluation of an elective course for undergraduate students. *Nurse Education in Practice, 11*, 146–152.

Van Sant-Smith, D. (2015). Supporting the integrative health care curriculum in schools of nursing. *Holistic Nursing Practice, 28*, 312.

Yeh, Y., & Chung, U. (2007). An investigation into competence in TCM of BSN graduates from technological universities in Taiwan. *Journal of Nursing Research, 15*, 310–317.

Yildirim, Y., Parlar, S., Eyigor, S., Sertoz, O., Eyigor, C., Fadiloglu, C., & Uyar, M. (2010). An analysis of nursing and medical students' attitudes towards and knowledge of complementary and alternative medicine. *Journal of Clinical Nursing, 19*, 1157–1166.

28

Integrating Complementary Therapies Into Nursing Practice

SUSANNE M. CUTSHALL AND ELIZABETH L. PESTKA

Complementary therapies are increasingly being offered across the continuum of healthcare. Nurses are essential leaders for maximizing use of complementary and integrative therapies that support holistic healthcare. Holistic healthcare in nursing recognizes the humanistic, caring, healing nature of interventions and often uses many modalities to support the mind–body–spirit on its healing journey (Clark, 2012).

This chapter provides examples of strategies that nurses have used to incorporate complementary therapies into their practices. Three healthcare settings in the Midwest are used to demonstrate the integration of complementary therapies into both inpatient and outpatient hospital nursing practice. The hospitals include one small health campus, Woodwinds Health Campus; one large medical center, Abbott Northwestern Hospital; and one very large healthcare provider, Mayo Clinic. In addition to traditional nursing roles in hospital settings, examples of nurses incorporating complementary and integrative therapies into community-based care, holistic health and wellness centers, and care provided to military veterans shows the breadth of opportunities for integration into nursing practice.

Healthcare facilities in the United States are not alone in integrating complementary therapies; this is being done across the world as well. Sidebar 28.1 illustrates the use of complementary therapies in Brazil.

MEDICAL CENTER SETTINGS

As complementary therapies become more widely used in the United States, many nurses want strategies to incorporate them. Three different healthcare settings in the Midwest—Woodwinds Health Campus, Abbott Northwestern Hospital, and Mayo Clinic—all use holistic nursing care in addition to traditional Western medicine.

SIDEBAR 28.1 USE OF COMPLEMENTARY THERAPIES IN BRAZIL

Milena Flória-Santos

Healthcare in Brazil includes some traditional medicine that is part of indigenous and popular practices performed by healers and medicine men. Most of these practices provide a search for self-knowledge and focus on the spiritual aspects of culture, religion, and traditions of its users. Brazilian people use these practices because they are easily accessible, have demonstrated relative effectiveness, are congruent with their cultural beliefs, and access to biomedicine is often scarce and expensive in some areas of the country. In western Brazil, traditional practices are undergoing a process of becoming more scientific, specialized, and performed by skilled professionals because they are gradually being disconnected from their traditional cultural context. The use of homeopathy, medicinal plants/phytotherapy, acupuncture, traditional Chinese medicine, anthroposophy medicine, and thermal water therapy are included in the Public Health Unified System.

Spiritist psychiatric hospitals are one example of complementary therapies integrated into care, combining conventional psychiatric treatment and complementary therapies (Lucchetti et al., 2012). These hospitals include voluntary-based spiritual approaches such as laying-on of hands (fluidotherapy), intercessory prayer, and spirit release therapy (disobsession). Nurses may be trained to provide these therapies. The optional nature of these spiritual complementary therapies seems to increase acceptance by patients and their family members. Outcomes from these interventions have not been scientifically studied.

A recent study found that Brazilian nurses, more so than physicians, are interested in complementary and integrative therapies (Thiago & Tesser, 2011). This is likely due to the belief that nurses use more nonpharmacological interventions to deliver care to patients. For both groups of professionals, acupuncture and homeopathy were the preferred complementary strategies, and acceptance was associated with previous contact with the therapies. Acupuncture was more widely used at public health services, where nurses and physical therapists, in addition to physicians, were allowed to use this intervention. The 177 healthcare professionals who responded to the survey identified the following therapies that are included in practice: homeopathy, Chinese and Ayurvedic medicine, acupuncture, auriculotherapy, massage, chiropractic and phytotherapy, yoga, biodance, relaxation, meditation, dance, and tai chi chuan.

Nurses can take elective courses at Brazilian universities and independent courses offered by private organizations to become qualified to use complementary and integrative therapies in their care. More use of these therapies offers growing possibilities for the Brazilian people from individual, healthcare professional, and health services perspectives.

Woodwinds Health Campus

Located in Woodbury, Minnesota, Woodwinds Health Campus is an 86-bed, not-for-profit facility that opened in 2000. The philosophy of care is based on the creation of an unprecedented healing environment that revolves around the needs of patients and their families, including extensive use of complementary therapies (HealthEast, 2017b). The vision for the Woodwinds campus of the HealthEast Care System was to transform the patient care experience and create compassionate service, holistic care, and a patient-centered care model (Lincoln, 2003). From the spacious main entry to the convenient layout, patients in need of care are easily guided to the area of service they require as quickly and comfortably as possible.

According to Lincoln and Johnson (2009), critical aspects of a healing environment are the relationships and attitudes of healthcare professionals and administrators in addition to the architectural design elements. The vision of Woodwinds' healing healthcare model is to be innovative, unique, and a preferred resource for healthcare. Leadership as well as staff nurses and other employees personally and professionally commit to supporting the principles of holistic care (Lincoln & Johnson, 2009).

Woodwinds Health Campus offers a variety of healing arts therapies that are meant to complement medical care and meet the diverse needs of each patient. These healing arts therapies, also known as *integrative therapies* or *complementary therapies*, are designed to enhance, not replace, traditional therapeutic measures ordered by a primary provider such as medications, exercise, and therapy. Therapies offered include essential oils, Healing Touch or energy-based therapies, guided imagery, healing music, acupuncture, acupressure, and massage therapy (HealthEast, 2017a).

In addition to complementary therapies offered by the staff at Woodwinds Health Campus, an ongoing outpatient partnership with Northwestern Health Sciences University provides additional therapies and services such as chiropractic, acupuncture, massage, and naturopathy at the Natural Care Center. This broadens the range of complementary therapies available so that each patient can select options that will help most in the healing process (HealthEast, 2017a).

Nurses play an integral role in providing complementary therapies at Woodwinds. Holistic nursing principles are integrated into the vision for the hospital. Woodwinds Health Campus includes components of holistic nursing in job descriptions and ongoing performance evaluations for nursing staff. The facility continues to attract highly skilled nurses that have a passion for holistic nursing care. The care environment is collaborative, and individual contributions are honored, with nurses providing input on how the holistic care model continues to be implemented (Lincoln, 2003). Woodwinds established a Holistic Practice Council that includes nurses from various patient care units to better understand the needs of staff nurses in providing care and to strengthen participation in evidence-based practice (Lincoln & Johnson, 2009).

Education for all nurses at Woodwinds includes holistic nursing-related courses: one focusing on Healing Touch and the second including training in other complementary and alternative modalities such as music therapy, guided imagery, and use of essential oils. In addition, nurses are required to complete educational contact hours annually in holistic nursing. Nurses are expected to include what they have learned in these courses in the care provided to each patient (Lincoln, 2003). The "Woodwinds way" requires nurses to take personal and professional steps to practice from a place of healing, compassion, and love while performing with high clinical competence (Lincoln & Johnson, 2009). Nurses have been involved in evaluating these practices that add to the literature. An example of this is a retrospective analysis of the impact of Healing Touch with Healing Harp on inpatient acute care pain. This analysis demonstrated the effectiveness of using concomitant Healing Touch and Healing Harp to significantly reduce moderate to severe pain and anxiety for inpatient acute care patients (Lincoln, et al. 2014).

Nurses are encouraged to use complementary therapies themselves for self-care. They are able to use the many healing spaces in the integrative services area at Woodwinds to enhance their own well-being. They can take "spirit breaks" to rejuvenate themselves during their work shifts. For nurses employed at Woodwinds, using integrative therapies becomes an aspect of their own lives (Lincoln, 2003).

Woodwinds' impact goes beyond its own campus and into the surrounding community. The facility has formed wellness initiatives with local corporations such as 3M and Medtronic. Medtronic has created an Integrative Health Council and invited staff from Woodwinds to conduct a Healing Harp seminar on their premises (Olson, 2010). This model of offering integrative services has spread to other HealthEast medical centers in the health system, with nurses leading these efforts (HealthEast, 2017a).

Abbott Northwestern Hospital

Abbott Northwestern Hospital, a part of the Allina Health System, is a 674-bed, tertiary care, not-for-profit hospital in Minneapolis, Minnesota. The nursing department's philosophy at Abbott Northwestern is based on advocacy through caring. In 1999, a complementary and alternative medicine program for cardiovascular inpatients was initiated and has grown into a nationally recognized model for providing integrative care (Sendelbach, Carole, Lapensky, & Kshettry, 2003).

Abbott Northwestern Hospital, in collaboration with the Minneapolis Heart Institute, identified a mission to provide an exceptional healthcare experience for patients with cardiovascular disorders, and to support this initiative, they established a holistic nursing framework for practice. The prevalence of the public's use of complementary and alternative therapies identified in the literature, along with an increasing number of patient and family requests for these interventions, motivated Abbott Northwestern Hospital to initiate its original innovative program, which was called *Healing the Hearts* and which include therapeutic interventions such as music and massage (Sendelbach et al., 2003).

Nursing involvement has been critical to the ongoing success of integrative therapies. An Integrative Practice Advisory Board was established in 2001, and one of the three key areas identified for growth was to further develop holistic nursing to complement the interventions received by patients. The interventions were assessed to be congruent with the nursing department's philosophy and the cornerstones of the patient care model. Work was also focused on enhancing a total healing environment that includes developing positive and collaborative relationships between nurses and physicians because this has been shown to influence patient outcomes (Sendelbach et al., 2003).

With initial success and institutional support, along with continuing education for providers, the inpatient cardiovascular integrative therapy program developed into a national model for not only inpatient care but also outpatient care, research, and education. The Penny George Institute for Health and Healing (a part of Abbott Northwestern) is a role model for enhancing health through an integrative approach. The mission of this innovative program is to transform health-care locally by providing outstanding integrative care and to transform healthcare nationally through the dissemination of integrative practices that enhance quality and safety, and reduce costs. The Penny George Institute has been recognized as one of the best practices for enhancing care through integrative services (Allina Health, 2017; Bravewell Collaborative, 2015).

The Penny George Institute for Health and Healing offers inpatient services that include acupressure/acupuncture; aromatherapy; energy-based healing; healing arts; Korean hand therapy; mind/body therapies, including relaxation response, guided imagery, and biofeedback; music therapy; reflexology; and therapeutic massage (Allina Health, 2017). Outpatient services include Oriental medicine/acupuncture; Ayurveda; energy healing; healing coaching; herbal consultations; integrative medicine physician consultations; integrative nutrition counseling; mind/body therapies, spiritual coaching; massage therapy; therapeutic yoga; classes and workshops on aromatherapy; drum circle; and healing through the arts. Integrative therapy practitioners have provided more than 900 interventions to patients in the inpatient setting, as well as 700 appointments that include comple-mentary therapies in the outpatient clinic per month. More than 60,000 inpatients have benefited from these services since the beginning of the program in 2003 (Allina Health, 2017).

The holistic nurse clinicians and other members of the integrative therapy team provide ongoing education to the staff. Together with the Bravewell Collaborative, Abbott Northwestern Hospital sponsors physician and nurse practitioner train-ing in integrative medicine and advocates for integrative health in healthcare reform. Education programs are focused on integrative therapies, promotion of self-managed health and wellness, community education classes, transformative nurse training programs, and local healthcare conferences. Ongoing classes and programs for the community on topics such as yoga, stress reduction, nutrition, and fitness provide up-to-date information to thousands of participants a year (Allina Health, 2017).

Research to measure patient outcomes and identify best practices is also a key to expanding this innovative model. Nurses are involved with ongoing clinical trials using integrative therapies and data analysis to provide evidence for integrating com-plementary and alternative therapies into clinical practice. The impact of integrative therapies has been documented to provide immediate and beneficial effects on pain among hospitalized patients. Following integrative therapy interventions, the aver-age pain reduction was over 55% (Dusek, Finch, Plotnikoff, & Knutson, 2010).

Mayo Clinic

Mayo Clinic, located in Rochester, Minnesota, is a large tertiary medical center with almost 2,000 hospital beds. Mayo Clinic has other medical campuses in Phoenix, Arizona, and Jacksonville, Florida, as well as affiliated facilities around the nation. Mayo Clinic defines *quality* as a comprehensive look at all aspects of a patient's experience (Mayo Clinic, 2017f). Mayo strives toward a vision to provide an unparalleled experience as a trusted partner in healthcare (Mayo Clinic, 2016).

The Mayo Clinic Nursing Care Model is based on the nursing theory of human caring proposed by Dr. Jean Watson, which honors every patient as a unique person with the potential to heal holistically and is nurtured by the intentional presence of a nurse who connects with the patient in the moment, expressing care through words, actions, and empathy (Mayo Clinic, 2017b). Nurses across the continuum of care include complementary therapies as part of the holistic healing process.

All nurses, both inpatient and outpatient, are encouraged to include complementary therapies as part of ongoing pain management. One of the policy statements in the institution's procedure guideline on pain management states that complementary interventions such as relaxation techniques, imagery, and music therapy are incorporated in the pain management plan when appropriate (Mayo Clinic, 2017e). A pain menu lists several complementary interventions for patients to consider for ongoing treatment. Identification of resources to support the use of complementary therapies for pain management has been included in departmental orientation for nurses new to the organization, within the nurse residency program, and in ongoing staff-development sessions. A class in complementary therapies for pain management is offered for nurses to learn more about specific evidence-based practices. The course reviews mind–body modalities, energy-based therapies, biologically based approaches, and manipulative-based methods. A holistic nursing toolkit is available on the Rochester Nursing home page that summarizes resource guidelines, education materials, and videos that nurses can use to support their practice.

As part of patient education, a brochure that nurses provide to patients in many specialties is *Using Relaxation Skills to Relieve Your Symptoms* (Mayo Foundation for Medical Education and Research, 2015b). This handout focuses on the importance of relaxation to eliminate tension in the body and mind. It describes the complementary therapies of relaxed breathing, guided imagery, and muscle relaxation. The nurse uses this resource to introduce complementary therapies to assist a patient with holistic healing and to emphasize that learning relaxation skills may improve symptom management and quality of life.

Other strategies nurses use to integrate complementary therapies into a patient's care include a television channel with continuous relaxing music in each patient's room; CD players and CDs available for patient use through the patient library for music listening; CDs with audio-guided imagery that a patient can use in the hospital and take home at discharge; journals available for patients to write in; a chaplain service that can be requested to provide spirituality support; and the ongoing basics of nursing presence, touch, and humor. Humanities in Medicine programs, including music, arts, and narrative writing at the bedside, are offered through the Dolores Jean Lavins Center for Humanities in Medicine (Mayo Clinic, 2017d).

The Mayo Clinic Cancer Education Center supports a model of nurses providing leadership and education on complementary and integrative therapies. A nurse coordinates a creative renewal program in collaboration with the Humanities in Medicine program that provides patients, visitors, and staff with an opportunity to explore integrative/complementary medicine approaches and creative expression. Several nurses also teach classes to oncology patients on aromatherapy, mindfulness, and yoga. Other integrative medicine and community-based practitioners present on topics such as acupuncture, mandalas, and music therapy. These free educational programs enhance self-care and support the experience of holistic healing.

Healing Enhancement Program

The Healing Enhancement Program was initiated in the inpatient setting based on patient feedback and review of the patient experience for cardiovascular surgery patients. A team, including nurses and led by a clinical nurse specialist, was formed to address the needs of patients that often occur with and after cardiac surgery: managing pain, anxiety, tension, stress, sleeplessness, and nausea. When the team realized that initial orders focused on pain medications were not enough, a trial of massage and music therapies targeted at reducing patients' complaints of musculoskeletal pain and decreasing anxiety and tension after surgery was initiated. Studies confirmed positive findings (Cutshall et al., 2007).

Nurses educate patients and their family members about complementary and alternative therapy resources and coordinate the delivery of services. Nurses promote patient use of a wide array of opportunities. Massage therapy is available to provide treatment for back, neck, and shoulder pain. CD players are available in each of the cardiac surgical rooms for music therapy with a small CD library available on each unit and additional CDs in the patient library. The Patient Education Section made guided-imagery selections available on each patient's television, as well provided as other CD resources for passive muscle relaxation, stress management, and additional imageries. Patient education classes on stress and wellness and healing movement are offered on an ongoing basis. Live, soothing music is sometimes available in clinical areas; patients are able to select art pieces for their hospital room; and some hospital volunteers are trained to offer hand massage to patients, family members, and staff (Cutshall et al., 2007).

The success of the Healing Enhancement Program has led to replication in other practices across Mayo Clinic in Rochester, Minnesota. Recognizing the benefits to patients, nurses continue to collaborate with other healthcare providers and the outpatient Integrative Medicine and Health Program to expand resources and opportunities for additional services and patient populations. An advanced practice nurse/integrative health specialist is available to assist patients regarding incorporating integrative therapies into their plan of care. There is also an inpatient consult service for integrative therapies that includes massage therapy, acupuncture, animal-assisted therapy and integrative health specialist nurse (Cutshall et al., 2015). The Integrative Medicine Healing Enhancement program also partners with volunteer services to expand integrative services to patients to provide Caring Hands massage, Reiki and Healing Touch (Mayo Clinic, 2017g).

Pain Rehabilitation Center

Mayo Clinic Pain Rehabilitation Center (PRC) is an exemplary outpatient model of nurses integrating complementary and alternative therapies into their practice (Mayo Foundation for Medical Education and Research, 2015a). It was among the first pain-rehabilitation programs in the United States, established in 1974, and is now one of the largest interdisciplinary pain-rehabilitation programs. The PRC focuses on functional restoration with a cognitive behavioral basis and extensive use of complementary therapies (Bruce & Harrison, 2013).

A team of healthcare professionals, with nurses as integral members of the group, delivers care to patients in the program. Patients are provided education on medication management, cognitive behavioral therapy, complementary therapies, stress and emotional management, physical therapy, occupational therapy, biofeedback, sleep hygiene, and lifestyle management. Complementary therapies have been carefully researched and proved to be helpful: these include biofeedback, deep diaphragmatic breathing, guided imagery, yoga, tai chi, music, art, exercise, and humor.

The PRC tapers patients off opioid medications because there is evidence that these individuals can experience significant and sustained improvement in pain severity and functioning following participation in a comprehensive pain-rehabilitation program without these medications (Townsend et al., 2008). Many people who have lived with chronic pain for much of their lives inform the nurses they are skeptical that if large dosages of medication have not helped their pain, nonpharmacological methods such as complementary therapies are unlikely to be effective. Program outcomes data support not only overwhelming patient satisfaction with the program (94%), but also a reduction in depressive symptoms (79%), a gain in activity level (75%), and a reduction in pain severity in 73% of the patients (Bruce & Harrison, 2013). Program participants credit complementary therapies as one of the most effective elements of their pain-rehabilitation program and improved quality of life.

Evidence-Based Practice Related to the Use of Integrative Therapies

Research to provide evidence for integrative therapies is supported at Mayo Clinic. Investigators have conducted numerous clinical trials of various complementary therapies for treating a variety of conditions and symptoms. Nurses have been involved or led many of these studies on specific therapies, such as massage therapy (including introduction of massage therapy into busy surgical practices; Cutshall et al., 2010). Nurses are also conducting research on how complementary therapies provide a resource for nurses' self-care. An example is a study on resilience training with new nurses. This study is the first in a series finding that it is feasible to incorporate a specific stress-management and resilience program into a nurse residency program, with an improvement in mindfulness and resilience scores over time (Chesak et al., 2015). Nurse are also involved in quality-improvement projects related to integrating complementary therapies into clinical practice, such as the integration of aromatherapy into clinical practice (Conlon et al, 2016). This quality-improvement project highlighted the process and initial outcomes of introducing aromatherapy as a minimally invasive, independent, and integrative nursing intervention at a large Midwest medical center.

Mayo Clinic Healthy Living Center and Healthy Living Program

The Dan Abraham Healthy Living Center and Health Living Program at Mayo Clinic provides access to complementary and integrative health and wellness programs for staff and consumers. These include cooking demonstrations, group fitness classes, individual wellness evaluations, massage therapy, wellness coaching, small-group training, stress-management programs, massage therapy, Reiki, acupressure, acupuncture, yoga, tai chi, Alexander technique, and weight-loss programs. The Healthy Living Center has initiated a Wellness Champions Program to promote health and wellness activities for staff. Several nurses have volunteered to participate in this program and serve as leaders in their work locations. The department of nursing has a Wellness Champions Steering Group to help support nurse engagement in wellness offerings (Mayo Clinic, 2017a). The Mayo Healthy Living Program offers wellness consultation to patients and family members that are interested in an individualized wellness program. The main focus areas are nutrition, fitness, and resilience, but there is also a spa that offers skin and nail health, as well as massage and acupuncture services. Nurses are in roles such as resiliency specialist and may also be wellness coaches (Mayo Clinic, 2017c).

Mayo Clinic Affiliated Practices

Community services are sometimes part of larger healthcare networks. Nurses who work at Mayo Clinic Health Systems and Affiliated Practices are integrating complementary therapies into practice in local communities. Mayo Clinic Health System in Red Wing, Minnesota, has initiated a Healing Arts Program. The program offers guided imagery, essential oils, healing music, antinausea acupressure bands, Healing Touch, massage therapy, reflexology, and yoga in the community. Several nurses are trained in these healing arts practices and discuss the programs with patients (Carstensen, 2012).

Another extension of the Mayo Clinic system is the Center for Health and Healing Healthcare in Onalaska, Wisconsin. Patients and other interested people in the community are offered access to integrative therapies. The services provided in this center include healing oils, osteopathic medicine, qigong, massage therapy, guided imagery, and meditation. Nurses have been actively involved in the leadership of the center. Nurses are also leaders in providing education within the healthcare setting on the complementary and integrative therapies and providing guidance for nursing practice (Mayo Clinic Health System, 2016).

COMMUNITY-BASED HEALTHCARE SETTINGS

Complementary therapies are also included as part of patient care in other healthcare settings. The following examples show how some community-based hospices, clinics, and healing and wellness centers use holistic care in their programs.

Holy Redeemer Hospice

Holy Redeemer Hospice in southeastern Pennsylvania provides an innovative model with a team of nurses certified in complementary therapy modalities (Hansen, 2012). This approach enables experienced hospice nurses who are experts in hospice care to have another set of tools in their toolbox. Hospice care does not end when the patient who is being cared for dies because nurses continue to provide support to family members following the loss. Complementary therapies can help family members relax and address their stress level and cope more effectively.

Pillsbury House Integrated Health Clinic

The Pillsbury House Integrated Health Clinic uses student practitioners and serves patients living in south Minneapolis, Minnesota, and the surrounding communities. All services are at no cost and offered by appointment to the public. Patients are offered integrative care services and therapies from student interns who are supervised by licensed faculty. The care is planned and delivered by a team of students and providers from several disciplines. These providers and disciplines include chiropractic care, acupuncture, massage therapy, and health coaching. Nursing students from the University of Minnesota and the Center for Spirituality and Healing are involved in providing information at the Pillsbury House. Nurses may be involved in collaborative planning for patients, and nurses who are health-coaching students may also be offering services (Northwestern Health Sciences University, 2016).

Hermitage Farm Center for Healing

Nurses may work as instructors and practitioners in community-based holistic health and wellness centers. An example of such a community-based program initiated by nurses is the Hermitage Farm Center for Healing in Rochester, Minnesota. This center was founded by an advanced practice nurse, and several of the practitioners affiliated with the center are nurses with advanced skills in complementary and integrative therapies. These nurses interact and collaborate with other complementary and integrative health practitioners to provide a variety of services. The classes offered are related to energy healing, stress management, and mindfulness-based stress reduction. Practitioners also provide therapies such as Reiki, energy healing, acupuncture, homeopathy, health coaching, and massage (Hermitage Farm Center for Healing, 2017). The Southeast Minnesota chapter of the American Holistic Nurses Association meets at this location.

Pathways: A Healing Center

Pathways, in Minneapolis, Minnesota, is another example of a community-based holistic wellness center that provides classes focused on the mind, body, and spirit. More than 120 volunteers offer therapies free of charge. These providers include nurses who provide therapies and also teach classes. The Minnesota chapter of the American Holistic Nurses Association meets at this location and these meetings serve as an opportunity for networking and sharing resources for practice and self-care (Pathways, 2017).

VETERANS ADMINISTRATION

Complementary therapies are increasingly becoming part of care provided to military veterans. Results of a 2011 survey were presented at a meeting discussing complementary practice in the Department of Veterans Affairs (U.S. Department of Veterans Affairs, 2011). According to this survey, 89% of Veterans Administration (VA) facilities offered complementary therapies compared with 84% in 2002. The five most common therapies provided are meditation (72% of hospitals), stress management/relaxation therapy (66%), guided imagery (58%), progressive muscle relaxation (53%), and biofeedback (50%) (U.S. Department of Veterans Affairs, 2011).

There is significant interest in using complementary therapies to treat chronic pain and posttraumatic stress disorder (PTSD) because these are growing concerns in the VA. A July 2012 report from the Institute of Medicine estimated that 13% to 20% of the more than 2.6 million U.S. service members deployed to Iraq or Afghanistan since 2001 could develop PTSD (Kennedy, 2012). Review of research evidence showed that the highest quality evidence supported the use of acupuncture; however, strong conclusions cannot be drawn without further evidence. Findings in studies using forms of breathing and muscle relaxation were positive overall but also need more research (U.S. Department of Veterans Affairs, 2011). The U.S. Department of Veterans Affairs lists complementary treatments on its National Center for PTSD website and provides brochures that highlight the evidence (U.S. Department of Veterans Affairs, 2014, 2017). The VA is committed to maximizing roles that nurses play in comprehensive holistic care for veterans. The Office of Nursing developed the Clinical Practice Program to support nursing clinical practice. Ten specialty advisory committees consisting of a clinical nurse advisor and nurses actively involved in clinical practice focus on identifying and developing recommendations for best practice guidelines and patient care standards and policies (U.S. Department of Veterans Affairs, 2016a). Each of these specialty committees is examining evidence for integrating complementary therapies into comprehensive recommendations.

The VA is working for patient-driven care across its entire system through a Health for Life program. The VA's Whole Health model focuses on empowering the individual's self-healing mechanisms. This model is evidence based and makes use of all appropriate therapeutic approaches, including complementary and integrative health therapies along with traditional approaches to disease and injury management (U.S. Department of Veterans Affairs, 2016b). Nurses have led development and evaluation of Integrative Health Clinics for outcomes on chronic pain and stress, depression, anxiety and PTSD. One such clinic in Salt Lake City, Utah, concluded that an Integrative Health Clinic and Program was effective at improving chronic pain, stress-related depression, anxiety, and health-related quality of life for veterans. This program used complementary and alternative mind body skills and was an innovative treatment option that was acceptable to patients and providers and was low risk and low cost (Smeeding, Bradshaw, Kumpfer, Travithick, & Stoddard, 2010).

NURSES USING COMPLEMENTARY THERAPIES

Nurses are in a key position to help integrate complementary and alternative therapies into clinical practice. They are in a critical position to guide and impact the growth and use of complementary therapies in the continuum of healthcare environments. Nurses have a background and educational curriculum that focuses on holistic mind, body, and spiritual care. The nursing profession has long been a strong advocate of holistic nursing care.

A national survey of critical care nurses was conducted by Tracy et al. (2005) to determine attitudes, knowledge, perspectives, and use of complementary and alternative therapies. This study used a random sample of members of the American Association of Critical-Care Nurses, with 726 respondents. The results indicated that most of the respondents were using one or more complementary and alternative therapies in their clinical practice. The most common therapies mentioned were diet, exercise, relaxation techniques, and prayer. A majority of the nurses had some knowledge of more than half of the 28 therapies listed on the survey. A majority desired additional training for 25. The participants generally required more evidence before using or recommending conventional therapy than before using or recommending complementary and alternative therapies. Overall the respondents viewed complementary and alternative therapies positively, perceived them as legitimate and beneficial to patients for a variety of symptoms, and were open to their use (Tracy et al, 2005).

A majority of respondents desired increased availability of therapies for patients, families, and nursing staff. Respondents' professional use of the therapies was related to additional knowledge about them, perception of benefits from them, total number of therapies recommended to patients, personal use, and affiliation with a mainstream religion. This study concluded that the benefits of having educational programs that provide information about and evidence for the use of complementary and alternative therapies would increase the appropriate use of these therapies (Tracy et al., 2005).

Nursing as a profession is well rooted in understanding the supportive needs of patients to reduce stress to allow for healing from illness or disease. Nurses are exposed to stress in their own lives and in the work environment. They can benefit from stress-reducing complementary and integrative therapies for their own self-care and for preventing professional burnout. There is especially a great potential for stress and burnout among new nurses (Boychuk, Duchscher, & Cowin, 2006). In a study of new nurses with less than 2 years' tenure, 66% were found to have symptoms of burnout, mental exhaustion, and depression (Cho, Laschinger, & Wong, 2006). Complementary therapies aimed at stress reduction and relaxation may be helpful in allowing both new and experienced nurses to manage ongoing stressful activities and events.

A study by Tucker, Weymiller, Cutshall, Rhudy, and Lohse (2012) on stress ratings and health-promotion practices among more than 2,200 RNs, highlighted the importance of continued focus on the health of nurses and recognized a large opportunity for incorporating complementary therapies into nursing self-care. Study results indicated that although overall stress levels of nurses who participated were similar to the national average, the stress levels were inversely correlated with overall health-promotion behavior scores. Nurses with caregiver responsibilities outside of their nursing roles had higher stress and lower health-promoting behavior scores. In a multivariate analysis, health responsibility, spiritual growth, and stress management accounted for most of the variance in perceived stress scores. The findings support work-site interventions that promote nurses' health and wellness and a focus on reducing work and home stress using complementary relaxation and exercise strategies.

Another study examined the effects of a brief stress-management intervention for nurse leaders. Nurse leaders were assigned to a randomized controlled trial of a brief mindfulness meditation course or a leadership course. Results supported the preliminary effectiveness of a 4-week mindfulness meditation course in reducing self-reported stress symptoms, demonstrating positive results for this complementary therapy intervention (Pipe et al., 2009).

A related study evaluated results of HeartMath, an approach incorporating complementary therapies into an educational intervention, on the stress of health team members. The compelling imperative for the project was to find a positive and effective way to address the documented stress levels of healthcare workers. A pilot study of primarily nurses, including oncology staff ($n = 29$) and healthcare leaders ($n = 15$), explored the impact of a positive coping approach on Personal and Organizational Quality Assessment–Revised (POQA-R) scores (HeartMath Institute & Caring Management Consulting, 1999–2002) at baseline and at 7 months using paired t tests. Baseline measures of distress demonstrated that stress and its symptoms are problematic issues for hospital and ambulatory clinic staff nurses. This workplace intervention that included complementary therapies was feasible and effective in promoting positive strategies for coping and enhancing well-being, personally and organizationally (Pipe et al., 2011).

By gaining a greater appreciation of the value of complementary therapies for their own well-being, nurses can be very instrumental in further integration of these modalities into comprehensive holistic care. Nurses can continue serving as strong advocates for patients and families and communicate with interdisciplinary team members, promoting the use of complementary therapies. Motivated nurses influence standards, guidelines, and policies for using complementary therapies in clinical nursing. Nurses can also develop frameworks and practice models for hospital-based complementary alternative therapy services.

INTEGRATION IN HEALTHCARE SETTINGS

Nurses are integral healthcare leaders who provide support for integrating complementary therapies into healthcare practices. It is not easy to bring these practices into the current healthcare environment. There is still a level of skepticism about the evidence for such practices. Nurses need to be savvy about how to gather evidence by reviewing the literature and conducting research studies or evidence-based practice projects that can influence healthcare leaders.

The financial challenges in healthcare are great, and these services, although increasingly in demand by patients, are often not covered by insurance and are not seen as generating revenue. This is where nurse administrators and leaders can help meet the challenges of optimizing healing environments in an efficient manner to meet the challenges of an evolving healthcare landscape. This may involve developing clear business models for how these practices align with strategic goals within healthcare systems and benchmarking with other programs that have been able to sustain these models of care over time.

Nurses need to be able to create partnerships with other key leaders in the healthcare environment to be able to influence holistic models of care and highlight the evidence for complementary and integrative therapies. This may include partnering with physicians, administrators, specialty practice leaders, integrative medicine programs, quality-improvement specialists, patient experience leaders, volunteer services, and philanthropic or development leaders. Integrating these programs requires significant collaboration, and nurses must be able to establish buy-in across all disciplines.

Nurses need to be aware of their own state board of nursing statements and requirements for being able to integrate complementary therapies into their practice. They should advocate for the inclusion of use of such therapies in state board of nursing guidelines. Nurses should also be able to work within their own nursing departments for creating guidelines and resources so that nurses feel comfortable using complementary therapies. Embedding the use of these therapies into the electronic health record so that they can be assessed and included in the plan of care for patients is valuable. Nurses should also be aware of reliable and credible electronic applications and resources that can support patient use of complementary and integrative therapies and self-care practices.

Nurses and nurse leaders can garner support for incorporating these therapies into a model of the whole person/whole system perspective by aligning them with their healthcare facilities' values, missions, strategic initiatives, and priority areas, such as pain management and improvement of the patient experience, but nurses need to be at the table for these discussions. Nurses are on the front line of caring for patients daily and are the advocates for providing additional ways to address patients' needs beyond the typical medical management. Future consideration should be on expanding the data and research on the integration of complementary therapies into nursing practice and the creation of greater support for the inclusion of these practices as a standard for nursing education and practice for all nursing roles—entry level practice, advanced practice, and administration.

REFERENCES

Allina Health. (2017). *Penny George Institute for Health and Healing.* Retrieved from http://wellness.allinahealth.org/servicelines/802

Bravewell Collaborative. (2015). *Penny George Institute for Health and Healing.* Retrieved from http://www.bravewell.org/current_projects/clinical_network/institute_health_healing

Boychuk Duchscher, J. E., & Cowin, L. S. (2006). The new graduates' professional inheritance. *Nursing Outlook, 54*(3), 152–158.

Bruce, B. K. & Harrison, T. E. (Eds.). (2013). *Mayo Clinic guide to pain relief* (2nd ed.). Rochester, MN: Mayo Foundation for Medical Education and Research.

Carstensen, R. (2012). Fairview will soon offer "healing touch." *Red Wing Republican Eagle.* Retrieved from http://www.republican-eagle.com/retrieve/Fairview%20will%20soon%20offer%20"healing%20touch/1/relevance

Clark, C. S. (2012). Beyond holism: Incorporating an integral approach to support caring-healing-sustainable nursing practices. *Holistic Nursing Practice, 26*(2), 92–102.

Chesak, S. S., Bhagra, A., Schroeder, D. R., Foy, D. A., Cutshall, S. M., & Sood, A. (2015). Enhancing resilience among new nurses: Feasibility and efficacy of a pilot intervention. *The Ochsner Journal, 15*(1), 38–44.

Cho, J., Laschinger, H. K. S., & Wong, C. (2006). Workplace empowerment, work engagement and organizational commitment of new graduate nurses. *Canadian Journal of Nursing Leadership, 19*(3), 43–60.

Conlon, P. M., Haack, K. M., Rodgers, N. J., Dion, L. J., Cambern, K. L., Rohlik, G. M., ... Cutshall, S. M. (2016). Introducing essential oils into pediatric and other practices at an academic medical center. *Journal of Holistic Nursing, 35*(4), 389–396. doi:10.1177/0898010116677400.

Cutshall, S., Fenske, L., Kelly, R., Phillips, B., Sundt, T., & Bauer, B. (2007). Creation of a healing enhancement program at an academic medical center. *Complementary Therapies in Clinical Practice, 13,* 217–223.

Cutshall, S., Rodgers N. J., Dion, L. J., Dreyer, N. E., Thomley, B. S., Do, A., ... Bauer, B. A. (2015). A decade of offering a healing enhancement program at an academic medical center. *Complementary Therapies in Clinical Practice, 21*(4), 211–216.

Cutshall, S. M., Wentworth, L. J., Engen, D., Sundt, T. M., Kelly, R. F., & Bauer, B. A. (2010). Effect of massage therapy on pain, anxiety, and tension in cardiac surgical patients: A pilot study. *Complementary Therapies in Clinical Practice, 16*(2), 92–95.

Dusek, J. A., Finch, M., Plotnifkoff, G., & Knutson, L. (2010). The impact of integrative medicine on pain management in a tertiary hospital. *Journal of Patient Safety, 6*(1), 48–51.

Hansen, S. (2012). *Complementary therapy program at hospice puts nurses in unique role.* Retrieved from https://www.nurse.com/blog/2012/09/10/complementary-therapy-program-at-hospice-puts-nurses-in-unique-role-2

HealthEast. (2017a). *Integrative services.* Retrieved from https://www.healtheast.org/integrative-services.html

HealthEast. (2017b). *Woodwinds Health Campus.* Retrieved from http://www.healtheast.org/woodwinds-health-campus/about/about.html

HeartMath Institute & Caring Management Consulting. (1999–2002). *POQA-R personal and organizational quality assessment-revised.* Boulder Creek, CA: Author.

Hermitage Farm Center for Healing. (2017). Retrieved from http://www.hermitagefarm.org/about.html

Kennedy, M. S. (2012). The hidden wounds of war. *American Journal of Nursing, 112*(11), 7.

Lincoln, V. (2003). Creating an integrated hospital: Woodwinds Health Campus. *Integrative Nursing, 2*(1), 12–13.

Lincoln, V., & Johnson, M. (2009). Staff nurse perceptions of a healing environment. *Holistic Nursing Practice, 23*(3), 183–190.

Lincoln, V., Nowak, E. W., Schommer, B., Briggs, T., Fehrer, A., & Way, G. (2014). Impact of healing touch with Healing Harp on inpatient acute care pain: A retrospective review. *Holistic Nursing Practice, 28*(3), 164–170.

Lucchetti, G., Aguiar, P. R., Braghetta, C. C., Vallada, C. P., Moreira-Almeida, A., & Vallada, H. (2012). Spiritist psychiatric hospitals in Brazil: Integration of conventional psychiatric treatment and spiritual complementary therapy. *Culture, Medicine and Psychiatry, 36*(1), 124–135.

Mayo Clinic. (2017a). *Dan Abraham Healthy Living Center. About DAHLC.* Retrieved from http://dahlc.mayoclinic.org

Mayo Clinic. (2017b). *Mayo nursing care model.* Retrieved from http://www.mayo.edu/pmts/mc5100-mc5199/mc5150-13.pdf

Mayo Clinic. (2017c). *Mayo Clinic Healthy Living Program.* Retrieved from https://healthyliving.mayoclinic.org/home.php

Mayo Clinic. (2017d). *Center for Humanities in Medicine.* Retrieved from https://connect.mayoclinic.org/page/center-for-humanities-in-medicine/

Mayo Clinic. (2017e). *Procedural guideline: Pain management.* Retrieved from http://mayocontent.mayo.edu/mcnursing/DOCMAN-0000053838

Mayo Clinic. (2017f). *Quality and Mayo Clinic.* Retrieved from http://www.mayoclinic.org/quality

Mayo Clinic. (2107g). *Volunteering at Mayo: Integrative Healing Enhancements.* http://www.mayoclinic.org/about-mayo-clinic/volunteers/minnesota/service-areas/integrative-healing-enhancement

Mayo Clinic Health System. (2016). *Welcome to Mayo Clinic Health System - Franciscan healthcare - Onalaska.* Retrieved from http://mayoclinichealthsystem.org/locations/onalaska/medical-services/complementary-medicine/center-for-health-and-healing

Mayo Foundation for Medical Education and Research. (2015a). *Comprehensive Pain Rehabilitation Center: Program guide* [Brochure]. Rochester, MN. Retrieved from http://www.mayo.edu/pmts/mc1400-mc1499/mc1459-18.pdf

Mayo Foundation for Medical Education and Research. (2015b). *Using relaxation skills to relieve your symptoms.* [Brochure]. Rochester, MN: Author.

Northwestern Health Sciences University. (2016). *Pillsbury House Integrated Health Clinic.* Retrieved from https://www.nwhealth.edu/pillsbury-house

Olson, P. (2010). Woodwinds Health Campus supports integrative care. *The Edge: Holistic Living.* Retrieved from http://edgemagazine.net/2010/05/woodwinds-health-campus-supports-integrative-care

Pathways. (2017). *About Pathways.* Retrieved from http://www.pathwaysminneapolis.org/about_us

Pipe, T., Bortz, J., Dueck, A., Pendergast, D., Buchda, V., & Summers, J. (2009). Nurse leader mindfulness meditation program for stress management: A randomized controlled trial. *Journal of Nursing Administration, 39*(3), 130–137.

Pipe, T., Buchada, V., Launder, S., Hudak, B., Hulvey, L., Karns, K., & Pendergast, D. (2011). Building personal and professional resources of resilience and agility in the healthcare workplace. *Stress and Health, 28*(1), 11–22. doi:10.1002/smi.1396.

Sendelbach, S., Carole, L., Lapensky, J., & Kshettry, V. (2003). Developing an integrative therapies program in a tertiary care cardiovascular hospital. *Critical Care Nursing Clinic of North America, 15*, 363–372.

Smeeding, S. J., Bradshaw, D. H., Kumpfer, K., Travithick, S. & Stoddard, G. J. (2010, August). Outcome evaluation of the Veterans Affairs Salt Lake City Integrative Health Clinic for chronic pain and stress-related depression, anxiety, and post-traumatic stress disorder. *Journal of Alternative Complementary Medicine, 16*(8), 823–835.

Thiago, S. C. S., & Tesser, C. D. (2011). Family health strategy doctors and nurses' perceptions of complementary therapies. *Revista De Saude Publica, 45*(2), 1–8. Retrieved from http://www.scielo.br/rsp

Townsend, C. O., Kerkvliet, J. L., Bruce, B. K., Rome, J. D., Hooten, W. M., Luedtke, C. A., & Hodgson, J. E. (2008). A longitudinal study of the efficacy of a comprehensive pain rehabilitation program with opioid withdrawal: Comparison of treatment outcomes based on opioid status at admission. *Pain, 140*, 177–189.

Tracy, M. F., Lindquist, R., Savik, K., Watanuki, S., Sendelbach, S., Kreitzer, M. M., & Berman, B. (2005). Use of complementary and alternative therapies: A national survey of critical care nurses. *American Journal of Critical Care, 14*(5), 404–414.

Tucker, S. J., Weymiller, A. J., Cutshall, S. M., Rhudy, L. M., & Lohse, C. M. (2012). Stress ratings and health promotion practice among RN's at Mayo Rochester: A case for action. *Journal of Nursing Administration, 42*(5), 282–292.

U.S. Department of Veterans Affairs. (2011). *PTSD and complementary alternative medicine–Research opportunities.* Retrieved from http://www.research.va.gov/news/research_highlights/ptsd-cam-051711.cfm

U.S. Department of Veterans Affairs. (2014). *Complementary and integrative medicine: A resource for veterans, service members, and their families.* Retrieved from https://www.warrelatedillness.va.gov/education/factsheets/complementary-and-integrative-medicine.pdf

U.S. Department of Veterans Affairs. (2016a). *Office of Nursing Services. The clinical practice program.* Retrieved from https://www.va.gov/NURSING/Practice/cpp.asp

U.S. Department of Veterans Affairs. (2016b). *VA patient centered care.* Retrieved from https://www.va.gov/PATIENTCENTEREDCARE/features/Veterans_Focus_on_Health_for_Life_during_2016.asp

U.S. Department of Veterans Affairs. (2017). *Complementary and alternative medicine (CAM) for PTSD.* Retrieved from http://www.ptsd.va.gov/professional/treatment/overview/complementary_alternative_for_ptsd.asp

29

Perspectives on Future Research

YEOUNGSUK SONG, SOHYE LEE, AND RUTH LINDQUIST

Nursing's commitment to the generation of high-quality, cost-effective patient outcomes requires that a sound scientific basis for practice be established. Previous chapters have identified existing research related to the therapies reviewed; however, most chapters end with statements that more research is needed. The need for more evidence related to the safety, efficacy, timing, "dose," and specific indications for most therapies is clearly evident. As noted in those chapters, there is considerable interest in and use of complementary therapies by the public. In a large and comprehensive examination of the use of complementary and alternative therapies, the number of annual visits to providers was found to outnumber visits to primary care physicians (Institute of Medicine [IOM], 2005). Subsequently, the 2012 National Health Interview Survey, a comprehensive in-person survey of Americans regarding their health, found that 33.2% of adults and 11.6% of children surveyed in the United States reported use of a form of complementary and alternative medicine in the preceding 12 months (Black, Clarke, Barnes, Stussman, & Nahin, 2015; Clarke, Black, Stussman, Barnes, & Nahin, 2015). A 2010 U.S. phone survey of more than 1,000 people aged 50 years and older reported that more than half of the respondents used some form of complementary and alternative medicine; however, only a little more than half of those who reported use said that they had ever discussed it their use with their healthcare providers (AARP & National Center for Complementary and Alternative Medicine [NCCAM], 2011). A systematic review of literature comprising 16 studies identified the prevalence rates of the use of complementary and alternative medicine among the general population and health professionals to range from 5% to 74.8% in the countries investigated (Frass, Strassl, Friehs, Mullner, Kundi & Kaye, 2012). One of the most exhaustive data collection on the use of complementary, alternative, and traditional health practices across the globe was published by the WHO in 2005 (Bodeker, Ong, Grundy, Buford, & Shein, 2005); it showed a wide range of practices and variability in the degree of use of different therapies. The fascinating details of this report are beyond the scope of this chapter; however, the report confirms the large interest in and diverse use of complementary and alternative therapies around the world.

Interest in complementary therapies is encountered in a broad range of health-care practice settings. Along with public and patient interest, there is a concomitant interest on the part of nurses who not only want to deliver these therapies to patients, but also have an interest the same therapies for their own personal use (Lindquist, Tracy, & Savik, 2003). However, despite provider interest, the therapies most often used by patients are not those that providers are familiar with or that providers most understand (Zhang, Peck, Spalding, Jones, & Cook, 2012). In addition to the significant demand, common use, and lack of understanding of even commonly used therapies, there is an urgency to increase knowledge among providers and to expand the evidence base that supports the safe and efficacious use of complementary and alternative therapies.

The world is shrinking. "New" therapies or new uses for old therapies are shared across continents. Health providers and researchers are challenged to create and use a solid evidence base to undergird the broad range of complementary therapies used by substantial segments of the U.S. population and populations around the globe. There is an acute need to know and understand the benefits of therapies and whether they work according to the purpose for which they are used; there is also a need to ensure the safety and efficacy of complementary therapies and to understand their effects and interactions when used with other complementary and allopathic therapies. In this chapter, the need for more evidence to support the expanding use of complementary therapies in practice is presented, research designs appropriate for the study of complementary therapies are explored, the overall state of research on complementary therapies is described, and implications for the state of evidence and expanded use of complementary therapies on future nursing research are identified.

NEED TO EXPAND THE EVIDENCE BASE

The significant documented worldwide interest in and use of alternative and complementary therapies and alternative systems of care have caused healthcare providers to acknowledge the appeal of these therapies to consumers and to carefully consider their safety and efficacy. Concomitantly, questions regarding costs and cost-effectiveness need to be answered for third-party payors and for individuals paying out-of-pocket. Questions need to be answered through research related to which therapies to select for given conditions, how many treatment sessions are necessary, and what results from the treatment can be expected. The optimal mix and relative cost of the complementary or alternative therapies versus traditional Western treatments must be determined.

With widespread use of complementary and alternative therapies, there is reason for concern regarding the safety of their use and about their potential interactions with Western medicine. An example is the interaction of herbal remedies such as St. John's wort with prescribed pharmacotherapy, including psychotropic agents, in the family of selective serotonin reuptake inhibitors. Contributing to the difficulty is the lack of regulation of complementary and alternative therapies such as dietary supplements (Ventola, 2010), although increasing attention is being paid to this in an effort to provide guidance for use to better ensure patient safety (Research Council for Complementary Medicine, 2016). The creation of the WHO's guidelines for standardization of herbal drugs recognizes the value of herbal medicine and its increased use but also acknowledges the concerns about their safety and efficacy (Pradham, Gavali, & Waghmare, 2015). Indeed, scientific data in this area are needed by providers to inform their practice. Accurate and reliable knowledge is also needed by consumers who wish to make informed decisions regarding their own health practices.

There is a rising interest in, and indeed a mandate for, evidence-based practice (EBP). EBP has been defined as, "the use of the best available evidence together with a clinician's expertise and a patient's values and preferences in making healthcare decisions" (Agency for Healthcare Research and Quality [AHRQ], 2015). Nurses and other providers practicing in the context of conventional allopathic care rely on an evidence base. They are also relying on or requiring similar evidence in their use of complementary therapies. However, in a national survey, critical care nurses generally reported that they required more evidence for conventional allopathic remedies than they did for complementary and alternative therapies (Tracy et al., 2005).

Resources for accessing knowledge about complementary and alternative therapies must be identified, made available, and used by providers; this information needs to be shared with patients and their families. This is well illustrated by the National Cancer Institute (NCI, 2015), which provides informative, though cautionary data regarding the safety of complementary therapy approaches; the site reminds visitors that "natural does not mean safe." Research findings regarding the safety and efficacy of therapies must be disseminated broadly to practitioners, who need to be informed so that the safety of patients can be protected and the potential benefits of therapies realized. A number of smartphone–based resources provide access to authoritative information as a resource for professional practice. Databases of research findings, such as the Cochrane Database of Systematic Reviews (www.cochranelibrary.com/cochrane-database-of-systematic-reviews), are other good resources for synthesized research findings. As of May 2017, a simple search of "complementary and alternative therapies" on this online resource produced 690 results, including, but not limited to, 49 Cochrane reviews and 44 "other" reviews related to healing therapies such as Healing Touch, dietary products, acupuncture, reflexology, meditation, relaxation techniques, herbal medicine, manual therapies, mind–body therapies, hypnosis, aromatherapy, and homeopathy. These reviews are an excellent source of well-integrated research-based knowledge about what is known regarding the use of therapies for specific conditions. In addition, websites of government agencies, such as the NCCIH in the National Institutes of Health (NIH; https://nccih.nih.gov) and the Office of Cancer Complementary and Alternative Medicine (OCCAM https://cam.cancer.gov) within the NCI, provide other sources of information on a wide range of complementary and alternative therapies. The Natural Medicines Professional Database provides high-quality information regarding herbs, dietary supplements, natural products, and other complementary therapies used for specific health conditions (Therapeutic Research Center, 2017). The information is graded on a scale ranging from A to F to reflect the level of scientific evidence available.

The NCCIH supports investigator-initiated research and interdisciplinary research training initiatives (NCCIH, 2017a). With a special encouragement of research that focuses on complementary and alternative therapies commonly used by the American public, NCCIH has begun building a solid foundation from which therapies can be selected and delivered with growing confidence as to their safety and efficacy. However, there is much work to be done. The ideal evidence base for complementary therapies would support decision making in a broad range of complex patient situations. It would differentiate effects on and appropriateness for people with diverse characteristics (e.g., age, gender, body mass) from various cultures (accounting for dietary practices, social acceptability, cultural traditions, and so forth) and genetic makeup, and it would outline the potential differing effects and indications for individuals suffering the full range of pathologies and comorbidities.

There are legitimate safety concerns related to therapy selection, quality of product (the purity or technique of delivery), dose, timing, duration, and other considerations related to specific therapies such as herbal therapies, nutraceuticals, and supplements. For example, more research is needed to identify potentially adverse drug–herb interactions to answer questions related to whether particular drugs and herbs can be ingested simultaneously; if not, the half-life of herbs in the body, or their "wash-out" times, need to be determined. Research is also needed to provide data to document the relative risks and benefits of therapies such as the use of diet therapy for hypertension (as opposed to standard allopathic pharmacological therapies) or to consider the potential reduction of the side effects of an allopathic agent if it used at a reduced dose but with a complementary therapy.

The growing evidence base provides much needed information for the consumer and provider. However, additional research is needed to determine the potential beneficial outcomes of complementary therapies. Likewise, studies are necessary to generate findings that protect the public from harm or from needless, costly therapies that have no evidence to support them or no clear evidence of benefit. For example, therapies such as the use of laetrile to combat cancer caused concern among allopathic providers who feared that the false hope of cure would dissuade patients from seeking legitimate forms of cancer therapy; an additional concern that the therapy would\ bleed fortunes from desperate families, despite the fact that there was no basis for its claims of beneficial effects (NCI, 2015). Extramural funding opportunities and the peer review system of NIH ensure the continued accumulation of high-quality evidence and encourage investigators who have the ideas, curiosity, and scientific expertise to explore potential therapies for human use.

RESEARCH DESIGNS FOR THE STUDY OF COMPLEMENTARY THERAPIES

Most scientists would agree that the most rigorous design for testing complementary and alternative therapies is the randomized, placebo-controlled, double-blind design that has long been the standard for testing therapies and advancing fields of inquiry, but randomized controlled trials (RCTs) are not without their limitations (Bothwell, Greene, Podolsky, & Jones, 2016). However, this design is not the only one that provides useful information, and data generated from quantitative studies are not the only available evidence base for practice. Other designs and sources of evidence are also important and contribute to knowledge and understanding of patients' responses to therapies, both allopathic and nonallopathic.

Consumers may be increasingly reluctant to enroll in clinical trials; hence, alternative study designs and strategies for the conduct of clinical research to advance the field are needed (Gul & Ali, 2010). The Committee on the Use of Complementary and Alternative Medicine by the American Public was commissioned by the IOM, AHRQ, NCCAM, and 15 other agencies and institutes of the NIH to study and provide specific recommendations regarding complementary and alternative therapies. As part of their report (IOM, 2005), innovative alternative designs for providing information about the effectiveness of therapies were identified, including

- **Preference RCTs**—Trials that include randomized and nonrandomized arms, which then permit comparisons between patients who chose a particular treatment and those who were randomly assigned to it.
- **Observational and cohort studies**—Studies that involve the identification of patients who are eligible for study and who may receive a specified treatment as part of the study.
- **Case-control studies**—Studies that involve identifying patients who have good or bad outcomes, then "working back" to find aspects of treatment associated with those differing outcomes.
- **Studies of bundles of therapies**—Analyses of the effectiveness, as a whole, of particular packages of treatments.
- **Studies that specifically incorporate, measure, or account for placebo or expectation effects**—Patients' hopes, emotional states, energies, and other self-healing processes are not considered extraneous, but are included as part of the therapy's main "mechanism of action."
- **Attribute-treatment interaction analyses**—A way of accounting for differences in effectiveness outcomes among patients within a study and among different studies of varying design (p. 3).

Employing Innovative Research Designs

Complementary and integrative approaches are often criticized due to lack of scientific evidence. Building the scientific evidence base about the usefulness and safety of complementary and integrative approaches is critical for the decision making of healthcare professionals, including nurses (NCCIH, 2017b). However, it is difficult to investigate the safety, efficacy, and effectiveness of complementary therapies and integrative approaches to care. The NCCIH recently introduced flexible and innovative clinical trial designs to assess complementary and integrative approaches and to help researchers to conduct studies in "real-world" settings (NCCIH, 2017b). These flexible and innovative design will facilitate investigation of the roles of complementary and integrative healthcare strategies in preventing disease, improving health, and managing symptoms (NCCIH, 2016a). In early stages of clinical research, including pilot and feasibility studies, investigators can use these innovative designs to develop, optimize, and establish intervention protocols and to develop possible resources and strategies for recruiting participants, obtaining measurements, and implementing the study intervention. Larger efficacy or effectiveness studies can use these flexible and innovative designs to assess generalizability in the "real-world" setting.

Complementary and alternative therapies are viewed as whole systems of care (Verhoef et al., 2005). Whole systems research (WSR) was introduced as a nonhierarchical, cyclical, flexible, and adaptive approach for addressing a broad range of modalities and complexities of interventions. Variations of RCT designs, such as pragmatic trials, factorial designs, preference trials, n-of-1 trials, and mixed methods research, design to evaluate WSR for the patient (individual) centered approach (Verhoef et al., 2005).

Bayesian approaches are flexible and innovative statistical approaches often used for studying pharmacokinetics/pharmacodynamics, decision making, toxicity monitoring, efficacy monitoring, and dose-finding (Lee & Chu, 2012). Bayesian approaches are used, for example, when physicians decide their preferred option of the therapy to maximize the probability of success from published data, with solutions derived from analysis of past collective experiences (Woo, Laxer, & Sherry, 2007). Using such an approach, complementary therapies, including acupuncture, aromatherapy, massage, and relaxation techniques, were introduced for children with rheumatological problems (Woo et al., 2007).

Pragmatic clinical trials can be used to determine the effectiveness of interventions in a normal routine practice, whereas explanatory designs can be used to identify efficacy under the ideal setting (MacPherson, 2004). A pragmatic approach was used in a trial to investigate the effectiveness of acupuncture for patients with chronic low back pain (Witt et al., 2006). The pragmatic design allowed investigators to reflect on and incorporate the conditions comprising routine medical practice. A recent study also used a pragmatic randomized trial to compare the effectiveness between integral-based Hatha yoga and waitlist groups among sedentary adults with arthritis for the purpose of enhancing the RCT's external validity and allowing flexibility of intervention delivery in "real-world" settings (Moonaz, Bingham, Wissow, & Bartlett, 2015).

In an effort to identify major issues in research design in funding proposals submitted to a specific funding program for clinical trials of complementary and alternative medicine for cancer symptom management, a number of problems with scientific methodology were found (Buchanan et al., 2005). Common issues included "unwarranted assumptions about the consistency and standardization of CAM interventions, the need for data-based justifications for the study hypothesis, and the need to implement appropriate quality control and monitoring procedures during the course of the trial" (Buchanan et al., 2005, p. 6682). Such problems need to be addressed and resolved to ensure the rigor and merit of studies of therapies for management of cancer symptoms and symptoms of other conditions.

Addressing Potential Placebo Effects

Another important and challenging area for investigators involves the placebo effect and placebo/attention control groups (Gross, 2005). The placebo effect has been studied with respect to pain and analgesia, neuroimmunology, fear, anxiety, and pharmacotherapy and may have the capacity to stimulate dramatic healing (Harrington, 1997). The power of the placebo effect, and cautions that it should not be underestimated, have long been appreciated (NCCIH, 2017c; Turner, Deyo, Loesser, Von Korff, & Fordyce, 1994). Placebo effects may lead to improvements in well over 50% of subjects in trials of medical therapies. There is evidence that the placebo effect in clinical trials of CAM is similar to that in clinical trials of conventional medicine (Dorn et al., 2007). Methods for managing placebo effects must be carefully considered in research on complementary therapies. In addition, when assessing the overall effects of a therapy, the potential added impact of the healer and the therapeutic relationship on the outcome must be considered (Quinn, Smith, Ritenbaugh, Swanson, & Watson, 2003). Alternative designs for exploring some therapies are needed, as it is may be difficult to use sham therapy or to identify a suitable control group. For example, in the case of the study of aromatherapy to enhance sleep, will subjects remain blinded or will they detect the aroma? If a "sham" aroma is administered to the control group, may it also have undocumented effects beyond a placebo effect?

Simply knowing that a therapy may be beneficial is not enough. Questions such as the following need to be answered: What are the conditions under which the therapy is effective? What is the dose needed? What dose is too much? How often must a therapy be delivered to achieve a benefit? How long does the effect last? How much therapy should insurers cover? There is a need for studies on the cost-effectiveness of complementary therapies and for research that compares and contrasts complementary therapies with other conventional therapies. There is also a need to examine the safety and effectiveness of complementary therapies when used with or as adjuncts to other allopathic pharmacological or nonpharmacological interventions.

Cultural Considerations

Studies of therapies relevant to aging populations, populations at varied ages/developmental stages, and those having varied cultural backgrounds, are also needed. These populations present challenges for the design, recruitment, and implementation of studies. Older subjects often have multiple comorbidities and may be taking multiple medications. Language and lack of cultural understanding may pose barriers to the inclusion of new immigrants. Access to young children, adolescents, and vulnerable adults and the unique ethical issues surrounding their recruitment and participation may also be perceived as barriers to the inclusion of these groups.

Research methods and findings from one country can inform the design and implementation of studies in other countries. Findings may be relevant across the globe, or interesting nuances or differences can be identified. It is appropriate that native scholars build a culturally relevant evidence base of complementary and alternative therapies for use. The work of nurse scholars in South Korea described in Sidebar 29.1 illustrates this point.

Other outcomes are sought by healthcare consumers. That a therapy is shown to have beneficial health effects is not the only legitimate reason for its use. Immigrants tend to use complementary and alternative therapies first and then seek conventional medical help if these are not effective (Garcés, Scarinici, & Harrison, 2006). Such patterns and the use of complementary therapies as an alternative to conventional care may also be attributable, in part, to barriers to conventional care or lack of insurance (Zhang, 2011). Certain therapies may also have cultural significance or be intricately tied with healing traditions, may lead to patients' peace of mind, or may meet patient and family expectations or lead to their increased satisfaction. For patients who have come to the United States from other countries, the cultural belief in alternative or complementary medicine is not changed. In considering the use of complementary therapies, the costs, risks, and value to recipients must be carefully weighed.

SIDEBAR 29.1 FUTURE RESEARCH FOR COMPLEMENTARY AND ALTERNATIVE THERAPY IN KOREA

Sohye Lee

In South Korea, complementary and alternative therapies (CATs) based on Chinese medicine and folk remedies have been used since ancient times. Traditionally, certain types of therapy have been underestimated because of their uncertainty, their side effects, and a lack of scientific evidence. Recently, some types of therapy have been studied and experimentally demonstrated to be effective in the treatment of selected health conditions. Many patients who have chronic conditions, such as cancer, stroke, arthritis, cardiovascular disease, diabetes, and obesity, tend to seek CATs to reduce their pain and alleviate anxiety.

Complementary therapies are practiced by South Korean nurses in the provision of care in many clinical specialty areas. Back, hand, and foot massages, as well as patient position changes, are techniques used by nurses to help patients' body circulation and to prevent patient pressure injuries in many intensive care units. Nurse midwives and obstetrics and gynecological nurses use imagery therapy, aromatherapy, reflexology, or hand massage therapy to reduce patients' pain and anxiety. Anesthesia nurses offer music therapy, aromatherapy, or foot massage to relieve patients' pain and anxiety during and after surgery. Oncology nurses recommend mind therapy (meditation) to their cancer patients for alleviating symptoms and maintaining mental stability.

According to the Korean Nurses Association for Complementary and Alternative Therapy, there are many areas being developed: hand therapy, aromatherapy, foot therapy, alternative dietary therapy, hortitherapy, and hypogastric breathing. Even though the difficulties of applying CATs to patients without strong scientific foundations remain, nurse researchers are trying to develop and test these CATs within nursing's holistic view. They also want to develop these CATs as nursing interventions to help their patients in many areas.

A study reported on Korean research trends in CATs. They found primary articles on foot massage, hand therapy, aromatherapy, acupressure, moxibustion (heat therapy), or combined therapy. They found that foot massage and aromatherapy were effective for improving sleep quality (Kim et al., 2006). As authors asserted, more research is needed to find scientific evidence of these approaches.

CAT can be used for diseases prevention and health promotion. Koreans are getting more interested in healthy eating and physical activity nowadays after the economy has stabilized. Yoga and Pilates are very popular among young women for weight management, stress relief, or posture correction. Stretch exercises, such as Tai-chi has been implemented for elderly in the public community health center. The dietary therapies are broadly used for weight loss and management, enhancing the immune system, and maintaining a better health.

(continued)

For prevention, treatment, and rehabilitation, CATs have a huge potential to be developed in Korea. The efficacy and safety of these CATs should be examined in order to be used widely.

Reference

Kim, H. J., Lee, K. S., Lee, M. H., Jung, D. S., Yoo, J. S., Han, H. S., ... Park, M. S. (2006). An analysis of Korean research on complementary and alternative therapy. *Thesis Collection, 41*, 529–539.

Longitudinal Studies

Many studies have used small samples and examined the short-term effects of therapies. If we want to know the real risks and benefits of complementary and alternative therapies, we need longitudinal studies because we can determine the severity and occurrence of adverse events only when therapies are applied on a long-term basis. Although similar longitudinal studies using the same design are performed, different results may be obtained from people from different cultures. Therefore, it is important that we study complementary and alternative therapy using the same or similar designs in other countries and different cultures.

CURRENT STATE OF RESEARCH ON COMPLEMENTARY THERAPIES

As previously noted, chapter authors have included the most recent research and have identified where more research is needed to provide knowledge to guide practice. Specific research challenges include the need for data-based decision support resources for combination therapies. Such resources would include data related to potential adverse interactions or the potentiating effects of therapies when given in combination. There is a need for research with special populations, including children, frail older adults, and the critically ill. Research is needed to study the effects of complementary therapies in specific health conditions or disease states. Clearly, research lags behind the public's appetite for complementary therapies; knowledge of the putative mechanisms of action, the qualities of therapies, and the predictability of outcomes is uneven across therapies.

Insistence on the use of standard conventions of scientific inquiry has been helpful in increasing the amount of evidence systematically obtained to provide information for decision making in complementary therapies. However, information is lacking on the appropriate dose and timing of interventions and on those for whom the interventions may have the most beneficial effects. A solid evidence base for complementary therapies would support decision making in broad and complex patient situations. Complementary therapies may have different effects on people of diverse ethnic backgrounds and demographic characteristics. So, too, they may have potentially different indications and effects in people suffering from differing pathologies or medical conditions. The lack of such information is limiting to practitioners who rely on a more fully developed evidence base, and this may hinder the full integration of the use of complementary therapies in practice.

Often, studies have been done that have relatively small sample sizes; meta-analyses can be conducted to synthesize findings to estimate "effect size" of therapies when examined across studies. Also, large, multicenter studies may facilitate the recruitment of participants so that studies have overall larger sample sizes to enable testing of hypotheses; such studies are important for scientifically testing the effects of alternative and complementary therapies (Singendonk et al., 2013). Synthesis and review articles would also contribute to the availability of well-organized, available information.

The NCCAM was established by Congress in 1998; however, in 2015, the center's name was changed to the National Center for Complementary and Integrative Health (NCCIH, 2017d). NCCIH's mission is "to define, through rigorous scientific investigation, the usefulness and safety of complementary and integrative interventions and their roles in improving health and healthcare" (NCCIH, 2017d, para. 1). The NCCIH website provides an authoritative, up-to-date resource with summaries of a wide range of therapies (NCCIH, 2017e). The website also provides a listing of clinical trials that are alphabetized by the name of the therapies. NCCIH has played a vital role in promoting the generation, organization, and dissemination of data for practice and research. It has fostered a standard language and is a source for arguably the most definitive information and funding. As part of its efforts to achieve its mission, NCCIH has funded multidisciplinary research centers to foster more rapid development of the scientific knowledge base for the use of complementary and alternative therapies. These centers and their structure, functioning, and productivity have received intensive review, resulting in changes in the focus and mechanisms of funding over time (NCCIH, 2017a, 2017b). The work of NCCIH promises to increase the scientific evidence base and improve the context and delivery of therapies in the years to come.

IMPLICATIONS FOR NURSING RESEARCH

There is a great need for nurses and scientists in other disciplines to develop ongoing programs of research related to specific complementary therapies. As primary care providers, nurses are in an excellent position to address patients' need for complementary therapies. Nurses have a vested interest in generating information that can be used to build the knowledge database underlying the use of specific therapies that may benefit patients. They may also generate data that refute the use of therapies or reveal adverse risk/benefit ratios. Nurses have conducted research on a number of complementary therapies. Most nurse scientists are educated in both qualitative and quantitative designs. This gives them an understanding of multiple ways of constructing research studies to determine the effects of complementary therapies. The need for the expansion and dissemination of evidence and access to it has particular significance for the discipline of nursing and underlies recommendations for future directions in nursing research. As illustrated in the international sidebar and evidenced in the increasingly global contributions of health science researchers, we can draw on the diverse contributions and perspectives of international colleagues.

The need to generate information that can be used to build the evidence base for complementary therapies is compelling for nurse scientists. Specialized clinical expertise of nurse researchers can be used to select therapies to test and to target outcomes of importance to their patient populations. Specialized clinical knowledge has the potential to enhance the identification of instruments that are sensitive enough to assess potential effects of therapies (subjective, objective, or behavioral). Nurses play important roles in generating, disseminating, and using the evidence base for practice.

Interdisciplinary collaborations between nurse investigators and investigators from other disciplines who bring strengths from basic science, genetics, complementary therapies, or clinical practice may lead to growth of the knowledge base and its breadth, depth, and relevance, which should ultimately improve the quality of care for patients. Collaborations between scientists who are capable of conducting research across disciplines may lead to new breakthroughs with regard to complementary therapies and integrative health approaches.

Broadening the frames of reference of nurse scientists to include global perspectives, genetic breakthroughs, new technologies, and information from around the world will ensure an appropriate and comprehensive view of the field. The WHO launched a global strategic initiative in 2002 and updated strategies for 2014 to 2023 to assist countries in blending complementary therapies with the respective countries' established system(s) of healthcare (WHO, 2013).

Such global initiatives and updated strategies on traditional and complementary therapies should serve as catalysts in making information available to practitioners worldwide and should advance the field of complementary and alternative medicine. Electronic means of posting new knowledge, warnings, or updated information on clinical trials speeds the availability of information and has the potential to bring a world of information to bear on practice—but only if used. Electronic publishing speeds the transfer of research findings to practice settings. The mandate set forth by prominent medical publishers that requires investigators to enroll their studies in a registry of clinical trials for their results to be published in highly distinguished medical journals was a step in the right direction; there are worldwide listings of clinical trials (U.S. Department of Health and Human Services, 2015).

Clinical research is costly. Advanced research training may help hone nurse-investigators' grant-writing skills to pursue needed funds for investigative work to generate new knowledge in the field. Design skills that permit nurse investigators to rigorously test interventions and advance clinical knowledge about the use of complementary therapies are critical. However, studies conducted in nonclinical settings, including surveys of public use of complementary therapies, are also important. Nursing research is also needed to focus on the costs, relative cost-versus-benefits ratio, and ethical issues surrounding access to and delivery of therapies.

Nurses and other providers have responsibilities to provide the public with guidance in the use of complementary therapies, to interpret and share scientific information, and to contribute to the development of the knowledge base through investigation and research dissemination. Guidelines that are founded in the evidence base are clearly needed to set the standards for the appropriate use of complementary therapies.

Using available knowledge and methods to disseminate research electronically and making information available at the point of care are important. However, as noted in the concluding sections of the intervention chapters of this book, many questions remain to be answered for the application of therapies in general, as well as for populations and individuals with different cultures, ages, and comorbidities. More research is needed to answer the myriad questions that exist, and it is increasingly recognized that interdisciplinary, multicultural, and transglobal partnerships may be the most fruitful in answering these questions.

REFERENCES

AARP, & National Center for Complementary and Alternative Medicine. (2011, April). *Complementary and alternative medicine: What people aged 50 and older discuss with their health care providers. AARP & NCCAM Survey Report.* Retrieved from https://nccih.nih.gov/sites/nccam.nih.gov/files/news/camstats/2010/NCCAM_aarp_survey.pdf

Agency for Healthcare Research and Quality. (2015). *Evidence-based decisionmaking.* Retrieved from https://www.ahrq.gov/professionals/prevention-chronic-care/decision/index.html

Black, L. I., Clarke, T. C., Barnes, P. M., Stussman, B. J., & Nahin, R. L. (2015). Use of complementary health approaches among children aged 4–17 years in the United States: National Health Interview Survey, 2007–2012. *National Health Statistics Reports, 78,* 1–19.

Bodeker, G., Ong, C. K., Grundy, C., Burford, G., & Shein, K. (2005). *WHO global atlas of traditional complementary, and alternative medicine.* Kobe, Japan: World Health Organization. Retrieved from http://apps.who.int/iris/bitstream/10665/43108/1/9241562862_map.pdf

Bothwell, L. E., Greene, J. A., Podolsky, S. H., & Jones, D. S. (2016). Assessing the gold standard—Lessons from the history of RCTs. *New England Journal of Medicine, 374,* 2175–2181.

Buchanan, D. R., White, J. D., O'Mara, A. M., Kelaghan, J. W., Smith, W. B., & Minasian, L. M. (2005). Research-design issues in cancer-symptom-management trials using complementary and alternative medicine: Lessons from the National Cancer Institute Community Clinical Oncology Program experience. *Journal of Clinical Oncology, 23*(27), 6682–6689.

Clarke, T. C., Black, L. I., Stussman, B. J., Barnes, P. B., & Nahin, R. L. (2015). Trends in the use of complementary health approaches among adults: United States, 2002–2012. *National Health Statistics Reports, 79,* 1–16.

Dorn, S. D., Kaptchuk, T. J., Park, J. B., Nguyen, L. T., Canenguez, K., Nam, B. H., Lembo, A. J. (2007). A meta-analysis of the placebo response in complementary and alternative medicine trials of irritable bowel syndrome. *Neurogastroenterology & Motility, 19*(8), 630–637.

Frass, M., Strassl, R. P., Friehs, H., Mullner, M., Kundi, M., & Kaye, A. D. (2012). Use and acceptance of complementary and alternative medicine among the general population and medical personnel: A systematic review. *Ochsner Journal, 12*(1), 45–56.

Garcés, I. C., Scarinici, I. C., & Harrison, L. (2006). An examination of sociocultural factors associated with health and health care seeking among Latina immigrants. *Journal of Immigrant Health, 8,* 377–385.

Gross, D. (2005). On the merits of attention-control groups. *Research in Nursing & Health, 28,* 93–94.

Gul, R. B., & Ali, P. A. (2010). Clinical trials: The challenge of recruitment and retention of participants. *Journal of Clinical Nursing, 19,* 227–233.

Harrington, A. (1997). Introduction. In A. Harrington (Ed.), *The placebo effect: An interdisciplinary exploration* (pp. 1–11). Cambridge, MA: Harvard University Press.

Institute of Medicine, & Committee on the Use of Complementary and Alternative Medicine by the American Public. (2005). *Complementary and alternative medicine in the United States.* Washington, DC: National Academies Press. Retrieved from https://www.ncbi.nlm.nih.gov/books/NBK83799

Lee, J. J., & Chu, C. T. (2012). Bayesian clinical trials in action. *Statistics in Medicine*, *31*(25), 2955–2972.

Lindquist, R., Tracy, M. F., & Savik, K. (2003). Personal use of complementary and alternative therapies by critical care nurses. *Critical Care Nursing Clinics of North America*, *15*(3), 393–399.

MacPherson, H. (2004). Pragmatic clinical trials. *Complementary Therapies in Medicine*, *12*(2), 136–140.

Moonaz, S. H., Bingham, C. O., Wissow, L., & Bartlett, S. J. (2015). Yoga in sedentary adults with arthritis: Effects of a randomized controlled pragmatic trial. *Journal of Rheumatology*, *42*(7), 1194–1202.

National Cancer Institute. (2015). *Complementary and alternative medicine*. Retrieved from https://www.cancer.gov/about-cancer/treatment/cam

National Center for Complementary and Integrative Health. (2017a). *NCCIH clinical trial funding opportunity announcements*. Retrieved from https://nccih.nih.gov/grants/funding/clinicaltrials

National Center for Complementary and Integrative Health (2017b). Clinical trials utilizing innovative study designs to assess complementary health approaches and their integration into health care. Retrieved from https://nccih.nih.gov/about/strategic-plans/2016/Clinical-Trials-Utilizing-Innovative-Study-Designs

National Center for Complementary and Integrative Health. (2017c). *Placebo effect*. Retrieved from https://nccih.nih.gov/health/placebo

National Center for Complementary and Integrative Health. (2107d). *The NIH Almanac: National Center for Complementary and Integrative Health*. Retrieved from https://www.nih.gov/about-nih/what-we-do/nih-almanac/national-center-complementary-integrative-health-nccih

National Center for Complementary and Integrative Health (2017e). Home page. Retrieved from https://nccih.nih.gov

Quinn, J. F., Smith, M., Ritenbaugh, C., Swanson, K., & Watson, M. J. (2003). Research guidelines for assessing the impact of the healing relationship in clinical nursing. *Alternative Therapies in Health and Medicine*, *9*(Suppl. 3), A65–A79.

Pradham, N., Gavali, J., & Waghmare, N. (2015). WHO (World Health Organization) guidelines for standardization of herbal drugs. *International Ayurvedic Medical Journal*, *3*(8), 2238–2243.

Research Council for Complementary Medicine. (2016). *Evidence and best practice*. Retrieved from http://www.rccm.org.uk/node/23

Singendonk, M., Kaspers, G. J., Naafs-Wilstra, M., Meeteren, A. S., Loeffen, J., & Vlieger, A. (2013). High prevalence of complementary and alternative medicine use in the Dutch pediatric oncology population: A multicenter survey. *European Journal of Pediatrics*, *172*(1), 31–37.

Therapeutic Research Center. (2017). *Natural Medicines Professional Database*. Retrieved from https://naturalmedicines.therapeuticresearch.com/Login.aspx

Tracy, M. F., Lindquist, R., Savik, K., Watanuki, S., Sendelbach, S., Kreitzer, M. J., & Berman, B. (2005). Use of complementary and alternative therapies: A national survey of critical care nurses. *American Journal of Critical Care*, *14*(5), 404–414.

Turner, J., Deyo, R., Loesser, J., Von Korff, J., & Fordyce, W. E. (1994). The importance of placebo effects in pain treatment and research. *Journal of the American Medical Association*, *271*(10), 1609–1614.

U.S. Department of Health and Human Services. (2015). *Listing of clinical trial registries*. Retrieved from https://www.hhs.gov/ohrp/international/clinical-trial-registries

Ventola, C. L. (2010). Current issues regarding complementary and alternative medicine (CAM) in the United States. *Pharmacy & Therapeutics*, *35*(9), 514–522.

Verhoef, M. J., Lewith, G., Ritenbaugh, C., Boon, H., Fleishman, S., & Leis, A. (2005). Complementary and alternative medicine whole systems research: Beyond identification of inadequacies of the RCT. *Complementary Therapies in Medicine*, *13*(3), 206–212.

Witt, C. M., Jena, S., Selim, D., Brinkhaus, B., Reinhold, T., Wruck, K., ... Willich, S. N. (2006). Pragmatic randomized trial evaluating the clinical and economic effectiveness of acupuncture for chronic low back pain. *American Journal of Epidemiology*, *164*(5), 487–496.

Woo, P., Laxer, R. M., & Sherry, D. D. (2007). *Pediatric rheumatology in clinical practice*. London: Springer Science & Business Media.

World Health Organization. (2013). *WHO traditional medicine strategy: 2014–2024*. Geneva, Switzerland: Author. Retrieved from http://who.int/medicines/publications/traditional/trm_strategy14_23/en

Zhang, L. (2011). *Use of complementary and alternative medicine (CAM) in racial, ethnic and immigrant (REI) populations: Assessing the influence of cultural heritage and access to medical care* (Doctoral dissertation). Retrieved from http://conservancy.umn.edu/bitstream/104632/1/Zhang_umn_0130E_11782.pdf

Zhang, Y., Peck, K., Spalding, M., Jones, B. G., & Cook, R. L. (2012). Discrepancy between patients' use of and health providers' familiarity with CAM. *Patient Education and Counseling, 89*(3), 399–404.

Independent Personal Use of Complementary Therapies

Barbara Leonard and Mariah Snyder

There are several reasons people decide to explore use of a complementary therapy or compare the various therapies available for specific conditions. They may have a symptom or health problem that moves them to consider a complementary therapy. They may wish to improve their overall health. A health professional or a friend may suggest a therapy. Individuals may read about a therapy, view its use on television, or see an offering at a local site. Any of these possibilities may pique an interest in seeking more information to see if the practice would fit with a person's needs. In any case, the first action should be to acquire accurate information about the therapy or practice before trying to incorporate it.

ACCESSING INFORMATION

In the 21st century, the place many people begin seeking information about virtually anything is the Internet. The Internet is indeed a good starting point to learn about complementary practices and integrative health. Numerous websites contain credible information regarding the safety and efficacy of therapies.

An excellent place to begin the search for information about complementary therapies is the website for the National Center for Complementary and Integrative Health (NCCIH). One of NCCIH's objectives is to "define, through rigorous scientific investigation, the usefulness and safety of complementary and integrative health interventions and their roles in improving health and health care" (NCCIH, 2016). For people with minimal knowledge about complementary and integrative practices, the NCCIH website (https://nccih.nih.gov/about/ataglance) provides basic information on these practices. NCCIH is a comprehensive resource for current scientific information about common and less common therapies and the health conditions for which they are used. Research funded by NCCIH helps build evidence about whether complementary therapies and integrative health approaches are safe and effective. Information on the NCCIH website provides current, science-based, objective information on the risks and benefits of many complementary products and practices. Although this site provides guidance such as identifying credentials in the selection of practitioners, it does not make judgments about the use of specific therapies or practitioners.

Many other scientific-based resources exist to help individuals select a therapy for personal use. One of these is PubMed (2017), which is a service of the U. S. National Library of Medicine (NLM). PubMed provides access to information and summaries of articles from scientific and medical journals (www.nlm .nih.gov). Another resource from NLM that assists people in finding scientific information on complementary and integrative health practices is MedlinePlus (medlineplus.gov). This resource brings together authoritative information from the National Institutes of Health, governmental agencies, and other health-related organizations.

A source which synthesizes research on a therapy or practice is the Cochrane Database of Systematic Reviews (2017). This database includes comprehensive systematic reviews of specific complementary therapies and integrative health practices for a wide range of conditions (e.g., obesity, depression). Reviews must meet rigorous criteria before they are uploaded and made available in the database.

Nongovernmental websites such as Mayo Clinic (2017) provide information on common complementary and integrative practices. Four criteria for selecting or recommending complementary therapies are (a) safety, (b) standardization, (c) a need that conventional medicine cannot meet, and (d) evidence that the therapy has been shown to help patients.

Websites sponsored by organizations are another source of information. For example, the American Tai Chi and qigong Association (ATCQA, 2017) website has a section for consumers and assists in locating local tai chi instructors. In using organization-based websites, one must be cautious, remembering that the website is not free of bias. However, many have excellent information about the therapy and may include findings from studies that have been conducted.

When doing online research to locate information about a specific therapy or product, it is important to establish the credibility of the source. One must remember that no one judges the quality or accuracy of information of websites before the material is posted. In this era of "fake news," it is important for the user to approach all websites with a critical eye. Some sites on complementary and integrative health practices are created by experts or associations that are reputable, but numerous sites have information posted by individuals or companies whose intent is to sell their products; this is particularly true for natural products. The "CRAAP Test" provides useful criteria for evaluation of a website for the accuracy of website information. The CRAAP acronym stands for currency, relevance, authority, accuracy, and purpose (Bluford Library, 2017). The webpage has questions in each of those areas for the user to consider when seeking information: http://libguides. library.ncat.edu/content.php?pid=53820&sid=394505. After all 45 questions are answered, the score obtained can be used to determines whether content on a site is reliable and credible. Exhibit 30.1 provides an overview of the CRAAP evaluation guide.

Currency is important for deciding on information about products or practices. The source should provide recent references from reliable scientific journals. The authors of the site should have appropriate credentials related to the content. The purpose of the website should be clear. It may exist to sell products. Although some quality websites contain advertising, the website provides disclaimers that it

Exhibit 30.1   Parameters of the CRAAP Test for Evaluating Websites

Currency: The timeliness of the information.
When was the site developed? Updated? Are the sources cited current?
Relevance: The importance of the information for your needs
Does the site contain information that you can use? Is it at the level you need for your purpose?
Authority: The source of the information
Is the author or authors cited? After looking up their credentials, are they credible on the topic? Is the organization well known?
Accuracy: The reliability, truthfulness, and correctness of the content
Are sources for the information contained on the site documented? Is credit given to other persons or sources?
Purpose: The reason the information exists
Does the content appear to be truthful and honest? Does it seem to have a bias? What is the purpose of the website or its sponsor?

Source: Adapted from Bluford Library. (2017). Retrieved from http://libguides.library.ncat.edu/content.php?pid=53820&sid=394505

is not responsible for the advertisement claims. For example, Mayo Clinic's website contains a disclaimer, but it does present current information from relevant scientific sources.

The search for credible information for selecting complementary therapies, while akin to determining the efficacy of conventional treatments, can be a challenge. Since much of the research on complementary therapies has a shorter history, fewer scientific studies are available on many therapies. The "gold standard" double-blind, tightly controlled research studies are fewer than for many Western medicine treatments. Also, researchers are still developing study designs that are applicable for some therapies in which blinding subjects to the therapy is difficult.

Websites can serve as a readily available resource for finding information about books, CDs, smartphone apps, etc. for a specific therapy. A CD or YouTube video may guide individuals through practices such as imagery or meditation. Again, careful evaluation of the website should be done by consumers so that they can be confident the product has been developed and marketed by credible entities.

SELECTING A COMPLEMENTARY THERAPIST

Because a number of providers of complementary practices may not be licensed healthcare professionals, it is important to inquire about the practitioner's preparation or background. Chapter 1 presents information about licensing, credentialing, and certification. Also, NCCIH provides general information about this area. Another source of information is the professional organizations that have been established for a specific therapy. Many of the preceding chapters include websites for their specific therapy. For example, the International Association of Yoga

Therapists (2017) has as its goal to establish yoga as a recognized and respected therapy; the organization includes information about education and certification on its website. The association is intent on having only qualified instructors teach yoga.

States can regulate practitioners within their states. Therapies for which no licensing or certification exist pose a problem for consumers in determining the legitimacy and preparation of a practitioner of that therapy. Some states, like Minnesota, have a specific office for complementary and alternative therapies. Minnesota has developed a Patient Bill of Rights related to complementary therapies. It provides questions to ask practitioners before agreeing to have them administer a complementary therapy (Minnesota Statutes, 2017).

Hospitals and healthcare facilities offering integrative healthcare may have staff members who are practitioners for specific therapies, or they may have a list of qualified practitioners. The facility often establishes the requirements for complementary therapists practicing in their facility. At some point, the person desiring to use a therapy may seek assistance from the health provider to identify competent practitioners. Health insurers are another source for advice on practitioners, particularly if reimbursement for the therapy is available and desired. It is a good practice to keep healthcare providers updated on complementary or alternative therapies used so that interactions among conventional therapies and complementary or alternative therapies may be avoided.

Once a practitioner is found, the person needs to find out as much as possible about the therapist: What is the therapist's training, years of practice, licensing (where applicable), and certification? Is the therapist willing to cooperate with conventional health providers when necessary? It is important to know whether or not the practitioner has experience administering the therapy with a particular health condition. The provider should be aware of contraindications to use of the therapy. Although insurers are beginning to cover more complementary therapies, cost factors must also be addressed because consumers often have to pay out-of-pocket for the therapy.

There are, however, a number of complementary therapies for which a practitioner is not required, such as journaling, meditation, exercise, natural products, and dietary supplements. Individuals may read about the therapy or buy a DVD to guide them through the initial practices. Websites or smartphone apps may provide introductions to the therapy and allow the individual to compare several therapies for the best fit with personal characteristics and the purpose for which it is desired. People commonly seek complementary and integrative health practices for health promotion and illness prevention.

USING THERAPIES FOR HEALTH PROMOTION

Complementary and integrative practices may be incorporated into a person's life for a variety of reasons. Health promotion is one of the primary reasons. One has only to look at the number of people beginning exercise regimens or diets as New Year's resolutions to provide evidence for this. Health promotion encompasses the entire being: physical, mental, spiritual, and social. Social interaction is one of the reasons people often seek groups or classes for exercise, yoga, and other therapies. Not only does the group support help them adhere to the therapy, but also the camaraderie adds joy to their lives.

One of the purposes of NCCIH is to foster health promotion and disease prevention (NCCIH, 2017). Although many nurses include complementary therapies in their care of patients, incorporation of these therapies in their own lives may promote not only health, but also quality of life. Johnson, Ward, Knutson, and Sendelbach (2012) reported that healthcare workers used complementary practices more often than the general public.

For nurses, exploring and developing a personal health-promotion regimen is of high importance because nursing has been identified as one of the most stressful professions. Wakim (2014) identified the following as factors contributing to high stress: physical labor, encounters with human suffering, work hours that may include understaffing, and interpersonal relations. Other factors noted include shift work, lack of control, and poor reward structures (Roberts, Grubb, & Grosch, 2012). This list is not exhaustive, and many nurses can add their own work stressors in addition to ones in their personal lives, such as family and finances. Whatever the causes of stress, a stress-management program can promote the nurse's personal health and increase work efficiency.

If a nurse is not familiar with the wide scope of therapies that have been proved effective in preventing stress buildup and in reducing stress levels, the person should seek information. Nursing has stressed the holistic approach in patient care, and likewise, it is important when developing a personal health-promotion regimen to consider the physical, mental, and spiritual realms of therapies. Dietary supplements other than vitamins and minerals are the most commonly used, with fish oil being number one (NCCIH, 2017). Other commonly used therapies are deep breathing, meditation, massage, progressive muscle relaxation, and guided imagery. Practices such as music and exercise were not included because they have often not been included in surveys.

Sidebar 30.1 details the selection and use of one complementary therapy, aromatherapy, for health promotion by a Japanese nurse.

SIDEBAR 30.1 PERSONAL USE OF AROMATHERAPY IN JAPAN

Keiko Tanida

Aromatherapy has been widely accepted in Japan. Some nurses voluntary study aromatherapy and use the knowledge and techniques to help patients with relaxation and sleep promotion. However, offering aromatherapy as nursing care requires education that connects the knowledge of aromatherapy and the elements of practical nursing care. Recently, Yuka Aihara, an expert aromatherapist and nurse, has been working on constructing educational programs for satisfying this demand, and future development is expected. Aromatherapy attracts the attention of nurses and is adopted in their daily lives as well.

One thing that foreigners traveling to Japan find surprising is that many people in towns wear disposable facial masks. There are various reasons for

(continued)

wearing masks: I wear a mask to prevent catching a cold or infecting others, people with pollinosis do so to avoid pollen, and many women use the mask to conceal their faces when they go out without makeup. I use a mask habitually; however, after wearing the mask for a few hours, an unpleasant smell sometimes emanates. To avoid the smell, I spray small quantities of aroma oil on a gauze and put the gauze into the mask. Eucalyptus radiate oil not only has antibacterial properties, but also makes me feel refreshed. Japanese people, especially the young generations, prefer citrus fragrances such as sweet orange and grapefruit. A combination of lemon oil and eucalyptus is sometimes placed in masks. Although many Japanese people do not like the strong smell of perfumes or colognes, the aroma of the citrus oil can generate a comfortable smell for not only the person wearing the mask, but also for people surrounding them.

I use aroma oils in the bathroom as well. In Japan, the water used to bathe is sometimes also used for washing clothes; therefore, I put the aroma oil in the washbowl instead. When the weather is hot, I fill the washbowl with about a liter of hot water, put two drops of peppermint oil and stir well; then, I sprinkle the hot water on my feet. Since the oil has cooling effects, it prevents excessive heat-generation after bathing, and the aroma of peppermint makes me feel refreshed.

In these ways, I often use aroma oils with a mask and as a partial bath, expecting the antibacterial action and relaxation effect all in one.

The preceding chapters provide extensive information about many therapies that can be used in health promotion, of which reduction or prevention of stress is a paramount outcome. The relationship of high levels of stress to many health conditions has been documented. Lower levels of stress are associated with overall well-being. Since significant information is available on multitude therapies in the mind–body–spirit area, attention will focus on the spiritual realm.

SPIRITUAL DIRECTION

Spiritual direction is a time-honored tradition of accompanying other people as they seek to grow in their relationship with the sacred power in their lives (Barry, 2015). Spiritual direction is not psychotherapy or pastoral counseling, even though professional boundaries, ethics, and listening skills are common to all of them. All conversations are strictly confidential. Spiritual directors often state that a Higher Power is the director; the spiritual director listens for God's work in the directee's life. Spiritual direction does not try to fix problems, but instead helps directees find meaning and purpose in their life circumstances. Directors guide rather than direct. The term *spiritual direction* can be misunderstood as a rather authoritarian approach to helping another with spiritual questions and lived experience. Spiritual guidance and accompaniment are other names for spiritual direction. The direction is from the Higher Power, and the director is listening for it and helps the directee get in touch with it (Spiritual Directors International [SDI], 2016).

Some form of spiritual direction is found in many major religions of the world. Among traditional Native Americans, a medicine man/woman will guide a "vision quest" and interpret the dreams and visions of the seeker. A Zen master gives spiritual guidance to a seeker in the Buddhist tradition. In Christianity, spiritual direction has existed since the 4th century CE. Until fairly recently, spiritual direction was almost exclusive to those in religious life; laypersons rarely sought direction. Today, it is found in many Protestant denominations as well as in the Roman Catholic Church. People from other faith traditions or no faith tradition also seek spiritual direction. Today, large groups of young people consider themselves *nones* in terms of a specific religious group. They do, however, express interest in the spiritual.

The spiritual director has received education in the art and practice of spiritual direction and adheres to professional ethics such as those specified by the SDI (2016). SDI is a global organization of people from many faiths who share a common concern and passion for the practice of spiritual direction. Opportunities are available for sharing of resources and ideas online (www.sdiworld.org).

Those who seek spiritual direction do so to reflect on how the sacred is present in their lived experience. The focus of spiritual direction is on the inward movement of the sacred in the individual's life. A person may seek direction during a life transition or crisis or during ordinary time to gain a deeper relationship with the sacred. All of life's experiences can be brought to bear, but always at the discretion of the person seeking direction. In the course of receiving direction, some of the circumstances of one's life may appear unchanged, yet the inner transformation may be evident in professional work and personal relationships, even in one's environment. Problems may resolve as a benefit of direction.

A person may use the services of a spiritual director during a crisis or problematic time. For example, the person may seek direction during a time of loss. The spiritual deepening felt during this time may prompt a person to continue direction after the problem has been resolved. Spiritual direction may offer benefits for nurses whose working lives are spent in high-stress healthcare environments and dealing with life-and-death questions on a regular basis. Spiritual direction is about reflection on one's life in all of its complexity. At the heart of direction is one's unique relationship with the sacred. Direction can help nurses become more sensitive to the sacred in their work and the desire to give more attention to the sacred. Developing an awareness of this aspect of one's life provides a serenity that can help prevent emotional and spiritual burnout so that relationships with patients, families, colleagues, and oneself become healthy and healing (Fosarelli, 2012).

Selecting a Spritual Director

The SDI publishes a directory of spiritual directors, listing their members both in the United States and world-wide. The SDI does not vet the directors on the list. The SDI website provides a listing of directors by geographic area with contact information and religious affiliation, if any. This list is updated annually and is exclusive to SDI members.

Spiritual Direction With People From Other Cultures

The spiritual direction that grew in the west came largely from the Christian tradition. The SDI, however, has directors from many traditions, including Jewish, Muslim, and Christian. If spiritual seekers are reflective on their lives and open to developing spiritually, being in spiritual direction with a director from another religious tradition can and does work. Just as in the Alcoholics Anonymous tradition, a person participates in the 12 steps with an own understanding of a Higher Power, so too in spiritual direction, the directee proceeds from a religious/ spiritual tradition. For example, if a directee is considering divorce, the director asks questions that can help discover the directee's desire is about the divorce. The directee is always the decision maker.

The compatibility and trust of the director and the directee are more important than their respective religious backgrounds. Directors need to be willing to suspend judgment and listen and learn from any directee. This may take a bit more work with individuals from other cultures. Assumptions about the culture need to be set aside to learn how the directee identifies with his or her culture. Directors are taught to listen and develop an understanding of the person's spirituality. Asking for help in understanding how the directee is thinking is essential to building trust in their relationship. First and foremost, spiritual directors need to be culturally competent.

FUTURE RESEARCH

There are many areas in which additional knowledge will help people develop a personal health plan that includes complementary therapies. A few of these areas include:

1. Surveys of nurses to identify the complementary and integrative health practices that they and their patients find helpful for their personal use
2. Qualitative studies of people who use spiritual direction and the impact that it may or may not have had on their overall health
3. Surveys to identify where individuals seek information about complementary therapies they have incorporated into their personal health regimen

REFERENCES

American Tai Chi and qigong Association [ATCQA]. (2017). Retrieved from http://www .americantaichi.org/about/acp

Barry, W. A. (2015). What is spiritual direction? A retrospective reflection. *Presence: An International Journal of Spiritual Direction, 21*(2), 31–34.

Bluford Library. (2017). Retrieved from http://libguides.library.ncat.edu/content. php?pid=53820&sid=394505

Cochrane Database of Systematic Reviews. (2017). Retrieved from www.cochranelibrary.com/ cochrane-database-of-systematic-reviews

Fosarelli, P. (2012). Facilitating healing of the healers: Spiritual direction with physicians and other health professionals. *Presence: An International Journal of Spiritual Direction, 18*(6), 41–53.

International Association of Yoga Therapists. (2017). Retrieved from https://iayt.site-ym.com/ yoga/login.aspx

Johnson, P. J., Ward, A., Knutson, L., & Sendelbach, S. (2012). Personal use of complementary and alternative medicine (CAM) by U.S. health care workers. *Health Services Research, 47*, 211–227. doi:10.1111/j.1475-6773.2011.01304.x

Mayo Clinic. (2017). Complementary and alternative medicine. Retrieved from http://www .mayoclinic.org/complementary-integrative-medicine/complementary-integrative-medicine-program/overview

Minnesota Statutes. (2017). Retrieved from https://www.revisor.mn.gov/statutes/?id=146a.01

National Center for Complementary and Integrated Health. (2016). NCCIH facts-at-a-glance and mission. Retrieved from https://nccih.nih.gov/about/ataglance

National Center for Complementary and Integrated Health. (2017). Retrieved from https://nccih.nih.gov

PubMed. (2017). Retrieved from https://www.ncbi/nih/gov/pubmed

Roberts, R., Grubb, P. L., & Grosch, J. W. (2012). *Alleviating job stress in nurses*. Retrieved from http://www.medscape.com/viewarticle/765974_2

Spiritual Directors International. (2016). Retrieved from http://www.spiritualworld.org

Wakim, N. (2014). Occupational stressors. *Journal of Nursing Administration, 44*(12), 632–639.

Afterword: Creating a Preferred Future—Editors' Reflections

RUTH LINDQUIST, MARY FRAN TRACY, AND MARIAH SNYDER

There are countless trajectories of science and discovery that will continue to evolve to shape and change the future. Trajectories of change are particularly salient in healthcare, where areas such as precision medicine, genomics, and bionic organs and limbs promise to transform medical treatment options. However, new treatments and technologies do not themselves translate into more holistic care and greater satisfaction with care. Complementary therapies, as adjuncts to allopathic medicine, can enhance comfort, reduce pain, and help individuals adjust to illness, in addition to creating and maintaining well-being. Judging from their current popularity and extensive use by people around the world, complementary therapies will enjoy a prominent role in the future of healthcare. Professionals who use these therapies, including nurses, have an opportunity to create or contribute to a future in which complementary therapies are used for optimal benefits to the health and well-being of people around the world.

Forecasts and future views on science and healthcare can be extrapolations and forecasted trajectories of current trends, or they can be imaginative transformative "leaps" into the future based on desires and dreams in which we address the myriad problems of our present day, including, for example, the opioid epidemic, obesity epidemic, and other present or future pandemics. There are also future eventualities that are hard to imagine. For example, who imagined a driverless car? Or imagined virtual meetings through technologies with colleagues from across the globe? The future is an exciting mystery, full of potential change and opportunity. We can welcome the positive changes that enhance our lives and work to counter those that have the potential to harm our health.

Health is increasingly framed in global terms. The Internet has become a highly relevant source of updated information, connecting people around the globe. We can learn much from international perspectives on successful complementary therapies, holding possibilities that are yet untapped locally as they are adjusted to cultural nuances in local therapy implementation.

The contemporaneous access to information is unparalleled with the past. The technical advances that lie ahead are staggering as knowledge continues to increase at an unprecedented pace. New research informs us, opening up new possibilities in ways to care for individuals and populations with ever greater precision, and online dissemination of cutting-edge research findings can be accessed almost instantaneously. Technology helps us reach even the most geographically remote places. Nurses and other providers can readily contemplate and explore this evidence and its applicability to their practice, with the ultimate goal of translating the evidence into practice in a timelier manner. Likewise, laypersons around the world can also access, process, and apply knowledge related to these therapies.

It is a certainty that technology will evolve and be an ever-present part of daily life. The future will be increasingly portable, instantaneous, detailed, and digital. More information will be available "on-demand," and real-time monitoring will be widely available. We can only imagine. These changes will transform the nature of the work that we do. Much of what lies ahead will be nothing like we have seen before, so it is difficult to anticipate. However, decisions and actions made now will have consequences rippling forward. Therefore, decisions made that affect healthcare and the environment must be made with careful foresight, and the subsequent actions need clear stakeholder accountability, with thoughtful weighing of consequences.

In the future, the era of precision medicine and omics will be in full bloom— or be overshadowed by the next transformative discoveries. World metrics on longevity, morbidity, and mortality will continue to illuminate targets to address in an increasingly global world. The health of our earth and the global environment will be important. Global action and networks addressing health will become more prominent.

WE NEED TO THINK BEYOND

Solutions will need to come from a broad range of sources, with the need for thinking beyond even our global perspectives. The company, 100 Year Starship, is led by Mae Jemison, the first woman of color in the world to go into space. This company is founded on the belief that determinedly developing solutions for human travel beyond our solar system within the next 100 years will also contribute significantly to breakthroughs that will enhance the quality of life for humans on Earth today, including advances in the sciences and healthcare (100 Year Starship, 2013).

Renowned organizations have spent time and resources contemplating the future and making recommendations. The Rockefeller Foundation (2013) highlights that a change in the way we think is needed to break silos. In the future, equity and solidarity values will become increasingly important, fueled by efforts to promote the common good and to reach those with greatest need. Economic policies will need to align with ecological and health-related goals. Social and healthcare systems will need to be examined to sustain population health and well-being.

In the future, complementary therapies will continue to be used to promote health, enhance comfort and well-being, and improve satisfaction with healthcare. How will future changes in society and environment impact the availability and use of complementary therapies? In the future, scientific evidence underlying the use of complementary therapies will be increasingly important, in keeping with the mega-trends of value-based models and data sharing (Weber, 2016). With an eye on alignment of cost to outcomes and quality, the role and place of complementary therapies in healthcare will be determined; insurers will demand evidence to justify the costs of therapies.

Therapies that address the problems associated with aging and those that prevent and treat chronic illnesses will be in greater demand. Ways to integrate these therapies into healthcare will be sought. Integrative approaches will be at the forefront in the shift to preventive and chronic care (Schimpff, 2012).

As we continue to learn more about the safety and efficacy of therapies with specific populations and more specifically with individuals' response to therapies, the underlying knowledge base will grow stronger. We know that there is not always rigorous evidence for traditional allopathic and nursing interventions. However, just as we would not always assume allopathic interventions have only positive results or are without unintended consequences, we must carefully review the evidence available with supporting rationale, surveillance, and safety-monitoring precautions in determining when complementary therapies are used—while gathering more rigorous evidence. Health professionals have a role to play in reporting adverse events, as well as unique success in therapy application. Through remote monitoring and expert systems, clinical alerts can be in place, and practitioners who are practicing at the top of their license can better help people manage their health and disease conditions at home (Phillips, 2015). In the best future scenarios, complementary therapies will be delivered seamlessly alongside Western allopathic therapies in a context of truly culturally sensitive "integrative" healthcare delivered around the globe.

THE FUTURE: INTEGRATIVE HEALTHCARE

I see it as integrative medicine and the evidence-based fusion of conventional and alternative medicine—the common ground being evidence-based. Much of what we do in conventional medicine, as you know, is not evidence-based. Much of what we do in integrative medicine or alternative medicine *has as good, if not better, evidence base. So, we need to recognize our bias and move forward to get the two systems working together.*

—Kenneth R. Pelletier (2014)

The mission of the National Center of Complementary and Integrative Health (NCCIH) is, "to define, through rigorous scientific investigation, the usefulness and safety of complementary and integrative health interventions and their roles in improving health and health care" (NCCIH, 2017a). To accomplish this vision, the center has set forth a strategic plan, which is available on the center's website (NCCIH, 2017b). The strategic plan is outlined in Exhibit 31.1. The strategic plan and activities will go far in identifying evidence for best practices using complementary therapies and integrative health approaches.

Exhibit 31.1 The National Center for Complementary and Integrative Health 2016 Strategic Plan

Objective 1: Advance Fundamental Science and Methods Development
- Advance understanding of basic biological mechanisms of action of natural products, including prebiotics and probiotics.
- Advance understanding of the mechanisms through which mind and body approaches affect health, resiliency, and well-being.
- Develop new and improved research methods and tools for conducting rigorous studies of complementary health approaches and their integration into health care.

Objective 2: Improve Care for Hard-to-Manage Symptoms
- Develop and improve complementary health approaches and integrative treatment strategies for managing symptoms such as pain, anxiety, and depression.
- Conduct studies in "real world" clinical settings to test the safety and efficacy of complementary health approaches, including their integration into health care.

Objective 3: Foster Health Promotion and Disease Prevention
- Investigate mechanisms of action of complementary and integrative health approaches in health resilience and practices that improve health and prevent disease.
- Study complementary health approaches to promote health and wellness across the life span in diverse populations.
- Explore research opportunities to study and assess the safety and efficacy of complementary health approaches in nonclinical settings such as community and employer-based wellness programs.

Objective 4: Enhance the Complementary and Integrative Health Research Workforce
- Support research training and career development opportunities to increase the number and quality of scientists trained to conduct rigorous, cutting-edge research on complementary and integrative health practices.
- Foster interdisciplinary collaborations and partnerships.

Objective 5: Disseminate Objective Evidence-Based Information on Complementary and Integrative Health Interventions
- Disseminate evidence-based information on complementary and integrative health approaches.
- Develop methods and approaches to enhance public understanding of basic scientific concepts and biomedical research

NCCIH, National Center of Complementary and Integrative Health.
Source: From the National Center for Complementary and Integrative Health. (2017b). NCCIH 2016 strategic plan. Retrieved from https://nccih.nih.gov/about/strategic-plans/2016

The NCCIH framework provides a great foundation for the future of complementary therapies and integrative health approaches. What is significant about the strategic plan of NCCIH is how these objectives will work together to benefit all patients, with the potential to improve their health through safe, effective, and knowledgeable use of complementary therapies. The plan calls for more evidence and builds a knowledgeable public and provider workforce to effectively evaluate and use the evidence available in practice to improve the health and well-being of individuals and communities. Evidence is needed for practitioners to recommend or prescribe therapies and for insurers to pay. Meeting the objectives of the strategic plan will go far in ensuring the development of best practices and improving the quality of care delivered.

The first objective is to advance fundamental science and methods development. This objective will strengthen our understanding of how therapies work, including natural products and mind–body approaches. The development of new and improved research methods and tools to generate rigorous studies with robust findings bodes well for the future of healthcare.

The second objective, to improve care for hard-to-manage symptoms, is consistent with objectives stated in strategic plans of other institutes of the National Institutes of Health, since it is well known that hard-to-manage symptoms such as pain, anxiety, and depression are common in many acute and chronic illnesses. The focus of care moves beyond the treatment of disease to manage symptoms that affect function and health-related quality of life. Clinical studies that test these complementary therapies for symptom management will ensure appropriate use in clinical environments.

The third objective, focused on fostering health promotion and disease prevention, is important because it focuses on positive health states, and new ways of promoting health and well-being may be discovered. Furthermore, the safety and efficacy of complementary health approaches in nonclinical settings, including community- and employer-based wellness programs, are emphasized.

The fourth objective is to enhance the complementary and integrative health research workforce. In this objective of the strategic plan, support for building the future of research and science in complementary health programs is ensured through the development of human potential. This objective also promotes the development of effective interprofessional collaborations and partnerships.

Finally, the fifth objective of NCCIH's strategic plan is to disseminate objective evidence-based information on complementary and integrative health interventions. This is a vital objective for meeting the need for accurate information for the safe and informed use of complementary therapies by the public and providers. With the goal of disseminating key findings, we are assured that evidence-based information will be available, or that we will be alerted when evidence is not available to support claims about interventions of potential interest. A second point under this objective is the development of methods and approaches for enhancing public understanding of basic scientific concepts and biomedical research. In this objective, greater understanding of the nature of evidence underlying therapeutic benefits risks and safety concerns may be realized.

New findings, methods, workforce strengths, and strategies spawned by the strategic plan can transform healthcare as we know it, as well as our use of complementary therapies. These resonate with what Finkelstein (2016), a physician/blog columnist for the The Huffington Post, advocates as a "whole-being/whole-life approach to wellness." Furthermore, he believes that "by recognizing the many kinds of doctors and healers in our midst; by providing tools to unify these practitioners in collaborative teams; and by providing tools for consumers to access these teams, while also monitoring their own health on a daily basis, we truly do have the potential not only to evolve medicine, but to revolutionize it."

In essence, he is envisioning a preferred future.

DREAMING: CONSTRUCTING A PREFERRED FUTURE

From the editing of the chapters and gathering and processing the information published and presented over time, a bright future is envisioned, and reflections on a preferred future are offered by the editors. While dreaming of the future, when integrative health models of care become adapted, prevalent, and routine, consumers will be able to find credible practitioners easily and use their expertise in using integrative health therapies. In this preferred future for healthcare, complementary therapies have a well-integrated role, and nurses are on the front lines in the process of evaluation, research, and integration of these therapies. This section describes the preferred future as it relates to complementary therapies. In addition to the reflections of the editors, several international nurse leaders and educators from around the globe expand on the content as they share their reflections. These perspectives increase the depth and expand the geographical context of the vision of the preferred future and promise of its realization worldwide.

Editors' Perspectives and Optimism

The editors have rose-colored glasses as they envision the preferred future and place for complementary therapies in healthcare and for personal use. There are six elements agreed on and believed to be both ideal and obtainable in healthcare.

Ample Scientific Evidence

Ample evidence is available from multiple sites and countries to safely and effectively provide a broad array of complementary therapies with confidence according to the needs of the patient, dosage/frequency/amount required, and known effects. The knowledge base is expanded to include many ancient practices used by indigenous cultures. The large increase in the number of studies and ongoing investigations related to complementary therapies continues to generate data for practice. It is noted, however, that more data do not translate into more insight. Strong information workers will be needed to translate evidence into meaningful knowledge that can be applied to care. Thus, nurses have a significant role to play in healthcare envisioned in this future.

Integrative Approaches Taught in Curricula Across Professions

Professional education/curricula integrate content on the use of complementary therapies along with allopathic content at undergraduate and graduate levels across health disciplines. Students are familiar with and prepared to recommend and refer a broad range of therapies; they will develop expertise to administer selected therapies. Moreover, they will be prepared to educate and refer patients and consumers to sources of credible information concerning complementary therapies.

Well-Informed Consumers

Consumers will be well aware of how to find expert complementary therapy practitioners and will have the knowledge or resources to find evidence-based therapies. Currently, the NCCIH clearinghouse provides significant information on complementary and integrative health approaches; it is envisioned that this will be expanded to include publications and searches of federal databases of scientific and medical literature. Regular public/community forums will help patients/consumers to be cognizant of and understand new and ongoing evidence-based developments in complementary/integrative health that are relevant to them. With better understanding of complementary therapies and integrative health, individuals will take hold of their health in a well-educated, health literate society. Providers may educate patients about complementary care practices or refer them for instruction in complementary care practices, such as meditation, journaling, and nutrition. Complementary therapy classes will be available at businesses for their employees.

People across the life span, including young people, will have a greater understanding of how their bodies work and what is needed to maintain and optimize their health and vital functions. Complementary therapies, as part of self-compassion and self-care, will be taught at an early age. Lifestyle problems such as stress, addiction, diabetes, and obesity will be reduced through not only allopathic medicine, but also its integration with complementary therapies. Knowledge-empowered patients will be healthier patients. Greater consumer awareness and engagement will fuel the demand for the thorough integration of complementary therapies and integrative approaches in healthcare.

Complementary therapies will endure as care that honors humanity of both patients and providers. The therapies build and strengthen trust in therapeutic relationships and fosters the development of connecting bridges between human beings (see Sidebar 31.1).

SIDEBAR 31.1 FUTURE OF COMPLEMENTARY THERAPIES IN HEALTHCARE: TRENDS, TRAJECTORIES, AND VISIONS

Janice Post-White

Thirty years ago, a small collective of my colleagues and I sat together at our annual Oncology Nursing Society conference and brainstormed the future of complementary therapies and psychoneuroimmunology in cancer nursing. "We can do better than just manage symptoms," we concurred as we enthusiastically outlined strategies to support healing and wellness in our patients, despite their cancer. We set a decades-long agenda for measuring and studying outcomes of our massage, healing touch, Reiki, mindfulness, meditation, imagery, yoga, and other supportive therapies. Most important, we envisioned and created a healing therapies room at the conference—a model that still exists today—where colleagues can drop in and receive caring touch, healing energy,

(continued)

and respite from the task of always giving. We taught each other skills, gave each other permission, and learned compassion for each other and for ourselves. It wasn't any one therapy that empowered us, as it isn't any one therapy that heals a particular patient. It was the spirit of caring and compassion that connected us. When we accept our own humanness, our own vulnerability, our patients come to accept theirs, opening the way toward healing.

We knew then that complementary therapies and the integration of the body, mind, and spirit was missing from our healthcare system. In our practice and our research, we strove to integrate our care and to define and measure the effects of illness and wellness on the body, mind, and spirit. We envisioned and tirelessly advocated for change, for an awakening. We expected that data would eventually give us a platform. Many complementary therapies are now accepted into Western medicine, some with stronger evidence than others, most with case studies signifying their importance to at least some patients, and all with criticism of their scientific rigor. Has anything really changed in 30 years?

Care is still delivered from the top-down, rather than from a very real patient-centered model. The provider has goals. The insurer has goals. The system has goals. Has anyone asked what the patient's goals are? In most cases, they won't be the same as the patient care outcomes determined by the experts. Western medicine has brought many lifesaving advances to healthcare, but the care also needs to be meaningful to the patient.

Western countries continue to borrow practices from other cultures, traditions, and beliefs. While medical care is the standard first line of care in the United States, complementary therapies may be the first, or only, or preferred care, in developing countries. Worldwide, providing culturally sensitive care means honoring and respecting healing traditions and allowing and supporting these practices within the context of accessible and available medical care.

Faith and beliefs influence acceptance and adherence. Whether complementary therapies, traditional, or conventional medicine, patients need to have faith and trust in their treatment, their caregivers, and their own healing power. It's not just the intervention we offer—the one that's defined in the methods section of the study—but also the spirit and intention in which we administer the healing therapy, from one vulnerable and imperfect human to another.

Do we need more evidence or do we need more trust? What do you envision for humanity-centered, culturally respectful, personalized healing relationships and interventions?

Fully Integrated Healthcare

In the preferred future, there will be a better blend of care, incorporating allopathic and complementary therapies, resulting in improved, more patient-centered ("better") care. From the perspective of one international nurse leader, the preferred future of complementary therapies is one in which healthcare can use well-selected therapies intrinsically related to the natural intrinsic healing powers of the body in harmony alongside the best therapies that Western medicine can offer. This is captured in Sidebar 31.2.

SIDEBAR 31.2 COMPLEMENTARY THERAPIES UNMASK THE SELF-HEALING WISDOM OF THE BODY

Patrick J. Dean

Complementary therapies blend well with self-awareness: an awareness of one's human evolution toward natural healing and environmental health. Ideally we have within us an evolutionary inclination to restore our health spontaneously, to enhance the health of those around us, and an instinctive protectiveness of the world in which we live. Neglect of these naturally evolving, self-healing abilities may cause us to experience various diseases for which chosen remedies often contradict natural processes. Often labeled "natural," some complementary therapies may be ineffective and possibly harmful when combined with some allopathic medicines if deep self-awareness is not involved. Such deep awareness can be achieved through mindfulness and meditation or at least an ability to ponder on what is invited into our bodies, minds, and souls.

Perhaps the original, foundational element of complementary therapy is intentionality, essentially an inclination toward seeking and intending that an intervention is of benefit to self, other, and/or both. Within the past several decades, an evolving understanding of the power of intentionality, especially in terms of interpersonal human reciprocity with the natural environment, has been achieved through research within the discipline of caring science, and it portends to have an ever-greater influence over universal human activity in the future. Intentionality is, perhaps, the only means of human survival. Much of modern medicine originates from natural resources. However, a respect for, awareness of, and communion with those same natural resources appears to have been overshadowed by commercial interests. Such interests not only obscure access to natural remedies, but also cloud interpersonal human caring relationships, so essential to healing.

Born and raised in Bath, United Kingdom, I was exposed to complementary therapy at an early age. My dad once obtained from an herbalist a plant-derived anxiolytic for me to take prior to a piano recital. He sometimes used herbals to supplement typical medical remedies my mother would obtain from our family physician. My own willingness to combine valid complementary therapies with Western medical interventions has persisted to this day. For example, my current physician endorsed my use of cherry juice as an effective therapy for gouty arthritis and referred to his own coauthorship of research findings that cherry juice can be as effective as ibuprofen in relieving this type of pain.

There appears to be no doubt that a complementary relationship between natural and artificial medicines is essential and necessary. Natural evolution is perhaps a process of refinement, a process no less important than the evolution of modern medicine. However, nature does not appear to ignore and neglect its origins, since without direct access to its past, there would be no ability to return to a natural beginning from which alternative paths can be taken. In essence, complementary and alternative therapies provide a

(continued)

time-transcendent portal to return to the original gifts of nature and self-healing in a never-ending process of discovery and rediscovery. An ongoing evolution of complementary therapies with modern medicines is full of promise for the future, especially in a greater potential synergy of subjective patient self-awareness pertaining to what is suggested by the wisdom of nature and its skilled interpreters, as well as in research that evolves from objective assessments of group responses to large-scale organized medicine.

The ability to routinely receive complementary therapies and allopathic treatments in one integrated healthcare system will result in more seamless healthcare and greater consumer satisfaction. Providers with disparate expertise will work together within the same systems and share information. In such systems, patients' needs will be fully assessed, with treatments selected from a menu of options and drawn together in plan of care with the "right" blend of allopathic and complementary therapies. The plan of care crafted with precision to meet the needs according to the patient's satisfaction and preferences. The result of the full integration of allopathic, complementary therapies and integrative health approaches will be a "better blend" of therapies in the delivery of true patient-centered care. Precision medicine, inclusive of complementary therapies, will take individual differences and characteristics into account in the plan of care/treatment to better match needs of the individual. Needs can be met with a range of therapies that are culturally sensitive and tailored to patient preferences—appropriate for and aligned with consumers' needs and lifestyles. Such a system should result in consumers' greater satisfaction with healthcare, and greater health and well-being. The integration of complementary therapies into mainstream healthcare around the globe is viewed as a win-win situation in which the best of all worlds can be enjoyed (see Sidebar 31.3).

Insurance Coverage

Coverage/payment for evidence-based complementary therapies and integrative approaches will be available and offered across insurance plans and national health insurance programs. Coverage ensures that there is greater access to therapies across subpopulations and sociodemographic circumstances. For example, therapies could be even more available and used to promote the health of elders, who consume the largest portion of healthcare dollars.

Global Networks

In the preferred future, there will be a global network of integrative healthcare practitioners and researchers who will easily be able to share expertise, methodologies, research, evidence, and learnings in a shared global healthcare environment. Indeed, as Sidebar 31.4 illustrates, complementary therapies are important components of healthcare systems are being embraced in countries and continents across the globe. There will be abundant training and career-development opportunities for building expertise and quality in practitioners and scientists. This will not only promote interprofessional collaboration but also enable professionals to share expertise and conduct leading-edge research on complementary and integrative health practices. This aligns well with the futuristic research-related objectives of the NCCIH strategic plan.

In summary, the optimism reflected in the views of the editors is obvious; the preferred future is attainable. So, how can we optimize the use of complementary therapies in a preferred future? An inspiring call to action and direction for leadership in the work of creating our preferred future is provided by Dr. Daniel Pesut (see Sidebar 31.5).

SIDEBAR 31.3 COMPLEMENTARY AND ALTERNATIVE THERAPIES ENHANCE CARE BECAUSE THEY ARE MALLEABLE AND CULTURALLY SENSITIVE WHEN OFFERED AS PART OF MAINSTREAM HEALTHCARE AROUND THE GLOBE

Jehad Adwan

Growing up in Palestine, I had had many arguments with my older brother, Ra'ed, about his passion for herbal medicine and home remedies for common ailments. As I was nearing graduation from the nursing program, I had been thinking that our American teachers, our textbooks printed in the United States, and the western medicine/healthcare we had been learning were all there were to have safe and effective healthcare services anywhere in the world.

Typically, he would tell me about a new recipe for headache made of ginger, lemon, and honey; I would counter with "why not 500 or even a 1,000 milligrams of Paracetamol?" The ensuing argument about side effects and damage to the human body that these chemicals was encountered by a fierce defense of the scientific method and its robustness in finding the best evidence about the effectiveness and safety of these drugs. We had never settled that age-long argument.

Seeing healthcare around the world today, especially political ideologies and politics in the 21st century, I am starting to think that the current, unaffordable, Western-style, technology-heavy healthcare is not a sustainable choice for healing broken bones and shattered psyches resulting from the everyday struggles of the layperson. Affordable healthcare is going to be the main struggle among millions of Americans and many other millions across the globe.

Working in the emergency department at Gaza's main Shifa Hospital in Palestine in the mid-late 1990s, a simple x-ray or a blood test would be ordered if the physician suspected a fracture or anemia/bleeding, respectively. Currently, an MRI and a slew of other blood tests are standard practice for diagnosing and treating the same problems.

In this day and age, a quantum leap forward is needed in the healthcare field to recognize the centrality of the various modalities of complementary and alternative therapies that can be as effective as traditional Western-style therapies. Complementary and alternative therapies can be as evidence-based as

---

(continued)

any other treatment modalities. Are complementary and alternative therapies always safe and effective? Maybe not! Western-style therapies aren't either. Are complementary and alternative therapies going to take over and replace traditional Western-style healthcare? Of course not! Complementary and alternative therapies complement, augment, and synergize the current healthcare system. When complementary and alternative therapies are strategically and thoughtfully implemented in the mainstream healthcare system, they can become an integral part of the current system and provide great benefit and value to the consumers. Above all, complementary and alternative therapies will make the current obscenely unaffordable healthcare services with sky-rocketing costs, all the more palatable and accessible to more people around the world.

Finally, a great advantage of implementing complementary and alternative therapies in mainstream healthcare around the globe is their malleability and cultural sensitivity. What is appropriate in one country or region can be adapted and properly used without insulting or compromising the culture or the belief systems of the recipients of health services. In other words, it's a win-win situation.

SIDEBAR 31.4 USE OF COMPLEMENTARY THERAPIES IN AUSTRALIA: PAST, PRESENT, AND FUTURE

Juliana Christina

The use of complementary therapy (CT) is very popular in Australia. Natural products, naturopathy, chiropractic care, yoga, massage therapy, and acupuncture are the most popular CTs used as adjunct therapy to support conventional treatments (Armstrong, Thiebaut, & Binod Nepal, 2011; Australia Bureau Statistic, 2008; Australian Government/Cancer Australia, 2010; Conrady & Bonney, 2017). Studies have shown that over the last few decades, the number of CT practice visits by health consumers are almost similar to the number of visits to general practitioners for conventional treatments (Australia Bureau Statistic, 2008). The Australian National Health Survey, from 2004 to 2005, reported that approximately 24% (1.3 million) of Australian adults with a chronic condition have used at least one form of CT (Armstrong et al., 2011). Contributing to increased use of CT are personal beliefs toward CT, (particularly in the area of women's reproductive health), and use within the ageing population (Conrady & Bonney, 2017; Reid, Steel, Wardle, Trubody, & Adams, 2016).

Research shows that the use of CT in Australia is increasing alongside the aging population and with the increasing incidence of chronic diseases (Armstrong et al., 2011; Conrady & Bonney, 2017; Reid et al., 2016). To achieve optimal healing outcomes, elderly Australians living with chronic conditions, including osteoporosis, arthritis, diabetes, heart disease, asthma, and cancer, integrate conventional medicine with CT (Reid et al., 2016). Some chronic disease treatments may cause debilitating symptoms such as pain, nausea,

(continued)

anorexia, and insomnia, which results in the use of CT to reduce those symptoms and improve quality of life (Reid et al., 2016).

Research has found that the majority of the CT users in Australia are middle-aged Caucasian women with high income and high education levels (Australian Government/Cancer Australia, 2017). More than 80% of breast cancer patients in this country had used at least four types of CT (Australian Government/Cancer Australia, 2017; Kremser et al., 2008; Phillips & Dunne, 2010). Furthermore, 90% of Australian women reported using CT to reduce uncomfortable menopausal symptoms such as hot flashes, night sweats, and vaginal dryness (Gartoulla, Davis, Worseley, & Bell, 2015; McLaughlin, Lui, & Adams, 2012). In addition, one in six Australian couples have reported difficulty conceiving, and CT such as acupuncture is often considered as a solution to enhance fertility (The Fertility Society of Australia, 2016; Rayner, Willis, & Burgess, 2011).

Personal beliefs toward CT also contribute to the use of CT in Australia. Many Australians perceive CT use to be safe because they are natural therapies (Armstrong et al., 2011; Conrady & Bonney, 2017). Australians believe that CT can be used to improve physical and mental well-being, as well as to treat and prevent illnesses (Australian Government/Cancer Australia, 2017). Studies have shown that those who are unsatisfied with conventional medical treatment view that CT provides hope to cure diseases (Gartoulla et al., 2015; Kremser etal., 2008; McLaughlin et al., 2012; Phillips & Dunne, 2010). Interestingly, some Australians found that CT practitioners are more supportive than other healthcare providers, thus encouraging them to seek further CT options (Gartoulla et al., 2015; McLaughlin et al., 2012; Reid et al., 2016).

CT use is an important and emerging component of Australian healthcare adjunct treatments. Increasing annual revenue of CT companies in Australia shows that the interest and spending in CT use is growing (Access Economics, 2010; Complementary Medicine Australia, 2014). This situation shows that the use of CT could be beneficial to Australians, other healthcare providers, and the government because the integration of CT and conventional treatments could improve personal well-being, support achievement of successful conventional treatments, and reduce healthcare costs (Access Economics, 2010; Complementary Medicine Australia, 2014). Accordingly, more research investigating the efficacy and safety of CT should be included in strategic plans, policies, and programs (Access Economics, 2010; Armstrong et al., 2011; Australia Bureau Statistic, 2008; Australian Government/Cancer Australia, 2010; Complementary Medicine Australia, 2014; Conrady & Bonney, 2017; Reid et al., 2016). Education on and regulation of CT need to be continuously developed to ensure that health literacy surrounding CT is promoted at all levels and that use is evidence based.

References

Access Economics. (2010). Cost effectiveness of complementary medicines. Report to the National Institute of Complementary Medicine, Sydney, Australia. Retrieved from http://www.cmaustralia.org.au

Armstrong, A. R., Thiebaut, S. P., & Binod Nepal, L. J. B. (2011). Australian adults use complementary and alternative medicine in the treatment of chronic illness: A national study. *Australian and New Zealand Journal of Public Health, 35*(4), 380–390.

(continued)

Australia Bureau Statistic. (2008). *Complementary therapies*. Retrieved from http://www.abs.gov.au

Australian Government/Cancer Australia. (2010). *Complementary and alternative therapies*. Retrieved from http://www.canceraustralia.gov.au/publications-and-resources/positions-statements/complementary-and-alternative-therapies

Australian Government/Cancer Australia. (2017). *Complementary and alternative therapies*. Retrieved from https://canceraustralia.gov.au/affected-cancer/cancer-types/breast-cancer/treatment/what-does-treatment-breast-cancer-involve/complementary

Complementary Medicine Australia. (2014). a. Retrieved from http://www.cmaustralia.org.au

Conrady, D. M. V., & Bonney, A. (2017). Patterns of complementary and alternative use and health literacy in general practice patients in urban and regional Australia. *Australian Family Physician, 46*(5), 316–320.

The Fertility Society of Australia. (2016). *The role of complementary therapies and medicines to improve fertility and emotional well-being*. Retrieved from http://www.yourfertility.org.au

Gartoulla, P., Davis, S. R., Worseley, R., & Bell, R. J. (2015). Use of complementary and alternative medicines for menopausal symptoms in Australian women aged 40-65 years. *Medical Journal of Australia, 203*(3), 384–390.

Kremser, T., Evans, A., Moore, A., Luxford, K., Begbie, S., Bensoussan, A., ... Zorbas, H. (2008). Use of complementary therapies by Australian women with breast cancer. *Breast, 17*(4), 387–394.

McLaughlin, D., Lui, C. W., & Adams, J. (2012). Complementary and alternative medicine use among older Australian women—A qualitative analysis. *Complementary and Alternative Medicine, 12*(34), 12–34.

Phillips, C., & Dunne, A. (2010). Complementary and alternative medicine: Representation in popular magazines. *Australian Family Physician, 39*(9), 671–674.

Rayner, J. A., Willis, K., & Burgess, R. (2011). Women's use of complementary and alternative medicine for fertility enhancement: A review of the literature. *Journal of Alternative and Complementary Medicine, 17*(8), 685–690.

Reid, R., Steel, A., Wardle, J., Trubody, A., & Adams, J. (2016). Complementary medicine use by the Australian population: A critical mixed studies systematic review of utilisation, perceptions and factors associated with use. *Complementary and Alternative Medicine, 16*, 176–199.

SIDEBAR 31.5. CREATE THE FUTURE WITH FORESIGHT

Daniel J. Pesut

To create a preferred future for the use of complementary and alternative therapies in healthcare, we need nurse leaders and practitioners with foresight. We need clinical scholars who act on values that support their visions. We need individuals who commit time, energy, and talents to looking ahead and are willing to be futurists. Such practitioners are lifetime learners, attuned to emerging trends, who are resilient, curious, creative, and courageous. The interdependence of people in the world necessitates a holistic perspective and a transdisciplinary approach for the organization of knowledge for decision making and social action.

(continued)

Effective leaders who are capable of looking ahead are likely to subscribe to some of the following beliefs and assumptions that provide a foundation for future studies (Bell, 2003). To create the future with foresight, one should consider embracing some of Bell's values and assumptions, such as new beliefs foster renewal and creation. The consequences of action always lie in the future. There are no facts about the future. The future is not totally predetermined. The future is uncertain and represents freedom, power, and hope. Clinicians and leaders need to know how the past and present produce future effects. Future-thinking is essential for human action. To a greater or lesser degree, future outcomes are influenced by individual and collective action. To act effectively in the world, humans need to estimate consequences of a given action and to guard against unintended and unanticipated consequences. A preferable future is one that you would like to have happen. There is a difference between assessing the likely future and creating a preferred one.

Smyre and Richardson (2016) describe additional principles and practices for creating the future. Many of the characteristic expected of transformational foresight leaders are also true of integrative health practitioners committed to the use of alternative and complementary therapies. Characteristics include patience, caring, openness, truth, interdependence, self-reliance, and awareness of the importance of diversity. Creating the future with foresight requires clinicians and leaders who attend to long- versus short-term effects, as well as leaders who can anticipate what may emerge using trends and weak signals. We need leaders who have nonlinear and adaptive planning skills, which focus on networks, and alternatives based on feedback. We need leaders who are open to new ideas and choices. We need leaders who have concern for how action affects others and the ecosystem under consideration. We need leaders and clinicians who appreciate, value, and nurture nested service–designed systems. The future will unfold if we activate and cultivate the future consciousness that is connected to our caring practices.

References

Bell, W. (2003). *Foundations of future studies: Volume I: History, purposes knowledge.* New York: NY: Taylor & Francis.

Smyre, R. & Richardson, N. (2016). *Preparing for a world that does not exist-yet.* Alresford, England: Changemaker Books, John Hunt Publishers.

CLOSING REMARKS

Imagine the future with a full and robust new culture of care, one that is open and that offers a full menu of patient-centered care that is grounded in a well-established evidence base and inclusive of a well-honed set of complementary therapies alongside Western allopathic therapies, a future world where care is viewed through the lens of the patient experience and integrates the best of Western medicine with the best of available nonallopathic remedies. Imagine care informed by the best knowledge from a global perspective, care that truly has the potential to be "the best in the world," because what is available in the world is well known. The exploration of therapeutic options includes the consideration of allopathic and nonallopathic remedies by patients and their providers, followed by the evaluation of the outcomes of the therapies selected, and revisions made, doses and duration closely tailored to the need and guided by research evidence.

With the exploding increase in the use of complementary therapies, there will be new and interesting therapies explored and adopted based on evidence that supports their efficacy. Imagination aside, new information regarding the health practices of immigrant groups, increased global sharing of healing practices, and the globally expressed appetite for new ways to achieve better health, to effect cures, or to forestall aging, all guarantee that the future of the use of complementary therapies by nurses, healthcare providers, and the public will always be fresh and interesting. We can see it already … now, we just need to create it. In this work, nurses have a critical role.

REFERENCES

100 Year Starship. (2013). Purpose—take the next giant leap forward. Retrieved from https://100yss.org/mission/purpose

National Center for Complementary and Integrative Health. (2017a). NCCIH facts-at-a-glance and mission. Retrieved from https://nccih.nih.gov/about/ataglance

National Center for Complementary and Integrative Health. (2017b). NCCIH 2016 strategic plan. Retrieved from https://nccih.nih.gov/about/strategic-plans/2016

Pelletier, K. R. (2014, August 26). *The Blog: Slow medicine is the medicine of the future.* Interview by M. Finkelstein. *The Huffington Post.* Retrieved from http://www.huffingtonpost.com/michael-finkelstein-md/slow-medicine-is-the-medi_b_5705923.html

Phillips, L. (2015). What will health care look like in 5-15 years? *Healthcare Financial Management Association E-Bulletins.* Retrieved from http://www.hfma.org/Leadership/E-Bulletins/2015/April/What_Will_Health_Care_Look_Like_in_5-15_Years_

Rockefeller Foundation. (2013). *Dreaming the future of health for the next 100 years. White paper from the Global Health Summit Beijing China, January 26-27, 2013.* Retrieved from https://assets.rockefellerfoundation.org/app/uploads/20130126182958/1b8843cc-0d4c-4d5e-bf35-4c7b2fbbb63d-the.pdf

Schimpff, S. C. (2012) *The future of healthcare delivery: Why it must change and how it will affect you.* Dulles, VA: Potomac Books.

Weber, M. (2016). Healthcare innovations and technologies news and views—Looking ahead: The future of healthcare delivery in 2017 and beyond. *HIT Leaders and News.* Retrieved from https://hitleadersandnews.com/blog/2016/12/27/looking-ahead-the-future-of-healthcare-delivery-in-2017-and-beyond

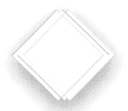

Index

Printed in the United States
By Bookmasters